Anatomy and Physiology Terminology

Ehrlich | Schroeder

CENGAGE Learning

Australia • Brazil • Japan • Korea • Mexico • Singapore • Spain • United Kingdom • United States

CENGAGE Learning

Anatomy and Physiology Terminology

Senior Project Development Manager:
Linda deStefano

Market Development Manager:
Heather Kramer

Senior Production/Manufacturing Manager:
Donna M. Brown

Production Editorial Manager:
Kim Fry

Sr. Rights Acquisition Account Manager:
Todd Osborne

Medical Terminology for Health Professions, 7th Edition
Ehrlich | Schroeder

ISBN-13: 978-1-285-56471-5

ISBN-10: 1-285-56471-5

Cengage Learning
5191 Natorp Boulevard
Mason, Ohio 45040
USA

Cengage Learning is a leading provider of customized learning solutions with office locations around the globe, including Singapore, the United Kingdom, Australia, Mexico, Brazil, and Japan. Locate your local office at:
international.cengage.com/region.

Cengage Learning products are represented in Canada by Nelson Education, Ltd.

For your lifelong learning solutions, visit **www.cengage.com/custom.**
Visit our corporate website at **www.cengage.com.**

Printed in the United States of America

Table of Contents

CHAPTER 1

Introduction to Medical Terminology

Overview of INTRODUCTION TO MEDICAL TERMINOLOGY

Primary Medical Terms	Primary terms enable you to prioritize terms in your study of medical terminology. These are the words that are shown in boldface.
Word Parts Are the Key	An introduction to medical word parts and how they are used to create complex medical terms.
Word Roots	The word parts that usually, but not always, indicate the part of the body involved.
Combining Form	A combining form is a word root that has had a vowel, usually the letter "o," added to the end.
Suffixes	The word part attached at the end of a word that usually, but not always, indicates the procedure, condition, disorder, or disease.
Prefixes	The word part attached at the beginning of a word that usually, but not always, indicates location, time, number, or status.
Determining Meanings on the Basis of Word Parts	Knowledge of word parts helps decipher medical terms.
Medical Dictionary Use	Guidelines to make the use of a medical dictionary easier.
Pronunciation	Use the easy-to-use "sounds-like" pronunciation system.
Spelling Is Always Important	A one-letter spelling error can change the entire meaning of a term.
Singular and Plural Endings	Unusual singular and plural endings used in medical terms.
Basic Medical Terms	Terms used to describe disease conditions.
Look-Alike, Sound-Alike Terms and Word Parts	Clarification of confusing terms and word parts that look or sound alike.
Using Abbreviations	Caution is always important when using abbreviations.

Vocabulary Related to **THE INTRODUCTION TO MEDICAL TERMINOLOGY**

This list contains essential word parts and medical terms for this chapter. These terms are pronounced in the StudyWARE™ and Audio CDs that are available for use with this text. These and the other important **primary terms** are shown in boldface throughout the chapter. *Secondary terms*, which appear in *orange* italics, clarify the meaning of primary terms.

Word Parts

- ☐ **-algia** pain, painful condition
- ☐ **dys-** bad, difficult, or painful
- ☐ **-ectomy** surgical removal, cutting out
- ☐ **hyper-** excessive, increased
- ☐ **hypo-** deficient, decreased
- ☐ **-itis** inflammation
- ☐ **-osis** abnormal condition, disease
- ☐ **-ostomy** the surgical creation of an artificial opening to the body surface
- ☐ **-otomy** cutting, surgical incision
- ☐ **-plasty** surgical repair
- ☐ **-rrhage** bleeding, abnormal excessive fluid discharge
- ☐ **-rrhaphy** surgical suturing
- ☐ **-rrhea** flow or discharge
- ☐ **-rrhexis** rupture
- ☐ **-sclerosis** abnormal hardening

Medical Terms

- ☐ **abdominocentesis** (ab-**dom**-ih-noh-sen-**TEE**-sis)
- ☐ **acronym** (**ACK**-roh-nim)
- ☐ **acute**
- ☐ **angiography** (**an**-jee-**OG**-rah-fee)
- ☐ **appendectomy** (**ap**-en-**DECK**-toh-mee)
- ☐ **arteriosclerosis** (ar-**tee**-ree-oh-skleh-**ROH**-sis)
- ☐ **arthralgia** (ar-**THRAL**-jee-ah)
- ☐ **colostomy** (koh-**LAHS**-toh-mee)
- ☐ **cyanosis** (**sigh**-ah-**NOH**-sis)
- ☐ **dermatologist** (**der**-mah-**TOL**-oh-jist)
- ☐ **diagnosis** (**dye**-ag-**NOH**-sis)
- ☐ **diarrhea** (**dye**-ah-**REE**-ah)
- ☐ **edema** (eh-**DEE**-mah)
- ☐ **endarterial** (**end**-ar-**TEE**-ree-al)
- ☐ **eponym** (**EP**-oh-nim)
- ☐ **erythrocyte** (eh-**RITH**-roh-sight)
- ☐ **fissure** (**FISH**-ur)
- ☐ **fistula** (**FIS**-tyou-lah)
- ☐ **gastralgia** (gas-**TRAL**-jee-ah)
- ☐ **gastritis** (gas-**TRY**-tis)
- ☐ **gastroenteritis** (**gas**-troh-en-ter-**EYE**-tis)
- ☐ **gastrosis** (gas-**TROH**-sis)
- ☐ **hemorrhage** (**HEM**-or-idj)
- ☐ **hepatomegaly** (**hep**-ah-toh-**MEG**-ah-lee)
- ☐ **hypertension** (**high**-per-**TEN**-shun)
- ☐ **hypotension** (**high**-poh-**TEN**-shun)
- ☐ **infection** (in-**FECK**-shun)
- ☐ **inflammation** (**in**-flah-**MAY**-shun)
- ☐ **interstitial** (**in**-ter-**STISH**-al)
- ☐ **intramuscular** (**in**-trah-**MUS**-kyou-lar)
- ☐ **laceration** (**lass**-er-**AY**-shun)
- ☐ **lesion** (**LEE**-zhun)
- ☐ **malaise** (mah-**LAYZ**)
- ☐ **mycosis** (my-**KOH**-sis)
- ☐ **myelopathy** (my-eh-**LOP**-ah-thee)
- ☐ **myopathy** (my-**OP**-ah-thee)
- ☐ **myorrhexis** (**my**-oh-**RECK**-sis)
- ☐ **natal** (**NAY**-tal)
- ☐ **neonatology** (**nee**-oh-nay-**TOL**-oh-jee)
- ☐ **neurorrhaphy** (new-**ROR**-ah-fee)
- ☐ **otorhinolaryngology** (**oh**-toh-**rye**-noh-**lar**-in-**GOL**-oh-jee)
- ☐ **palpation** (pal-**PAY**-shun)
- ☐ **palpitation** (**pal**-pih-**TAY**-shun)
- ☐ **pathology** (pah-**THOL**-oh-jee)
- ☐ **phalanges** (fah-**LAN**-jeez)
- ☐ **poliomyelitis** (**poh**-lee-oh-**my**-eh-**LYE**-tis)
- ☐ **prognosis** (prog-**NOH**-sis)
- ☐ **pyoderma** (**pye**-oh-**DER**-mah)
- ☐ **pyrosis** (pye-**ROH**-sis)
- ☐ **remission**
- ☐ **sign**
- ☐ **supination** (**soo**-pih-**NAY**-shun)
- ☐ **suppuration** (**sup**-you-**RAY**-shun)
- ☐ **supracostal** (**sue**-prah-**KOS**-tal)
- ☐ **symptom** (**SIMP**-tum)
- ☐ **syndrome** (**SIN**-drohm)
- ☐ **tonsillitis** (**ton**-sih-**LYE**-tis)
- ☐ **trauma** (**TRAW**-mah)
- ☐ **triage** (tree-**AHZH**)
- ☐ **viral** (**VYE**-ral)

LEARNING GOALS

On completion of this chapter, you should be able to:

1. Identify the roles of the four types of word parts used in forming medical terms.
2. Use your knowledge of word parts to analyze unfamiliar medical terms.
3. Describe the steps in locating a term in a medical dictionary.
4. Define the commonly used word roots, combining forms, suffixes, and prefixes introduced in this chapter.
5. Use the "sounds-like" pronunciation system to correctly pronounce the primary terms introduced in this chapter.
6. Recognize the importance of spelling medical terms correctly.
7. State why caution is important when using abbreviations.
8. Recognize, define, spell, and correctly pronounce the primary terms introduced in this chapter.

PRIMARY MEDICAL TERMS

In this book, you will be introduced to many medical terms; however, mastering them will be easier than you anticipate because this book has many features to make learning easier:

- **Primary terms** appear in boldface. Learning these terms should be your highest priority as only primary terms are used as correct answers in the Learning Exercises and tests.
- *Secondary terms* appear in *orange* italics. Some of these terms are the "also known as" names for conditions or procedures. Other secondary terms clarify words used in the definitions of primary terms.

WORD PARTS ARE THE KEY

Learning medical terminology is much easier once you understand how word parts work together to form medical terms (Figure 1.1). This book includes many aids to help you continue reinforcing your word-building skills.

- The types of word parts and the rules for their use are explained in this chapter. Learn these rules and follow them.
- When a term is made up of recognizable word parts, these word parts and their meanings are included with the definition of that term. These word parts appear in **magenta**.

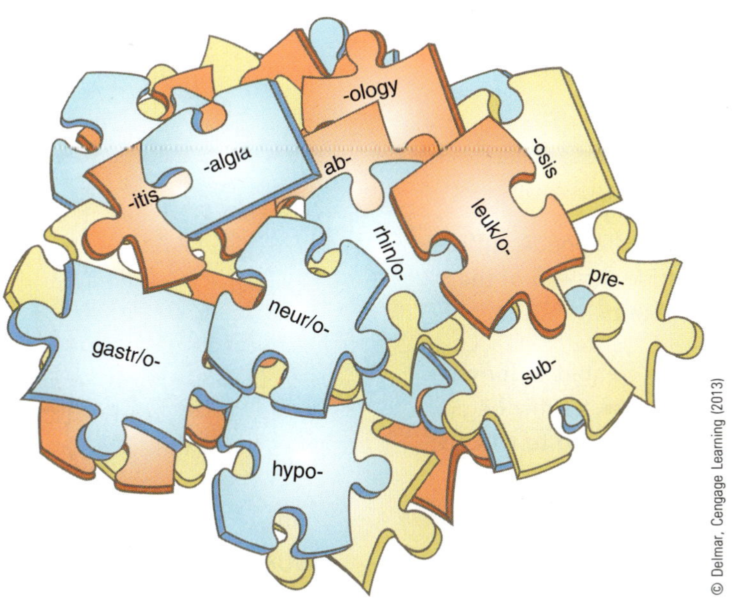

FIGURE 1.1 Word parts (word roots, combining forms, suffixes, and prefixes) make up most medical terms.

- The Learning Exercises for each chapter include a "Challenge Word Building" section to help develop your skills in working with word parts.
- The Word Part Review follows Chapter 2. This section provides additional word part practice and enables you to evaluate your progress toward mastering the meaning of these word parts.

The Four Types of Word Parts

The four types of word parts used to create medical terms are: **word roots**, **combining forms**, **suffixes**, and **prefixes**. Guidelines for their use are shown in Table 1.1.

1. A **word root** contains the basic meaning of the term. In medical terminology, this word part usually, *but not always*, indicates the involved body part. For example, the word root meaning stomach is **gastr**.
2. A **combining form** is a word root with a combining vowel added at the end. For example, the combining form meaning stomach is **gastr/o**. This form is used when a suffix beginning with a consonant is added. When a combining form appears alone, it is shown with a back slash (/) between the word root and the combining vowel.
3. A **suffix** usually, *but not always*, indicates the procedure, condition, disorder, or disease.

- A suffix always comes at the end of the word.
- You'll know a word part is a suffix when it is shown with a hyphen (-) preceding it. For example, the suffix **-itis** means inflammation.

4. A **prefix** usually, *but not always*, indicates location, time, number, or status.

- A prefix always comes at the beginning of a word.

TABLE 1.1
Word Part Guidelines

- A word root cannot stand alone. A suffix must always be added at the end of the word to complete the term.
- The rules for creating a combining form by adding a vowel apply when a suffix beginning with a consonant is added to a word root.
- When a prefix is added, it is *always* placed at the beginning of the word.

- You'll know a word part is a prefix when it is shown followed by a hyphen (-). For example, **hyper-** means excessive or increased.

WORD ROOTS

Word roots act as the foundation for most medical terms. They usually, *but not always*, describe the part of the body that is involved (Figure 1.2). As shown in Table 1.2, some word roots indicate color.

StudyWARE™ CONNECTION

Play an interactive game labeling word parts on your StudyWARE™.

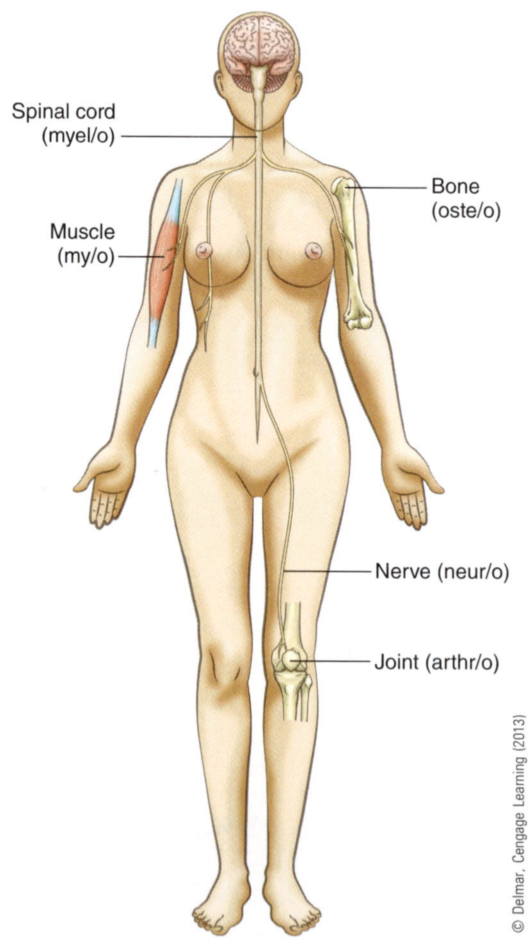

FIGURE 1.2 Word roots, shown here as combining forms, usually indicate the involved body part.

TABLE 1.2
Word Roots and Combining Forms Indicating Color

cyan/o means blue	**Cyanosis** (**sigh**-ah-**NOH**-sis) is blue discoloration of the skin caused by a lack of adequate oxygen in the blood (**cyan** means blue, and **-osis** means abnormal condition or disease).
erythr/o means red	An **erythrocyte** (eh-**RITH**-roh-sight) is a mature red blood cell (**erythr/o** means red, and **-cyte** means cell).
leuk/o means white	A **leukocyte** (**LOO**-koh-sight) is a white blood cell (**leuk/o** means white, and **-cyte** means cell).
melan/o means black	**Melanosis** (**mel**-ah-**NOH**-sis) is any condition of unusual deposits of black pigment in body tissues or organs (**melan** means black, and **-osis** means abnormal condition or disease).
poli/o means gray	**Poliomyelitis** (**poh**-lee-oh-**my**-eh-**LYE**-tis) is a viral infection of the gray matter of the spinal cord (**poli/o** means gray, **myel** means spinal cord, and **-itis** means inflammation).

Combining Forms Vowels

A combining form includes the vowel that has been added to the end of a word root. For example, **gastr/o** is the combining form of the word root for stomach. The letter *"o"* is the most commonly used combining vowel, and under certain conditions, this is added to make the resulting medical term easier to pronounce. The rules for the use of a combining vowel are:

- When two word roots are joined, a combining vowel is always added to the first word root. A combining vowel is used with the second word root *only if the suffix begins with a consonant.*
- For example, the term **gastroenteritis** combines two word roots with a suffix: when **gastr/o** (stomach) is joined with **enter/o** (small intestine), the combining vowel is used with **gastr/o**.
- The word root **enter** is joined to **–itis** *without a combining vowel* because this suffix begins with a vowel. **Gastroenteritis** (**gas**-troh-en-ter-**EYE**-tis) is an inflammation of the stomach and small intestine.

SUFFIXES

A suffix is *always* added at the end of a word to complete that term. In medical terminology, suffixes usually, *but not always*, indicate a procedure, condition, disorder, or disease.

A combining vowel is used when the suffix begins with a consonant. For example, when **neur/o** (nerve) is joined with the suffix **-plasty** (surgical repair) or **-rrhaphy** (surgical suturing), the combining vowel "o" *is used* because **-plasty** and **-rrhaphy** both begin with a consonant.

- **Neuroplasty** (**NEW**-roh-**plas**-tee) is the surgical repair of a nerve.
- **Neurorrhaphy** (new-**ROR**-ah-fee) is suturing together the ends of a severed nerve.

A combining vowel is *not* used when the suffix begins with a consonant. For example, the word root **tonsill** means tonsils. The suffix that is added to complete the term tells what is happening to the tonsils (Figure 1.3).

- **Tonsillitis** (**ton**-sih-**LYE**-tis) is an inflammation of the tonsils (**tonsill** means tonsils, and **-itis** means inflammation).
- A **tonsillectomy** (**ton**-sih-**LECK**-toh-mee) is the surgical removal of the tonsils (**tonsill** means tonsils, and **-ectomy** means surgical removal).

Suffixes as Noun Endings

A *noun* is a word that is the name of a person, place, or thing. In medical terminology, some suffixes change the word root into a noun. For example, the **cranium** (**KRAY**-nee-um) is the portion of the skull that encloses the brain (**crani** means skull, and **-um** is a noun ending). Other suffixes complete the term by changing the word root into a noun. Suffixes that are commonly used as noun endings are shown in Table 1.3.

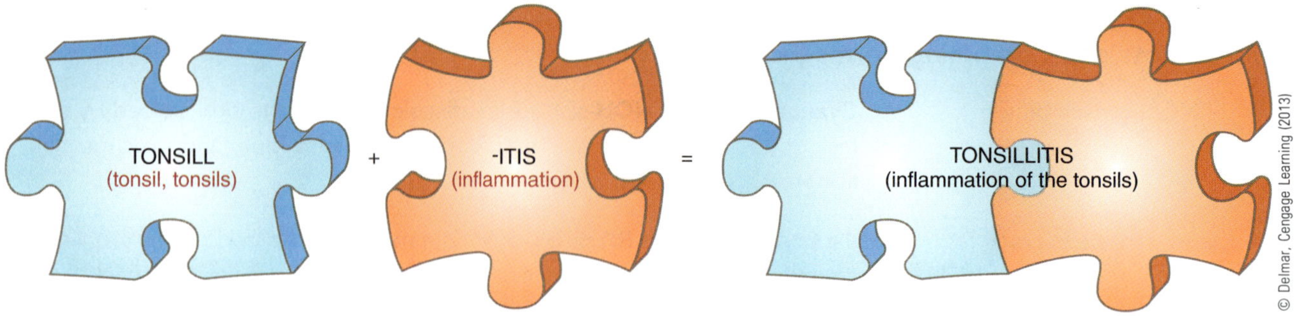

FIGURE 1.3 The term *tonsillitis* is created by adding the suffix **-itis** to the word root **tonsill**.

TABLE 1.3
Suffixes as Noun Endings

-a	-um	-y
-e	-us	

Suffixes Meaning "Pertaining To"

An ***adjective*** is a word that defines or describes a thing. In medical terminology, many suffixes meaning "pertaining to" are used to change the meaning of the word root into an adjective. For example, the term **cardiac** (**KAR**-dee-ack) is an adjective that means pertaining to the heart (**cardi** means heart, and **-ac** means pertaining to). Commonly used suffixes meaning "pertaining to" are shown in Table 1.4.

TABLE 1.4
Suffixes Meaning "Pertaining To"

-ac	-eal	-ior
-al	-ical	-ory
-an	-ial	-ous
-ar	-ic	-tic
-ary	-ine	

Suffixes Meaning "Abnormal Condition"

In medical terminology, many suffixes, such as **-osis**, mean "abnormal condition or disease." For example, **gastrosis** (gas-**TROH**-sis) means any disease of the stomach (**gastr** means stomach, and **-osis** means abnormal condition or disease). Commonly used suffixes meaning "abnormal condition or disease" are shown in Table 1.5.

TABLE 1.5
Suffixes Meaning "Abnormal Condition"

-ago	-iasis	-osis
-esis	-ion	
-ia	-ism	

Suffixes Related to Pathology

Pathology (pah-**THOL**-oh-jee) is the study of all aspects of diseases (**path** means disease, and **-ology** means study of). Suffixes related to pathology describe specific disease conditions.

- **-algia** means pain and suffering. **Gastralgia** (gas-**TRAL**-jee-ah), also known as a ***stomachache***, means pain in the stomach (**gastr** means stomach, and **-algia** means pain).
- **-dynia** also means pain. **Gastrodynia** (**gas**-troh-**DIN**-ee-ah) also means pain in the stomach (**gastr/o** means stomach, and **-dynia** means pain). Although **-dynia** has the same meaning as **-algia**, it is not used as commonly. (Figure 1.4.)
- **-itis** means inflammation. **Gastritis** (gas-**TRY**-tis) is an inflammation of the stomach (**gastr** means stomach, and **-itis** means inflammation).
- **-megaly** means enlargement. **Hepatomegaly** (**hep**-ah-toh-**MEG**-ah-lee) is abnormal enlargement of the liver (**hepat/o** means liver, and **-megaly** means enlargement).
- **-malacia** means abnormal softening. **Arteriomalacia** (ar-**tee**-ree-oh-mah-**LAY**-shee-ah) is the abnormal

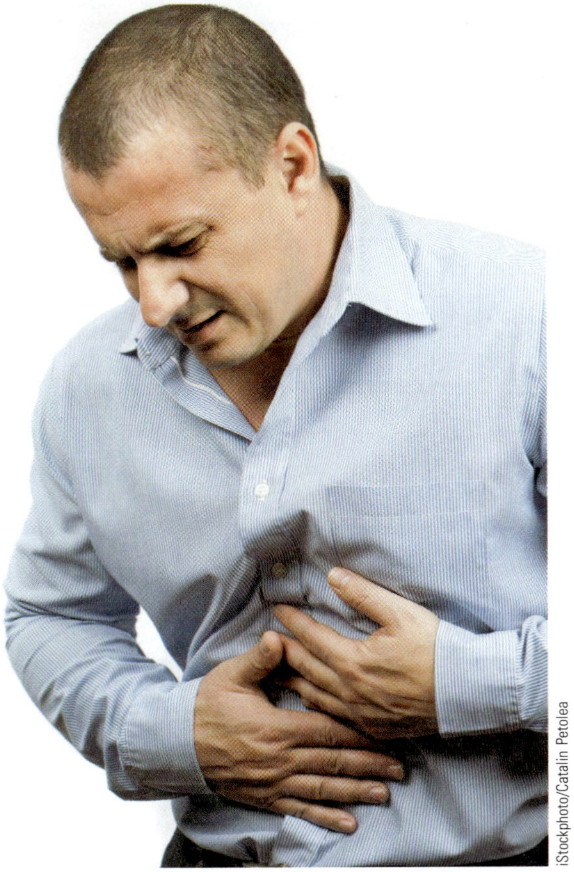

FIGURE 1.4 *Gastrodynia* and *gastralgia* are both terms meaning stomach pain.

softening of the walls of an artery or arteries (**arteri/o** means artery, and **-malacia** means abnormal softening). Notice that **-malacia** is the opposite of **-sclerosis**.

- **-necrosis** means tissue death. **Arterionecrosis** (ar-**tee**-ree-oh-neh-**KROH**-sis) is the tissue death of an artery or arteries (**arteri/o** means artery, and **-necrosis** means tissue death).
- **-sclerosis** means abnormal hardening. **Arteriosclerosis** (ar-**tee**-ree-oh-skleh-**ROH**-sis) is the abnormal hardening of the walls of an artery or arteries (**arteri/o** means artery, and **-sclerosis** means abnormal hardening). Notice that **-sclerosis** is the opposite of **-malacia**.
- **-stenosis** means abnormal narrowing. **Arteriostenosis** (ar-**tee**-ree-oh-steh-**NOH**-sis) is the abnormal narrowing of an artery or arteries (**arteri/o** means artery, and **-stenosis** means abnormal narrowing).

Suffixes Related to Procedures

Some suffixes identify the procedure that is performed on the body part identified by the word root.

- **-centesis** is a surgical puncture to remove fluid for diagnostic purposes or to remove excess fluid. **Abdominocentesis** (ab-**dom**-ih-noh-sen-**TEE**-sis) is the surgical puncture of the abdominal cavity to remove fluid (**abdomin/o** means abdomen, and **-centesis** means a surgical puncture to remove fluid).
- **-graphy** means the process of producing a picture or record. **Angiography** (**an**-jee-**OG**-rah-fee) is the process of producing a radiographic (x-ray) study of blood vessels after the injection of a contrast medium to make these blood vessels visible (**angi/o** means blood vessel, and **-graphy** means the process of recording).
- **-gram** means a picture or record. An **angiogram** (**AN**-jee-oh-**gram**) is the resulting film that is produced by angiography (**angi/o** means blood vessel, and **-gram** means a picture or record).
- **-plasty** means surgical repair. **Myoplasty** (**MY**-oh-**plas**-tee) is the surgical repair of a muscle (**my/o** means muscle, and **-plasty** means surgical repair).
- **-scopy** means visual examination. **Arthroscopy** (ar-**THROS**-koh-pee) is the visual examination of the internal structure of a joint (**arthr/o** means joint, and **-scopy** means visual examination).

The "Double R" Suffixes

Suffixes beginning with two *r*s, often referred to as the "double Rs," can be particularly confusing. They are grouped together here to help you understand the word parts and to remember the differences.

- **-rrhage** and **-rrhagia** mean bleeding; however, they are most often used to describe sudden, severe bleeding. A **hemorrhage** (**HEM**-or-idj) is the loss of a large amount of blood in a short time (**hem/o** means blood, and **-rrhage** means abnormal excessive fluid discharge). This term also means to bleed.
- **-rrhaphy** means surgical suturing to close a wound and includes the use of sutures, staples, or surgical glue. **Myorrhaphy** (my-**OR**-ah-fee) is the surgical suturing of a muscle wound (**my/o** means muscle, and **-rrhaphy** means surgical suturing).
- **-rrhea** means flow or discharge and refers to the flow of most body fluids. **Diarrhea** (**dye**-ah-**REE**-ah) is the frequent flow of loose or watery stools (**dia-** means through, and **-rrhea** means flow or discharge).
- **-rrhexis** means rupture. **Myorrhexis** (**my**-oh-**RECK**-sis) is the rupture of a muscle (**my/o** means muscle, and **-rrhexis** means rupture).

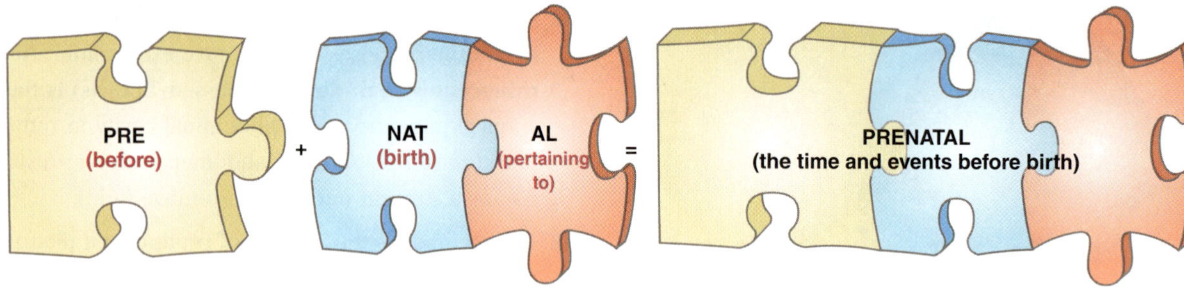

FIGURE 1.5 The term *prenatal* is created by joining the suffix **-al** to the word root **nat** and then adding the prefix **pre-**.

PREFIXES

A prefix is added to the beginning of a word to influence the meaning of that term. Prefixes usually, *but not always*, indicate location, time, or number. See Table 1.6 for a list of prefixes describing direction, quantity, size, and amount. The term **natal** (**NAY**-tal) means pertaining to birth (**nat** means birth, and **-al** means pertaining to). The following examples show how prefixes change the meaning of this term (Figures 1.5–1.8).

- **Prenatal** (pre-**NAY**-tal) means the time and events before birth (**pre-** means before, **nat** means birth, and **-al** means pertaining to).
- **Perinatal** (**pehr**-ih-**NAY**-tal) refers to the time and events surrounding birth (**peri-** means surrounding, **nat** means birth, and **-al** means pertaining to). This is the time just before, during, and just after birth.
- **Postnatal** (pohst-**NAY**-tal) refers to the time and events after birth (**post-** means after, **nat** means birth, and **-al** means pertaining to).

TABLE 1.6
Prefixes Describing Direction, Quantity, Size, and Amount

ab- away from, negative, absent	**ad-** toward, to, in the direction of
dextr/o right side	**sinistr/o** left side
ex- out of, outside, away from	**in-** in, into, not, without
macro- large, abnormal size, or long	**micr/o, micro-** small
mega-, megal/o large, great	**olig/o** scanty, few
pre- before	**post-** after, behind

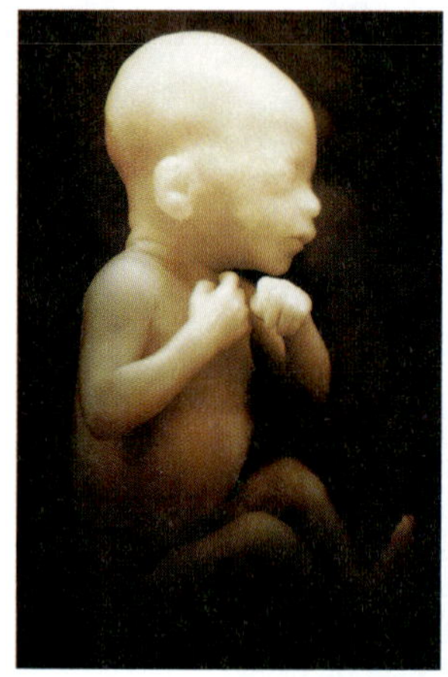

FIGURE 1.6 The *prenatal* development of a fetus (baby).

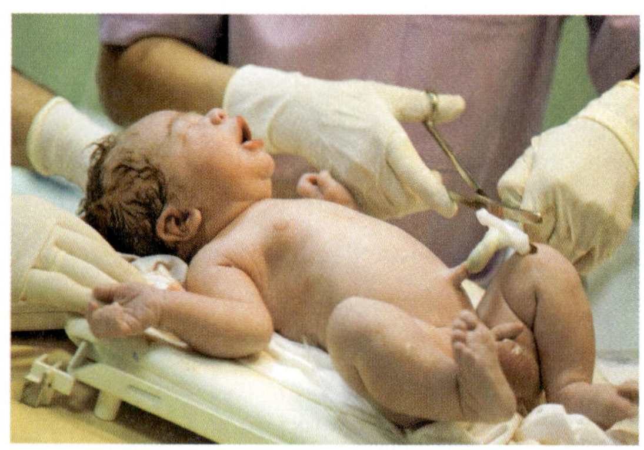

FIGURE 1.7 A *perinatal* event of the umbilical cord being cut immediately after the baby is born.

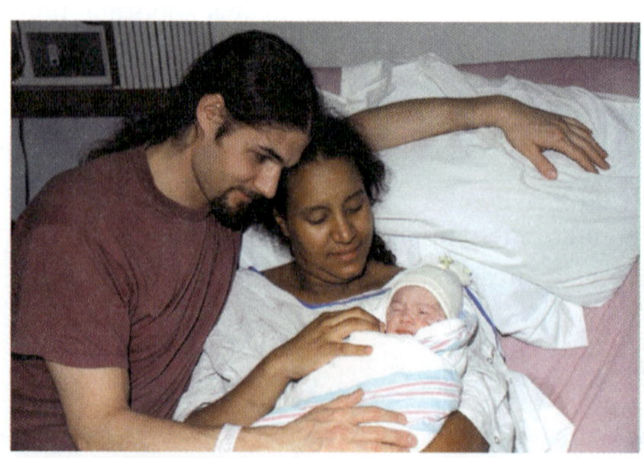

FIGURE 1.8 A joyful *postnatal* moment as the parents bond with their new baby.

TABLE 1.7
Contrasting Prefixes

ab- means away from. **Abnormal** means not normal or away from normal.	**ad-** means toward or in the direction of. **Addiction** means drawn toward or a strong dependence on a drug or substance.
dys- means bad, difficult, or painful. **Dysfunctional** means an organ or body part that is not working properly.	**eu-** means good, normal, well, or easy. **Eupnea** means easy or normal breathing.
hyper- means excessive or increased. **Hypertension** is higher-than-normal blood pressure.	**hypo-** means deficient or decreased. **Hypotension** is lower-than-normal blood pressure.
inter- means between or among. **Interstitial** means between, but not within, the parts of a tissue.	**intra-** means within or inside. **Intramuscular** means within the muscle.
sub- means under, less, or below. **Subcostal** means below a rib or ribs.	**super-**, **supra-** mean above or excessive. **Supracostal** means above or outside the ribs.

Contrasting and Confusing Prefixes

Some prefixes are confusing because they are similar in spelling, but opposite in meaning. The more common prefixes of this type are summarized in Table 1.7.

StudyWARE CONNECTION

Watch an animation on **How Word Parts Work Together** in the StudyWARE™.

DETERMINING MEANINGS ON THE BASIS OF WORD PARTS

Knowing the meaning of the word parts often makes it possible to figure out the definition of an unfamiliar medical term.

Taking Terms Apart

To determine a word's meaning by looking at the component pieces, you must first separate it into word parts.

- Always start at the end of the word, with the suffix, and work toward the beginning.
- As you separate the word parts, identify the meaning of each. Identifying the meaning of each part should give you a definition of the term.
- Because some word parts have more than one meaning, it also is necessary to determine the context in which the term is being used. As used here, ***context*** means to determine which body system this term is referring to.
- If you have any doubt, use your medical dictionary to double-check your definition.
- Be aware that not all medical terms are made up of word parts.

An Example to Take Apart

Look at the term **otorhinolaryngology** (oh-toh-**rye**-noh-**lar**-in-**GOL**-oh-jee) as shown in Figure 1.9. It is made up of two combining forms, a word root, and a suffix. This is how it looks when the word parts have been separated by working from the end to the beginning.

- The suffix **-ology** means the study of.
- The word root **laryng** means larynx or throat. The combining vowel *is not used* here, because the word root is joining a suffix that begins with a vowel.
- The combining form **rhin/o** means nose. The combining vowel *is used* here because the word root **rhin** is joining another word root.

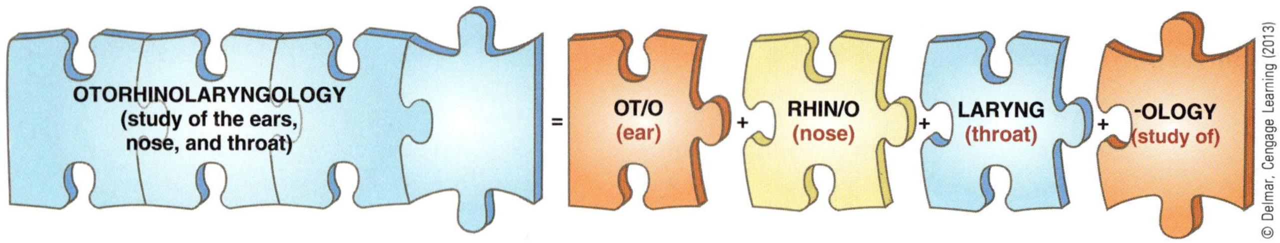

FIGURE 1.9 To determine the meaning of a medical term, the word parts are separated working from the end of the word toward the beginning.

- The combining form **ot/o** means ear. The combining vowel *is used* here because the word root **ot** is joining another word root.
- Together they form *otorhinolaryngology*, which is the study of the ears, nose, and throat (**ot/o** means ear, **rhin/o** means nose, **laryng** means throat, and **-ology** means study of). Note: **Laryng/o** also means larynx and is discussed in Chapter 7.
- Because this is such a long term, this specialty is frequently referred to as *ENT* (ears, nose, and throat).
- A shortened version of this term is **otolaryngology** (**oh**-toh-**lar**-in-**GOL**-oh-jee), which is the study of the ears and larynx or throat (**ot/o** means ears, **laryng** means larynx, and **-ology** means study of).

StudyWARE CONNECTION

Watch the **Combining Word Roots** animation in the StudyWARE™.

Guessing at Meanings

When you are able to guess at the meaning of a term on the basis of its word parts, you must always double-check for accuracy because some terms have more than one meaning. For example, look at the term **lithotomy** (lih-**THOT**-oh-mee):

- On the basis of word parts, a **lithotomy** is a surgical incision for the removal of a stone (**lith** means stone, and **-otomy** means a surgical incision). This meaning is discussed further in Chapter 9.
- However, **lithotomy** is also the name of an examination position in which the patient is lying on her back with her feet and legs raised and supported in stirrups. The term is used to describe this position because in the early days, this was the preferred position for lithotomy surgery. This term is discussed further in Chapter 15.
- This type of possible confusion is one of the many reasons why a medical dictionary is an important medical terminology tool.

MEDICAL DICTIONARY USE

Learning to use a medical dictionary and other resources to find the definition of a term is an important part of mastering the correct use of medical terms. The following tips for dictionary use apply whether you are working with a traditional book-form dictionary or with electronic dictionary software, websites, or applications on your computer or handheld device.

If You Know How to Spell the Word

When starting to work with an unfamiliar print dictionary, spend a few minutes reviewing its user guide, table of contents, and appendices. The time you spend reviewing now will be saved later when you are looking up unfamiliar terms.

- On the basis of the first letter of the word, start in the appropriate section of the dictionary. Look at the top of the page for clues. The top left word is the first term on the page. The top right word is the last term on that page.
- Next, look alphabetically for words that start with the first and second letters of the word you are researching. Continue looking through each letter until you find the term you are looking for.
- When you think you have found it, check the spelling very carefully, letter by letter, working from left to right. Terms with similar spellings have very different meanings.
- When you find the term, carefully check *all* of the definitions.

If You Do Not Know How to Spell the Word

Listen carefully to the term, and write it down. If you cannot find the word on the basis of your spelling, start looking for alternative spellings based on the beginning sound as shown in Table 1.8. Note: All of these examples are in this textbook. However, you could practice looking them up in the dictionary!

Look Under Categories

Most print dictionaries use categories such as *Diseases* and *Syndromes* to group disorders with these terms in their titles. For example:

- *Venereal disease* would be found under *Disease, venereal.*
- *Fetal alcohol syndrome* would be found under *Syndrome, fetal alcohol.*
- When you come across such a term and cannot find it listed by the first word, the next step is to look under the appropriate category.

Multiple-Word Terms

When you are looking for a term that includes more than one word, begin your search with the last term. If you do not find it there, move forward to the next word.

- For example, *congestive heart failure* is sometimes listed under *heart failure, congestive.* This term is discussed in Chapter 5.

Searching for Definitions on the Internet

Internet search engines are valuable resources in finding definitions and details about medical conditions and terms; however, it is important that you rely on a site, such as the National Institutes of Health (NIH) website (http://www.nih.gov), which is known to be a reputable information source.

- For better results, an Internet search should include visits to at least two reputable sites. If there is a major difference in the definitions, go on to a third site. Sometimes a search engine will recommend a site that is not appropriate but appears because it paid to be listed.
- Beware of suggested search terms. If you do not spell a term correctly, a website may guess what you were searching for. Make sure to double-check that the term you are defining is the intended term.

The same caution applies to medical dictionary applications on handheld devices. Make sure that the application comes from a reputable source, and always double-check that this definition is for the term that you intended to look up.

TABLE 1.8
Guidelines to Looking Up the Spelling of Unfamiliar Terms

If it sounds like	It may begin with	Example
F	F	**flatus** (**FLAY**-tus) [see Chapter 8]
	PH	**phlegm** (**FLEM**) [see Chapter 7]
J	G	**gingivitis** (**jin**-jih-**VYE**-tis) [see Chapter 8]
	J	**jaundice** (**JAWN**-dis) [see Chapter 8]
K	C	**crepitus** (**KREP**-ih-tus) [see Chapter 3]
	CH	**cholera** (**KOL**-er-ah) [see Chapter 8]
	K	**kyphosis** (kye-**FOH**-sis) [see Chapter 3]
	QU	**quadriplegia** (**kwad**-rih-**PLEE**-jee-ah) [see Chapter 4]
S	C	**cytology** (sigh-**TOL**-oh-jee) [see Chapter 2]
	PS	**psychologist** (sigh-**KOL**-oh-jist) [see Chapter 10]
	S	**serum** (**SEER**-um) [see Chapter 5]
Z	X	**xeroderma** (zee-roh-**DER**-mah) [see Chapter 12]
	Z	**zygote** (**ZYE**-goht) [see Chapter 14]

PRONUNCIATION

A medical term is easier to understand and remember when you know how to pronounce it properly. To help you master the pronunciation of new terms, a commonly accepted pronunciation of that word appears in parentheses next to the term. Audio for the terms on the vocabulary list is available in the student StudyWARE™.

The sounds-like pronunciation system is used in this textbook. Here the word is respelled using normal English letters to create sounds that are familiar. To pronounce a new word, just say it as it is spelled in the parentheses.

- The part of the word that receives the primary (most) emphasis when you say it is shown in uppercase boldface letters. For example, **edema** (eh-**DEE**-mah) is swelling caused by an abnormal accumulation of fluid in cells, tissues, or cavities of the body.
- A part of the word that receives secondary (less) emphasis when you say it is shown in boldface lowercase letters. For example, **appendicitis** (ah-**pen**-dih-**SIGH**-tis) means an inflammation of the appendix (**appendic** means appendix, and **-itis** means inflammation).

A Word of Caution

Frequently, there is more than one correct way to pronounce a medical term.

- The pronunciation of many medical terms is based on their Greek, Latin, or other foreign origin. However, there is a trend toward pronouncing terms as they would sound in English.
- The result is more than one "correct" pronunciation for a term. The text shows the most commonly accepted pronunciation.
- If your instructor prefers an alternative pronunciation, follow the instructions you are given.

SPELLING IS ALWAYS IMPORTANT

Accuracy in spelling medical terms is extremely important!

- Changing just one or two letters can completely change the meaning of a word—and this difference literally could be a matter of life or death for the patient.
- The section "Look-Alike, Sound-Alike Terms and Word Parts" later in this chapter will help you become aware of some terms and word parts that are frequently confused.
- The spelling shown in this text is commonly accepted in the U.S. You may encounter alternative spellings used in England, Australia, and Canada.

SINGULAR AND PLURAL ENDINGS

Many medical terms have Greek or Latin origins. As a result of these different origins, there are unusual rules for changing a singular word into a plural form. In addition, English endings have been adopted for some commonly used terms.

- Table 1.9 provides guidelines to help you better understand how these plurals are formed.
- Also, throughout the text, when a term with an unusual singular or plural form is introduced, both forms are included. For example, the **phalanges** (fah-**LAN**-jeez) are the bones of the fingers and toes (singular, *phalanx*) (Figure 1.10).

BASIC MEDICAL TERMS TO DESCRIBE DISEASES

Some of the medical terms that are used to describe diseases and disease conditions can easily be confusing. Some of the more common terms of this type are described in Table 1.10. You will find that studying the groups of three as they are shown in the table makes it easier to master these terms.

LOOK-ALIKE, SOUND-ALIKE TERMS AND WORD PARTS

This section highlights some frequently used terms and word parts that are confusing because they look and sound alike. However, their meanings are very different. It is important that you pay close attention to these terms and word parts as you encounter them in the text.

arteri/o, ather/o, and arthr/o

- **arteri/o** means artery. **Endarterial** (**end**-ar-**TEE**-ree-al) means pertaining to the interior or lining of an artery (**end-** means within, **arteri** means artery, and **-al** means pertaining to).
- **ather/o** means plaque or fatty substance. An **atheroma** (**ath**-er-**OH**-mah) is a fatty deposit within the wall

TABLE 1.9
Guidelines to Unusual Plural Forms

Guideline	Singular	Plural
If the singular term ends in the suffix **-a**, the plural is usually formed by changing the ending to **-ae**.	bursa vertebra	bursae vertebrae
If the singular term ends in the suffix **-ex** or **-ix**, the plural is usually formed by changing these endings to **-ices**.	appendix index	appendices indices
If the singular term ends in the suffix **-is**, the plural is usually formed by changing the ending to **-es**.	diagnosis metastasis	diagnoses metastases
If the singular term ends in the suffix **-itis**, the plural is usually formed by changing the **-is** ending to **-ides**.	arthritis meningitis	arthritides meningitides
If the singular term ends in the suffix **-nx**, the plural is usually formed by the **-x** ending to **-ges**.	phalanx meninx	phalanges meninges
If the singular term ends in the suffix **-on**, the plural is usually formed by changing the ending to **-a**.	criterion ganglion	criteria ganglia
If the singular term ends in the suffix **-um**, the plural usually is formed by changing the ending to **-a**.	diverticulum ovum	diverticula ova
If the singular term ends in the suffix **-us**, the plural is usually formed by changing the ending to **-i**.	alveolus malleolus	alveoli malleoli

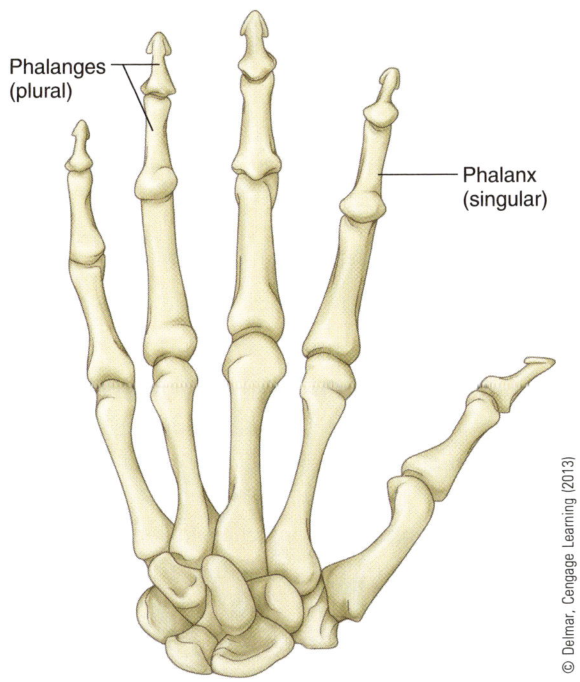

FIGURE 1.10 Singular and plural endings. A phalanx is one finger or toe bone. Phalanges are more than one finger or toe bones.

of an artery (**ather** means fatty substance, and **-oma** means tumor).

- **arthr/o** means joint. **Arthralgia** (ar-**THRAL**-jee-ah) means pain in a joint or joints (**arthr** means joint, and **-algia** means pain).

-ectomy, -ostomy, and -otomy

- **-ectomy** means surgical removal. An **appendectomy** (**ap**-en-**DECK**-toh-mee) is the surgical removal of the appendix (**append** means appendix, and **-ectomy** means surgical removal).
- **-ostomy** means the surgical creation of an artificial opening to the body surface. A **colostomy** (koh-**LAHS**-toh-mee) is the surgical creation of an artificial excretory opening between the colon and the body surface (**col** means colon, and **-ostomy** means the surgical creation of an artificial opening).
- **-otomy** means cutting or a surgical incision. A **colotomy** (koh-**LOT**-oh-mee) is a surgical incision into the colon (**col** means colon, and **-otomy** means a surgical incision).

TABLE 1.10
Basic Medical Terms to Describe Disease Conditions

A **sign** is objective evidence of disease such as a fever. *Objective* means the sign can be evaluated or measured by the patient or others.	A **symptom** (**SIMP**-tum) is subjective evidence of a disease, such as pain or a headache. *Subjective* means that it can be evaluated or measured only by the patient.	A **syndrome** (**SIN**-drohm) is a set of the signs and symptoms that occur together as part of a specific disease process.
A **diagnosis** (**dye**-ag-**NOH**-sis) (DX) is the identification of a disease (plural, *diagnoses*). To *diagnose* is the process of reaching a diagnosis.	A **differential diagnosis** (D/DX), also known as a *rule out* (R/O) is an attempt to determine which one of several diseases can be causing the signs and symptoms that are present.	A **prognosis** (prog-**NOH**-sis) is a prediction of the probable course and outcome of a disorder (plural, *prognoses*).
An **acute** condition has a rapid onset, a severe course, and a relatively short duration.	A **chronic** condition is of long duration. Although such diseases can be controlled, they are rarely cured.	A **remission** is the temporary, partial, or complete disappearance of the symptoms of a disease without having achieved a cure.
A **disease** is a condition in which one or more body parts are not functioning normally. Some diseases are named for their signs and symptoms. For example, *chronic fatigue syndrome* (CFS) is a persistent overwhelming fatigue of unknown origin (see Chapter 4).	An **eponym** (**EP**-oh-nim) is a disease, structure, operation, or procedure named for the person who discovered or described it first. For example, *Alzheimer's disease* is named for German neurologist Alois Alzheimer (see Chapter 10).	An **acronym** (**ACK**-roh-nim) is a word formed from the initial letter of the major parts of a compound term. For example, the acronym **laser** stands for **l**ight **a**mplification by **s**timulated **e**mission of **r**adiation (see Chapter 12).

Fissure and Fistula

- A **fissure** (**FISH**-ur) is a groove or crack-like sore of the skin (see Chapter 12). This term also describes normal folds in the contours of the brain.
- A **fistula** (**FIS**-tyou-lah) is an abnormal passage, usually between two internal organs or leading from an organ to the surface of the body. A fistula may be due to surgery, injury, or the draining of an abscess.

Ileum and Ilium

- The **ileum** (**ILL**-ee-um) is the last and longest portion of the small intestine. *Memory aid: ileum* is spelled with an ***e*** as in *intestine.*
- The **ilium** (**ILL**-ee-um) is part of the hip bone. *Memory aid: ilium* is spelled with an ***i*** as in *hip.* (Figure 1.11)

Infection and Inflammation

- Although the suffix **-itis** means inflammation, it also is commonly used to indicate infection.
- An **infection** (in-**FECK**-shun) is the invasion of the body by a pathogenic (disease-producing) organism. The infection can remain localized (near the point of entry) or can be systemic (affecting the entire body). Signs and symptoms of infection include malaise, chills and fever, redness, heat and swelling, or exudate from a wound.
- **Malaise** (mah-**LAYZ**) is a feeling of general discomfort or uneasiness that is often the first indication of an infection or other disease.
- An **exudate** (**ECKS**-you-dayt) is fluid, such as pus, that leaks out of an infected wound.

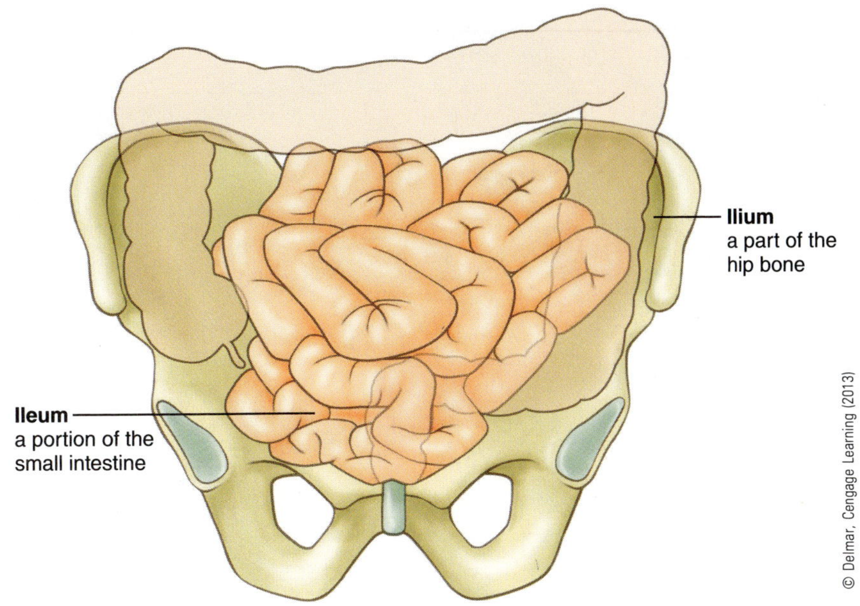

FIGURE 1.11 There is only one letter difference between *ileum* and *ilium*, but they are very different parts of the body.

- **Inflammation** (**in**-flah-**MAY**-shun) is a localized response to an injury or to the destruction of tissues. The key indicators of inflammation are (1) *erythema* (redness), (2) *hyperthermia* (heat), (3) *edema* (swelling), and (4) *pain*. These are caused by extra blood flowing into the area as part of the healing process.

Laceration and Lesion

- A **laceration** (**lass**-er-**AY**-shun) is a torn or jagged wound or an accidental cut wound.
- A **lesion** (**LEE**-zhun) is a pathologic change of the tissues due to disease or injury.

Mucous and Mucus

- The adjective **mucous** (**MYOU**-kus) describes the specialized membranes that line the body cavities.
- The noun **mucus** (**MYOU**-kus) is the name of the fluid secreted by these mucous membranes.

myc/o, myel/o, and my/o

- **myc/o** means fungus. **Mycosis** (my-**KOH**-sis) describes any abnormal condition or disease caused by a fungus (**myc** means fungus, and **-osis** means abnormal condition or disease).
- **myel/o** means bone marrow *or* spinal cord. The term **myelopathy** (my-eh-**LOP**-ah-thee) describes any pathologic change or disease in the spinal cord (**myel/o** means spinal cord or bone marrow, and **-pathy** means disease).
- **my/o** means muscle. The term **myopathy** (my-**OP**-ah-thee) describes any pathologic change or disease of muscle tissue (**my/o** means muscle, and **-pathy** means disease).

-ologist and -ology

- **-ologist** means specialist. A **dermatologist** (**der**-mah-**TOL**-oh-jist) is a physician who specializes in diagnosing and treating disorders of the skin (**dermat** means skin, and **-ologist** means specialist).
- **-ology** means the study of. **Neonatology** (**nee**-oh-nay-**TOL**-oh-jee) is the study of disorders of the newborn (**neo-** means new, **nat** means birth, and **-ology** means study of).

Palpation and Palpitation

- **Palpation** (pal-**PAY**-shun) is an examination technique in which the examiner's hands are used to feel the texture, size, consistency, and location of certain body parts.
- **Palpitation** (**pal**-pih-**TAY**-shun) is a pounding or racing heart.

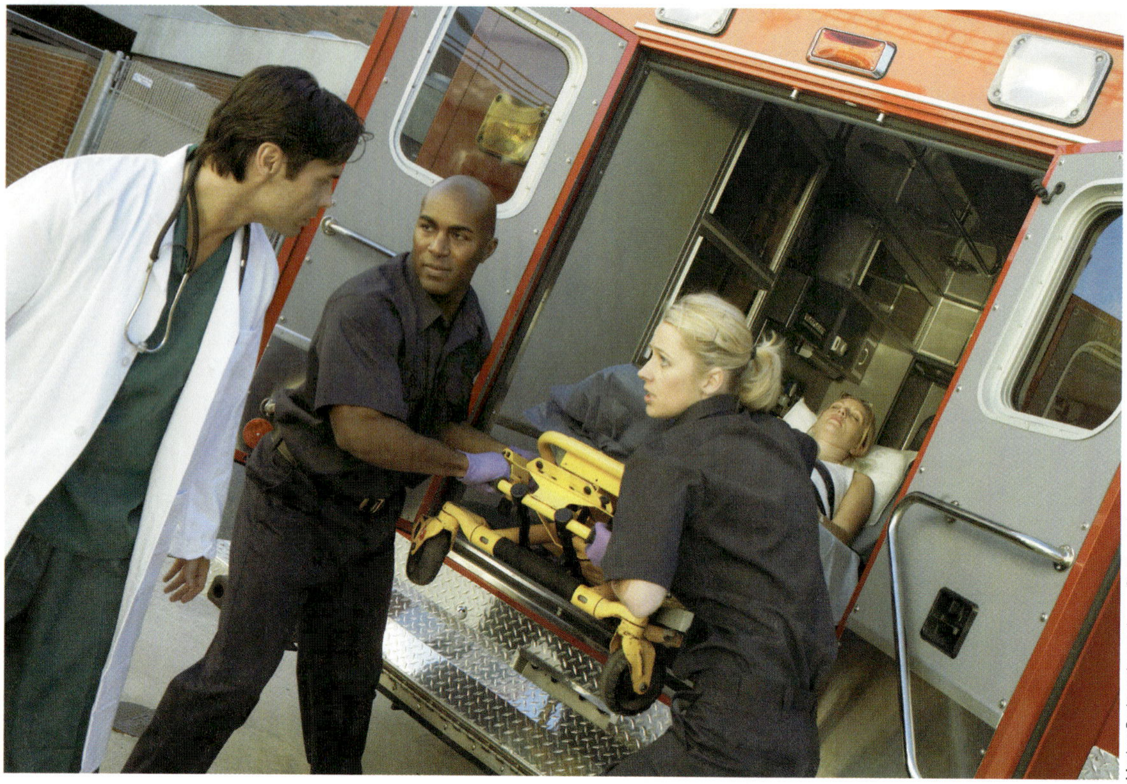

FIGURE 1.12 Triage describes the process through which emergency personnel arriving on an accident scene identify which of the injured require care first and where they can be treated most effectively.

pyel/o, py/o, and pyr/o

- **pyel/o** means renal pelvis, which is part of the kidney. **Pyelitis** (**pye**-eh-**LYE**-tis) is an inflammation of the renal pelvis (**pyel** means renal pelvis, and **-itis** means inflammation).
- **py/o** means pus. **Pyoderma** (**pye**-oh-**DER**-mah) is any acute, inflammatory, pus-forming bacterial skin infection such as impetigo (**py/o** means pus, and **-derma** means skin).
- **pyr/o** means fever or fire. **Pyrosis** (pye-**ROH**-sis), also known as ***heartburn***, is discomfort due to the regurgitation of stomach acid upward into the esophagus (**pyr** means fever or fire, and **-osis** means abnormal condition or disease).

Supination and Suppuration

- **Supination** (**soo**-pih-**NAY**-shun) is the act of rotating the arm so that the palm of the hand is forward or upward.
- **Suppuration** (**sup**-you-**RAY**-shun) is the formation or discharge of pus.

Triage and Trauma

- **Triage** (tree-**AHZH**) is the medical screening of patients to determine their relative priority of need and the proper place of treatment. (Figure 1.12)
- **Trauma** (**TRAW**-mah) means wound or injury. These are the types of injuries that might occur in an accident, shooting, natural disaster, or fire.

Viral and Virile

- **Viral** (**VYE**-ral) means pertaining to a virus (**vir** means virus or poison, and **-al** means pertaining to).
- **Virile** (**VIR**-ill) means having the nature, properties, or qualities of an adult male.

USING ABBREVIATIONS

Abbreviations are frequently used as a shorthand way to record long and complex medical terms; Appendix B contains an alphabetized list of many of the more commonly used medical abbreviations.

- Abbreviations can also lead to confusion and errors! Therefore, it is important that you be very careful when using or interpreting an abbreviation.
- For example, the abbreviation *BE* means both "below elbow" (as in amputation) and "barium enema." Just imagine what a difference a mix-up here would make for the patient!
- Most clinical agencies have policies for accepted abbreviations. It is important to follow this list for the facility where you are working.
- If there is any question in your mind about which abbreviation to use, always follow this rule: ***When in doubt, spell it out.***

TABLE 1.11
Examples of Abbreviations Not to Be Used

Abbreviation	Potential Problem
MS	can mean either morphine sulfate *or* magnesium sulfate
QD and QOD	mean daily and every other day, sometimes mistaken for each other
U	means unit, sometimes mistaken for 0 or 4

Some abbreviations should never be used (as decided by the *Joint Commission,* an organization founded in 1910 to standardize medical practices). See Table 1.11 for examples. The Joint Commission's latest standards are available at http://www.jointcommission.org. Many medical facilities have their own suggested "do not use" abbreviation list.

StudyWARE™ CONNECTION

For more practice and to test your mastery of this material, go to the StudyWARE™ to play interactive games and complete the quiz for this chapter.

Workbook Practice

Go to your workbook, and complete the exercises for this chapter.

Downloadable audio is available for selected medical terms in this chapter to enhance your learning of medical terminology.

CHAPTER 1 LEARNING EXERCISES

MATCHING WORD PARTS 1

Write the correct answer in the middle column.

	Definition	Correct Answer	Possible Answers
1.1.	bad, difficult, painful	________	-algia
1.2.	excessive, increased	________	dys-
1.3.	enlargement	________	-ectomy
1.4.	pain, suffering	________	-megaly
1.5.	surgical removal	________	hyper-

MATCHING WORD PARTS 2

Write the correct answer in the middle column.

	Definition	Correct Answer	Possible Answers
1.6.	abnormal condition or disease	________	hypo-
1.7.	abnormal softening	________	-itis
1.8.	deficient, decreased	________	-malacia
1.9.	inflammation	________	-necrosis
1.10.	tissue death	________	-osis

MATCHING WORD PARTS 3

Write the correct answer in the middle column.

	Definition	Correct Answer	Possible Answers
1.11.	bleeding, bursting forth	________	-ostomy

1.12.	surgical creation of an artificial opening to the body surface	______________	**-otomy**
1.13.	surgical incision	______________	**-plasty**
1.14.	surgical repair	______________	**-rrhage**
1.15.	surgical suturing	______________	**-rrhaphy**

MATCHING WORD PARTS 4

Write the correct answer in the middle column.

	Definition	Correct Answer	Possible Answers
1.16.	visual examination	______________	**-rrhea**
1.17.	rupture	______________	**-rrhexis**
1.18.	abnormal narrowing	______________	**-sclerosis**
1.19.	abnormal hardening	______________	**-scopy**
1.20.	flow or discharge	______________	**-stenosis**

DEFINITIONS

Select the correct answer, and write it on the line provided.

1.21. The term ______________ describes any pathologic change or disease in the spinal cord.

myelopathy   myopathy   pyelitis   pyrosis

1.22. The medical term for higher-than-normal blood pressure is ______________.

hepatomegaly   hypertension   hypotension   supination

1.23. The term ______________ means pertaining to birth.

natal   perinatal   postnatal   prenatal

1.24. Pain is classified as a ______________.

diagnosis   sign   symptom   syndrome

1.25. In the term *myopathy*, the suffix **-pathy** means ______________.

abnormal condition   disease   inflammation   swelling

MATCHING TERMS AND DEFINITIONS 1

Write the correct answer in the middle column.

Definition	Correct Answer	Possible Answers
1.26. white blood cell	__________	acute
1.27. prediction of the probable course and outcome of a disorder	__________	edema
1.28. swelling caused by an abnormal accumulation of fluid in cells, tissues, or cavities of the body	__________	leukocyte
1.29. rapid onset	__________	prognosis
1.30. turning the palm of the hand upward	__________	supination

MATCHING TERMS AND DEFINITIONS 2

Write the correct answer in the middle column.

Definition	Correct Answer	Possible Answers
1.31. examination procedure	__________	laceration
1.32. fluid, such as pus, that leaks out of an infected wound	__________	lesion
1.33. pathologic tissue change	__________	palpitation
1.34. pounding heart	__________	palpation
1.35. torn or jagged wound, or an accidental cut wound	__________	exudate

WHICH WORD?

Select the correct answer, and write it on the line provided.

1.36. The medical term __________ describes an inflammation of the stomach.

gastritis gastrosis

1.37. The formation of pus is called __________.

supination suppuration

1.38. The term meaning wound or injury is ________________________.

trauma triage

1.39. The term ________________________ means pertaining to a virus.

viral virile

1.40. A/an ________________________ is the surgical removal of the appendix.

appendectomy appendicitis

SPELLING COUNTS

Find the misspelled word in each sentence. Then write that word, spelled correctly, on the line provided.

1.41. A disease named for the person who discovered it is known as an enaponym. ________________________

1.42. A localized response to injury or tissue destruction is called inflimmation. ________________________

1.43. A fisure of the skin is a groove or crack-like sore of the skin. ________________________

1.44. The medical term meaning suturing together the ends of a severed nerve is neurorraphy. ________________________

1.45. The medical term meaning inflammation of the tonsils is tonsilitis. ________________________

MATCHING TERMS

Write the correct answer in the middle column.

Definition	Correct Answer	Possible Answers
1.46. abnormal condition or disease of the stomach	________________________	syndrome
1.47. a set of signs and symptoms	________________________	gastralgia
1.48. rupture of a muscle	________________________	gastrosis
1.49. stomach pain	________________________	pyoderma
1.50. any acute, inflammatory, pus-forming bacterial skin infection	________________________	myorrhexis

TERM SELECTION

Select the correct answer, and write it on the line provided.

1.51. The abnormal hardening of the walls of an artery or arteries is called ______________________.

arteriosclerosis arteriostenosis arthrostenosis atherosclerosis

1.52. A fever is considered to be a ______________________.

prognosis sign symptom syndrome

1.53. An inflammation of the stomach and small intestine is known as ______________________.

gastralgia gastroenteritis gastritis gastrosis

1.54. The term meaning pain in a joint or joints is ______________________.

arthralgia arthritis arthrocentesis atherosclerosis

1.55. A ______________________ is a physician who specializes in diagnosing and treating diseases and disorders of the skin.

dermatologist dermatology neurologist neurology

SENTENCE COMPLETION

Write the correct term on the line provided.

1.56. Lower-than-normal blood pressure is called ______________________.

1.57. The process of recording a radiographic study of the blood vessels after the injection of a contrast medium is known as ______________________.

1.58. The term meaning above or outside the ribs is ______________________.

1.59. A/An ______________________ diagnosis is also known as a rule out.

1.60. A/An ______________________ is an abnormal passage, usually between two internal organs or leading from an organ to the surface of the body.

TRUE/FALSE

If the statement is true, write **True** on the line. If the statement is false, write **False** on the line.

1.61. ______________________ An erythrocyte is commonly known as a red blood cell.

1.62. ______________________ Arteriomalacia is abnormal hardening of blood vessels of the walls of an artery or arteries.

1.63. ______________________ A colostomy is the surgical creation of an artificial opening between the colon and the body surface.

1.64. ______________________ Malaise is often the first symptom of inflammation.

1.65. ______________________ An infection is the invasion of the body by a disease-producing organism.

WORD SURGERY

Divide each term into its component word parts. Write these word parts, in sequence, on the lines provided. When necessary, use a slash (/) to indicate a combining vowel. (You may not need all of the lines provided.)

1.66. **Otorhinolaryngology** is the study of the ears, nose, and throat.

__________ __________ __________ __________

1.67. The term **mycosis** means any abnormal condition or disease caused by a fungus.

__________ __________ __________ __________

1.68. **Poliomyelitis** is a viral infection of the gray matter of the spinal cord.

__________ __________ __________ __________

1.69. **Neonatology** is the study of disorders of the newborn.

__________ __________ __________ __________

1.70. The term **endarterial** means pertaining to the interior or lining of an artery.

__________ __________ __________ __________

CLINICAL CONDITIONS

Write the correct answer on the line provided.

1.71. Miguel required a/an ______________________ injection. This term means that the medication was placed directly within the muscle.

1.72. Mrs. Tillson underwent ______________________ to remove excess fluid from her abdomen.

1.73. The term ***laser*** is a/an ______________________. This means that it is a word formed from the initial letters of the major parts of a compound term.

1.74. In an accident, Felipe Valladares broke several bones in his fingers. The medical term for these injuries is fractured ______________________.

1.75. In case of a major disaster Cheng Lee, who is a trained paramedic, helps perform ________________________. This is the screening of patients to determine their relative priority of need and the proper place of treatment.

1.76. Gina's physician ordered laboratory tests that would enable him to establish a differential ________________________ to identify the cause of her signs and symptoms.

1.77. Jennifer plans to go to graduate school so she can specialize in ________________________. This specialty is concerned with the study of all aspects of diseases.

1.78. John Randolph's cancer went into ________________________. Although this is not a cure, his symptoms disappeared and he felt much better.

1.79. Mr. Jankowski describes that uncomfortable feeling as heartburn. The medical term for this condition is ________________________.

1.80. Phyllis was having great fun traveling until she ate some contaminated food and developed ________________________. She felt miserable and needed to stay in her hotel because of the frequent flow of loose or watery stools.

WHICH IS THE CORRECT MEDICAL TERM?

Select the correct answer, and write it on the line provided.

1.81. The term ________________________ describes the surgical repair of a nerve.

neuralgia neurorrhaphy neurology neuroplasty

1.82. The term ________________________ means loss of a large amount of blood in a short time.

diarrhea hemorrhage hepatorrhagia otorrhagia

1.83. The term ________________________ means the tissue death of an artery or arteries.

arteriomalacia arterionecrosis arteriosclerosis arteriostenosis

1.84. The term ________________________ means between, but not within, the parts of a tissue.

interstitial intrastitial intermuscular intramuscular

1.85. The term ________________________ means enlargement of the liver.

hepatitis hepatomegaly nephromegaly nephritis

CHALLENGE WORD BUILDING

These terms are *not* found in this chapter; however, they are made up of the following familiar word parts. If you need help in creating the term, refer to your medical dictionary.

neo- = new	**arteri/o** = artery	**-algia** = pain and suffering
	arthr/o = joint	**-itis** = inflammation
	cardi/o = heart	**-ologist** = specialist
	nat/o = birth	**-otomy** = a surgical incision
	neur/o = nerve	**-rrhea** = flow or discharge
	rhin/o = nose	**-scopy** = visual examination

1.86. A medical specialist concerned with the diagnosis and treatment of heart disease is a/an ______________________.

1.87. The term meaning a runny nose is ______________________.

1.88. The term meaning the inflammation of a joint or joints is ______________________.

1.89. A medical specialist in disorders of the newborn is a/an ______________________.

1.90. The term meaning a surgical incision into a nerve is a/an ______________________.

1.91. The term meaning inflammation of the heart is ______________________.

1.92. The term meaning pain in the nose is ______________________.

1.93. The term meaning pain in a nerve or nerves is ______________________.

1.94. The term meaning a surgical incision into the heart is a/an ______________________.

1.95. The term meaning an inflammation of the nose is ______________________.

CHAPTER 2

The Human Body in Health and Disease

Overview of THE HUMAN BODY IN HEALTH AND DISEASE

Anatomic Reference Systems	Terms used to describe the location of body planes, directions, and cavities.
Structures of the Body	The cells, tissues, and glands that form the body systems that work together to enable the body to function properly.
Genetics	The genetic components that transfer characteristics from parents to their children.
Tissues	A group of similarly specialized cells that work together to perform specific functions.
Glands	A group of specialized cells that is capable of producing secretions.
Body Systems and Related Organs	Organs are somewhat independent parts of the body that perform specific functions. Organs with related functions are organized into body systems.
Pathology	The study of the nature and cause of disease that involve changes in structure and function.

Vocabulary Related to **THE HUMAN BODY IN HEALTH AND DISEASE**

This list contains essential word parts and medical terms for this chapter. These terms are pronounced in the StudyWARE™ and Audio CDs that are available for use with this text. These and the other important **primary terms** are shown in boldface throughout the chapter. *Secondary terms*, which appear in *orange* italics, clarify the meaning of primary terms.

Word Parts

- ☐ **aden/o** gland
- ☐ **adip/o** fat
- ☐ **anter/o** before, front
- ☐ **caud/o** lower part of body, tail
- ☐ **cephal/o** head
- ☐ **cyt/o**, **-cyte** cell
- ☐ **end-**, **endo-** in, within, inside
- ☐ **exo-** out of, outside, away from
- ☐ **hist/o**, **histi/o** tissue
- ☐ **-ologist** specialist
- ☐ **-ology** the science or study of
- ☐ **path/o**, **-pathy** disease, suffering, feeling, emotion
- ☐ **plas/i**, **plas/o**, **-plasia** development, growth, formation
- ☐ **poster/o** behind, toward the back
- ☐ **-stasis**, **-static** control, maintenance of a constant level

Medical Terms

- ☐ **abdominal cavity** (ab-**DOM**-ih-nal)
- ☐ **adenectomy** (**ad**-eh-**NECK**-toh-mee)
- ☐ **adenocarcinoma** (**ad**-eh-noh-**kar**-sih-**NOH**-mah)
- ☐ **adenoma** (**ad**-eh-**NOH**-mah)
- ☐ **adenomalacia** (**ad**-eh-noh-mah-**LAY**-shee-ah)
- ☐ **adenosclerosis** (**ad**-eh-noh-skleh-**ROH**-sis)
- ☐ **anaplasia** (**an**-ah-**PLAY**-zee-ah)
- ☐ **anatomy** (ah-**NAT**-oh-mee)
- ☐ **anomaly** (ah-**NOM**-ah-lee)
- ☐ **anterior** (an-**TEER**-ee-or)
- ☐ **aplasia** (ah-**PLAY**-zee-ah)
- ☐ **bloodborne transmission**
- ☐ **caudal** (**KAW**-dal)
- ☐ **cephalic** (seh-**FAL**-ick)
- ☐ **chromosomes** (**KROH**-moh-sohmes)
- ☐ **communicable disease** (kuh-**MEW**-nih-kuh-bul)
- ☐ **congenital disorder** (kon-**JEN**-ih-tahl)
- ☐ **cytoplasm** (**SIGH**-toh-plazm)
- ☐ **distal** (**DIS**-tal)
- ☐ **dorsal** (**DOR**-sal)
- ☐ **dysplasia** (dis-**PLAY**-see-ah)
- ☐ **endemic** (en-**DEM**-ick)
- ☐ **endocrine glands** (**EN**-doh-krin)
- ☐ **epidemic** (**ep**-ih-**DEM**-ick)
- ☐ **epigastric region** (**ep**-ih-**GAS**-trick)
- ☐ **etiology** (**ee**-tee-**OL**-oh-jee)
- ☐ **exocrine glands** (**ECK**-soh-krin)
- ☐ **functional disorder**
- ☐ **genetic disorder**
- ☐ **geriatrician** (**jer**-ee-ah-**TRISH**-un)
- ☐ **hemophilia** (**hee**-moh-**FILL**-ee-ah)
- ☐ **histology** (hiss-**TOL**-oh-jee)
- ☐ **homeostasis** (**hoh**-mee-oh-**STAY**-sis)
- ☐ **hyperplasia** (**high**-per-**PLAY**-zee-ah)
- ☐ **hypertrophy** (high-**PER**-troh-fee)
- ☐ **hypogastric region** (**high**-poh-**GAS**-trick)
- ☐ **hypoplasia** (**high**-poh-**PLAY**-zee-ah)
- ☐ **iatrogenic illness** (eye-**at**-roh-**JEN**-ick)
- ☐ **idiopathic disorder** (**id**-ee-oh-**PATH**-ick)
- ☐ **infectious disease** (in-**FECK**-shus)
- ☐ **inguinal** (**ING**-gwih-nal)
- ☐ **medial** (**MEE**-dee-al)
- ☐ **mesentery** (**MESS**-en-**terr**-ee)
- ☐ **midsagittal plane** (mid-**SADJ**-ih-tal)
- ☐ **nosocomial infection** (**nos**-oh-**KOH**-mee-al in-**FECK**-shun)
- ☐ **pandemic** (pan-**DEM**-ick)
- ☐ **pelvic cavity** (**PEL**-vick)
- ☐ **peritoneum** (**pehr**-ih-toh-**NEE**-um)
- ☐ **peritonitis** (**pehr**-ih-toh-**NIGH**-tis)
- ☐ **phenylketonuria** (**fen**-il-**kee**-toh-**NEW**-ree-ah)
- ☐ **physiology** (**fiz**-ee-**OL**-oh-jee)
- ☐ **posterior** (pos-**TEER**-ee-or)
- ☐ **proximal** (**PROCK**-sih-mal)
- ☐ **retroperitoneal** (**ret**-roh-**pehr**-ih-toh-**NEE**-al)
- ☐ **stem cells**
- ☐ **thoracic cavity** (thoh-**RAS**-ick)
- ☐ **transverse plane** (trans-**VERSE**)
- ☐ **umbilicus** (um-**BILL**-ih-kus)
- ☐ **vector-borne transmission**
- ☐ **ventral** (**VEN**-tral)

LEARNING GOALS

On completion of this chapter, you should be able to:

1. Define anatomy and physiology and the uses of anatomic reference systems to identify the anatomic position plus body planes, directions, and cavities.
2. Recognize, define, spell, and pronounce the primary terms related to cells and genetics.
3. Recognize, define, spell, and pronounce the primary terms related to the structure, function, pathology, and procedures of tissues and glands.
4. Identify the major organs and functions of the body systems.
5. Recognize, define, spell, and pronounce the primary terms used to describe pathology, the modes of transmission, and the types of diseases.

ANATOMIC REFERENCE SYSTEMS

Anatomic reference systems are used to describe the locations of the structural units of the body. The simplest anatomic reference is the one we learn in childhood: our right hand is on the right, and our left hand on the left.

In medical terminology, there are several additional ways to describe the location of different body parts. These anatomical reference systems include:

- Body planes
- Body directions
- Body cavities
- Structural units

When body parts work together to perform a related function, they are grouped together and are known as a body system.

Anatomy and Physiology Defined

- **Anatomy** (ah-**NAT**-oh-mee) is the study of the structures of the body.
- **Physiology** (**fiz**-ee-**OL**-oh-jee) is the study of the functions of the structures of the body (**physi** means nature or physical, and **-ology** means study of).

The Anatomic Position

The **anatomic position** describes the body standing in the standard position. This includes:

- Standing up straight so that the body is erect and facing forward
- Holding the arms at the sides with the hands turned so that the palms face toward the front.

The Body Planes

Body planes are imaginary vertical and horizontal lines used to divide the body into sections for descriptive purposes (Figure 2.1). These planes are aligned to a body standing in the anatomic position.

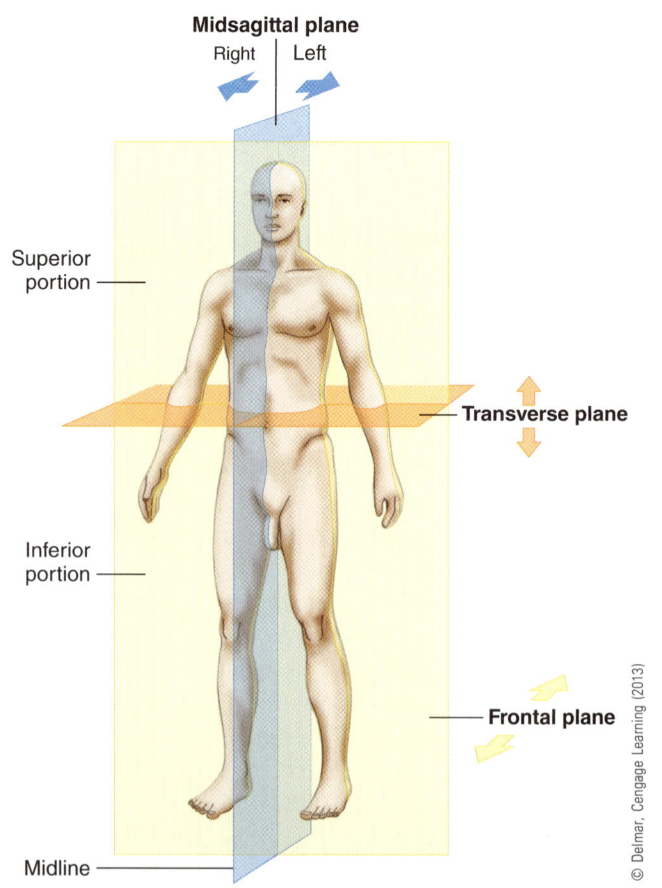

FIGURE 2.1 Body planes: the midsagittal plane divides the body into equal left and right halves. The transverse plane divides the body into superior (upper) and inferior (lower) portions. The frontal plane divides the body into anterior (front) and posterior (back) portions.

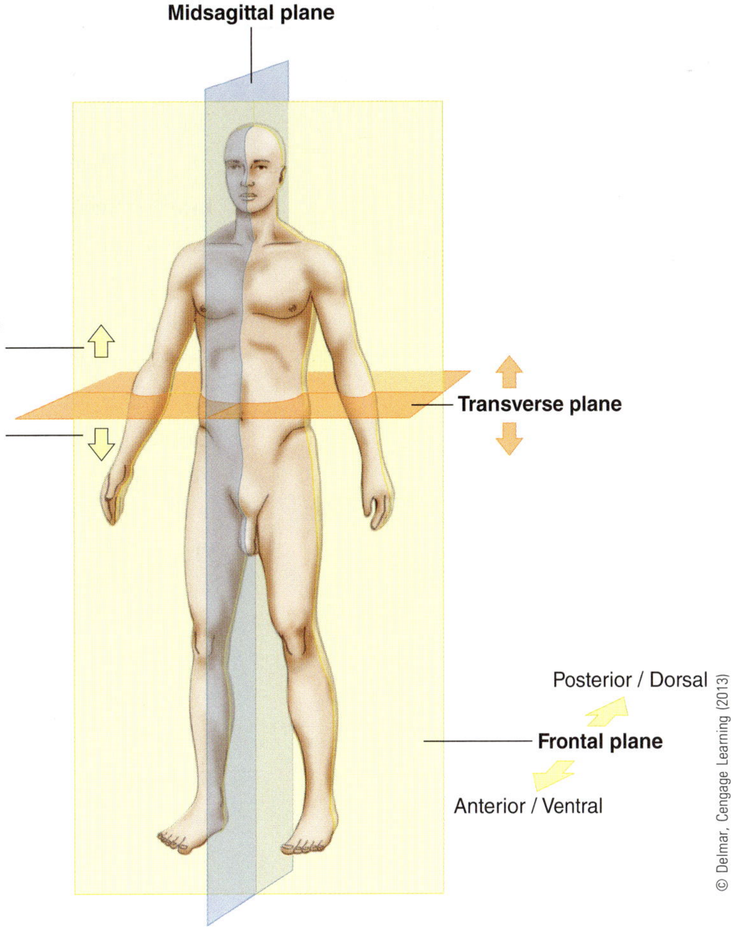

FIGURE 2.2 Body directions: Cephalic means toward the head, and caudal means toward the feet. Anterior means toward the front, and the front of the body is known as the ventral surface. Posterior means toward the back, and the back of the body is known as the dorsal surface.

The Vertical Planes

A **vertical plane** is an up-and-down plane that is a right angle to the horizon.

- A **sagittal plane** (**SADJ**-ih-tal) is a vertical plane that divides the body into *unequal* left and right portions.
- The **midsagittal plane** (mid-**SADJ**-ih-tal), also known as the ***midline***, is the sagittal plane that divides the body into *equal* left and right halves (Figure 2.1).
- A **frontal plane** is a vertical plane that divides the body into anterior (front) and posterior (back) portions. Also known as the ***coronal plane***, it is located at right angles to the sagittal plane (Figure 2.1).

The Horizontal Plane

A **horizontal plane** is a flat crosswise plane, such as the horizon.

- A **transverse plane** (trans-**VERSE**) is a horizontal plane that divides the body into superior (upper) and inferior (lower) portions. A transverse plane can be at the waist or at any other level across the body (Figure 2.1).

StudyWARE CONNECTION

Watch the **Body Planes** animation on the StudyWARE™.

Body Direction Terms

The relative location of sections of the body or of an organ can be described through the use of pairs of contrasting body direction terms. These terms are illustrated in Figures 2.2 and 2.3.

- **Ventral** (**VEN**-tral) refers to the front, or belly side, of the organ or body (**ventr** means belly side of the body, and **-al** means pertaining to). Ventral is the opposite of *dorsal*.

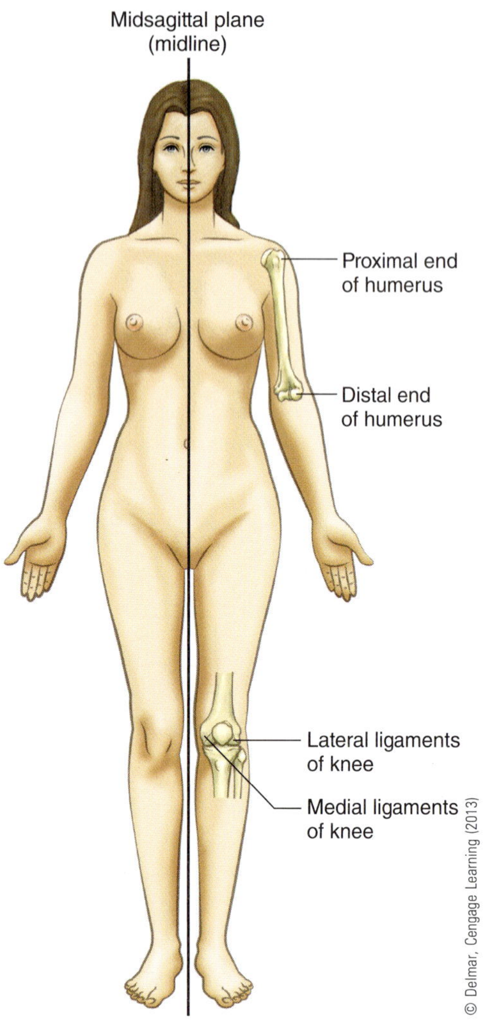

FIGURE 2.3 Body directions: Proximal means situated nearest the midline, and distal means situated farthest from the midline. Medial means toward or nearer the midline, and lateral means toward the side and away from the midline.

- **Dorsal** (**DOR**-sal) refers to the back of the organ or body (**dors** means back of the body, and **-al** means pertaining to). Dorsal is the opposite of *ventral.*
- **Anterior** (an-**TEER**-ee-or) means situated in the front. It also means on the front or forward part of an organ (**anter** means front or before, and **-ior** means pertaining to). For example, the stomach is located anterior to (in front of) the pancreas. *Anterior* is also used in reference to the ventral surface of the body. *Anterior* is the opposite of *posterior.*
- **Posterior** (pos-**TEER**-ee-or) means situated in the back. It also means on the back part of an organ (**poster** means back or toward the back, and **-ior** means pertaining to). For example, the pancreas is located posterior to (behind) the stomach. The term *posterior* is also used in reference to the dorsal surface of the body. *Posterior* is the opposite of *anterior.*
- **Superior** means uppermost, above, or toward the head. For example, the lungs are located superior to (above) the diaphragm. *Superior* is the opposite of *inferior.*
- **Inferior** means lowermost, below, or toward the feet. For example, the stomach is located inferior to (below) the diaphragm. *Inferior* is the opposite of *superior.*
- **Cephalic** (seh-**FAL**-ick) means toward the head (**cephal** means head, and **-ic** means pertaining to). *Cephalic* is the opposite of *caudal.*
- **Caudal** (**KAW**-dal) means toward the lower part of the body (**caud** means tail or lower part of the body, and **-al** means pertaining to). *Caudal* is the opposite of *cephalic.*
- **Proximal** (**PROCK**-sih-mal) means situated nearest the midline or beginning of a body structure. For example, the proximal end of the humerus (bone of the upper arm) forms part of the shoulder. *Proximal* is the opposite of *distal.*
- **Distal** (**DIS**-tal) means situated farthest from the midline or beginning of a body structure. For example, the distal end of the humerus forms part of the elbow (Figure 2.3). *Distal* is the opposite of *proximal.*
- **Medial** (**MEE**-dee-al) means the direction toward, or nearer, the midline. For example, the medial ligament of the knee is near the inner surface of the leg (Figure 2.3). *Medial* is the opposite of *lateral.*
- **Lateral** means the direction toward, or nearer, the side of the body, away from the midline. For example, the lateral ligament of the knee is near the side of the leg. *Lateral* is the opposite of *medial.* ***Bilateral*** means relating to, or having, two sides.

Major Body Cavities

The two major **body cavities**, which are the dorsal (back) and the ventral (front) cavities, are spaces within the body that contain and protect internal organs (Figure 2.4).

The Dorsal Cavity

The **dorsal cavity**, which is located along the back of the body and head, contains organs of the nervous system that coordinate body functions and is divided into two portions:

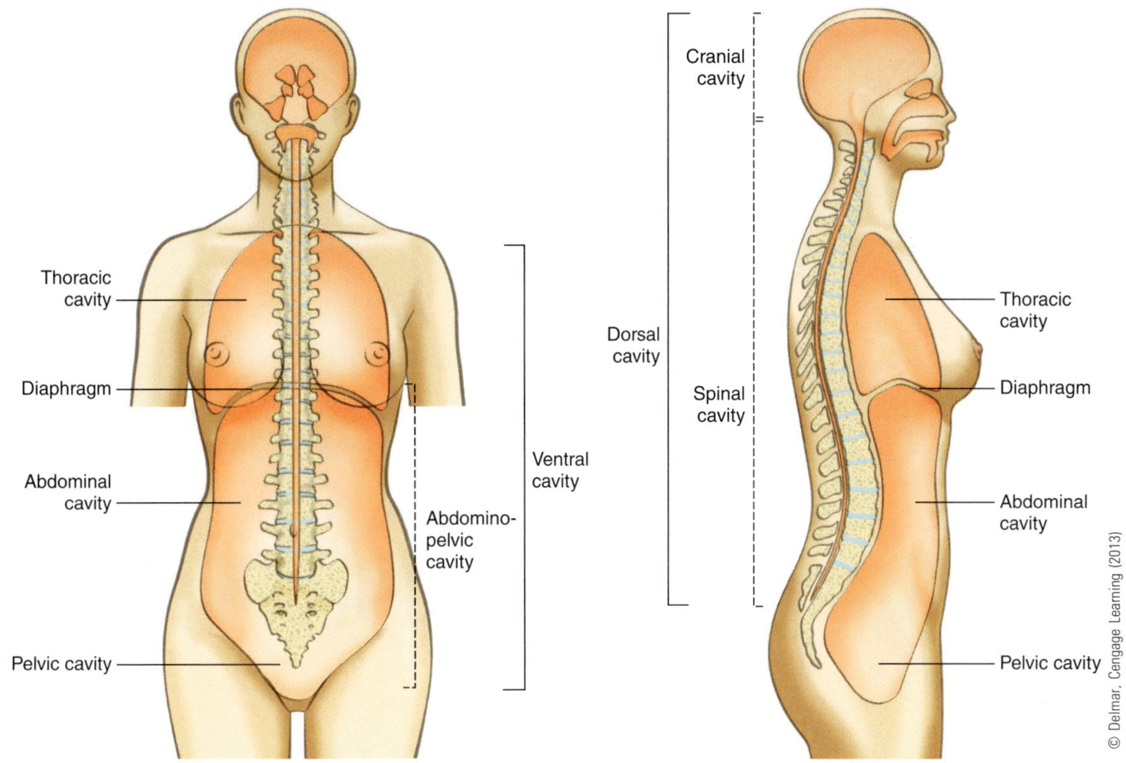

FIGURE 2.4 The major body cavities.

- The **cranial cavity**, which is located within the skull, surrounds and protects the brain. ***Cranial*** means pertaining to the skull.
- The **spinal cavity**, which is located within the spinal column, surrounds and protects the spinal cord.

The Ventral Cavity

The **ventral cavity**, which is located along the front of the body, contains the body organs that sustain homeostasis. **Homeostasis** (**hoh**-mee-oh-**STAY**-sis) is the processes through which the body maintains a constant internal environment (**home/o** means constant, and **-stasis** means control). The ventral cavity is divided into the following portions:

- The **thoracic cavity** (thoh-**RAS**-ick), also known as the ***chest cavity*** or ***thorax***, surrounds and protects the heart and the lungs. The ***diaphragm*** is a muscle that separates the thoracic and abdominal cavities.
- The **abdominal cavity** (ab-**DOM**-ih-nal) contains primarily the major organs of digestion. This cavity is frequently referred to simply as the **abdomen** (**AB**-doh-men).
- The **pelvic cavity** (**PEL**-vick) is the space formed by the hip bones and contains primarily the organs of the reproductive and excretory systems.

There is no physical division between the abdominal and pelvic cavities. The term **abdominopelvic cavity** (ab-**dom**-ih-noh-**PEL**-vick) refers to these two cavities as a single unit (**abdomin/o** means abdomen, **pelv** means pelvis, and **-ic** means pertaining to).

The term **inguinal** (**ING**-gwih-nal), which means relating to the groin, refers to the entire lower area of the abdomen. This includes the ***groin***, which is the crease at the junction of the trunk with the upper end of the thigh.

Regions of the Thorax and Abdomen

Regions of the thorax and abdomen are a descriptive system that divides the abdomen and lower portion of the thorax into nine parts (Figure 2.5). These parts are:

- The **right and left hypochondriac regions** (**high**-poh-**KON**-dree-ack) are covered by the lower ribs (**hypo-** means below, **chondr/i** means cartilage, and **-ac** means pertaining to). As used here, the term ***hypochondriac*** means below the ribs. This term also describes an individual with an abnormal concern about his or her health.
- The **epigastric region** (**ep**-ih-**GAS**-trick) is located above the stomach (**epi-** means above, **gastr** means stomach, and **-ic** means pertaining to).

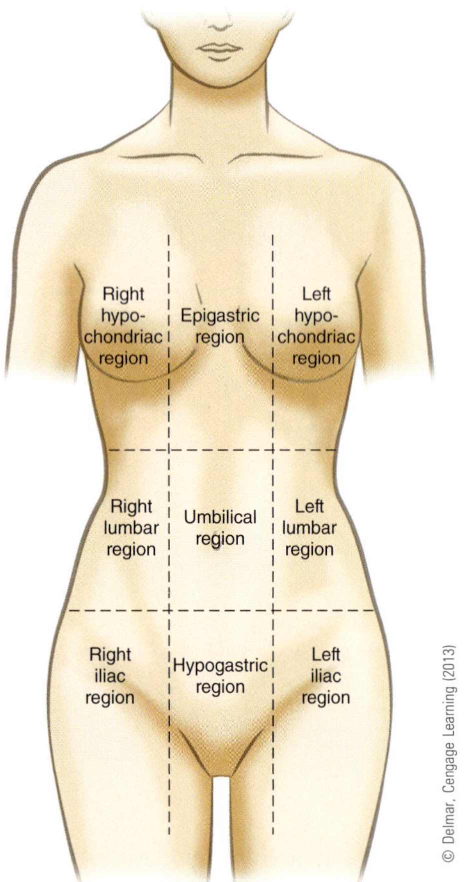

FIGURE 2.5 Regions of the thorax and abdomen.

- The **right and left lumbar regions** (**LUM**-bar) are located near the inward curve of the spine (**lumb** means lower back, and **-ar** means pertaining to). The term ***lumbar*** describes the part of the back between the ribs and the pelvis.
- The **umbilical region** (um-**BILL**-ih-kal) surrounds the **umbilicus** (um-**BILL**-ih-kus), which is commonly known as the ***belly button*** or ***navel***. This pit in the center of the abdominal wall marks the point where the umbilical cord was attached before birth.
- The **right and left iliac regions** (**ILL**-ee-ack) are located over the hip bones (**ili** means hip bone, and **-ac** means pertaining to).
- The **hypogastric region** (**high**-poh-**GAS**-trick) is located below the stomach (**hypo-** means below, **gastr** means stomach, and **-ic** means pertaining to).

Quadrants of the Abdomen

Describing where an abdominal organ or pain is located is made easier by dividing the abdomen into four imaginary quadrants. The term **quadrant** means divided into four. As shown in Figure 2.6 the quadrants of the abdomen are:

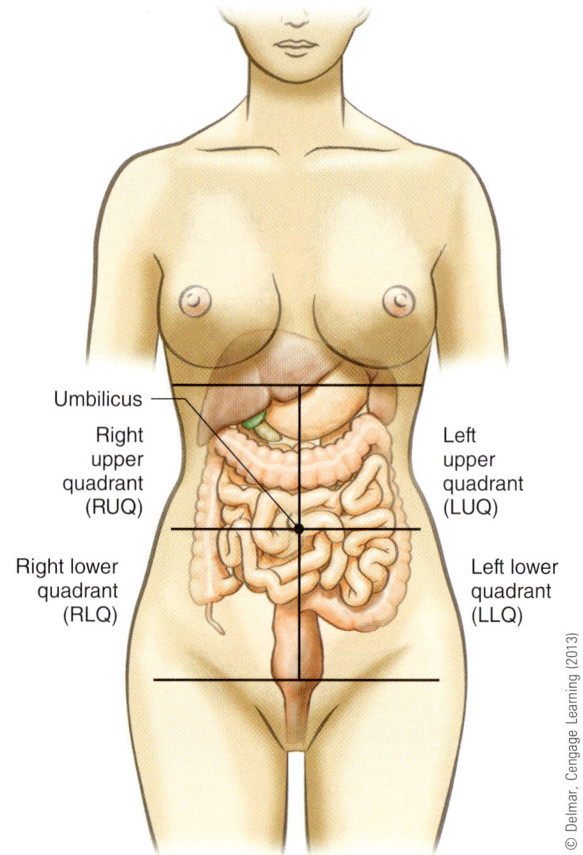

FIGURE 2.6 Division of the abdomen into quadrants.

- Right upper quadrant (RUQ)
- Left upper quadrant (LUQ)
- Right lower quadrant (RLQ)
- Left lower quadrant (LLQ)

The Peritoneum

The **peritoneum** (**pehr**-ih-toh-**NEE**-um) is a multilayered membrane that protects and holds the organs in place within the abdominal cavity. A ***membrane*** is a thin layer of tissue that covers a surface, lines a cavity, or divides a space or organ.

- The **parietal peritoneum** (pah-**RYE**-eh-tal **pehr**-ih-toh-**NEE**-um) is the outer layer of the peritoneum that lines the interior of the abdominal wall. ***Parietal*** means cavity wall.
- The **mesentery** (**MESS**-en-**terr**-ee) is a fused double layer of the parietal peritoneum that attaches parts of the intestine to the interior abdominal wall.

- The **visceral peritoneum** (**VIS**-er-al **pehr**-ih-toh-**NEE**-um) is the inner layer of the peritoneum that surrounds the organs of the abdominal cavity. *Visceral* means relating to the internal organs.

Retroperitoneal (**ret**-roh-**pehr**-ih-toh-**NEE**-al) means located behind the peritoneum (**retro-** means behind, **periton** means peritoneum, and **-eal** means pertaining to). For example, the location of the kidneys is retroperitoneal with one on each side of the spinal column. **Peritonitis** (**pehr**-ih-toh-**NIGH**-tis) is inflammation of the peritoneum.

STRUCTURES OF THE BODY

The body is made up of increasingly larger and more complex structural units. From smallest to largest, these are cells, tissues, organs, and the body systems (Figure 2.7). Working together, these structures form the complete body and enable it to function properly.

CELLS

Cells are the basic structural and functional units of the body. Cells are specialized and grouped together to form tissues and organs.

- **Cytology** (sigh-**TOL**-oh-jee) is the study of the anatomy, physiology, pathology, and chemistry of the cell (**cyt** means cell, and **-ology** means study of).
- A **cytologist** (sigh-**TOL**-oh-jist) is a specialist in the study and analysis of cells (**cyt** means cell, and **-ologist** means specialist).

The Structure of Cells

- The **cell membrane** (**MEM**-brain) is the tissue that surrounds and protects the contents of the cell by separating them from its external environment (Figure 2.8).
- **Cytoplasm** (**SIGH**-toh-plazm) is the material within the cell membrane that is *not* part of the nucleus (**cyt/o** means cell, and **-plasm** means formative material of cells).
- The **nucleus** (**NEW**-klee-us), which is surrounded by the nuclear membrane, is a structure within the cell. It has two important functions: it controls the activities of the cell, and it helps the cell divide.

Stem Cells

Stem cells differ from other kinds of cells in the body because of two characteristics:

- **Stem cells** are unspecialized cells that are able to renew themselves for long periods of time by cell

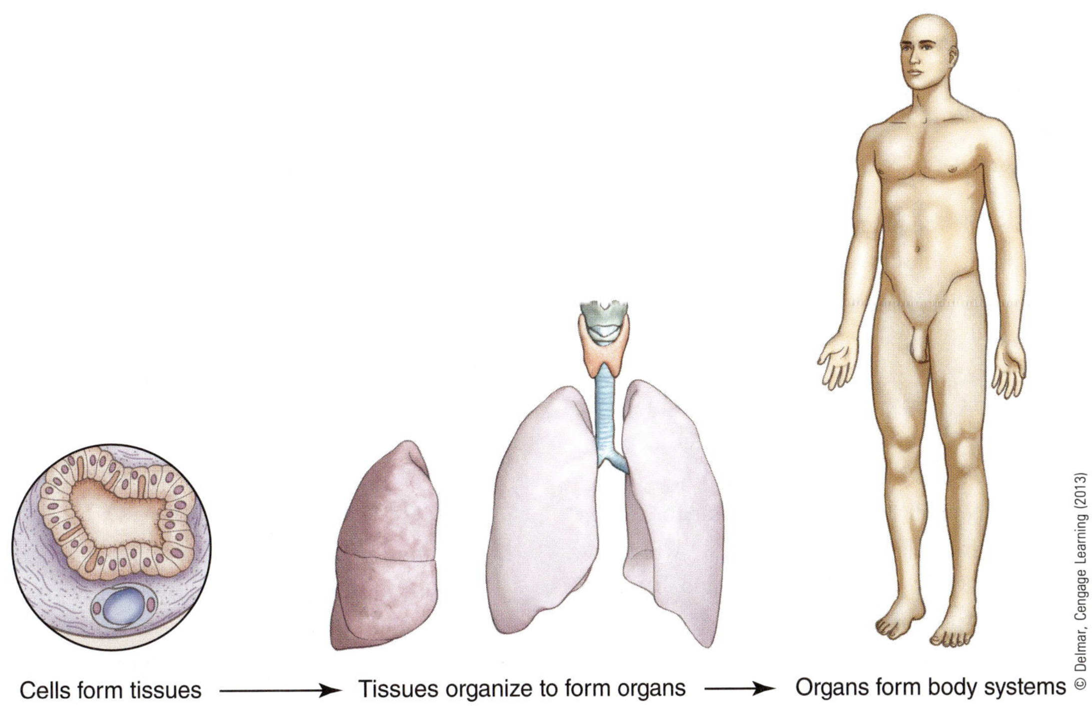

FIGURE 2.7 The human body is highly organized, from the single cell to the total organism.

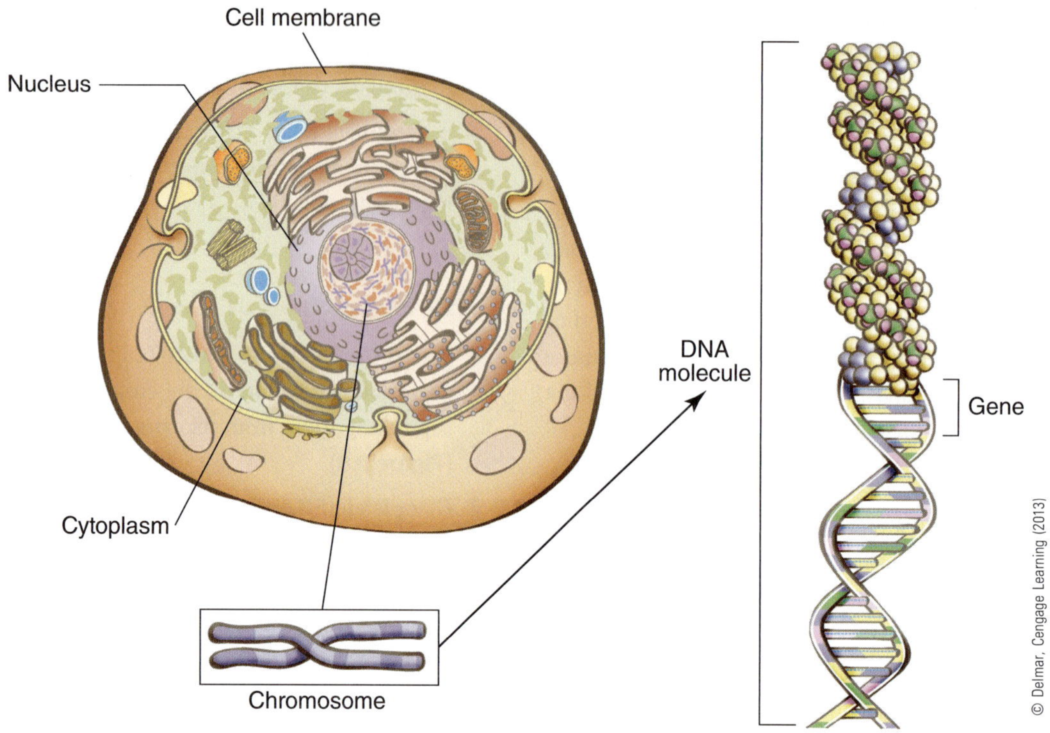

FIGURE 2.8 A basic cell and DNA molecule.

division. This is in contrast to other types of cells that have a specialized role and die after a determined life span.

- Under certain conditions stem cells can be transformed into cells with special functions such as the cells of the heart muscle that make the heartbeat possible or the specialized cells of the pancreas that are capable of producing insulin.

Adult Stem Cells

Adult stem cells, also known as ***somatic stem cells***, are undifferentiated cells found among differentiated cells in a tissue or organ. Normally the primary role of these cells is to maintain and repair the tissue in which they are found. The term ***undifferentiated*** means not having a specialized function or structure. In contrast the term ***differentiated*** means having a specialized function or structure.

Stem cells potentially have many therapeutic uses, including being transplanted from one individual to another. Cells for this purpose are harvested from the ***hemopoietic*** (blood forming) tissue of the donor's bone marrow. However, unless there is an excellent match between the donor and recipient, there is the possibility of rejection known as ***graft-versus-host disease***.

Embryonic Stem Cells

Embryonic stem cells are undifferentiated cells that are unlike any specific adult cell; however, they have the important ability to form *any* adult cell.

- These cells can proliferate (grow rapidly) indefinitely in a laboratory and could therefore potentially provide a source for adult muscle, liver, bone, or blood cells.
- Because these cells are more primitive than adult stem cells, an embryonic stem cell transplant does not require as perfect a match between the patient and donor as the transplantation of adult stem cells.
- Embryonic stem cells come from the ***cord blood*** found in the umbilical cord and placenta of a newborn infant. Embryonic stem cells from cord blood can be harvested at the time of birth without danger to mother or child. These cells are kept frozen until needed for treatment purposes.
- Embryonic stem cells can also be obtained from surplus embryos produced by in vitro (test tube) fertilization. With the informed consent of the donor couple, stem cells obtained in this manner are being used for medical and scientific research.

GENETICS

A **gene** is a fundamental physical and functional unit of heredity. Genes control hereditary disorders and all physical traits such as hair, skin, and eye color.

Genetics is the study of how genes are transferred from parents to their children and the role of genes in health and disease (**gene** means producing, and **-tics** means pertaining to). A specialist in this field is known as a **geneticist** (jeh-**NET**-ih-sist).

Dominant and Recessive Genes

Each newly formed individual receives two genes of each genetic trait: one from the father and one from the mother.

- When a **dominant gene** is inherited from either parent, the offspring *will* inherit that genetic condition or characteristic. For example, freckles are a physical trait that is transmitted by a dominant gene. So, too, is the hereditary disorder Huntington's disease.
- When the same **recessive gene** is inherited from both parents, the offspring *will have* that condition. For example, ***sickle cell anemia*** is a group of inherited red blood cell disorders that are transmitted by a recessive gene. When this gene is transmitted by both parents, the child *will have* sickle cell anemia.
- When a **recessive gene** is inherited from only one parent, and a normal gene is inherited from the other parent, the offspring *will not have* the condition. Although this child will not develop sickle cell anemia, he or she will have the *sickle cell anemia trait.* People with this trait can transmit the sickle cell gene to their offspring.

The Human Genome

A **genome** (**JEE**-nohm) is the complete set of genetic information of an organism. The Human Genome Project studied this genetic code for individual people and found that it is more than 99 percent identical among humans throughout the world. The first complete mapping of the *human genome,* which took 13 years to complete, was published in 2003.

Having access to this data is a very important step in studying the use of genetics in health and science. Scientists have begun to take the next step: attempting to understand the proteins encoded by the sequence of the 30,000 genes.

Chromosomes

Chromosomes (**KROH**-moh-sohmes) are the genetic structures located within the nucleus of each cell (Figure 2.8). These chromosomes are made up of the DNA molecules containing the body's genes. Packaging genetic information into chromosomes helps a cell keep a large amount of genetic information neat, organized, and compact. Each chromosome contains about 100,000 genes.

- A ***somatic cell*** is any cell in the body except the gametes (sex cells). ***Somatic*** means pertaining to the body in general. Somatic cells contain 46 chromosomes arranged into 23 pairs. There are 22 identical pairs of chromosomes, plus another pair. In a typical female, this remaining pair consists of XX chromosomes. In a typical male, this pair consists of an XY chromosome pair. This chromosome pair determines the sex of the individual.
- A ***sex cell*** (sperm or egg), also known as a ***gamete***, is the only type of cell that *does not* contain 46 chromosomes. Instead, each ovum (egg) or sperm has 23 single chromosomes. In a female, one of these will be an X chromosome. In a male, one of these will be either an X or a Y chromosome. When a sperm and ovum join, the newly formed offspring receives 23 chromosomes from each parent, for a total of 46.
- It is the X or Y chromosome from the father that determines the gender of the child.
- A defect in chromosomes can lead to birth defects. For example, individuals with Down syndrome have 47 chromosomes instead of the usual 46.

DNA

The basic structure of the **DNA** molecule, which is located on the pairs of chromosomes in the nucleus of each cell, is the same for all living organisms. Human DNA contains thousands of genes that provide the information essential for heredity, determining physical appearance, disease risks, and other traits (Figure 2.8).

- DNA is packaged in a chromosome as two spiraling strands that twist together to form a double helix. A ***helix*** is a shape twisted like a spiral staircase. A ***double helix*** consists of two of these strands twisted together.
- DNA, which is an abbreviation for *deoxyribonucleic acid,* is found in the nucleus of all types of cells except erythrocytes (red blood cells). The difference here is due to the fact that erythrocytes do not have a nucleus.

- The DNA for each individual is different, and no two DNA patterns are exactly the same. The only exception to this rule is identical twins, which are formed from one fertilized egg that divides. Although their DNA is identical, these twins do develop characteristics that make each of them unique, such as fingerprints.
- A very small sample of DNA, such as from human hair or tissue, can be used to identify individuals in instances such as criminal investigations, paternity suits, or genealogy research.

Genetic Mutation

A **genetic mutation** is a change of the sequence of a DNA molecule. Potential causes of genetic mutation include exposure to radiation or environmental pollution.

- A ***somatic cell mutation*** is a change within the cells of the body. These changes affect the individual but *cannot* be transmitted to the next generation.
- A ***gametic cell mutation*** is a change within the genes in a gamete (sex cell) that *can* be transmitted by a parent to his or her children.
- ***Genetic engineering*** is the manipulating or splicing of genes for scientific or medical purposes. The production of human insulin from modified bacteria is an example of one result of genetic engineering.

Genetic Disorders

A **genetic disorder**, also known as a ***hereditary disorder***, is a pathological condition caused by an absent or defective gene. Some genetic disorders are obvious at birth. Others may manifest (become evident) at any time in life. The following are examples of genetic disorders:

- **Cystic fibrosis** (CF), a genetic disorder that is present at birth and affects both the respiratory and digestive systems (See Chapter 7).
- **Down syndrome** (DS), a genetic variation that is associated with a characteristic facial appearance, learning disabilities, and physical abnormalities such as heart valve disease (Figure 2.9).
- **Hemophilia** (**hee**-moh-**FILL**-ee-ah), a group of hereditary bleeding disorders in which a blood-clotting factor is missing. This blood coagulation disorder is characterized by spontaneous hemorrhages or severe bleeding following an injury.

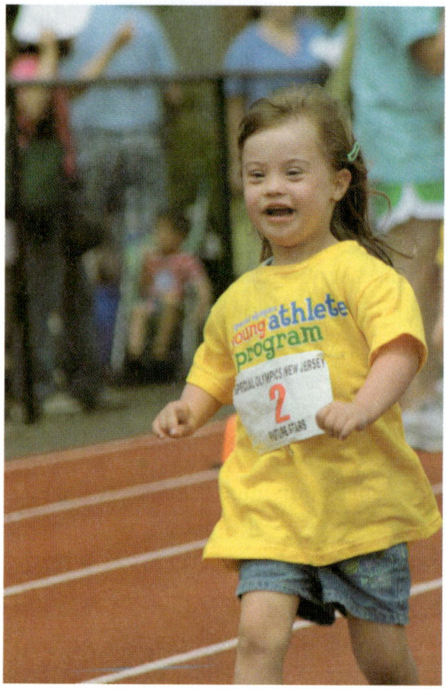

Used with permission from Special Olympics New Jersey.

FIGURE 2.9 Down syndrome is a genetic disorder that causes learning disabilities, developmental delays, and a characteristic facial appearance.

- **Huntington's disease** (HD), a genetic disorder that is passed from parent to child. Each child of a parent with the gene for Huntington's disease has a 50-50 chance of inheriting this defective gene. This condition causes nerve degeneration with symptoms that most often appear in midlife. (***Degeneration*** means worsening condition.) This damage eventually results in uncontrolled movements and the loss of some mental abilities.
- **Muscular dystrophy** (**DIS**-troh-fee), a group of genetic diseases that are characterized by progressive weakness and degeneration of the skeletal muscles that control movement.
- **Phenylketonuria** (**fen**-il-**kee**-toh-**NEW**-ree-ah), a genetic disorder in which the essential digestive enzyme *phenylalanine hydroxylase* is missing. This is commonly known as ***PKU***. PKU can be detected by a blood test performed on infants at birth. With careful dietary supervision, children born with PKU can lead normal lives. Without early detection and treatment, PKU causes severe mental retardation.

- **Tay-Sachs disease** (**TAY SAKS**), a fatal genetic disorder in which harmful quantities of a fatty substance buildup in tissues and nerve cells in the brain. Both parents must carry the mutated gene to have an affected child. The most common form of the disease affects babies who appear healthy at birth and seem to develop normally for the first few months. Development then slows, and a relentless deterioration of mental and physical abilities results in progressive blindness, paralysis, and early death.

TISSUES

A **tissue** is a group or layer of similarly specialized cells that join together to perform certain specific functions. **Histology** (hiss-**TOL**-oh-jee) is the study of the structure, composition, and function of tissues (**hist** means tissue, and **-ology** means a study of). A **histologist** (hiss-**TOL**-oh-jist) is a specialist in the study of the organization of tissues at all levels (**hist** means tissue, and **-ologist** means specialist). The four main types of tissue are:

- Epithelial tissues
- Connective tissues
- Muscle tissue
- Nerve tissue

Epithelial Tissues

Epithelial tissues (**ep**-ih-**THEE**-lee-al) form a protective covering for all of the internal and external surfaces of the body. These tissues also form glands.

- **Epithelium** (**ep**-ih-**THEE**-lee-um) is the specialized epithelial tissue that forms the epidermis of the skin and the surface layer of mucous membranes (see Chapter 12).
- **Endothelium** (**en**-doh-**THEE**-lee-um) is the specialized epithelial tissue that lines the blood and lymph vessels, body cavities, glands, and organs.

Connective Tissues

Connective tissues support and connect organs and other body tissues. The four kinds of connective tissue are:

- **Dense connective tissues**, such as bone and cartilage, form the joints and framework of the body.
- **Adipose tissue**, also known as *fat*, provides protective padding, insulation, and support (**adip** means fat, and **-ose** means pertaining to).
- **Loose connective tissue** surrounds various organs and supports both nerve cells and blood vessels.
- **Liquid connective tissues**, which are blood and lymph, transport nutrients and waste products throughout the body.

Muscle Tissue

Muscle tissue contains cells with the specialized ability to contract and relax.

Nerve Tissue

Nerve tissue contains cells with the specialized ability to react to stimuli and to conduct electrical impulses.

Pathology of Tissue Formation

Disorders of the tissues, which are frequently due to unknown causes, can occur before birth as the tissues are forming or appear later in life.

Incomplete Tissue Formation

- **Aplasia** (ah-**PLAY**-zee-ah) is the defective development, or the congenital absence, of an organ or tissue (**a-** means without, and **-plasia** means formation). Compare aplasia with *hypoplasia.*
- **Hypoplasia** (**high**-poh-**PLAY**-zee-ah) is the incomplete development of an organ or tissue usually due to a deficiency in the number of cells (**hypo-** means deficient, and **-plasia** means formation). Compare hypoplasia with *aplasia.*

Abnormal Tissue Formation

- **Anaplasia** (**an**-ah-**PLAY**-zee-ah) is a change in the structure of cells and in their orientation to each other (**ana-** means backward, and **-plasia** means formation). This abnormal cell development is characteristic of tumor formation in cancers. Contrast anaplasia with *hypertrophy.*
- **Dysplasia** (dis-**PLAY**-see-ah) is the abnormal development or growth of cells, tissues, or organs (**dys-** means bad, and **-plasia** means formation).

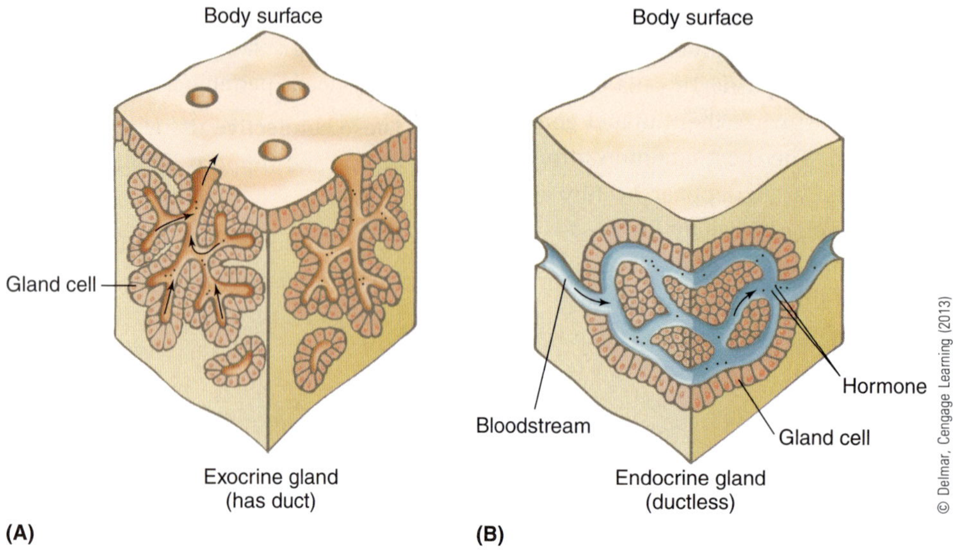

FIGURE 2.10 A. Exocrine glands secrete their chemical substances into ducts that lead either to other organs or out of the body. B. Endocrine glands pour their secretions directly into the bloodstream.

- **Hyperplasia** (**high**-per-**PLAY**-zee-ah) is the enlargement of an organ or tissue because of an abnormal increase in the number of cells in the tissues (**hyper-** means excessive, and **-plasia** means formation). Contrast hyperplasia with *hypertrophy*.
- **Hypertrophy** (high-**PER**-troh-fee) is a general increase in the bulk of a body part or organ that is due to an increase in the size, but not in the number, of cells in the tissues (**hyper-** means excessive, and **-trophy** means development). This enlargement is not due to tumor formation. Contrast hypertrophy with *anaplasia* and *hyperplasia*.

GLANDS

A **gland** is a group of specialized epithelial cells that are capable of producing secretions. A ***secretion*** is the substance produced by a gland. The two major types of glands are (Figure 2.10):

- **Exocrine glands** (**ECK**-soh-krin) secrete chemical substances into ducts that lead either to other organs or out of the body, such as sweat glands (**exo-** means out of, and **-crine** means to secrete) (See Chapter 12).
- **Endocrine glands** (**EN**-doh-krin), which produce hormones, do not have ducts (**endo-** means within, and **-crine** means to secrete). These hormones are secreted directly into the bloodstream, and are then transported to organs and structures throughout the body (See Chapter 13).

StudyWARE CONNECTION

Watch the **Exocrine and Endocrine Glands** animation on the StudyWARE™.

Pathology and Procedures of the Glands

- **Adenitis** (**ad**-eh-**NIGH**-tis) is the inflammation of a gland (**aden** means gland, and **-itis** means inflammation).
- An **adenocarcinoma** (**ad**-eh-noh-**kar**-sih-**NOH**-mah) is a malignant tumor that originates in glandular tissue (**aden/o** means gland, **carcin** means cancerous, and **-oma** means tumor). ***Malignant*** means harmful, capable of spreading, and potentially life threatening.
- An **adenoma** (**ad**-eh-**NOH**-mah) is a benign tumor that arises in or resembles glandular tissue (**aden** means gland, and **-oma** means tumor). ***Benign*** means not life threatening.
- **Adenomalacia** (**ad**-eh-noh-mah-**LAY**-shee-ah) is the abnormal softening of a gland (**aden/o** means gland, and **-malacia** means abnormal softening). *Adenomalacia* is the opposite of *adenosclerosis*.

- **Adenosis** (**ad**-eh-**NOH**-sis) is any disease or condition of a gland (**aden** means gland, and **-osis** means an abnormal condition or disease).
- **Adenosclerosis** (**ad**-eh-noh-skleh-**ROH**-sis) is the abnormal hardening of a gland (**aden/o** means gland, and **-sclerosis** means abnormal hardening). *Adenosclerosis* is the opposite of *adenomalacia*.
- An **adenectomy** (**ad**-eh-**NECK**-toh-mee) is the surgical removal of a gland (**aden** means gland, and **-ectomy** means surgical removal).

BODY SYSTEMS AND RELATED ORGANS

A body **organ** is a somewhat independent part of the body that performs a specific function. For purposes of description, the related tissues and organs are described as being organized into *body systems* with specialized functions. These body systems are explained in Table 2.1.

PATHOLOGY

Pathology (pah-**THOL**-oh-jee) is the study of disease: the nature and cause as well as the produced changes in structure and function. *Pathology* also means a condition produced by disease. The word root (combining form) **path/o** and the suffix **-pathy** mean disease; however, they also mean suffering, feeling, and emotion.

- A **pathologist** (pah-**THOL**-oh-jist) specializes in the laboratory analysis of tissue samples to confirm or establish a diagnosis (**path** means disease, and **-ologist** means specialist). These tissue specimens can be removed in biopsies, during operations, or in postmortem examinations.
- **Etiology** (**ee**-tee-**OL**-oh-jee) is the study of the causes of diseases (**eti-** means cause, and **-ology** means study of).

Disease Transmission

A **pathogen** is a disease-producing microorganism such as a virus. *Transmission* is the spread of a disease. *Contamination* means that a pathogen is possibly present. Contamination occurs through a lack of proper hygiene standards or by failure to take appropriate infection control precautions.

- A **communicable disease** (kuh-**MEW**-nih-kuh-bul), also known as a *contagious disease*, is any condition that is transmitted from one person to another either by direct or by indirect contact with contaminated objects. *Communicable* means capable of being transmitted.
- **Indirect contact transmission** refers to situations in which a susceptible person is infected by contact with a contaminated surface.
- **Bloodborne transmission** is the spread of a disease through contact with blood or other body fluids that are contaminated with blood. Examples include human immunodeficiency virus (HIV), hepatitis B, and most sexually transmitted diseases (STDs).
- **Airborne transmission** occurs through contact with contaminated respiratory droplets spread by a cough or sneeze. Examples include tuberculosis, flu, colds, and measles.
- **Food-borne and waterborne transmission**, also known as *fecal-oral transmission*, is caused by eating or drinking contaminated food or water that has not been properly treated to remove contamination or kill any pathogens present.
- **Vector-borne transmission** is the spread of certain disease due to the bite of a vector. As used here, the term *vector* describes insects or animals such as flies, mites, fleas, ticks, rats, and dogs that are capable of transmitting a disease. Mosquitoes are the most common vectors, and the diseases they transmit include malaria and West Nile virus.

Outbreaks of Diseases

An **epidemiologist** (**ep**-ih-**dee**-mee-**OL**-oh-jist) is a specialist in the study of outbreaks of disease within a population group (**epi-** means above, **dem/i** means population, and **-ologist** means specialist).

- **Endemic** (en-**DEM**-ick) refers to the ongoing presence of a disease within a population, group, or area (**en-** means within, **dem** means population, and **-ic** means pertaining to). For example, the common cold is endemic because it is always present within the general population.
- An **epidemic** (**ep**-ih-**DEM**-ick) is a sudden and widespread outbreak of a disease within a specific population group or area (**epi-** means above, **dem** means population, and **-ic** means pertaining to). For example, a sudden widespread outbreak of measles is an epidemic.

TABLE 2.1
Major Body Systems

Body System	Major Structures	Major Functions
Skeletal System (Chapter 3)	bones, joints, and cartilage	Supports and shapes the body. Protects the internal organs. Forms some blood cells and stores minerals.
Muscular System (Chapter 4)	muscles, fascia, and tendons	Holds the body erect. Makes movement possible. Moves body fluids and generates body heat.
Cardiovascular System (Chapter 5)	heart, arteries, veins, capillaries, and blood	Blood circulates throughout the body to transport oxygen and nutrients to cells, and to carry waste products to the kidneys where waste is removed by filtration.
Lymphatic System (Chapter 6)	lymph, lymphatic vessels, and lymph nodes	Removes and transports waste products from the fluid between the cells. Destroys harmful substances such as pathogens and cancer cells in the lymph nodes. Returns the filtered lymph to the bloodstream where it becomes plasma again.
Immune System (Chapter 6)	tonsils, spleen, thymus, skin, and specialized blood cells	Defends the body against invading pathogens and allergens.
Respiratory System (Chapter 7)	nose, pharynx, trachea, larynx, and lungs	Brings oxygen into the body for transportation to the cells. Removes carbon dioxide and some water waste from the body.
Digestive System (Chapter 8)	mouth, esophagus, stomach, small intestine, large intestine, liver, and pancreas	Digests ingested food so it can be absorbed into the bloodstream. Eliminates solid waste.
Urinary System (Chapter 9)	kidneys, ureters, urinary bladder, and urethra	Filters blood to remove waste. Maintains the electrolyte and fluid balance within the body.
Nervous System (Chapter 10)	nerves, brain, and spinal cord	Coordinates the reception of stimuli. Transmits messages throughout the body.
Special Senses (Chapter 11)	eyes and ears	Receive visual and auditory information, and transmit it to the brain.
Integumentary System (Chapter 12)	skin, sebaceous glands, and sweat glands	Protects the body against invasion by bacteria. Aids in regulating the body temperature and water content.
Endocrine System (Chapter 13)	adrenal glands, gonads, pancreas, parathyroids, pineal, pituitary, thymus, and thyroid	Integrates all body functions.
Reproductive Systems (Chapter 14)	*Male:* penis and testicles; *Female:* ovaries, uterus, and vagina	Produces new life.

- **Pandemic** (pan-**DEM**-ick) refers to an outbreak of a disease occurring over a large geographic area, possibly worldwide (**pan-** means entire, **dem** means population, and **-ic** means pertaining to). For example, the worldwide spread of acquired immunodeficiency syndrome (AIDS) is pandemic.

Types of Diseases

- A **functional disorder** produces symptoms for which no physiological or anatomical cause can be identified. For example, a panic attack is a functional disorder (see Chapter 10).
- An **iatrogenic illness** (eye-**at**-roh-**JEN**-ick) is an unfavorable response due to prescribed medical treatment. For example, severe burns resulting from radiation therapy are iatrogenic.
- An **idiopathic disorder** (**id**-ee-oh-**PATH**-ick) is an illness without known cause (**idi/o** means peculiar to the individual, **path** means disease, and **-ic** means pertaining to). ***Idiopathic*** means without known cause.
- An **infectious disease** (in-**FECK**-shus) is an illness caused by living pathogenic organisms such as bacteria and viruses (see Chapter 6).
- A **nosocomial infection** (**nos**-oh-**KOH**-mee-al in-**FECK**-shun) is a disease acquired in a hospital or clinical setting. For example, MRSA infections are often spread in hospitals (see Chapter 6). *Nosocomial* comes from the Greek word for hospital.
- An **organic disorder** (or-**GAN**-ick) produces symptoms caused by detectable physical changes in the body. For example, chickenpox, which has a characteristic rash, is an organic disorder caused by a virus (see Chapter 6).

Congenital Disorders

A **congenital disorder** (kon-**JEN**-ih-tahl) is an abnormal condition that exists at the time of birth. ***Congenital*** means existing at birth. These conditions can be caused by a developmental disorder before birth, prenatal influences, premature birth, or injuries during the birth process.

Developmental Disorders

A **developmental disorder**, also known as a ***birth defect***, can result in an anomaly or malformation such as the absence of a limb or the presence of an extra toe. An **anomaly** (ah-**NOM**-ah-lee) is a deviation from what is regarded as normal.

- The term **atresia** (at-**TREE**-zee-ah) describes the congenital absence of a normal body opening or the failure of a structure to be tubular. For example, anal atresia is the congenital absence of the opening at the bottom end of the anus; pulmonary atresia is the absence of a pulmonary valve.

Prenatal Influences

Prenatal influences are the mother's health, behavior, and the prenatal medical care she does or does not receive before delivery.

- An example of a problem with the mother's health is a ***rubella*** infection (see Chapter 6). Birth defects often develop if a pregnant woman contracts this viral infection early in her pregnancy.
- An example of a problem caused by the mother's behavior is **fetal alcohol syndrome** (FAS), which is caused by the mother's consumption of alcohol during the pregnancy. This resulting condition of the baby is characterized by physical and behavioral traits, including growth abnormalities, mental retardation, brain damage, and socialization difficulties.
- Examples of problems caused by lack of adequate prenatal medical care are premature delivery or a low birth-weight baby.

Premature Birth and Birth Injuries

- ***Premature birth***, which is a birth that occurs earlier than 37 weeks of development, can cause serious health problems because the baby's body systems have not had time to form completely. Breathing difficulties and heart problems are common in premature babies.
- ***Birth injuries*** are congenital disorders that were not present before the events surrounding the time of birth. For example, ***cerebral palsy***, which is the result of brain damage, can be caused by premature birth or inadequate oxygen to the brain during the birth process.

AGING AND DEATH

Aging is the normal progression of the life cycle that will eventually end in death. During the latter portion of life, individuals become increasingly at higher risk of developing health problems that are chronic or eventually fatal. As the average life span is becoming longer, a larger

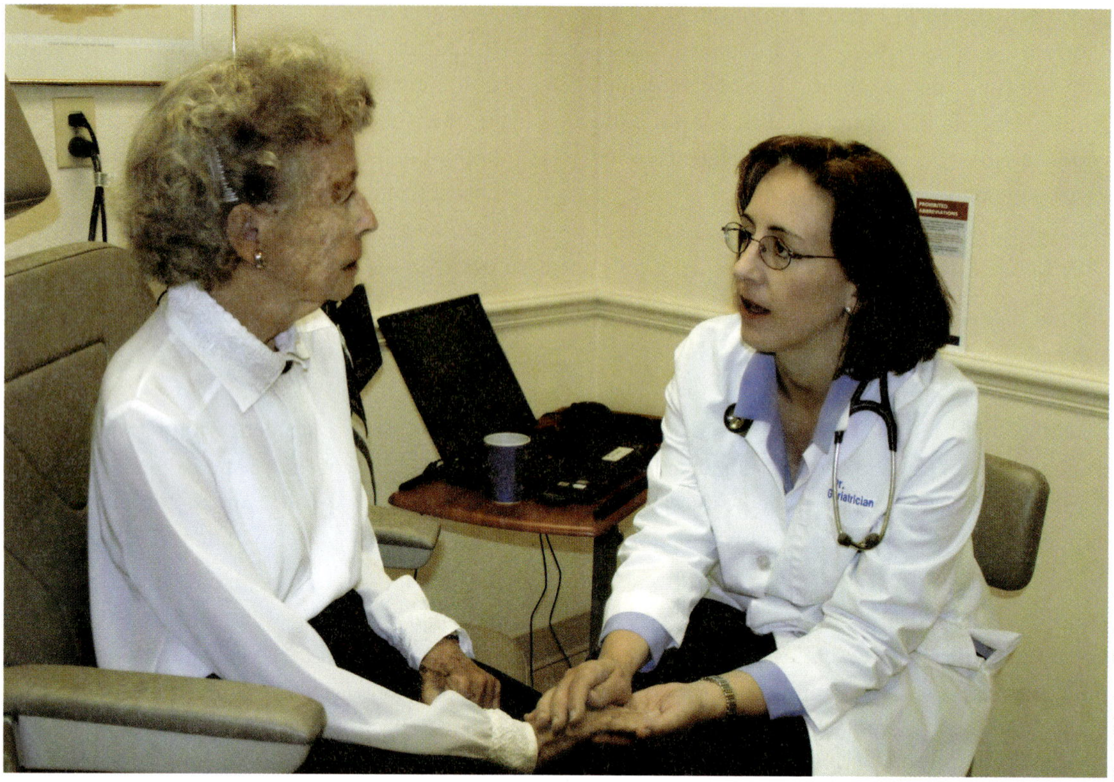

Dennis Sabo/www.Shutterstock.com

FIGURE 2.11 A geriatrician specializes in problems related to aging, and in the diagnosis, treatment, and prevention of disease in older people.

portion of the population are affected by such disorders related to aging.

- The study of the medical problems and care of older people is known as **geriatrics** (jer-ee-**AT**-ricks) or as ***gerontology***.
- ***Postmortem*** means after death. A postmortem examination is also known as an **autopsy** (**AW**-top-see).

GENERAL MEDICAL SPECIALTIES RELATING TO HEALTH AND DISEASE

Physicians caring for the well-being of patients during their lifetime include the following specialists:

- A **general practitioner** (GP), or ***family practice physician***, provides ongoing care for patients of all ages.
- An **internist** is a physician who specializes in diagnosing and treating diseases and disorders of the internal organs and related body systems.
- A **pediatrician** (**pee**-dee-ah-**TRISH**-un) is a physician who specializes in diagnosing, treating, and preventing disorders and diseases of infants and children. This specialty is known as ***pediatrics***.
- A **geriatrician** (**jer**-ee-ah-**TRISH**-un), or ***gerontologist***, is a physician who specializes in the care of older people (Figure 2.11).
- A **hospitalist** focuses on the general medical care of hospitalized patients.

ABBREVIATIONS RELATED TO THE HUMAN BODY IN HEALTH AND DISEASE

Table 2.2 presents an overview of the abbreviations related to the terms introduced in this chapter. Note: To avoid errors or confusion, always be cautious when using abbreviations.

TABLE 2.2

Abbreviations Related to the Human Body in Health and Disease

anatomy and physiology = A & P	**A & P** = anatomy and physiology
communicable disease = CD	**CD** = communicable disease
chromosome = CH, chr	**CH, chr** = chromosome
deoxyribonucleic acid = DNA	**DNA** = deoxyribonucleic acid
epidemic = epid	**epid** = epidemic
general practitioner = GP	**GP** = general practitioner
Huntington's disease = HD	**HD** = Huntington's disease
left lower quadrant = LLQ	**LLQ** = left lower quadrant
left upper quadrant = LUQ	**LUQ** = left upper quadrant
phenylketonuria = PKU	**PKU** = phenylketonuria
right lower quadrant = RLQ	**RLQ** = right lower quadrant
right upper quadrant = RUQ	**RUQ** = right upper quadrant

StudyWARE CONNECTION

For more practice and to test your mastery of this material, go to the StudyWARE™ to play interactive games and complete the quiz for this chapter.

Workbook Practice

Go to your workbook and complete the exercises for this chapter.

Downloadable audio is available for selected medical terms in this chapter to enhance your learning of medical terminology.

CHAPTER 2

LEARNING EXERCISES

MATCHING WORD PARTS 1

Write the correct answer in the middle column.

	Definition	Correct Answer	Possible Answers
2.1.	fat	______________	**aden/o**
2.2.	front	______________	**adip/o**
2.3.	gland	______________	**anter/o**
2.4.	specialist	______________	**-ologist**
2.5.	study of	______________	**-ology**

MATCHING WORD PARTS 2

Write the correct answer in the middle column.

	Definition	Correct Answer	Possible Answers
2.6.	cell	______________	**caud/o**
2.7.	head	______________	**cephal/o**
2.8.	lower part of the body	______________	**cyt/o**
2.9.	out of	______________	**endo-**
2.10.	within	______________	**exo-**

MATCHING WORD PARTS 3

Write the correct answer in the middle column.

	Definition	Correct Answer	Possible Answers
2.11.	back	______________	**hist/o**
2.12.	control	______________	**path/o**

2.13. disease, suffering, emotion ________________ **-plasia**

2.14. formation ________________ **poster/o**

2.15. tissue ________________ **-stasis**

DEFINITIONS

Select the correct answer, and write it on the line provided.

2.16. A/An ________________ is acquired in a hospital setting.

iatrogenic illness | idiopathic disorder | nosocomial infection | organic disorder

2.17. When a ________________ is inherited from only one parent, the offspring will have that genetic condition or characteristic.

dominant gene | genome | recessive gene | recessive trait

2.18. The ________________ contains the major organs of digestion.

abdominal cavity | cranial cavity | dorsal cavity | pelvic cavity

2.19. The term ________________ means the direction toward or nearer the midline.

distal | lateral | medial | proximal

2.20. The primary role of the undifferentiated ________________ cells is to maintain and repair the tissue in which they are found.

adult stem | cord blood | embryonic stem | hemopoietic

2.21. The genetic disorder in which an essential digestive enzyme is missing is known as ________________.

Down syndrome | Huntington's disease | phenylketonuria | Tay-Sachs disease

2.22. The inflammation of a gland is known as ________________.

adenectomy | adenitis | adenoma | adenosis

2.23. The ________________ is the outer layer of the peritoneum that lines the interior of the abdominal wall.

mesentery | parietal peritoneum | retroperitoneum | visceral peritoneum

2.24. A ______________________ is a fundamental physical and functional unit of heredity.

cell gamete gene genome

2.25. The study of the structure, composition, and function of tissues is known as ______________________.

anatomy cytology histology physiology

MATCHING REGIONS OF THE THORAX AND ABDOMEN

Write the correct answer in the middle column.

Definition	Correct Answer	Possible Answers
2.26. above the stomach	______________________	epigastric region
2.27. belly button area	______________________	hypochondriac region
2.28. below the ribs	______________________	hypogastric region
2.29. below the stomach	______________________	iliac region
2.30. hip bone area	______________________	umbilical region

WHICH WORD?

Select the correct answer, and write it on the line provided.

2.31. The term ______________________ refers to the entire lower area of the abdomen.

inguinal umbilicus

2.32. The study of how genes are transferred from parents to their children and the role of genes in health and disease is known as ______________________.

cytology genetics

2.33. A specialist in the study of the outbreaks of disease is a/an ______________________.

epidemiologist pathologist

2.34. The ______________________ secrete chemical substances into ducts.

endocrine glands exocrine glands

2.35. The location of the stomach is ______________________ to the diaphragm.

inferior superior

SPELLING COUNTS

Find the misspelled word in each sentence. Then write that word, spelled correctly, on the line provided.

2.36. The mesantry is a fused double layer of the parietal peritoneum. ________________

2.37. Hemaphilia is a group of hereditary bleeding disorders in which a blood-clotting factor is missing. ________________

2.38. Hypretrophy is a general increase in the bulk of a body part or organ due to an increase in the size, but not in the number, of cells in the tissues. ________________

2.39. The protective covering for all of the internal and external surfaces of the body is formed by epithealial tissues. ________________

2.40. An abnomolly is any deviation from what is regarded as normal. ________________

ABBREVIATION IDENTIFICATION

Write the correct terms for the abbreviations on the lines provided.

2.41. **HD** ________________

2.42. **CD** ________________

2.43. **GP** ________________

2.44. **LUQ** ________________

2.45. **CH** ________________

TERM SELECTION

Select the correct answer, and write it on the line provided.

2.46. The term meaning situated nearest the midline or beginning of a body structure is ________________.

distal lateral medial proximal

2.47. The term meaning situated in the back is ________________.

anterior posterior superior ventral

2.48. The body is divided into anterior and posterior portions by the ________________ plane.

frontal horizontal sagittal transverse

2.49. The body is divided into equal vertical left and right halves by the ______________ plane.

coronal midsagittal sagittal transverse

2.50. Part of the elbow is formed by the ______________ end of the humerus.

distal lateral medial proximal

SENTENCE COMPLETION

Write the correct term or terms on the lines provided.

2.51. ______________ is a genetic variation that is associated with characteristic facial appearance, learning disabilities, and physical abnormalities such as heart valve disease.

2.52. The study of the functions of the structures of the body is known as ______________.

2.53. The heart and the lungs are surrounded and protected by the ______________ cavity.

2.54. An unfavorable response to prescribed medical treatment, such as severe burns resulting from radiation therapy, is known as a/an ______________ illness.

2.55. The genetic structures located within the nucleus of each cell are known as ______________. These structures are made up of the DNA molecules containing the body's genes.

WORD SURGERY

Divide each term into its component word parts. Write these word parts, in sequence, on the lines provided. When necessary use a slash (/) to indicate a combining vowel. (You may not need all of the lines provided.)

2.56. An **adenectomy** is the surgical removal of a gland.

__________ __________ __________ __________

2.57. Hormones are secreted directly into the bloodstream by the **endocrine** glands.

__________ __________ __________ __________

2.58. A **histologist** is a specialist in the study of the organization of tissues at all levels.

__________ __________ __________ __________

2.59. The term **retroperitoneal** means located behind the peritoneum.

__________ __________ __________ __________

2.60. A **pathologist** specializes in the laboratory analysis of tissue samples to confirm or establish a diagnosis.

________ ________ ________ ________

2.61. The study of the causes of diseases is known as **etiology**.

________ ________ ________ ________

2.62. The term **homeostasis** refers to the processes through which the body maintains a constant internal environment.

________ ________ ________ ________

2.63. A **pandemic** is an outbreak of a disease occurring over a large geographic area, possibly worldwide.

________ ________ ________ ________

2.64. The **epigastric** region is located above the stomach.

________ ________ ________ ________

2.65. An **idiopathic** disorder is an illness without known cause.

________ ________ ________ ________

CLINICAL CONDITIONS

Write the correct answer on the line provided.

2.66. Mr. Tseng died of cholera during a sudden and widespread outbreak of this disease in his village. Such an outbreak is described as being a/an ________________.

2.67. Brenda Farmer's doctor could not find any physical changes to explain her symptoms. The doctor refers to this as a/an ________________ disorder.

2.68. Gerald Carlson was infected with hepatitis B through ________________ transmission.

2.69. To become a specialist in the study and analysis of cells, Lee Wong signed up for courses in ________________.

2.70. Malaria and West Nile virus are spread by mosquitoes. This is known as ________________ transmission.

2.71. Jose Ortega complained of pain in the lower right area of his abdomen. Using the system that divides the abdomen into four sections, his doctor recorded the pain as being in the lower right ________________.

2.72. Ralph Jenkins was very sick after drinking contaminated water during a camping trip. His doctor says that he contracted the illness through ________________________ transmission.

2.73. Tracy Ames has a bladder inflammation. This organ of the urinary system is located in the ________________________ cavity.

2.74. Mrs. Reynolds was diagnosed as having inflammation of the peritoneum. The medical term for this condition is ________________________.

2.75. Ashley Goldberg is fascinated by genetics. She wants to specialize in this field and is studying to become a/an ________________________.

WHICH IS THE CORRECT MEDICAL TERM?

Select the correct answer, and write it on the line provided.

2.76. Debbie Sanchez fell against a rock and injured her left hip and upper leg. This area is known as the left ________________________ region.

hypochondriac   iliac   lumbar   umbilical

2.77. A ________________________ is the complete set of genetic information of an organism.

cell   gamete   gene   genome

2.78. An ________________________ is a malignant tumor that originates in glandular tissue.

adenocarcinoma   adenitis   adenoma   adenosis

2.79. Nerve cells and blood vessels are surrounded and supported by ________________________ connective tissue.

adipose   epithelial   liquid   loose

2.80. A mother's consumption of alcohol during pregnancy can cause ________________________.

cerebral palsy   Down syndrome   fetal alcohol syndrome   genetic disorders

CHALLENGE WORD BUILDING

These terms are *not* found in this chapter; however, they are made up of the following familiar word parts. If you need help in creating the term, refer to your medical dictionary.

gastr/o	**my/o**
laryng/o	**nephr/o**
neur/o	**-itis**
-algia	**-osis**
-ectomy	**-plasty**

2.81. The term meaning the surgical repair of a muscle is ________________.

2.82. The term meaning muscle pain is ________________.

2.83. The term meaning an abnormal condition of the stomach is ________________.

2.84. The term meaning inflammation of the larynx is ________________.

2.85. The term meaning the surgical removal of part of a muscle is a/an ________________.

2.86. The term meaning pain in the stomach is ________________.

2.87. The term meaning surgical removal of the larynx is ________________.

2.88. The term meaning an abnormal condition of the kidney is ________________.

2.89. The medical term meaning surgical repair of a nerve is ________________.

2.90. The term meaning inflammation of the kidney is ________________.

LABELING EXERCISES

Identify the numbered items in the accompanying figures.

2.91. This is the right ________________ region.

2.92. This is the ________________ region.

2.93. This is the ________________ region.

2.94. This is the left ________________ region.

2.95. This is the left ________________ region.

2.96. This is the ________________ plane, which is also known as the midline.

2.97. This is the ________________ surface, which is also known as the ventral surface.

2.98. This arrow is pointing in a/an ________________ direction.

2.99. This is the ________________ surface, which is also known as the dorsal surface.

2.100. This is the ________________ plane, which is a horizontal plane.

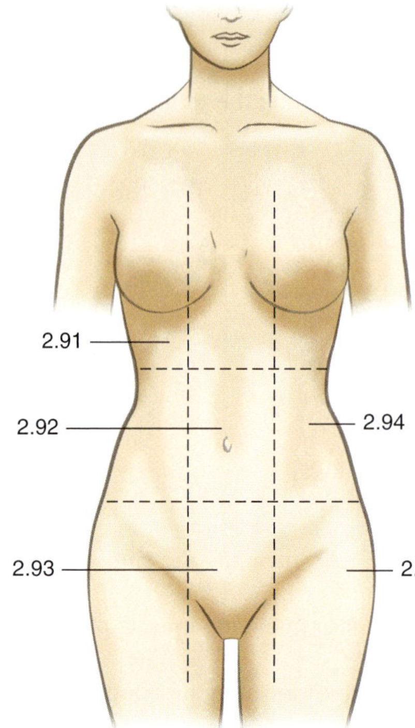

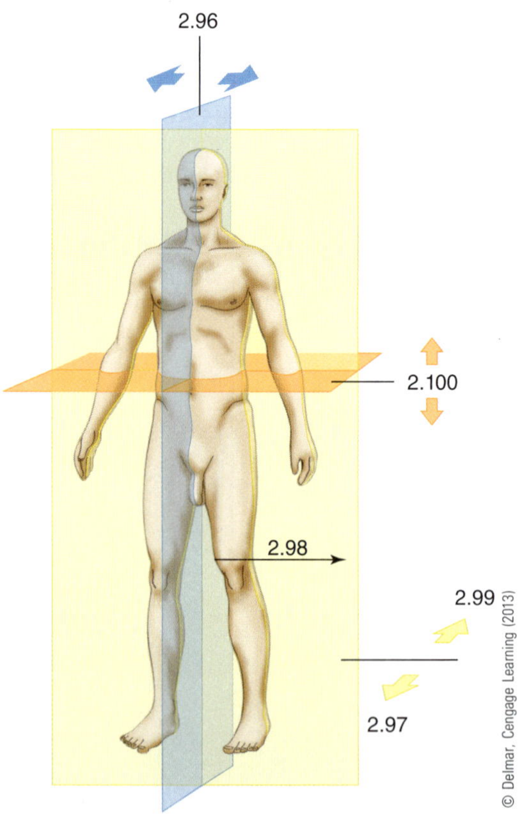

CHAPTER 3

The Skeletal System

Overview of STRUCTURES, COMBINING FORMS, AND FUNCTIONS OF THE SKELETAL SYSTEM

Major Structures	Related Combining Forms	Primary Functions
Bones	**oss/e**, **oss/i**, **oste/o**, **ost/o**	Act as the framework for the body, protect the internal organs, and store the mineral calcium.
Bone Marrow	**myel/o** (also means spinal cord)	Red bone marrow forms some blood cells. Yellow bone marrow stores fat.
Cartilage	**chondr/o**	Creates a smooth surface for motion within the joints and protects the ends of the bones.
Joints	**arthr/o**	Work with the muscles to make a variety of motions possible.
Ligaments	**ligament/o**	Connect one bone to another.
Synovial Membrane	**synovi/o**, **synov/o**	Forms the lining of synovial joints and secretes synovial fluid.
Synovial Fluid	**synovi/o**, **synov/o**	Lubricant that makes smooth joint movements possible.
Bursa	**burs/o**	Cushions areas subject to friction during movement.

Vocabulary Related to **THE SKELETAL SYSTEM**

This list contains essential word parts and medical terms for this chapter. These terms are pronounced in the StudyWARE™ and Audio CDs that are available for use with this text. These and the other important **primary terms** are shown in boldface throughout the chapter. *Secondary terms*, which appear in *orange* italics, clarify the meaning of primary terms.

Word Parts

- ☐ **ankyl/o** crooked, bent, stiff
- ☐ **arthr/o** joint
- ☐ **chondr/i**, **chondr/o** cartilage
- ☐ **cost/o** rib
- ☐ **crani/o** skull
- ☐ **-desis** to bind, tie together
- ☐ **kyph/o** bent, hump
- ☐ **lord/o** curve, swayback, bent
- ☐ **-lysis** loosening or setting free
- ☐ **myel/o** spinal cord, bone marrow
- ☐ **oss/e**, **oss/i**, **ost/o**, **oste/o** bone
- ☐ **scoli/o** curved, bent
- ☐ **spondyl/o** vertebrae, vertebral column, backbone
- ☐ **synovi/o**, **synov/o** synovial membrane, synovial fluid
- ☐ **-um** singular noun ending

Medical Terms

- ☐ **acetabulum** (**ass**-eh-**TAB**-you-lum)
- ☐ **allogenic** (**al**-oh-**JEN**-ick)
- ☐ **ankylosing spondylitis** (**ang**-kih-**LOH**-sing **spon**-dih-**LYE**-tis)
- ☐ **arthrodesis** (**ar**-throh-**DEE**-sis)
- ☐ **arthrolysis** (ar-**THROL**-ih-sis)
- ☐ **arthroscopy** (ar-**THROS**-koh-pee)
- ☐ **autologous** (aw-**TOL**-uh-guss)
- ☐ **chondroma** (kon-**DROH**-mah)
- ☐ **chondromalacia** (**kon**-droh-mah-**LAY**-shee-ah)
- ☐ **comminuted fracture** (**KOM**-ih-**newt**-ed)
- ☐ **compression fracture**
- ☐ **costochondritis** (**kos**-toh-kon-**DRIGH**-tis)
- ☐ **craniostenosis** (**kray**-nee-oh-steh-**NOH**-sis)
- ☐ **crepitation** (**krep**-ih-**TAY**-shun)
- ☐ **dual x-ray absorptiometry** (ab-**sorp**-shee-**OM**-eh-tree)
- ☐ **fibrous dysplasia** (dis-**PLAY**-see-ah)
- ☐ **hallux valgus** (**HAL**-ucks **VAL**-guss)
- ☐ **hemarthrosis** (**hem**-ar-**THROH**-sis)
- ☐ **hemopoietic** (**hee**-moh-poy-**ET**-ick)
- ☐ **internal fixation**
- ☐ **juvenile rheumatoid arthritis** (**ROO**-mah-toyd ar-**THRIGH**-tis)
- ☐ **kyphosis** (kye-**FOH**-sis)
- ☐ **laminectomy** (**lam**-ih-**NECK**-toh-mee)
- ☐ **lordosis** (lor-**DOH**-sis)
- ☐ **lumbago** (lum-**BAY**-goh)
- ☐ **malleolus** (mal-**LEE**-oh-lus)
- ☐ **manubrium** (mah-**NEW**-bree-um)
- ☐ **metacarpals** (met-ah-**KAR**-palz)
- ☐ **metatarsals** (met-ah-TAHR-salz)
- ☐ **myeloma** (**my**-eh-**LOH**-mah)
- ☐ **open fracture**
- ☐ **orthopedic surgeon** (**or**-thoh-**PEE**-dick)
- ☐ **orthotic** (or-**THOT**-ick)
- ☐ **osteitis** (**oss**-tee-**EYE**-tis)
- ☐ **osteoarthritis** (**oss**-tee-oh-ar-**THRIGH**-tis)
- ☐ **osteochondroma** (**oss**-tee-oh-kon-**DROH**-mah)
- ☐ **osteoclasis** (**oss**-tee-**OCK**-lah-sis)
- ☐ **osteomalacia** (**oss**-tee-oh-mah-**LAY**-shee-ah)
- ☐ **osteomyelitis** (**oss**-tee-oh-**my**-eh-**LYE**-tis)
- ☐ **osteonecrosis** (**oss**-tee-oh-neh-**KROH**-sis)
- ☐ **osteopenia** (**oss**-tee-oh-**PEE**-nee-ah)
- ☐ **osteoporosis** (**oss**-tee-oh-poh-**ROH**-sis)
- ☐ **osteoporotic hip fracture** (**oss**-tee-oh-pah-**ROT**-ick)
- ☐ **osteorrhaphy** (**oss**-tee-**OR**-ah-fee)
- ☐ **Paget's disease** (**PAJ**-its)
- ☐ **pathologic fracture**
- ☐ **percutaneous vertebroplasty** (**per**-kyou-**TAY**-nee-us **VER**-tee-broh-**plas**-tee)
- ☐ **periostitis** (**pehr**-ee-oss-**TYE**-tis)
- ☐ **podiatrist** (poh-**DYE**-ah-trist)
- ☐ **prosthesis** (pros-**THEE**-sis)
- ☐ **rheumatoid arthritis** (**ROO**-mah-toyd ar-**THRIGH**-tis)
- ☐ **rickets** (**RICK**-ets)
- ☐ **scoliosis** (**skoh**-lee-**OH**-sis)
- ☐ **spina bifida** (**SPY**-nah **BIF**-ih-dah)
- ☐ **spiral fracture**
- ☐ **spondylolisthesis** (**spon**-dih-loh-liss-**THEE**-sis)
- ☐ **spondylosis** (**spon**-dih-**LOH**-sis)
- ☐ **subluxation** (**sub**-luck-**SAY**-shun)
- ☐ **synovectomy** (sin-oh-**VECK**-toh-mee)
- ☐ **vertebrae** (**VER**-teh-bray)

LEARNING GOALS

On completion of this chapter, you should be able to:

1. Identify and describe the major functions and structures of the skeletal system.
2. Describe three types of joints.
3. Differentiate between the axial and appendicular skeletons.
4. Identify the medical specialists who treat disorders of the skeletal system.
5. Recognize, define, spell, and pronounce the primary terms related to the pathology and the diagnostic and treatment procedures of the skeletal system.

STRUCTURES AND FUNCTIONS OF THE SKELETAL SYSTEM

The skeletal system consists of the bones, bone marrow, cartilage, joints, ligaments, synovial membrane, synovial fluid, and bursa. This body system has many important functions:

- Bones act as the framework of the body.
- Bones support and protect the internal organs.
- Joints work in conjunction with muscles, ligaments, and tendons, making possible the wide variety of body movements. (Muscles and tendons are discussed in Chapter 4.)
- Calcium, which is required for normal nerve and muscle function, is stored in bones.
- Red bone marrow, which has an important function in the formation of blood cells, is located within spongy bone.

The Formation of Bones

A baby's skeleton begins as fragile membranes and cartilage, but after three months it starts turning into bone in a process called **ossification** (**oss**-us-fih-**KAY**-shun), which continues through adolescence.

Even after growth is completed, this process of new bone formation continues as *osteoclasts* break down old or damaged bone and *osteoblasts* help rebuild the bone. Ossification repairs the minor damage to the skeletal system that occurs during normal activity and also repairs bones after injuries such as fractures.

THE STRUCTURE OF BONES

Bone is the form of connective tissue that is the second hardest tissue in the human body. Only dental enamel is harder than bone.

The Tissues of Bone

Although it is a dense and rigid tissue, bone is also capable of growth, healing, and reshaping itself (Figure 3.1).

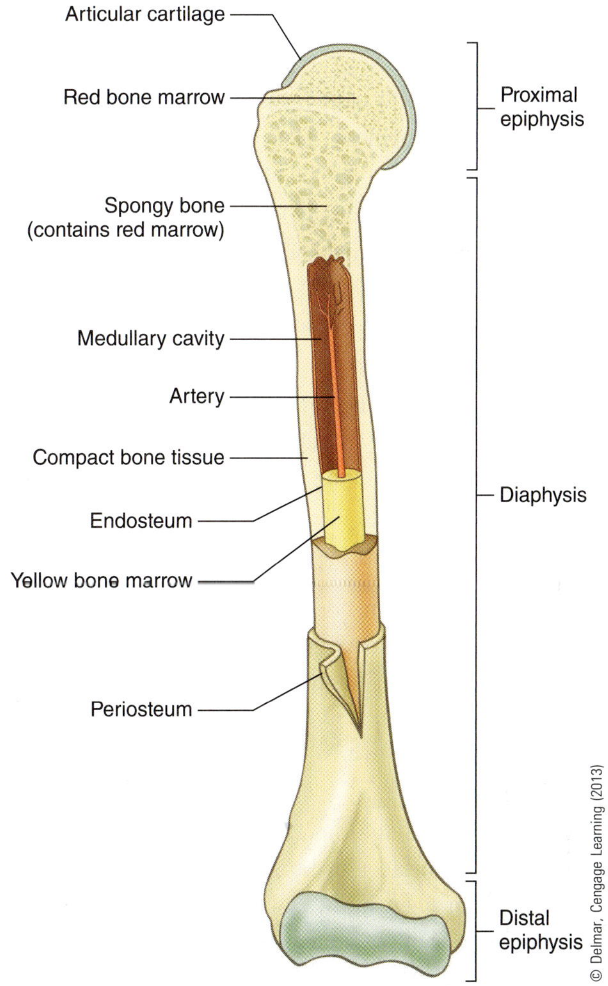

FIGURE 3.1 Anatomic features of a typical long bone.

- **Periosteum** (**pehr**-ee-**OSS**-tee-um) is the tough, fibrous tissue that forms the outermost covering of bone (**peri-** means surrounding, **oste** means bone, and **-um** is a noun ending).
- **Compact bone**, also known as ***cortical bone***, is the dense, hard, and very strong bone that forms the protective outer layer of bones.
- **Spongy bone**, also known as ***cancellous bone***, is lighter and not as strong as compact bone. This type of bone is commonly found in the ends and inner portions of long bones such as the femur. Red bone marrow is located within this spongy bone.
- The **medullary cavity** (**MED**-you-**lehr**-ee) is the central cavity located in the shaft of long bones where it is surrounded by compact bone. It is here that red and yellow bone marrow are stored. ***Medullary*** means pertaining to the inner section.
- The **endosteum** (en-**DOS**-tee-um) is the tissue that lines the medullary cavity (**end-** means within, **oste** means bone, and **-um** is a noun ending).

Bone Marrow

- **Red bone marrow**, which is located within the spongy bone, is a hemopoietic tissue that manufactures red blood cells, hemoglobin, white blood cells, and thrombocytes. These types of cells are discussed in Chapter 5.
- **Hemopoietic** (**hee**-moh-poy-**ET**-ick) means pertaining to the formation of blood cells (**hem/o** means blood, and **-poietic** means pertaining to formation). This term is also spelled ***hematopoietic***.
- **Yellow bone marrow** functions as a fat storage area. It is composed chiefly of fat cells and is located in the medullary cavity of long bones.

Cartilage

- **Cartilage** (**KAR**-tih-lidj) is the smooth, rubbery, blue-white connective tissue that acts as a shock absorber between bones. Cartilage, which is more elastic than bone, also makes up the flexible parts of the skeleton such as the outer ear and the tip of the nose.
- **Articular cartilage** (ar-**TICK**-you-lar **KAR**-tih-lidj) covers the surfaces of bones where they come together to form joints. This cartilage makes smooth joint movement possible and protects the bones from rubbing against each other (Figures 3.1 and 3.3).
- The **meniscus** (meh-**NIS**-kus) is the curved fibrous cartilage found in some joints, such as the knee and the temporomandibular joint of the jaw (Figure 3.3).

Anatomic Landmarks of Bones

- The **diaphysis** (dye-**AF**-ih-sis) is the shaft of a long bone (Figure 3.1).
- The **epiphyses** (ep-**PIF**-ih-seez) are the wider ends of long bones such as the femurs of the legs (singular *epiphysis*). Each epiphysis is covered with articular cartilage to protect it. The ***proximal epiphysis*** is the end of the bone located nearest to the midline of the body. The ***distal epiphysis*** is the end of the bone located farthest away from the midline of the body.
- A **foramen** (foh-**RAY**-men) is an opening in a bone through which blood vessels, nerves, and ligaments pass (plural, *foramina*). For example, the spinal cord passes through the ***foramen magnum*** of the occipital bone at the base of the skull.
- A **process** is a normal projection on the surface of a bone that most commonly serves as an attachment for a muscle or tendon For example, the ***mastoid process*** is the bony projection located on temporal bones just behind the ears (Figure 3.6).

JOINTS

Joints, which are also known as ***articulations***, are the place of union between two or more bones. Joints are classified either according to their construction or based on the degree of movement they allow.

Fibrous Joints

Fibrous joints, consisting of inflexible layers of dense connective tissue, hold the bones tightly together. In adults these joints, which are also known as ***sutures***, do not allow any movement (Figure 3.6). In newborns and very young children, some fibrous joints are movable before they have solidified.

- The **fontanelles** (**fon**-tah-**NELLS**), also known as the ***soft spots***, are normally present on the skull of a newborn. These flexible soft spots facilitate the passage of the infant through the birth canal. They also allow for the growth of the skull during the first year. As the child matures, and the sutures close, the fontanelles gradually harden.

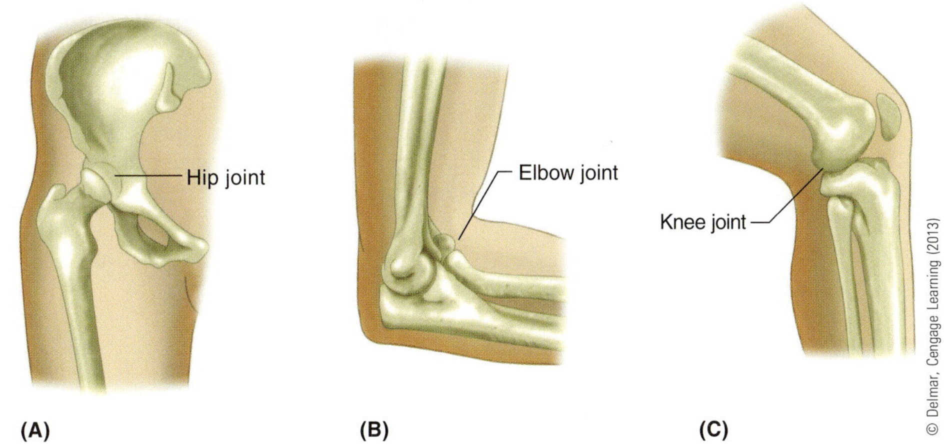

FIGURE 3.2 Examples of *synovial joints*. (A) Ball-and-socket joint of the hip. (B) Hinge joint of the elbow. (C) Hinge joint of the knee.

Cartilaginous Joints

Cartilaginous joints (**kar**-tih-**LADJ**-ih-nus) allow only slight movement and consist of bones connected entirely by cartilage. For example:

- Where the ribs connect to the sternum (breast bone), shown in Figure 3.8, these joints allow movement during breathing.
- The **pubic symphysis** (**PEW**-bick **SIM**-fih-sis) allows some movement to facilitate childbirth. This joint is located between the pubic bones in the anterior (front) of the pelvis as shown in Figure 3.12.

Synovial Joints

A **synovial joint** (sih-**NOH**-vee-al) is created where two bones articulate to permit a variety of motions. As used here, the term ***articulate*** means to come together. These joints are also described based on their type of motion (Figure 3.2).

- ***Ball-and-socket joints***, such as the hips and shoulders, allow a wide range of movement in many directions (Figure 3.2A).
- ***Hinge joints***, such as the knees and elbows, are synovial joints that allow movement primarily in one direction or plane (Figure 3.2B and 3.2C).

Components of Synovial Joints

Synovial joints consist of several components that make complex movements possible (Figure 3.3).

- The **synovial capsule** is the outermost layer of strong fibrous tissue that resembles a sleeve as it surrounds the joint.
- The **synovial membrane** lines the capsule and secretes synovial fluid.
- **Synovial fluid**, which flows within the synovial cavity, acts as a lubricant to make the smooth movement of the joint possible.
- **Ligaments** (**LIG**-ah-mentz) are bands of fibrous tissue that form joints by connecting one bone to another bone or by joining a bone to cartilage. Complex hinge joints, such as the knee as shown in Figures 3.2 and 3.3, are made up of a series of ligaments that permit movement in different directions.

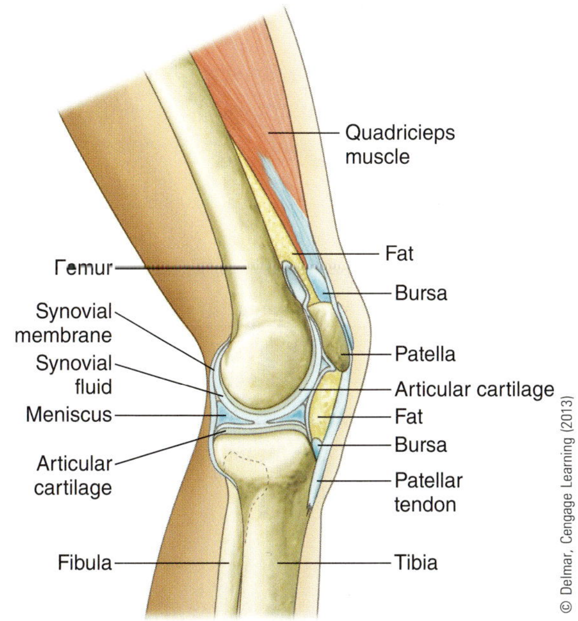

FIGURE 3.3 A lateral view of the knee showing the structures of a *synovial joint* and *bursa*.

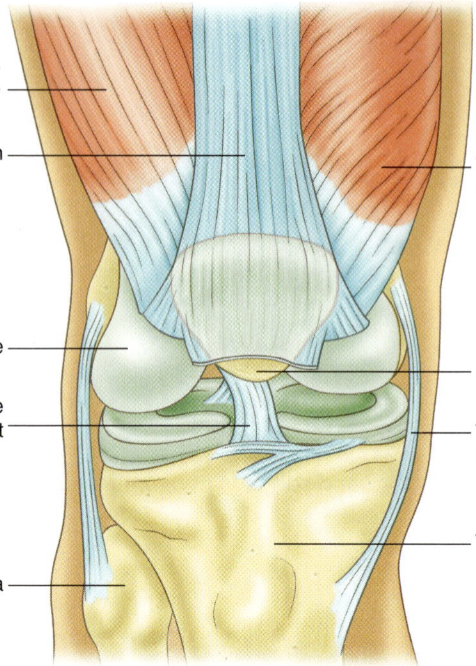

FIGURE 3.4 Major ligaments of the knee. This anterior view of the knee shows the complex system of ligaments that make its movements possible.

- A **bursa** (**BER**-sah) is a fibrous sac that acts as a cushion to ease movement in areas that are subject to friction, such as in the shoulder, elbow, and knee joints where a tendon passes over a bone (plural, *bursae*).

THE SKELETON

The typical adult human skeleton consists of approximately 206 bones, as shown in Figure 3.5. Depending upon the age of the individual, the exact number of bones ranges from 206 to 350. For descriptive purposes, the skeleton is divided into the axial and appendicular skeletal systems.

Axial Skeleton

The **axial skeleton** protects the major organs of the nervous, respiratory, and circulatory systems. In the human, the axial skeleton consists of the 80 bones of the head and body that are organized into five parts. These are (1) the bones of the skull, (2) the ossicles (bones) of the middle ear, (3) the hyoid bone, located on the throat between the chin and the thyroid, (4) the rib cage, and (5) the vertebral column.

Appendicular Skeleton

The **appendicular skeleton** makes body movement possible and also protects the organs of digestion, excretion, and reproduction. In the human, the appendicular skeleton consists of 126 bones that are organized into: (1) the *upper extremities* (shoulders, arms, forearms, wrists, and hands) and (2) the *lower extremities* (hips, thighs, legs, ankles, and feet).

An *appendage* is anything that is attached to a major part of the body and the term *appendicular* means referring to an appendage. An *extremity* is the terminal end of a body part such as an arm or leg.

Bones of the Skull

The **skull** consists of the 8 bones that form the cranium, 14 bones that form the face, and 6 bones in the middle ear. As you study the following bones of the skull, refer to Figures 3.6 and 3.7.

The Bones of the Cranium

The **cranium** (**KRAY**-nee-um), which is made up of the following eight bones, is that portion of the skull that encloses and protects the brain (**crani** means skull, and **-um** is a noun ending). These cranial bones are joined by jagged fibrous joints that are often referred to as **sutures.**

- The **frontal bone** is the anterior portion of the cranium that forms the forehead. This bone houses the frontal sinuses and forms the roof of the ethmoid sinuses, the nose and part of the socket that protects the eyeball.
- The **parietal bones** (pah-**RYE**-eh-tal) are two of the largest bones of the skull. Together they form most of the roof and upper sides of the cranium.

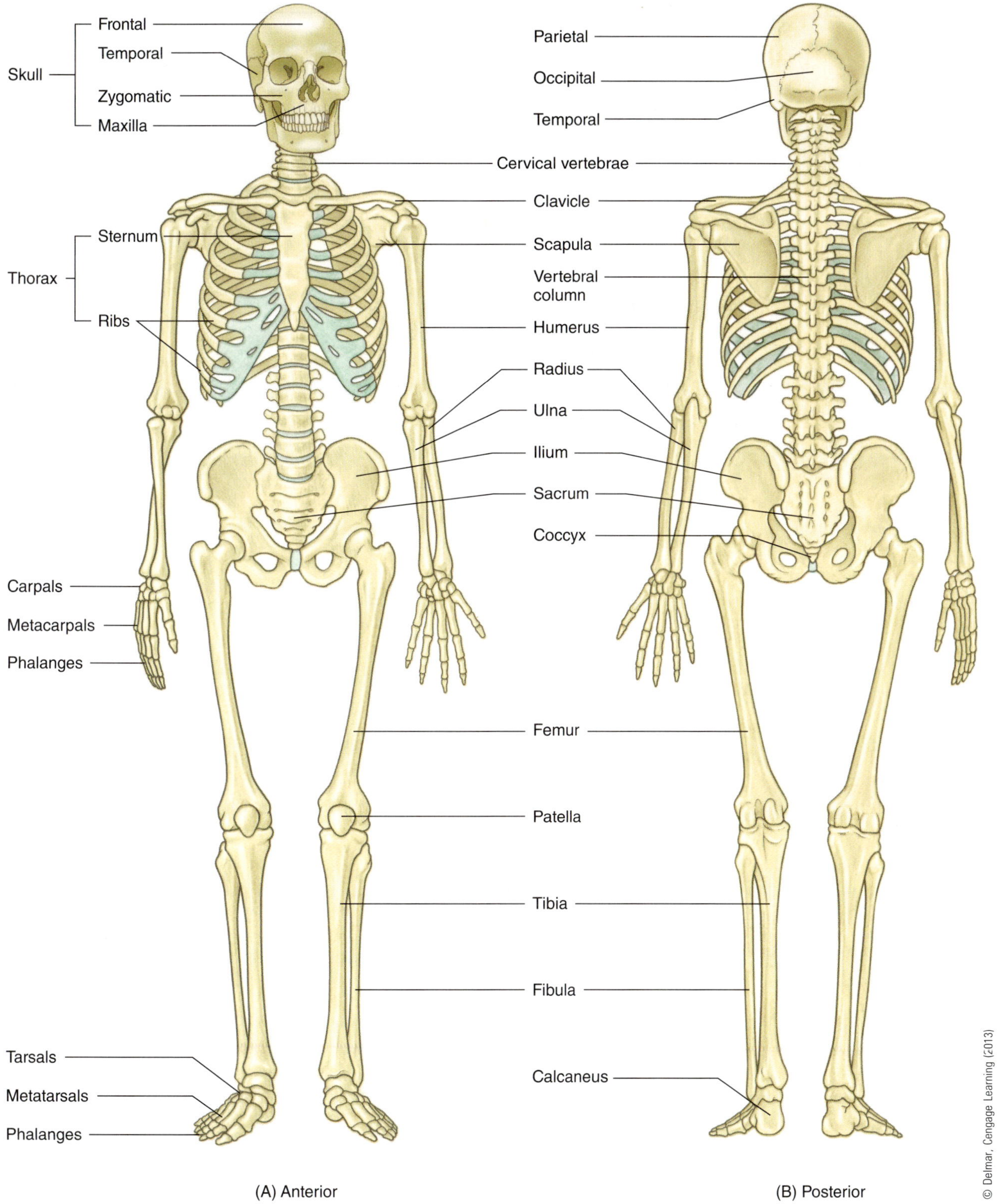

FIGURE 3.5 Anterior and posterior views of the human skeleton.

- The **occipital bone** (ock-**SIP**-ih-tal) forms the back part of the skull and the base of the cranium.
- The two **temporal bones** form the sides and base of the cranium.
- The **external auditory meatus** (mee-**AY**-tus) is the opening of the external auditory canal of the outer ear. This canal is located within the temporal bone on each side of the skull. A *meatus* is the external opening of a canal.

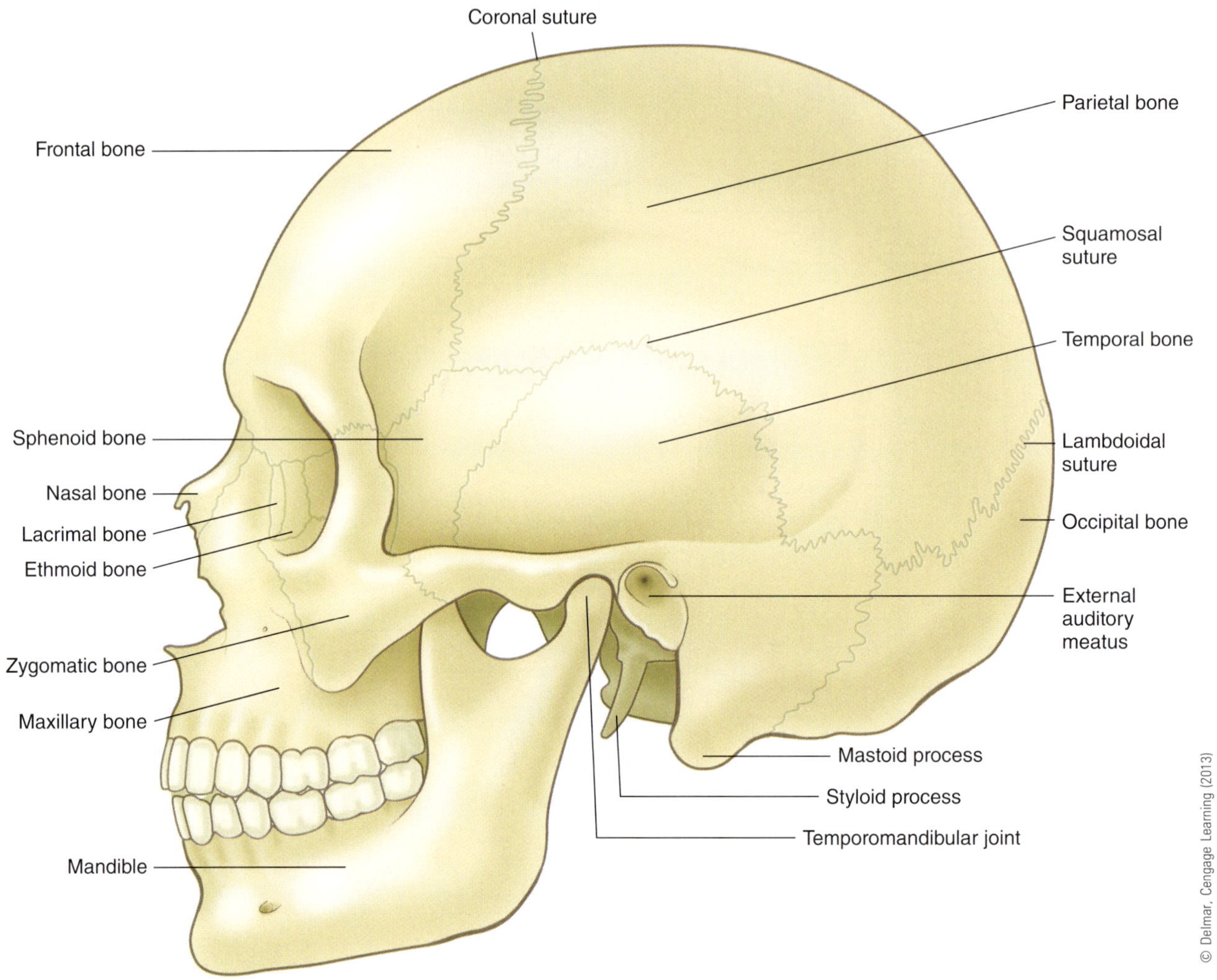

FIGURE 3.6 Lateral view of the adult human skull.

- The **sphenoid bone** (**SFEE**-noid) is an irregular, wedge-shaped bone at the base of the skull. This bone makes contact with all of the other cranial bones and helps form the base of the cranium, the sides of the skull, and the floors and sides of the eye sockets.
- The **ethmoid bone** (**ETH**-moid) is light, spongy bone located at the roof and sides of the nose. Here it separates the nasal cavity from the brain, and it also forms a portion of each orbit. An ***orbit*** is the bony socket that surrounds and protects each eyeball.

The Auditory Ossicles

The **auditory ossicles** (**OSS**-ih-kulz) are the three tiny bones located in each middle ear. These bones, known as the ***malleus***, ***incus***, and ***stapes***, are discussed in Chapter 11.

The Bones of the Face

- The face is made up of the following 14 bones. Some of these bones contain air-filled cavities known as sinuses. Among the purposes of these sinuses is to lighten the weight of the skull. (These sinuses are discussed in Chapter 7.)
- The two **nasal bones** form the upper part of the bridge of the nose.
- The two **zygomatic bones** (**zye**-goh-**MAT**-ick), also known as the ***cheekbones***, articulate with the frontal bone that makes up the forehead. The term *articulate* means to join together with.
- The two **maxillary bones** (**MACK**-sih-**ler**-ee) form most of the upper jaw (singular, *maxilla*). These bones are also known as the ***maxillae.***
- The two **palatine bones** (**PAL**-ah-tine) form the anterior (front) part of the hard palate of the mouth and the floor of the nose.
- The two **lacrimal bones** (**LACK**-rih-mal) make up part of the orbit (socket of the eye) at the inner angle.

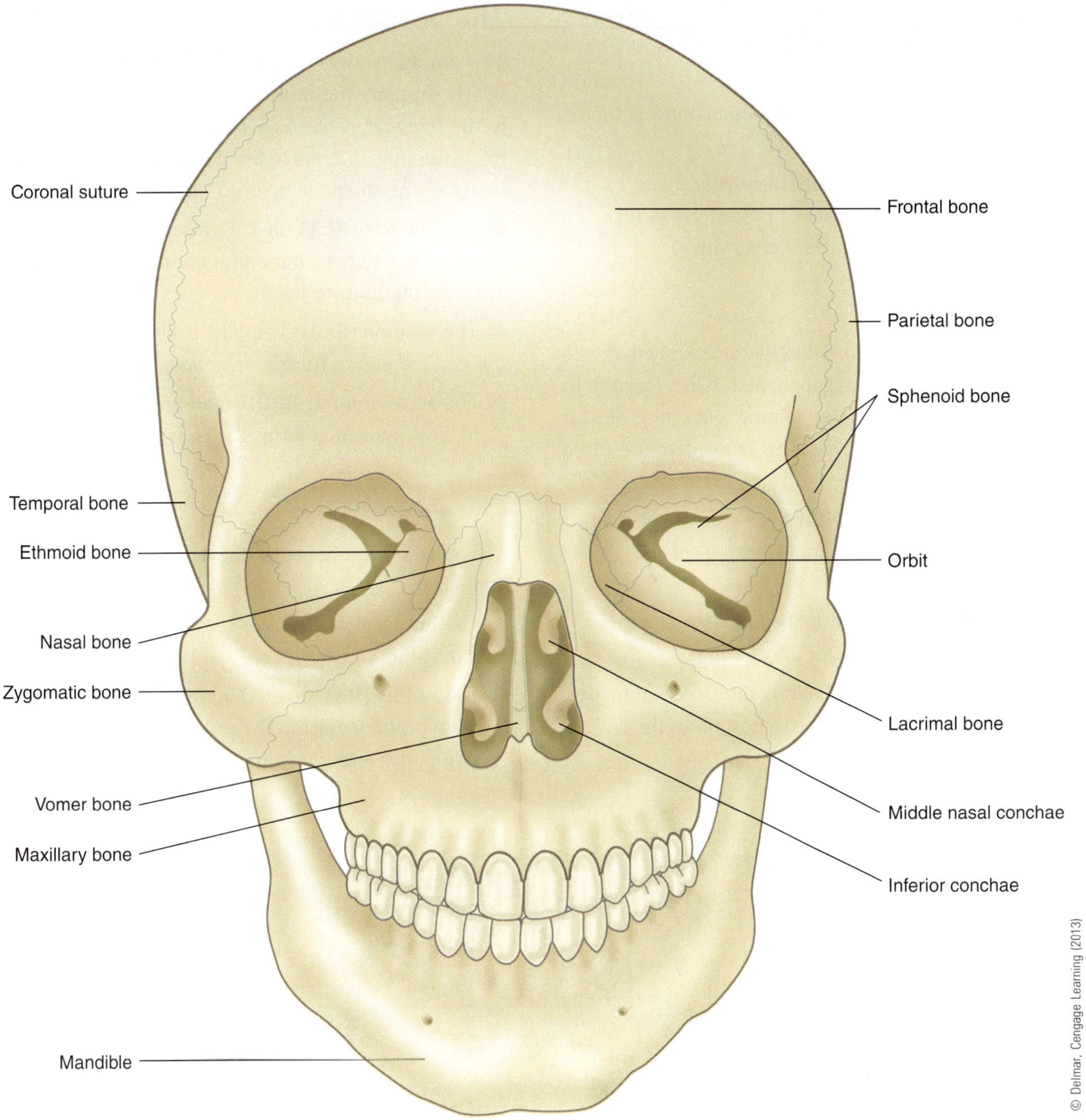

FIGURE 3.7 Anterior view of the adult human skull.

- The two **inferior conchae** (**KONG**-kee *or* **KONG**-kay) are the thin, scroll-like bones that form part of the interior of the nose (singular, *concha*).
- The **vomer bone** (**VOH**-mer) forms the base for the nasal septum. The ***nasal septum*** is the cartilage wall that divides the two nasal cavities.
- The **mandible** (**MAN**-dih-bul), also known as the ***jawbone***, is the only movable bone of the skull. The mandible is attached to the skull at the **temporomandibular joint** (**tem**-poh-roh-man-**DIB**-you-lar), which is commonly known as the ***TMJ*** (Figure 3.6).

Thoracic Cavity

The **thoracic cavity** (thoh-**RAS**-ick), also known as the ***rib cage***, is the bony structure that protects the heart and lungs. It consists of the ribs, sternum, and upper portion of the spinal column extending from the neck to the diaphragm, but not including the arms.

The Ribs

The 12 pairs of **ribs**, which are also known as ***costals***, attach posteriorly to the thoracic vertebrae (**cost** means rib, and **-al** means pertaining to) (Figure 3.8).

- The first seven pairs of ribs are called *true ribs*, and they attach anteriorly to the sternum.
- The next three pairs of ribs are called *false ribs*, and they attach anteriorly to cartilage that connects them to the sternum.
- The last two pairs of ribs are called *floating ribs*, because they are only attached posteriorly to the vertebrae but are not attached anteriorly.

The Sternum

The **sternum** (**STER**-num), which is also known as the *breast bone*, is a flat, dagger-shaped bone located in the middle of the chest. By joining with the ribs, it forms the front of the rib cage. This is divided into three parts (Figure 3.8).

- The **manubrium** (mah-**NEW**-bree-um) is the bony structure that forms the upper portion of the sternum.
- The **body of the sternum** is the bony structure that forms the middle portion of the sternum.
- The **xiphoid process** (**ZIF**-oid) is the structure made of cartilage that forms the lower portion of the sternum.

The Shoulders

The shoulders form the **pectoral girdle** (**PECK**-toh-rahl), which supports the arms and hands. This is also known as the *shoulder girdle.* As used here, the term *girdle* refers to a structure that encircles the body. As you study the bones of the shoulder, refer to Figures 3.5 and 3.8.

- The **clavicle** (**KLAV**-ih-kul), also known as the *collar bone*, is a slender bone that connects the manubrium of the sternum to the scapula.
- The **scapula** (**SKAP**-you-lah) is also known as the *shoulder blade* (plural, *scapulae*).
- The **acromion** (ah-**KROH**-mee-on) is an extension of the scapula that forms the high point of the shoulder.

The Arms

As you study the bones of the arms, refer to Figures 3.5 and 3.8.

- The **humerus** (**HEW**-mer-us) is the bone of the upper arm (plural, *humeri*).
- The **radius** (**RAY**-dee-us) is the smaller and shorter bone in the forearm. The radius runs up the thumb side of the forearm (plural, *radius bones*).

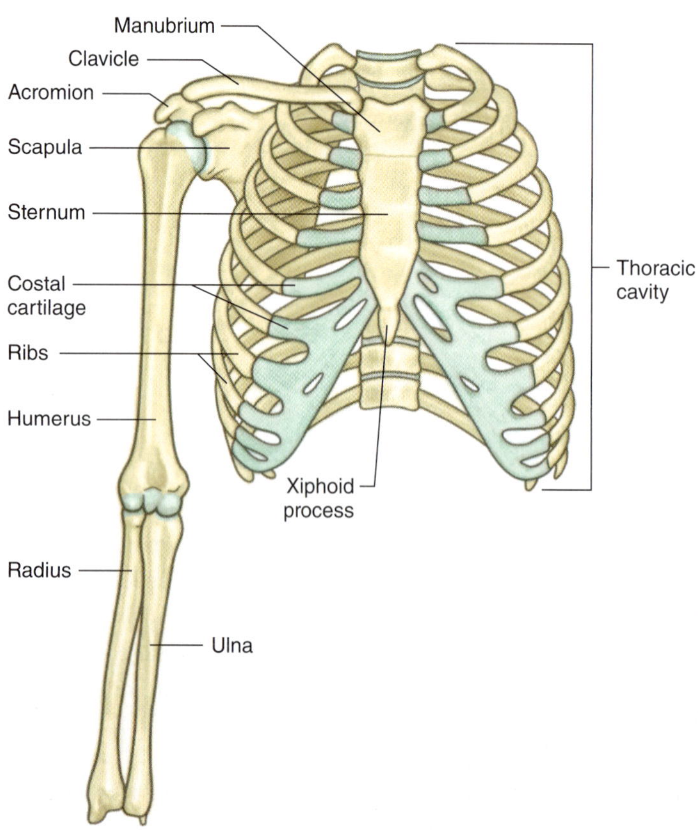

FIGURE 3.8 Anterior view of the ribs, shoulder, and arm. (Cartilaginous structures are shown in blue.)

- The **ulna** (**ULL**-nah) is the larger and longer bone of the forearm (plural, *ulnae*). The proximal end of the ulna articulates with the distal end of the humerus to form the elbow joint.
- The **olecranon process** (oh-**LEK**-rah-non), commonly known as the ***funny bone***, is a large projection on the upper end of the ulna. This forms the point of the elbow and exposes a nerve that tingles when struck.

The Wrists, Hands, and Fingers

As you study these bones, refer to Figure 3.9.

- The eight **carpals** (**KAR**-palz) are the bones that form the wrist (singular, *carpal*). These bones form a narrow bony passage known as the *carpal tunnel*. The median nerve and the tendons of the fingers pass through this tunnel to reach the hand. *Carpal tunnel syndrome* is described in Chapter 4.
- The **metacarpals** (met-ah-**KAR**-palz) are the five bones that form the palms of the hand.
- The **phalanges** (fah-**LAN**-jeez) are the 14 bones of the fingers (singular, *phalanx*). The bones of the toes are also known as phalanges.
- Each of the four fingers has three bones. These are the distal (outermost), middle, and proximal (nearest the hand) phalanges.
- The thumb has two bones. These are the distal and proximal phalanges.

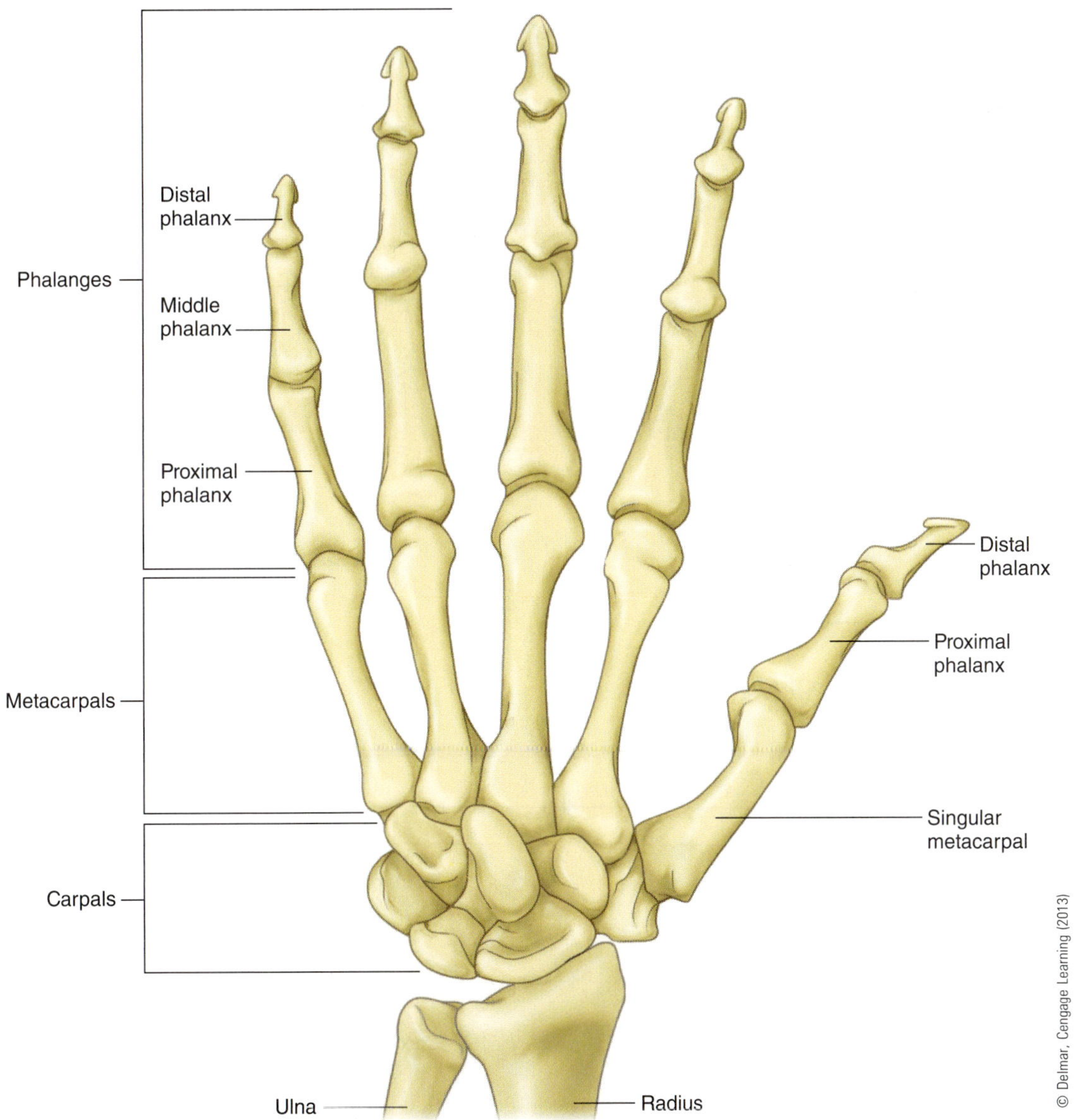

FIGURE 3.9 Superior view of the bones of the lower left arm, wrist, and hand.

The Spinal Column

The **spinal column,** which is also known as the ***vertebral column***, protects the spinal cord and supports the head and body. The spinal column consists of 26 **vertebrae** (**VER**-teh-bray). Each of these bony units is known as a **vertebra** (**VER**-teh-bruh), and the term ***vertebral*** means pertaining to the vertebrae.

The Structures of Vertebrae

As you study the structures of a vertebra, refer to Figure 3.10.

- The anterior portion of the vertebra is solid to provide strength and is known as the ***body of the vertebra.***
- The posterior portion of a vertebra is known as the **lamina** (**LAM**-ih-nah) (plural, *laminae*). The transverse and spinous processes extend from this area and serve as attachments for muscles and tendons.
- The ***vertebral foramen*** is the opening in the middle of the vertebra. This opening allows the spinal cord to pass through and to protect the spinal cord.

Intervertebral Disks

Intervertebral disks (**in**-ter-**VER**-teh-bral), which are made of cartilage, separate and cushion the vertebrae from each other. They also act as shock absorbers and allow for movement of the spinal column (Figure 3.18A).

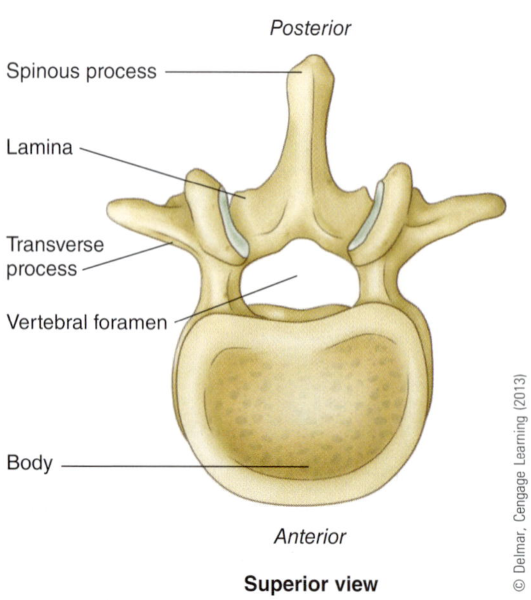

FIGURE 3.10 Characteristics of a typical vertebra.

The Types of Vertebrae

As you study the types of vertebrae, refer to Figure 3.11A & B.

- The **cervical vertebrae** (**SER**-vih-kal) are the first set of 7 vertebrae, and they form the neck. The term ***cervical*** means pertaining to the neck, and these vertebrae are also known as **C1** through **C7**.
- The **thoracic vertebrae** (thoh-**RASS**-ick), known as **T1** through **T12**, are the second set of 12 vertebrae.

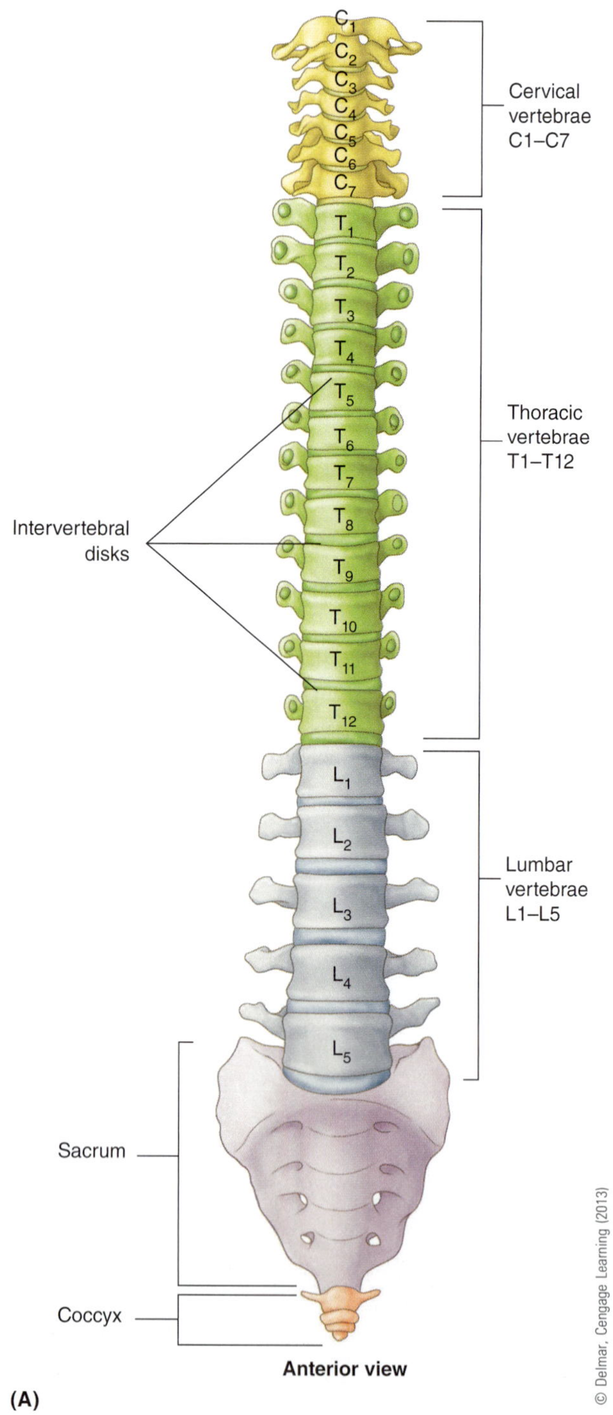

FIGURE 3.11A Anterior view of the vertebral column.

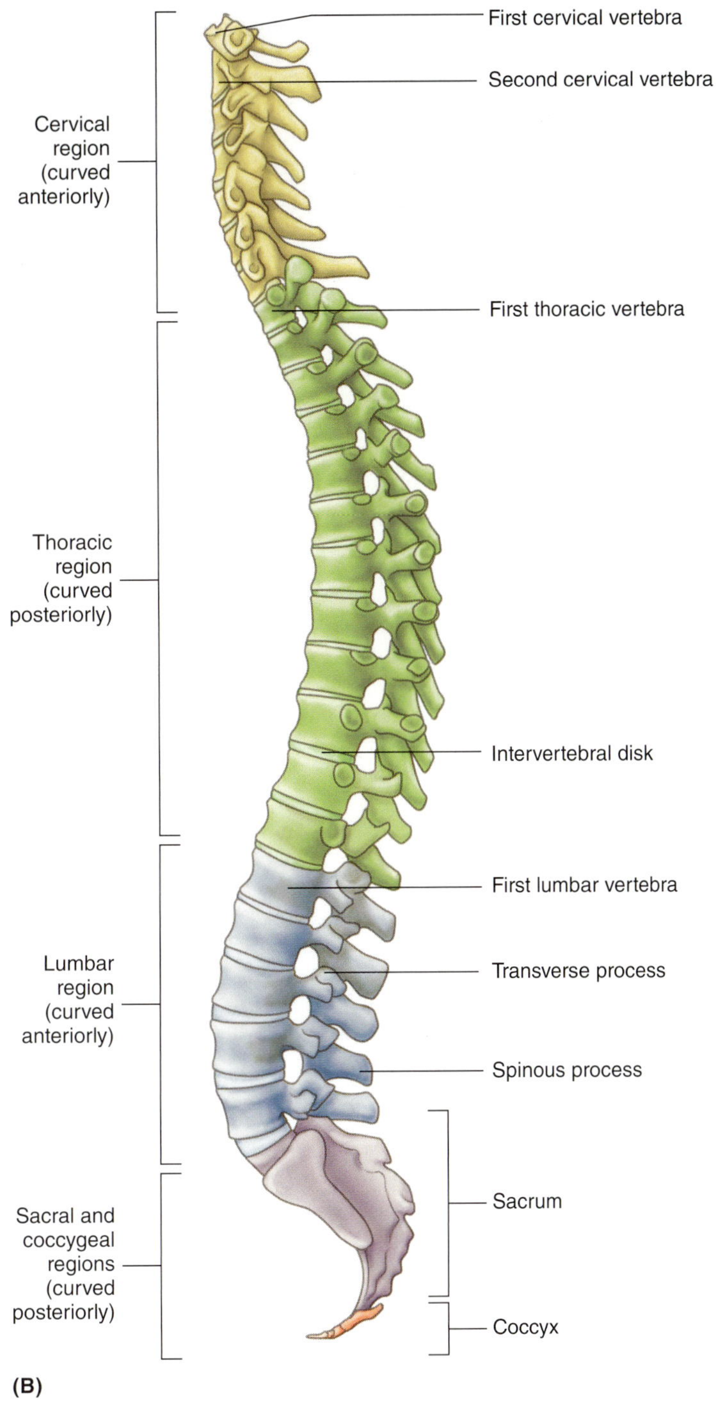

FIGURE 3.11B Lateral view of the vertebral column.

Each of these vertebra has a pair of ribs attached to it, and together they form the outward curve of the spine. *Thoracic* means pertaining to the thoracic cavity.

- The **lumbar vertebrae** (**LUM**-bar), known as **L1** through **L5**, make up the third set of 5 vertebrae, and together they form the inward curve of the lower spine. These are the largest and strongest of the vertebrae, and they bear most of the body's weight. *Lumbar* means relating to the part of the back and sides between the ribs and the pelvis.

The remaining two vertebrae are the sacrum and the coccyx. As you study these structures, refer to Figure 3.11.

- The **sacrum** (**SAY**-krum) is the slightly curved, triangular-shaped bone near the base of the spine that forms the lower portion of the back. At birth, the sacrum is composed of five separate bones; however in the young child, they fuse together to form a single bone.
- The **coccyx** (**KOCK**-sicks), which is also known as the *tailbone*, forms the end of the spine and is actually made up of four small vertebrae that are fused together.

The Pelvic Girdle

The **pelvic girdle** protects internal organs and supports the lower extremities. It is commonly known as the ***pelvis*** or ***hips***. The pelvis is a cup-shaped ring of bone at the lower end of the trunk, and it consists of the *ilium, ischium,* and *pubis* (Figures 3.12 and 3.14).

- The **ilium** (**ILL**-ee-um) is the broad blade-shaped bone that forms the back and sides of the pubic bone.
- The **sacroiliac** (**say**-kroh-**ILL**-ee-ack) is the slightly movable articulation between the sacrum and posterior portion of the ilium (**sacr/o** means sacrum, **ili** means ilium, and **-ac** means pertaining to).
- The **ischium** (**ISS**-kee-um), which forms the lower posterior portion of the pubic bone, bears the weight of the body when sitting.
- The **pubis** (**PEW**-bis), which forms the anterior portion of the pubic bone, is located just below the urinary bladder.
- At birth the *ilium, ischium,* and *pubis* are three separate bones. As the child matures, these bones fuse to form the left and right **pubic bones**, which are held securely together by the pubic symphysis.
- The **pubic symphysis** is the cartilaginous joint that unites the left and right pubic bones. A *cartilaginous joint* allows slight movement between bones.
- The **acetabulum** (**ass**-eh-**TAB**-you-lum), also known as the ***hip socket***, is the large circular cavity in each side of the pelvis that articulates with the head of the femur to form the hip joint (Figures 3.12 and 3.14).

The Legs and Knees

As you study these bones, refer to Figures 3.13 and 3.14.

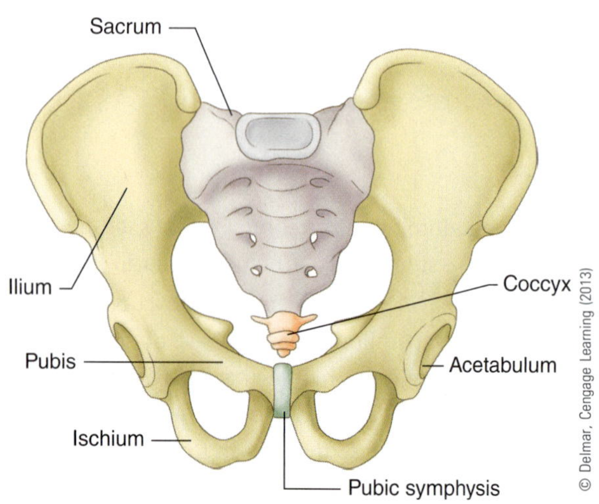

FIGURE 3.12 Anterior view of the pelvis.

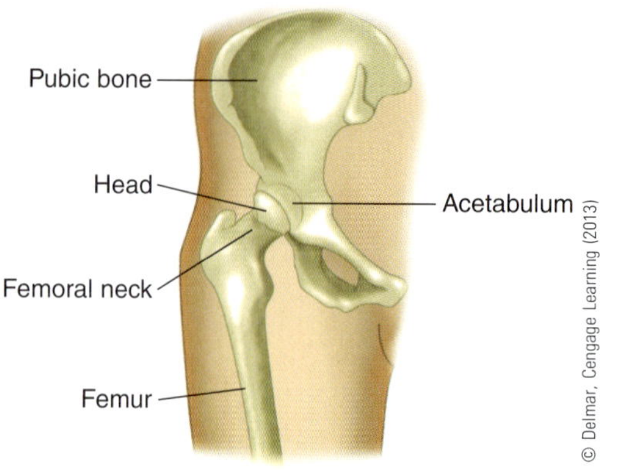

FIGURE 3.13 Structures of the proximal end of the femur and the acetabulum (hip socket).

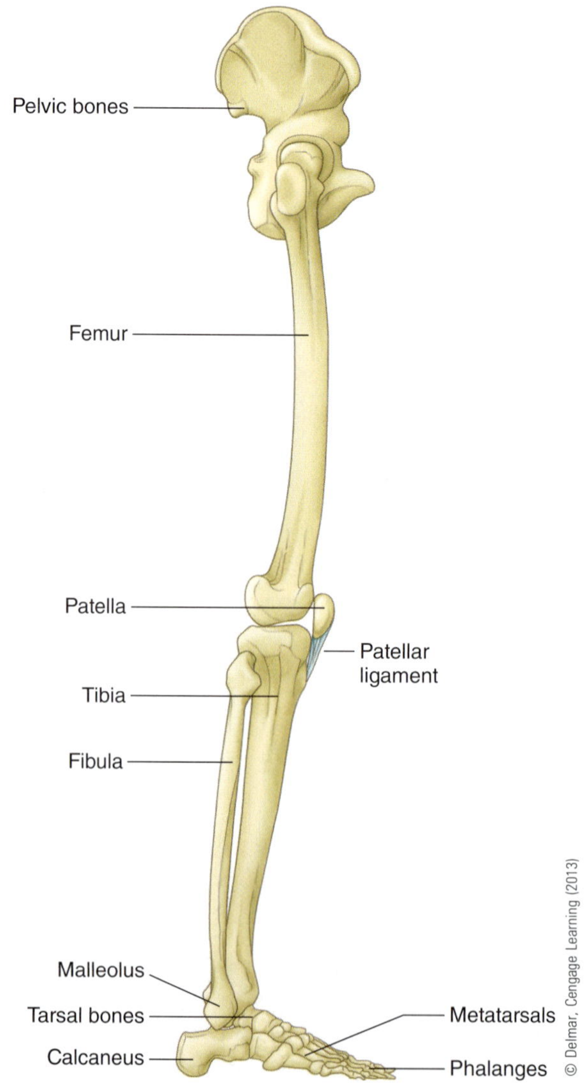

FIGURE 3.14 Lateral view of bones of the lower extremity.

The Femurs

- The **femurs** (**FEE**-murz) are the largest bones in the body. ***Femoral*** means pertaining to the femur.
- These bones are also known as ***thigh bones***.
- The ***head of the femur*** articulates with the acetabulum (hip socket).
- The ***femoral neck*** is the narrow area just below the head of the femur.

The Knees

- The **patella** (pah-**TEL**-ah), also known as the ***kneecap***, is the bony anterior portion of the knee.
- The term **popliteal** (pop-**LIT**-ee-al) describes the posterior space behind the knee where the ligaments, vessels, and muscles related to this joint are located.
- The **cruciate ligaments** (**KROO**-shee-ayt), which are shown in Figure 3.4, make possible the movements of the knee. These are known as the ***anterior*** and ***posterior cruciate ligaments*** because they are shaped like a cross.

The Lower Legs

The lower leg is made up of the *tibia* and the *fibula* (Figure 3.14).

- The **tibia** (**TIB**-ee-ah), also known as the ***shinbone***, is the larger anterior weight-bearing bone of the lower leg.
- The **fibula** (**FIB**-you-lah) is the smaller of the two bones of the lower leg.

The Ankles

- The **ankles** are the joints that connect the lower leg and foot and make the necessary movements possible.
- Each ankle is made up of seven short **tarsal** (**TAHR**-sal) bones. These bones are similar to the bones of the wrists; however, they are much larger in size (Figure 3.15).
- The **malleolus** (mal-**LEE**-oh-lus) is a rounded bony projection on the tibia and fibula on the sides of each ankle joint (plural, *malleoli*).
- The **talus** (**TAY**-luss) is the ankle bone that articulates with the tibia and fibula (Figures 3.15 and 3.17).
- The **calcaneus** (kal-**KAY**-nee-uss), also known as the ***heel bone***, is the largest of the tarsal bones (Figures 3.14 and 3.15).

The Feet and Toes

The feet and toes are made up of the following bones as shown in Figure 3.15.

- The five **metatarsals** (met-ah-**TAHR**-salz) form that part of the foot to which the toes are attached.
- The **phalanges** are the bones of the toes. The great toe has two phalanges. Each of the other toes has three phalanges. The bones of the fingers are also called phalanges.

MEDICAL SPECIALTIES RELATED TO THE SKELETAL SYSTEM

- A **chiropractor** (**KYE**-roh-**prack**-tor) holds a Doctor of Chiropractic (DC) degree and specializes in the manipulative treatment of disorders originating from misalignment of the spine. ***Manipulative treatment*** involves manually adjusting the positions of the bones.
- An **orthopedic surgeon** (**or**-thoh-**PEE**-dick), also known as an ***orthopedist***, is a physician who specializes in diagnosing and treating diseases and disorders involving the bones, joints, and muscles.
- An **osteopath** (**oss**-tee-oh-**PATH**) holds a Doctor of Osteopathy (DO) degree and uses traditional forms of medical treatment in addition to specializing in treating health problems by spinal manipulation (**oste/o** means bone, and **-path** means disease). This type of medical practice is known as ***osteopathy***; however, that term is also used to mean any bone disease.
- A **podiatrist** (poh-**DYE**-ah-trist) holds a Doctor of Podiatry (DP) or Doctor of Podiatric Medicine (DPM) degree and specializes in diagnosing and treating disorders of the foot (**pod** mean foot, and **-iatrist** means specialist).
- A **rheumatologist** (roo-mah-**TOL**-oh-jist) is a physician who specializes in the diagnosis and treatment of arthritis and disorders such as osteoporosis, fibromyalgia, and tendinitis that are characterized by inflammation in the joints and connective tissues.

PATHOLOGY OF THE SKELETAL SYSTEM

Joints

- **Ankylosis** (**ang**-kih-**LOH**-sis) is the loss or absence of mobility in a joint due to disease, injury, or a surgical procedure (**ankyl** means crooked, bent, or stiff, and

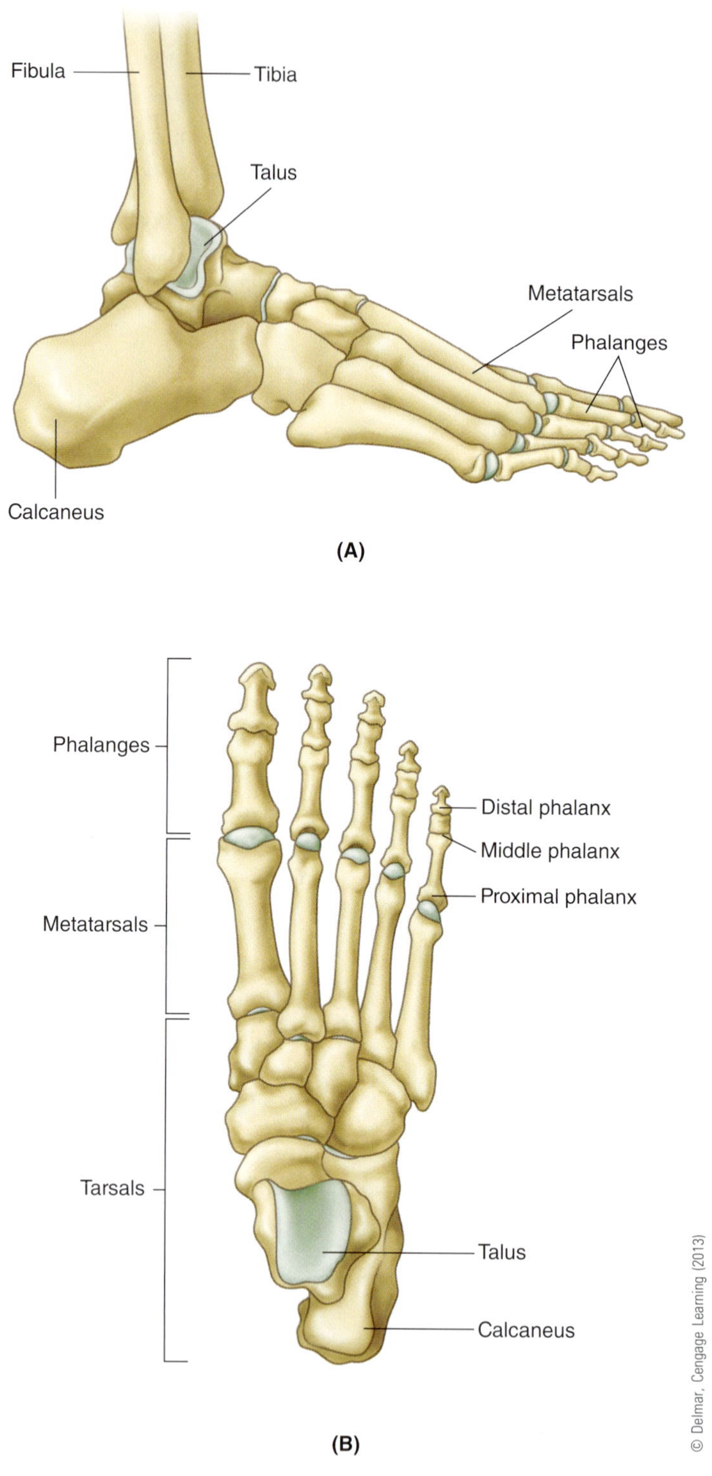

FIGURE 3.15 Bones of the right ankle and foot. (A) Lateral view. (B) Superior view.

-osis means abnormal condition or disease). ***Mobility*** means being capable of movement.

- **Arthrosclerosis** (**ar**-throh-skleh-**ROH**-sis) is stiffness of the joints, especially in the elderly (**arthr/o** means joint, and **-sclerosis** means abnormal hardening).
- **Bursitis** (ber-**SIGH**-tis) is an inflammation of a bursa (**burs** means bursa, and **-itis** means inflammation).
- **Chondromalacia** (**kon**-droh-mah-**LAY**-shee-ah) is the abnormal softening of cartilage (**chondr/o** means cartilage, and **-malacia** means abnormal softening).

- A **chondroma** (kon-**DROH**-mah) is a slow-growing benign tumor derived from cartilage cells (**chondr** means cartilage, and **-oma** means tumor).
- **Costochondritis** (**kos**-toh-kon-**DRIGH**-tis) is an inflammation of the cartilage that connects a rib to the sternum (**cost/o** means rib, **chondr** means cartilage, and **-itis** means inflammation).
- **Hallux valgus** (**HAL**-ucks **VAL**-guss), also known as a ***bunion***, is an abnormal enlargement of the joint at the base of the great toe (*hallux* means big toe, and *valgus* means bent).
- **Hemarthrosis** (**hem**-ar-**THROH**-sis) is blood within a joint (**hem** means blood, **arthr** means joint, and **-osis** means abnormal condition or disease). This condition is frequently due to a joint injury. It also can occur spontaneously in patients taking blood-thinning medications or those having a blood clotting disorder such as hemophilia (see Chapters 2 and 5).
- **Polymyalgia rheumatica** (PMR) (pol-ee-my-**AL**-jah roo-**MA**-tih-kah) is a geriatric inflammatory disorder of the muscles and joints characterized by pain and stiffness in the neck, shoulders, upper arms, and hips and thighs (**poly-** means many, **my** means muscle, and **-algia** means pain). *Rheumatica* is the Latin word for ***rheumatism***, an obsolete term for arthritis and other disorders causing pain in the joints and supporting tissue.
- A ***sprain*** occurs when a ligament that connects bones to a joint is wrenched or torn (see Chapter 4).
- **Synovitis** (sin-oh-**VYE**-tiss) is inflammation of the synovial membrane that results in swelling and pain of the affected joint (**synov** means synovial membrane, and **-itis** means inflammation). This condition can be caused by arthritis, trauma, infection, or irritation produced by damaged cartilage.

Dislocation

- **Dislocation**, also known as ***luxation*** (luck-**SAY**-shun), is the total displacement of a bone from its joint (Figure 3.16).
- **Subluxation** (**sub**-luck-**SAY**-shun) is the partial displacement of a bone from its joint.

Arthritis

Arthritis (ar-**THRIGH**-tis) is an inflammatory condition of one or more joints (**arthr** means joint, and **-itis** means inflammation). There are more than 100 types of arthritis with many different causes. Some of the more common types of arthritis follow.

Osteoarthritis

Osteoarthritis (OA) (**oss**-tee-oh-ar-**THRIGH**-tis), also known as ***wear-and-tear arthritis***, is most commonly associated with aging (**oste/o** means bone, **arthr** means joint, and **-itis** means inflammation) (Figure 3.17).

- OA is known as a ***degenerative joint disease*** because it is characterized by the wearing away of the articular cartilage within the joints. ***Degenerative*** means the breaking down or impairment of a body part.
- It is also characterized by hypertrophy of bone and the formation of **osteophytes** (**OSS**-tee-oh-fites), also known as bone spurs.

Spondylosis (**spon**-dih-**LOH**-sis) is also known as ***spinal osteoarthritis.*** This degenerative disorder can cause the loss of normal spinal structure and function (**spondyl** means vertebrae, and **-osis** means abnormal condition or disease).

Gouty Arthritis

Gouty arthritis (**GOW**-tee ar-**THRIGH**-tis), also known as ***gout***, is a type of arthritis characterized by deposits of uric

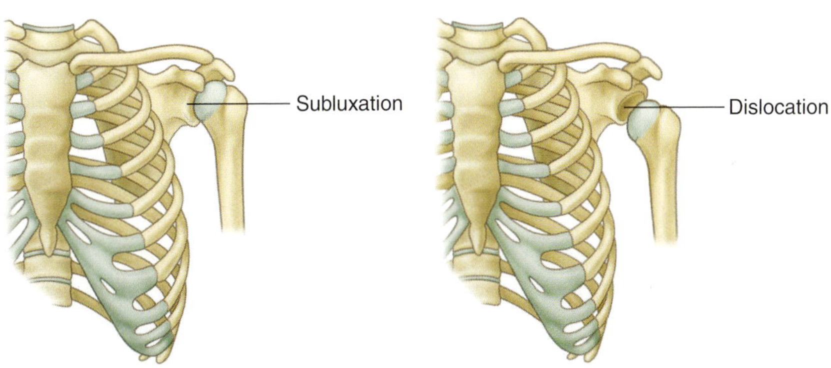

FIGURE 3.16 *Subluxation* and *dislocation* shown on an anterior view of the left shoulder.

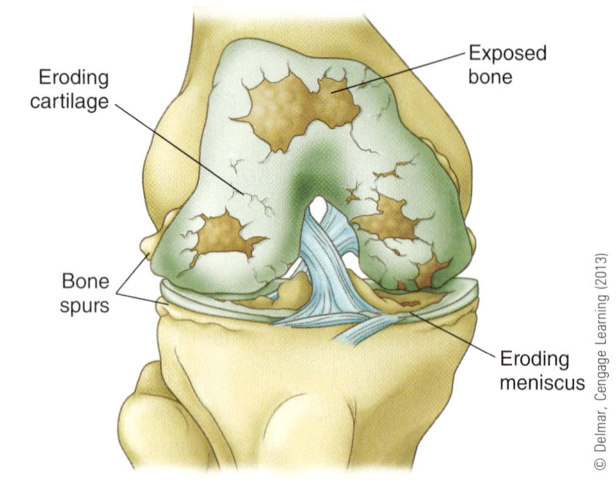

FIGURE 3.17 Damage to the knee joint caused by *osteoarthritis*.

acid in the joints. ***Uric acid*** is a by-product that is normally excreted by the kidneys. Gout develops when excess uric acid, which is present in the blood, forms crystals in the joints of the feet and legs.

Rheumatoid Arthritis

Rheumatoid arthritis (**ROO**-mah-toyd ar-**THRIGH**-tis), commonly known as ***RA***, is a chronic autoimmune disorder in which the joints and some organs of other body systems are attacked. ***Autoimmune disorders*** are described in Chapter 6.

- As RA progressively attacks the synovial membranes, they become inflamed and thickened so that the joints are increasingly swollen, painful, and immobile.

Ankylosing Spondylitis

Ankylosing spondylitis (**ang**-kih-**LOH**-sing **spon**-dih-**LYE**-tis) is a form of rheumatoid arthritis that primarily causes inflammation of the joints between the vertebrae. ***Ankylosing*** means the progressive stiffening of a joint or joints, and ***spondylitis*** means inflammation of the vertebrae.

Juvenile Rheumatoid Arthritis

Juvenile rheumatoid arthritis is an autoimmune disorder that affects children ages 16 years or less with symptoms that include stiffness, pain, joint swelling, skin rash, fever, slowed growth, and fatigue.

The Spinal Column

- A **herniated disk** (**HER**-nee-**ayt**-ed), also known as a ***slipped*** or ***ruptured disk***, is the breaking apart of an intervertebral disk that results in pressure on spinal nerve roots (Figure 3.18B).
- **Lumbago** (lum-**BAY**-goh), also known as ***low back pain***, is pain of the lumbar region of the spine (**lumb** means lumbar, and **-ago** means diseased condition).
- **Spondylolisthesis** (**spon**-dih-loh-liss-**THEE**-sis) is the forward slipping movement of the body of one of the lower lumbar vertebrae on the vertebra or sacrum below it (**spondyl/o** means vertebrae, and **-listhesis** means slipping).
- **Spina bifida** (**SPY**-nah **BIF**-ih-dah) is a congenital defect that occurs during early pregnancy when the spinal canal fails to close completely around the spinal

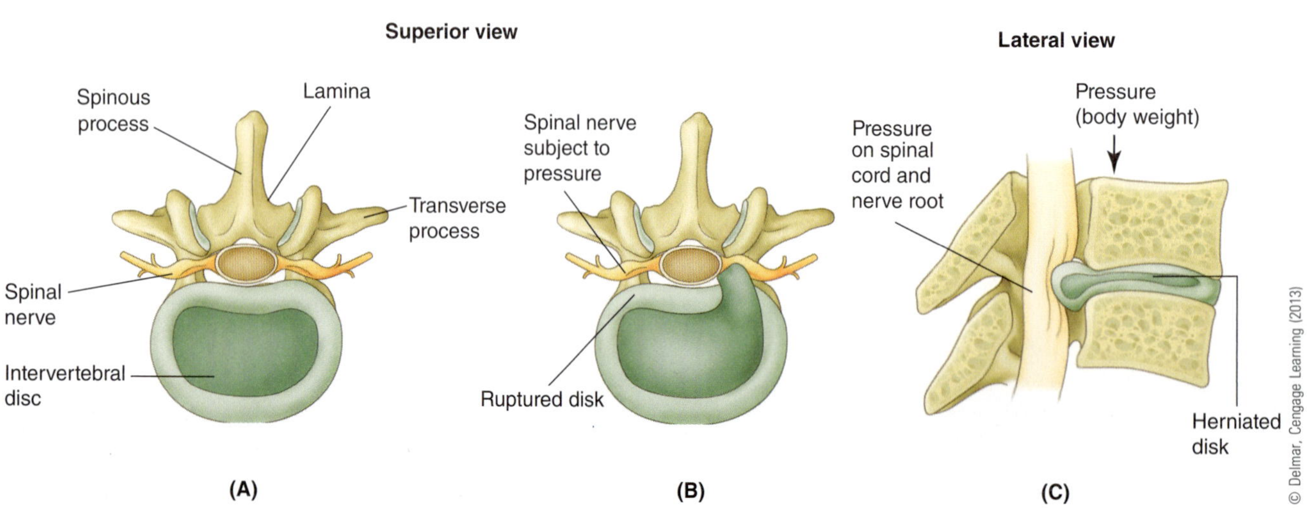

FIGURE 3.18 (A) Superior view of a normal intervertebral disk. (B) Superior and (C) lateral views of a ruptured disk causing pressure on a spinal nerve.

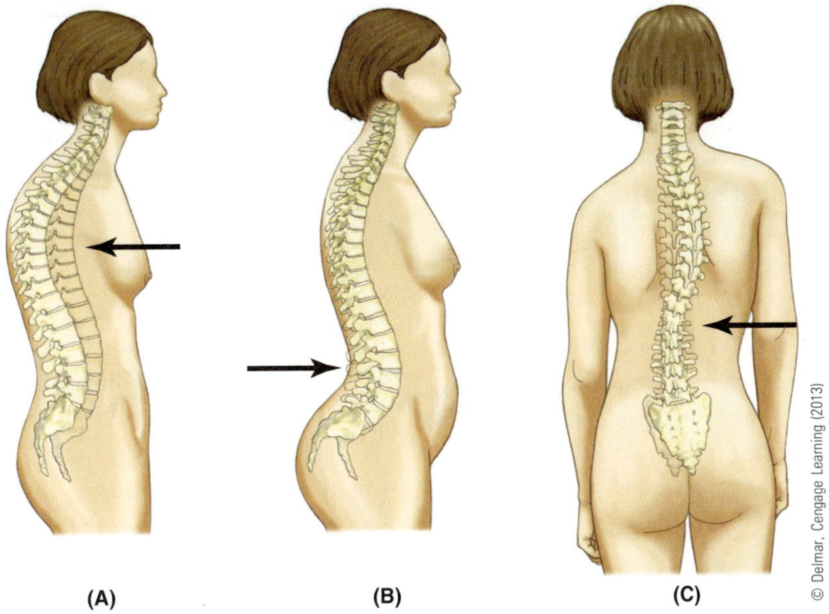

FIGURE 3.19 Abnormal curvatures of the spine. (A) *Kyphosis*. (B) *Lordosis*. (C) *Scoliosis*. (Normal curvatures are shown in shadow.)

cord to protect it. ***Spina*** means pertaining to the spine. ***Bifida*** means split. Some cases of spina bifida are due to a lack of the nutrient folic acid during the early stages of pregnancy.

Curvatures of the Spine

- **Kyphosis** (kye-**FOH**-sis) is an abnormal increase in the outward curvature of the thoracic spine as viewed from the side (**kyph** means hump, and **-osis** means abnormal condition or disease). This condition, also known as ***humpback*** or ***dowager's hump***, is frequently associated with aging (Figure 3.19A).
- **Lordosis** (lor-**DOH**-sis) is an abnormal increase in the forward curvature of the lumbar spine (**lord** means bent backward, and **-osis** means abnormal condition or disease). This condition is also known as ***swayback*** (Figure 3.19B).
- **Scoliosis** (**skoh**-lee-**OH**-sis) is an abnormal lateral (sideways) curvature of the spine (**scoli** means curved, and **-osis** means abnormal condition or disease) (Figure 3.19C).

StudyWARE CONNECTION

View the **Curvatures of the Spine** animation in the StudyWARE™.

Bones

- **Craniostenosis** (**kray**-nee-oh-steh-**NOH**-sis) is a malformation of the skull due to the premature closure of the cranial sutures (**crani/o** means skull, and **-stenosis** means abnormal narrowing).
- **Fibrous dysplasia** (dis-**PLAY**-see-ah) is a bone disorder of unknown cause that destroys normal bone structure and replaces it with fibrous (scarlike) tissue. This leads to uneven growth, brittleness, and deformity of the affected bones.
- **Ostealgia** (**oss**-tee-**AL**-jee-ah), also known as ***osteodynia***, means pain in a bone (**oste** means bone, and **-algia** means pain).
- **Osteitis** (**oss**-tee-**EYE**-tis), also spelled ***ostitis***, is an inflammation of a bone (**oste** means bone, and **-itis** means inflammation).
- **Osteomalacia** (**oss**-tee-oh-mah-**LAY**-shee-ah), also known as ***adult rickets***, is abnormal softening of bones in adults (**oste/o** means bone, and **-malacia** means abnormal softening). This condition is usually caused by a deficiency of vitamin D, calcium, and/or phosphate. Compare with *rickets*, below.
- **Osteomyelitis** (**oss**-tee-oh-**my**-eh-**LYE**-tis) is an inflammation of the bone marrow and adjacent bone (**oste/o** means bone, **myel** means bone marrow, and **-itis** means inflammation). The bacterial infection that causes osteomyelitis often originates in another part of the body and spreads to the bone via the blood.

- **Osteonecrosis** (**oss**-tee-oh-neh-**KROH**-sis) is the death of bone tissue due to insufficient blood supply (**oste/o** means bone, and **-necrosis** means tissue death).
- **Paget's disease** (**PAJ**-its), also known as ***osteitis deformans***, is a bone disease of unknown cause. This condition is characterized by the excessive breakdown of bone tissue, followed by abnormal bone formation. The new bone is structurally enlarged, but weakened and filled with new blood vessels.
- **Periostitis** (**pehr**-ee-oss-**TYE**-tis) is an inflammation of the periosteum (**peri-** means surrounding, **ost** means bone, and **-itis** means inflammation). This condition is often associated with shin splints, which are discussed in Chapter 4.
- **Rickets** (**RICK**-ets), also known as ***infantile osteomalacia***, is a deficiency disease occurring in children. This condition, which is characterized by defective bone growth, results from a vitamin D deficiency that is sometimes due to insufficient exposure to sunlight.
- **Short stature**, formerly known as ***dwarfism***, is a condition resulting from the failure of the bones of the limbs to grow to an appropriate length compared to the size of the head and trunk. The average adult height is no more than 4 feet 10 inches, and these individuals now prefer to be referred to as ***little people***.
- The term **talipes** (**TAL**-ih-peez), which is also known as ***clubfoot***, describes any congenital deformity of the foot involving the talus (ankle bones).

Bone Tumors

- **Primary bone cancer** is a relatively rare malignant tumor that originates in a bone. ***Malignant*** means becoming progressively worse and life-threatening. As an example, ***Ewing's sarcoma*** is a tumor that occurs in the bones of the upper arm, legs, pelvis, or rib. The peak incidence for the development of this condition is between ages 10 and 20 years.
- The term **secondary bone cancer** describes tumors that have metastasized (spread) to bones from other organs such as the breasts and lungs. Additional malignancies, sarcomas, and tumors are discussed in Chapter 6.
- A **myeloma** (**my**-eh-**LOH**-mah) is a type of cancer that occurs in blood-making cells found in the red bone marrow (**myel** means bone marrow, and **-oma** means tumor). This condition can cause pathologic fractures and is often fatal.
- An **osteochondroma** (**oss**-tee-oh-kon-**DROH**-mah) is a benign bony projection covered with cartilage (**oste/o** means bone, **chondr** means cartilage, and **-oma** means tumor). ***Benign*** means something that is not life-threatening and does not recur. This type of tumor is also known as an ***exostosis*** (plural, *exostoses*).

Osteoporosis and Osteopenia Compared

Osteoporosis (**oss**-tee-oh-poh-**ROH**-sis) (OP) is a marked loss of bone density and an increase in bone porosity that is frequently associated with aging (**oste/o** means bone, **por** means small opening, and **-osis** means abnormal condition or disease).

Osteopenia (**oss**-tee-oh-**PEE**-nee-ah) is thinner-than-average bone density (**oste/o** means bone, and **-penia** means deficiency). This term is used to describe the condition of someone who does not yet have osteoporosis, but is at risk for developing it.

Osteoporosis-Related Fractures

Osteoporosis is primarily responsible for three types of fractures:

- A **compression fracture**, also known as a ***vertebral crush fracture***, occurs when the bone is pressed together (compressed) on itself. These fractures are sometimes caused by the spontaneous collapse of weakened vertebrae or can be due to an injury. This results in pain, loss of height, and development of the spinal curvature known as ***dowager's hump***.
- A **Colles' fracture**, which is named for the Irish surgeon Abraham Colles, is also known as a *fractured wrist*. This fracture occurs at the lower end of the radius when a person tries to stop a fall by landing on his or her hands. The impact of this fall causes the bone weakened by osteoporosis to break (Figure 3.20).

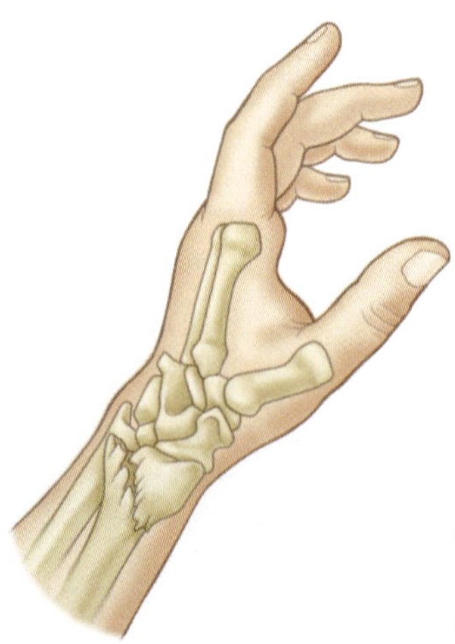

FIGURE 3.20 A *Colles' fracture* of the left wrist.

- An **osteoporotic hip fracture** (**oss**-tee-oh-pah-**ROT**-ick), also known as a ***broken hip***, is usually caused by weakening of the bones due to osteoporosis and can occur either spontaneously or as the result of a fall. Complications from these fractures can result in the loss of function, mobility, independence, or death. *Osteoporotic* means pertaining to or caused by the porous condition of bones.

Fractures

A **fracture**, which is a ***broken bone***, is described in terms of its complexity. As you study this section, follow Figure 3.21.

- A **closed fracture**, also known as a ***simple fracture*** or a ***complete fracture***, is one in which the bone is broken, but there is no open wound in the skin (see also Figure 3.22).
- An **open fracture**, also known as a ***compound fracture***, is one in which the bone is broken and there is an open wound in the skin.
- A **comminuted fracture** (**KOM**-ih-**newt**-ed) is one in which the bone is splintered or crushed. Comminuted means crushed into small pieces.
- A **greenstick fracture**, or ***incomplete fracture***, is one in which the bone is bent and only partially broken. This type of fracture occurs primarily in children.
- An **oblique fracture** occurs at an angle across the bone.
- A **pathologic fracture** occurs when a weakened bone breaks under normal strain. This is due to bones being weakened by osteoporosis or a disease process such as cancer.

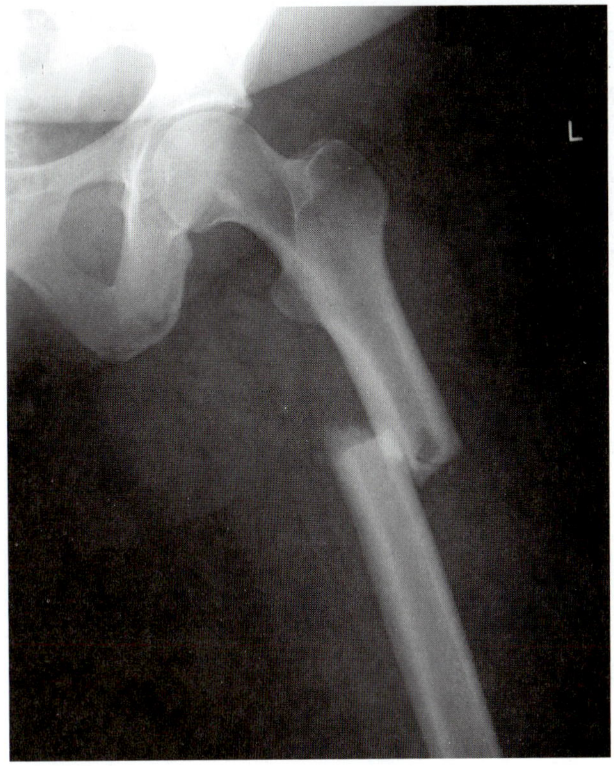

FIGURE 3.22 A radiograph showing an anteroposterior (AP) view of a closed fracture of the femur.

- A **spiral fracture** is a fracture in which the bone has been twisted apart. This type of fracture occurs as the result of a severe twisting motion such as in a sports injury.
- A **stress fracture**, which is an overuse injury, is a small crack in the bone that often develops from chronic,

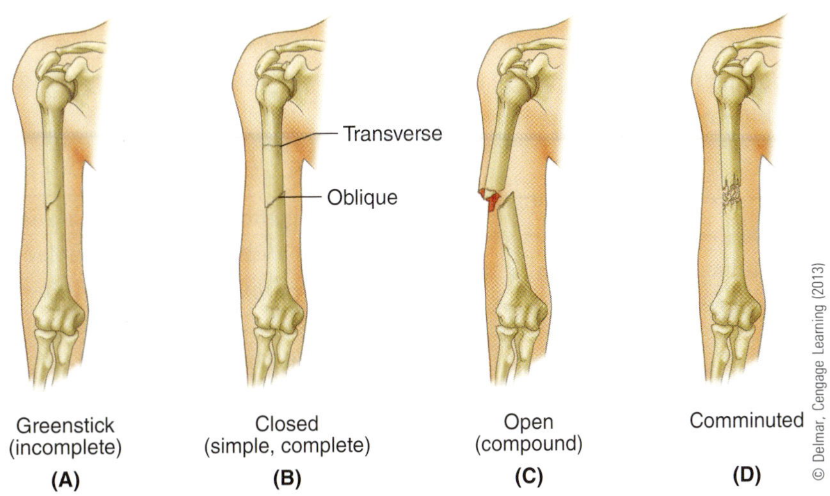

FIGURE 3.21 Types of bone fractures. (A) Greenstick (incomplete) (B) Closed (simple, complete) (C) Open (compound) (D) Comminuted

excessive impact. Additional overuse and sports injuries are discussed in Chapter 4.

- A **transverse fracture** occurs straight across the bone.

Additional Terms Associated with Fractures

- A **fat embolus** (**EM**-boh-lus) can form when a long bone is fractured and fat cells from yellow bone marrow are released into the blood. An ***embolus*** is any foreign matter circulating in the blood that can become lodged and block the blood vessel.
- **Crepitation** (**krep**-ih-**TAY**-shun), also known as ***crepitus***, is the grating sound heard when the ends of a broken bone move together. This term also describes the crackling sound heard in lungs affected with pneumonia and the clicking sound heard in the movements of some joints.
- As the bone heals, a **callus** (**KAL**-us) forms as a bulging deposit around the area of the break. This tissue eventually becomes bone. A ***callus*** is also a thickening of the skin caused by repeated rubbing.

DIAGNOSTIC PROCEDURES OF THE SKELETAL SYSTEM

- A **radiograph**, also known as an ***x-ray***, is the use of x-radiation to visualize bone fractures and other abnormalities (Figure 3.22).
- **Arthroscopy** (ar-**THROS**-koh-pee) is the visual examination of the internal structure of a joint (**arthr/o** means joint, and **-scopy** means visual examination) using an ***arthroscope***.
- A **bone marrow biopsy** is a diagnostic test that may be necessary after abnormal types or numbers of red or white blood cells are found in a complete blood count test.
- ***Bone marrow aspiration*** is the use of a syringe to withdraw the liquid bone marrow. This procedure is used to obtain tissue for diagnostic purposes or to collect bone marrow for medical procedures such as stem cell transplantation.
- **Magnetic resonance imaging** (MRI) is used to image soft tissue structures such as the interior of complex joints. It is not the most effective method of imaging hard tissues such as bone.
- ***Bone scans*** and ***arthrocentesis***, which are additional diagnostic procedures, are discussed in Chapter 15.

Bone Density Testing

Bone density testing (BDT) is used to determine losses or changes in bone density. These tests are used to diagnose conditions such as osteoporosis, osteomalacia, osteopenia, and Paget's disease.

- **Ultrasonic bone density testing** is a screening test for osteoporosis or other conditions that cause a loss of bone mass. In this procedure, sound waves are used to take measurements of the calcaneus (heel) bone. If the results indicate risks, more definitive testing is indicated.
- **Dual x-ray absorptiometry** (ab-**sorp**-shee-**OM**-eh-tree) is a low-exposure radiographic measurement of the spine and hips to measure bone density. This test produces more accurate results than ultrasonic bone density testing.

TREATMENT PROCEDURES OF THE SKELETAL SYSTEM

Bone Marrow Transplants

A **bone marrow transplant** (BMT) is used to treat certain types of cancers, such as leukemia and lymphomas, which affect bone marrow. Leukemia is discussed in Chapter 5, and lymphomas are discussed in Chapter 6.

- In this treatment, initially both the cancer cells and the patient's bone marrow are destroyed with high-intensity radiation and chemotherapy.
- Next, healthy bone marrow stem cells are transfused into the recipient's blood. These cells migrate to the spongy bone, where they multiply to form cancer-free red bone marrow. ***Stem cells*** produced by the bone marrow eventually develop into blood cells. (See Chapter 2 for more information on stem cells.)

Types of Bone Marrow Transplants

An **allogenic bone marrow transplant** uses healthy bone marrow cells from a compatible donor, often a sibling. However, unless this is a perfect match, there is the danger that the recipient's body will reject the transplant. **Allogenic** (**al**-oh-**JEN**-ick) means originating within another.

In an **autologous bone marrow transplant**, the patient receives his own bone marrow cells, which have been harvested, cleansed, treated, and stored before the remaining bone marrow in the patient's body is destroyed. **Autologous** (aw-**TOL**-uh-guss) means originating within an individual.

Medical Devices

- An **orthotic** (or-**THOT**-ick) is a mechanical appliance, such as a leg brace or a splint, that is specially designed to control, correct, or compensate for impaired limb function.
- A **prosthesis** (pros-**THEE**-sis) is a substitute for a diseased or missing body part, such as a leg that has been amputated (plural, *prostheses*).

Joints

- **Arthrodesis** (**ar**-throh-**DEE**-sis), also known as ***surgical ankylosis***, is the surgical fusion (joining together) of two bones to stiffen a joint, such as an ankle, elbow, or shoulder (**arthr/o** means joint, and **-desis** means to bind, tie together). This procedure is performed to treat severe arthritis or a damaged joint. Compare with *arthrolysis*.
- **Arthrolysis** (ar-**THROL**-ih-sis) is the surgical loosening of an ankylosed joint (**arthr/o** means joint, and **-lysis** means loosening or setting free). Note: The suffix **-lysis** also means breaking down or destruction, and may indicate either a pathologic state or a therapeutic procedure. Compare with *arthrodesis*.
- **Arthroscopic surgery** (**ar**-throh-**SKOP**-ick) is a minimally invasive procedure for the treatment of the interior of a joint. For example, torn cartilage can be removed with the use of an arthroscope and instruments inserted through small incisions (Figure 3.23).
- **Chondroplasty** (**KON**-droh-**plas**-tee) is the surgical repair of damaged cartilage (**chondr/o** means cartilage, and **-plasty** means surgical repair).
- A **synovectomy** (sin-oh-**VECK**-toh-mee) is the surgical removal of a synovial membrane from a joint (**synov** means synovial membrane, and **-ectomy** means surgical removal). One use of this procedure, which can be performed endoscopically, is to repair joint damage caused by rheumatoid arthritis.
- **Viscosupplementations** (**vis**-ko **sup**-leh-men-**TAY**-shunz) are injections used to add a preparation of hyaluronic acid and related compounds to a joint, easing friction and making movement easier. This is often used to treat osteoarthritis, especially in the knees. *Synvisc* is one of the products used for this purpose.

Joint Replacements

Based on its word parts, the term **arthroplasty** (**AR**-throh-**plas**-tee) means the surgical repair of a damaged joint (**arthr/o** means joint, and **-plasty** means surgical repair); however, this term has come to mean the surgical placement of an artificial joint. These procedures are named for the involved joint and the amount of the joint that is replaced (Figures 3.24 and 3.25).

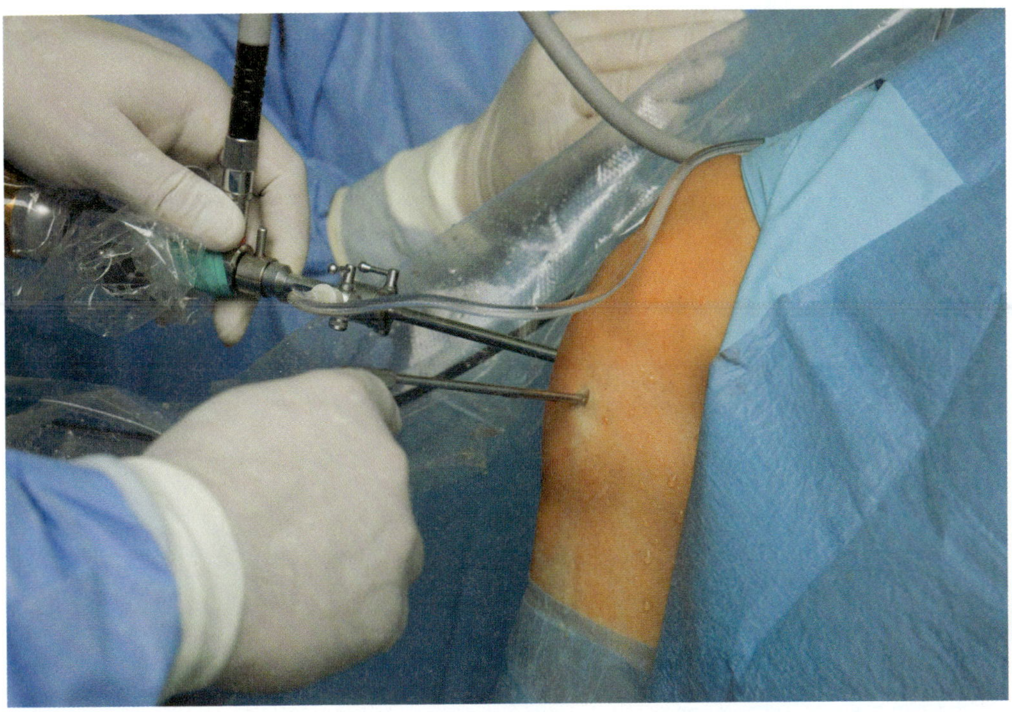

piotrwzk/www.Shutterstock.com

FIGURE 3.23 During arthroscopic surgery, the physician is able to view the interior of the knee on a monitor.

- The joint replacement part is a prosthesis that is commonly referred to as an ***implant***.
- A **total knee replacement** (TKR) means that all of the parts of the knee were replaced. This procedure is also known as a ***total knee arthroplasty*** (Figure 3.24).
- A **partial knee replacement** (PKR) describes a procedure in which only part of the knee is replaced.
- A **total hip replacement** (THR), also known as a ***total hip arthroplasty***, is performed to restore a damaged hip to full function. During the surgery, a plastic lining is fitted into the acetabulum to restore a smooth surface. The head of the femur is removed and replaced with a metal ball attached to a metal shaft that is fitted into the femur (see Figure 3.25). These smooth surfaces restore the function of the hip joint.
- **Hip resurfacing** is an alternative to removing the head of the femur. Function is restored to the hip by placing a metal cap over the head of the femur to allow it to move smoothly over a metal lining in the acetabulum.
- **Revision surgery** is the replacement of a worn or failed implant.

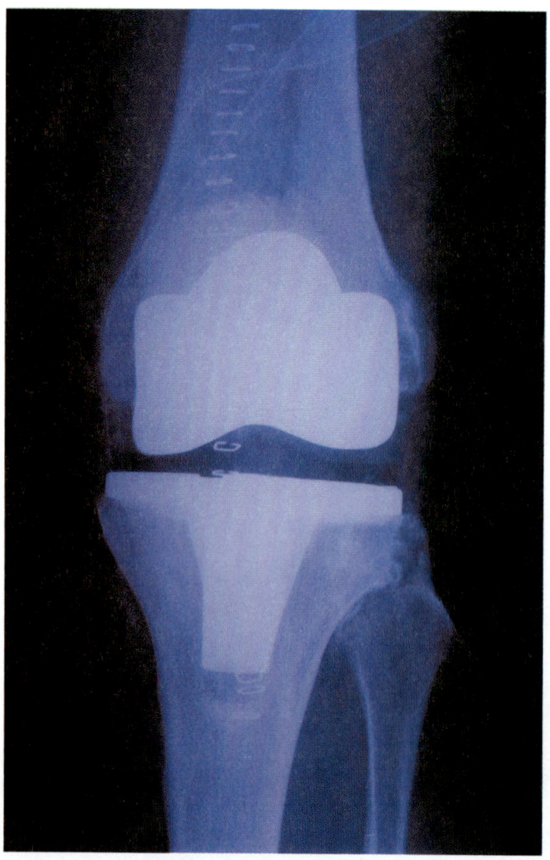

vadim kozlovsky/www.Shutterstock.com

FIGURE 3.24 Radiograph (x-ray) of a total knee replacement. On the film the metallic components appear brighter than the bone.

Spinal Column

- A **percutaneous diskectomy** (**per**-kyou-**TAY**-nee-us dis-**KECK**-toh-mee) is performed to treat a herniated intervertebral disk. In this procedure, a thin tube is inserted through the skin of the back to suction out the ruptured disk or to vaporize it with a laser. ***Percutaneous*** means performed through the skin.
- **Percutaneous vertebroplasty** (**per**-kyou-**TAY**-nee-us **VER**-tee-broh-**plas**-tee) is performed to treat osteoporosis-related compression fractures (**vertebr/o** means vertebra, and **-plasty** means surgical repair). In this minimally invasive procedure, bone cement is injected to stabilize compression fractures within the spinal column.
- A **laminectomy** (**lam**-ih-**NECK**-toh-mee) is the surgical removal of a lamina or posterior portion of a vertebra (**lamin** means lamina, and **-ectomy** means surgical removal).
- **Spinal fusion** is a technique to immobilize part of the spine by joining together (fusing) two or more vertebrae. ***Fusion*** means to join together.

Bones

- A **craniectomy** (**kray**-nee-**EK**-toh-mee) is the surgical removal of a portion of the skull (**crani** means skull, and **-ectomy** means surgical removal). This procedure is performed to treat craniostenosis or to relieve increased intracranial pressure due to swelling of the brain. The term ***intracranial pressure*** describes the amount of pressure inside the skull.

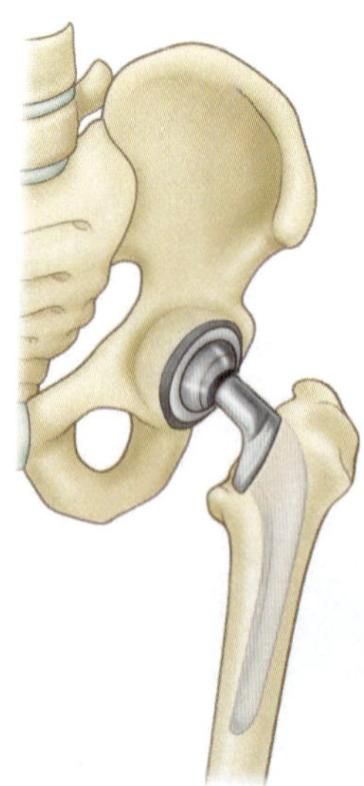

FIGURE 3.25 Total hip replacement (THR).

- A **craniotomy** (**kray**-nee-**OT**-oh-mee) is a surgical incision or opening into the skull (**crani** means skull, and **-otomy** means a surgical incision). This procedure is performed to gain access to the brain to remove a tumor, to relieve intracranial pressure, or to obtain access for other surgical procedures.
- A **cranioplasty** (**KRAY**-nee-oh-**plas**-tee) is the surgical repair of the skull (**crani/o** means skull, and **-plasty** means surgical repair).
- **Osteoclasis** (**oss**-tee-**OCK**-lah-sis) is the surgical fracture of a bone to correct a deformity (**oste/o** means bone, and **-clasis** means to break).
- An **ostectomy** (oss-**TECK**-toh-mee) is the surgical removal of bone (**ost** means bone, and **-ectomy** means the surgical removal).
- **Osteoplasty** (**OSS**-tee-oh-**plas**-tee) is the surgical repair of a bone or bones (**oste/o** means bone, and **-plasty** means surgical repair).
- **Osteorrhaphy** (**oss**-tee-**OR**-ah-fee) is the surgical suturing, or wiring together, of bones (**oste/o** means bone, and **-rrhaphy** means surgical suturing).
- **Osteotomy** (**oss**-tee-**OT**-oh-mee) is the surgical cutting of a bone (**oste** means bone, and **-otomy** means a surgical incision). This may include removing part or all of a bone, or cutting into or through a bone.
- A **periosteotomy** (**pehr**-ee-**oss**-tee-**OT**-oh-mee) is an incision through the periosteum to the bone (**peri-** means surrounding, **oste** means bone, and **-otomy** means surgical incision).

Treatment of Fractures

- **Closed reduction**, also known as ***manipulation***, is the attempted realignment of the bone involved in a fracture or joint dislocation. The affected bone is returned to its normal anatomic alignment by manually applied force and then is usually immobilized to maintain the realigned position during healing.
- When a closed reduction is not practical, a surgical procedure known as an ***open reduction*** is required to realign the bone parts.
- **Immobilization**, also known as ***stabilization***, is the act of holding, suturing, or fastening the bone in a fixed position with strapping or a cast.

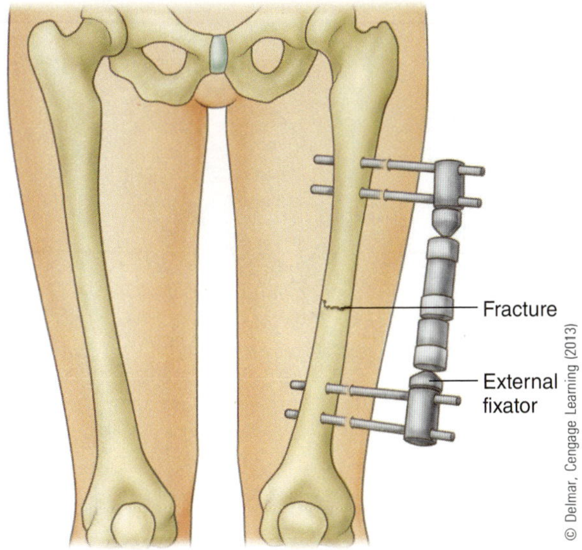

FIGURE 3.26 *External fixation* of the femur stabilizes the bone and is removed after the bone has healed.

- **Traction** is a pulling force exerted on a limb in a distal direction in an effort to return the bone or joint to normal alignment.

External and Internal Fixation

- **External fixation** is a fracture treatment procedure in which pins are placed through the soft tissues and bone so that an external appliance can be used to hold the pieces of bone firmly in place during healing. When healing is complete, the appliance is removed (Figure 3.26).
- **Internal fixation**, also known as ***open reduction internal fixation*** (ORIF), is a fracture treatment in which a plate or pins are placed directly into the bone to hold the broken pieces in place. This form of fixation is *not* usually removed after the fracture has healed (Figure 3.27).

ABBREVIATIONS RELATED TO THE SKELETAL SYSTEM

Table 3.1 presents an overview of the abbreviations related to the terms introduced in this chapter. Note: To avoid errors or confusion, always be cautious when using abbreviations.

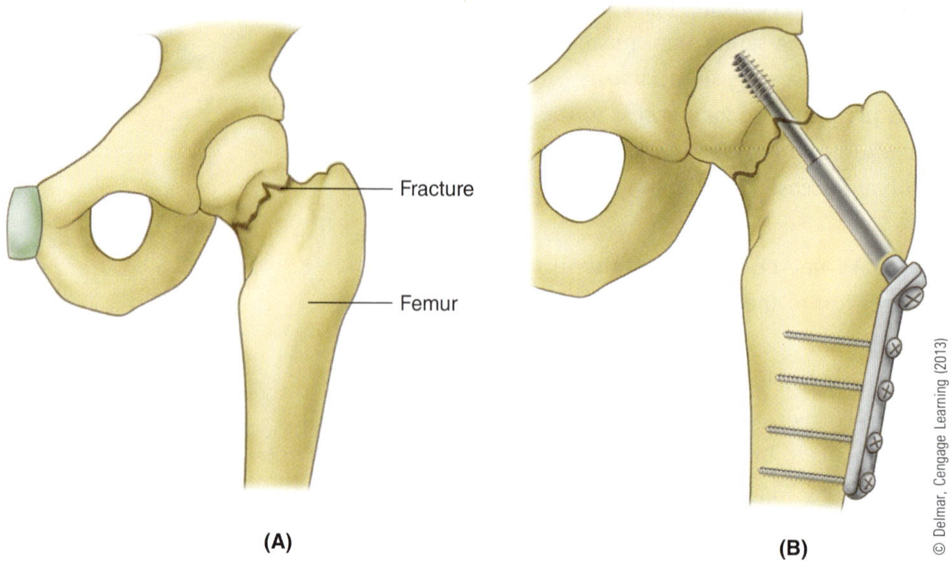

FIGURE 3.27 *Internal fixation* of fractured hip. (A) Fracture of the femoral neck. (B) *Internal fixation* pins are placed to stabilize the bone. These pins are not removed after the bone has healed.

TABLE 3.1
Abbreviations Related to the Skeletal System

bone density testing = BDT	**BDT** = bone density testing
closed reduction = CR	**CR** = closed reduction
fracture = Fx	**Fx** = fracture
osteoarthritis = OA	**OA** = osteoarthritis
osteoporosis = OP	**OP** = osteoporosis
partial knee replacement = PKR	**PKR** = partial knee replacement
polymyalgia rheumatica = PMR	**PMR** = polymyalgia rheumatica
rheumatoid arthritis = RA	**RA** = rheumatoid arthritis
total hip arthroplasty = THA	**THA** = total hip arthroplasty
total knee arthroplasty = TKA	**TKA** = total knee arthroplasty

StudyWARE CONNECTION

For more practice and to test your mastery of this material, go to the StudyWARE™ to play interactive games and complete the quiz for this chapter.

Workbook Practice

Go to your workbook and complete the exercises for this chapter.

DELMAR MOBILE MEDIA

Downloadable audio is available for selected medical terms in this chapter to enhance your learning of medical terminology.

CHAPTER 3

LEARNING EXERCISES

MATCHING WORD PARTS 1

Write the correct answer in the middle column.

	Definition	Correct Answer	Possible Answers
3.1.	hump	____________	**ankyl/o**
3.2.	cartilage	____________	**arthr/o**
3.3.	crooked, bent, stiff	____________	**-um**
3.4.	joint	____________	**kyph/o**
3.5.	singular noun ending	____________	**chondr/i, chondr/o**

MATCHING WORD PARTS 2

Write the correct answer in the middle column.

	Definition	Correct Answer	Possible Answers
3.6.	cranium, skull	____________	**cost/o**
3.7.	rib	____________	**crani/o**
3.8.	setting free, loosening	____________	**-desis**
3.9.	spinal cord, bone marrow	____________	**-lysis**
3.10.	to bind, tie together	____________	**myel/o**

MATCHING WORD PARTS 3

Write the correct answer in the middle column.

	Definition	Correct Answer	Possible Answers
3.11.	vertebrae	____________	**oste/o**
3.12.	curved	____________	**spondyl/o**

3.13.	swayback bent	____________________	**lord/o**
3.14.	synovial membrane	____________________	**synovi/o, synov/o**
3.15.	bone	____________________	**scoli/o**

DEFINITIONS

Select the correct answer, and write it on the line provided.

3.16. The shaft of a long bone is known as the ____________________.

diaphysis   distal epiphysis   endosteum   proximal epiphysis

3.17. Seven short ____________________ bones make up each ankle.

carpal   metatarsal   phalanx   tarsal

3.18. The upper portion of the sternum is the ____________________.

clavicle   mandible   manubrium   xiphoid process

3.19. A ____________________ is movable.

cartilaginous joint   fibrous joint   suture joint   synovial joint

3.20. The ____________________ bone is located just below the urinary bladder.

ilium   ischium   pubis   sacrum

3.21. The opening in a bone through which blood vessels, nerves, and ligaments pass is a ____________________.

foramen   foramina   process   symphysis

3.22. A/An ____________________ connects one bone to another bone.

articular cartilage   ligament   synovial membrane   phalange

3.23. The hip socket is known as the ____________________.

acetabulum   malleolus   patella   trochanter

3.24. The bones of the fingers and toes are known as the ____________________.

carpals   metatarsals   tarsals   phalanges

3.25. A normal projection on the surface of a bone that serves as an attachment for muscles and tendons is known as a/an ________________.

cruciate exostosis popliteal process

MATCHING STRUCTURES

Write the correct answer in the middle column.

Definition	Correct Answer	Possible Answers
3.26. breast bone	________________	clavicle
3.27. cheekbones	________________	olecranon process
3.28. collar bone	________________	sternum
3.29. kneecap	________________	patella
3.30. point of the elbow	________________	zygomatic

WHICH WORD?

Select the correct answer, and write it on the line provided.

3.31. The surgical procedure for loosening of an ankylosed joint is known as ________________.

arthrodesis arthrolysis

3.32. The bone disorder of unknown cause that destroys normal bone structure and replaces it with fibrous (scarlike) tissue is known as ________________.

fibrous dysplasia Paget's disease

3.33. An ________________ bone marrow transplant uses bone marrow from a donor.

allogenic autologous

3.34. A percutaneous ________________ is performed to treat osteoporosis-related compression fractures.

diskectomy vertebroplasty

3.35. The medical term for the form of arthritis that is commonly known as wear-and-tear arthritis is ________________.

osteoarthritis rheumatoid arthritis

SPELLING COUNTS

Find the misspelled word in each sentence. Then write that word, spelled correctly, on the line provided.

3.36. The medical term for the condition commonly known as low back pain is lumbaego. ____________________

3.37. The surgical fracture of a bone to correct a deformity is known as osteclasis. ____________________

3.38. Ankylosing spondilitis is a form of rheumatoid arthritis that primarily causes inflammation of the joints between the vertebrae. ____________________

3.39. An osterrhaphy is the surgical suturing, or wiring together, of bones. ____________________

3.40. Crepetation is the grating sound heard when the ends of a broken bone move together. ____________________

ABBREVIATION IDENTIFICATION

Write the correct answer on the line provided.

3.41. **BMT** ____________________

3.42. **CR** ____________________

3.43. **Fx** ____________________

3.44. **RA** ____________________

3.45. **TMJ** ____________________

TERM SELECTION

Select the correct answer, and write it on the line provided.

3.46. The term meaning the death of bone tissue is ____________________.

osteitis deformans osteomyelitis osteonecrosis osteoporosis

3.47. An abnormal increase in the forward curvature of the lumbar spine is known as ____________________.

kyphosis lordosis scoliosis spondylosis

3.48. The condition known as ____________________ is a congenital defect.

juvenile arthritis osteoarthritis rheumatoid arthritis spina bifida

3.49. A type of cancer that occurs in blood-making cells found in the red bone marrow is known as a/an ________________.

chondroma Ewing's sarcoma myeloma osteochondroma

3.50. The bulging deposit that forms around the area of the break during the healing of a fractured bone is a ________________.

callus crepitation crepitus luxation

SENTENCE COMPLETION

Write the correct term or terms on the lines provided.

3.51. A/An ________________ is performed to gain access to the brain or to relieve intracranial pressure.

3.52. The partial displacement of a bone from its joint is known as ________________.

3.53. The procedure that stiffens a joint by joining two bones is ________________. This is also known as surgical ankylosis.

3.54. The surgical placement of an artificial joint is known as ________________.

3.55. A medical term for the condition commonly known as a bunion is ________________.

WORD SURGERY

Divide each term into its component word parts. Write these word parts, in sequence, on the lines provided. When necessary, use a slash (/) to indicate a combining vowel. (You may not need all of the lines provided.)

3.56. **Hemarthrosis** is blood within a joint.

________ ________ ________ ________

3.57. An **osteochondroma** is a benign bony projection covered with cartilage.

________ ________ ________ ________

3.58. **Osteomalacia**, also known as adult rickets, is abnormal softening of bones in adults.

________ ________ ________ ________

3.59. **Periostitis** is an inflammation of the periosteum.

________ ________ ________ ________

3.60. **Spondylolisthesis** is the forward slipping movement of the body of one of the lower lumbar vertebrae on the vertebra or sacrum below it.

__________ __________ __________ __________

TRUE/FALSE

If the statement is true, write **True** on the line. If the statement is false, write **False** on the line.

3.61. ________________ Osteopenia is thinner-than-average bone density. This term is used to describe the condition of someone who does not yet have osteoporosis, but is at risk for developing it.

3.62. ________________ Paget's disease is caused by a deficiency of calcium and vitamin D in early childhood.

3.63. ________________ Costochondritis is an inflammation of the cartilage that connects a rib to the sternum.

3.64. ________________ Dislocation is the partial displacement of a bone from its joint.

3.65. ________________ Arthroscopic surgery is a minimally invasive procedure for the treatment of the interior of a joint.

CLINICAL CONDITIONS

Write the correct answer on the line provided.

3.66. When Bobby Kuhn fell out of a tree, the bone in his arm was bent and partially broken. Dr. Grafton described this as a/an ________________ fracture and told the family that this type of fracture occurs primarily in children.

3.67. Eduardo Sanchez was treated for an inflammation of the bone and bone marrow. The medical term for this condition is ________________.

3.68. Beth Hubert's breast cancer spread to her bones. These new sites are referred to as ________________ ________________ ________________.

3.69. Mrs. Morton suffers from dowager's hump. The medical term for this abnormal curvature of the spine is ________________.

3.70. Henry Turner wears a brace to compensate for the impaired function of his leg. The medical term for this orthopedic appliance is a/an ____________________.

3.71. As the result of a head injury in an auto accident, Sam Cheng required a/an ____________________ to relieve the rapidly increasing intracranial pressure.

3.72. Mrs. Gilmer has leukemia and requires a bone marrow transplant. Part of the treatment was the harvesting of her bone marrow so she could receive it later as a/an ____________________ bone marrow transplant.

3.73. Betty Greene has been running for several years; however, now her knees hurt. Dr. Morita diagnosed her condition as ____________________, which is an abnormal softening of the cartilage in these joints.

3.74. Patty Turner (age 7) has symptoms that include a skin rash, fever, slowed growth, fatigue, and swelling in the joints. She was diagnosed as having juvenile ____________________ arthritis.

3.75. Heather Lewis has a very sore shoulder. Dr. Plunkett diagnosed this as an inflammation of the bursa and said that Heather's condition is ____________________.

WHICH IS THE CORRECT MEDICAL TERM?

Select the correct answer, and write it on the line provided.

3.76. Rodney Horner is being treated for a ____________________ fracture in which the ends of the bones were crushed together.

Colles' comminuted compound spiral

3.77. Alex Jordon fell and injured her knee. Her doctor performed a/an ____________________ to surgically repair the damaged cartilage.

arthroplasty chondroma chondroplasty osteoplasty

3.78. Mrs. Palmer is at high risk for osteoporosis. To obtain a definitive evaluation of the status of her bone density, Mrs. Palmer's physician ordered a/an ____________________ test.

dual x-ray absorptiometry MRI x-ray ultrasonic bone density

3.79. In an effort to return a fractured bone to normal alignment, Dr. Wong ordered ______. This procedure exerts a pulling force on the distal end of the affected limb.

external fixation immobilization internal fixation traction

3.80. Baby Juanita was treated for ______, which is a congenital deformity of the foot involving the talus (ankle bones). Her family calls this condition clubfoot.

osteomalacia rickets scoliosis talipes

CHALLENGE WORD BUILDING

These terms are *not* found in this chapter; however, they are made up of the following familiar word parts. If you need help in creating the term, refer to your medical dictionary.

poly-	**arthr/o**	**-ectomy**
	chondr/o	**-itis**
	cost/o	**-malacia**
	crani/o	**-otomy**
	oste/o	**-pathy**
		-sclerosis

3.81. Abnormal hardening of bone is known as ______.

3.82. The surgical removal of a rib or ribs is a/an ______.

3.83. Any disease of cartilage is known as ______.

3.84. A surgical incision into a joint is a/an ______.

3.85. Inflammation of cartilage is known as ______.

3.86. The surgical removal of a joint is a/an ______.

3.87. Inflammation of more than one joint is known as ______.

3.88. Any disease involving the bones and joints is known as ______.

3.89. A surgical incision or division of a rib or ribs is a/an ______.

3.90. Abnormal softening of the skull is known as ______.

LABELING EXERCISES

Identify the numbered items on the accompanying figures.

3.91. ______________ vertebrae

3.92. ______________

3.93. ______________

3.94. ______________

3.95. ______________

3.96. ______________

3.97. ______________ bone

3.98. ______________ bone

3.99. ______________ bone

3.100. ______________

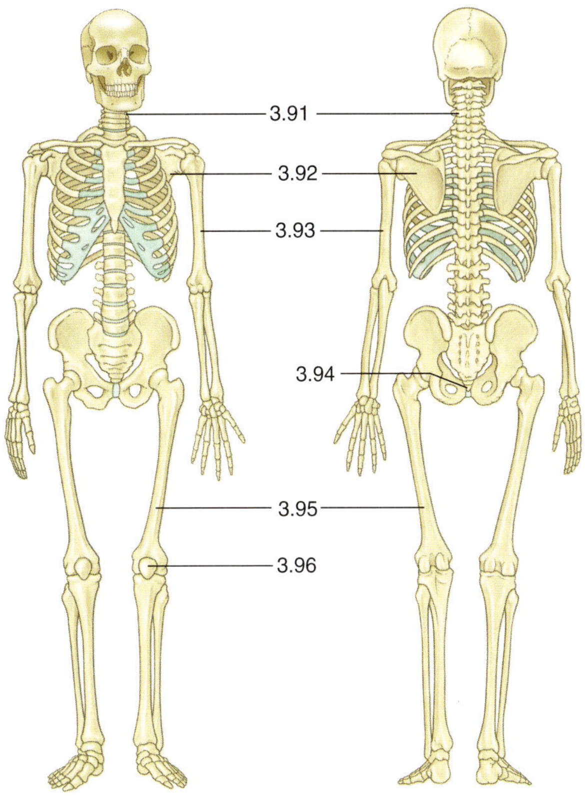

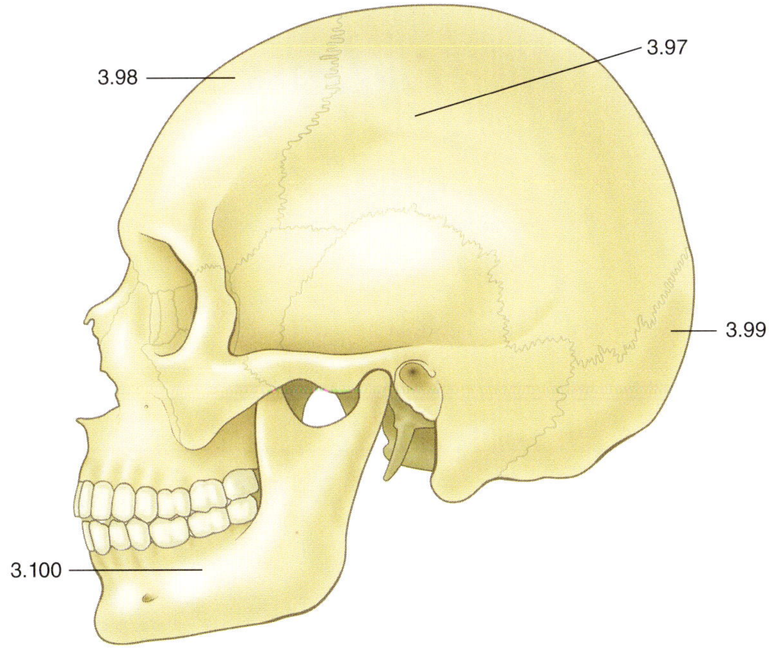

CHAPTER 4

The Muscular System

Overview of STRUCTURES, COMBINING FORMS, AND FUNCTIONS OF THE MUSCULAR SYSTEM

Major Structures	Related Combining Forms	Primary Functions
Muscles	**muscul/o**, **my/o**, **myos/o**	Make body movement possible, hold body erect, move body fluids, and produce body heat.
Fascia	**fasci/o**	Cover, support, and separate muscles.
Tendons	**ten/o**, **tend/o**, **tendin/o**	Attach muscles to bones.

Vocabulary Related to **THE MUSCULAR SYSTEM**

This list contains essential word parts and medical terms for this chapter. These terms are pronounced in the StudyWARE™ and Audio CDs that are available for use with this text. These and the other important **primary terms** are shown in boldface throughout the chapter. *Secondary terms*, which appear in *orange* italics, clarify the meaning of primary terms.

Word Parts

- ☐ **bi-** twice, double, two
- ☐ **-cele** hernia, tumor, swelling
- ☐ **dys-** bad, difficult, or painful
- ☐ **fasci/o** fascia, fibrous band
- ☐ **fibr/o** fibrous tissue, fiber
- ☐ **-ia** abnormal condition, disease, plural of **-ium**
- ☐ **-ic** pertaining to
- ☐ **kines/o**, **kinesi/o** movement
- ☐ **my/o** muscle
- ☐ **-plegia** paralysis, stroke
- ☐ **-rrhexis** rupture
- ☐ **tax/o** coordination, order
- ☐ **ten/o**, **tend/o**, **tendin/o** tendon, stretch out, extend, strain
- ☐ **ton/o** tone, stretching, tension
- ☐ **tri-** three

Medical Terms

- ☐ **abduction** (ab-**DUCK**-shun)
- ☐ **adduction** (ah-**DUCK**-shun)
- ☐ **adhesion** (ad-**HEE**-zhun)
- ☐ **ataxia** (ah-**TACK**-see-ah)
- ☐ **atonic** (ah-**TON**-ick)
- ☐ **atrophy** (**AT**-roh-fee)
- ☐ **bradykinesia** (**brad**-ee-kih-**NEE**-zee-ah)
- ☐ **carpal tunnel syndrome** (**KAR**-pul)
- ☐ **chronic fatigue syndrome**
- ☐ **circumduction** (**ser**-kum-**DUCK**-shun)
- ☐ **contracture** (kon-**TRACK**-chur)
- ☐ **dorsiflexion** (**dor**-sih-**FLECK**-shun)
- ☐ **dyskinesia** (**dis**-kih-**NEE**-zee-ah)
- ☐ **dystonia** (dis-**TOH**-nee-ah)
- ☐ **electromyography** (ee-**leck**-troh-my-**OG**-rah-fee)
- ☐ **epicondylitis** (**ep**-ih-**kon**-dih-**LYE**-tis)
- ☐ **ergonomics** (er-goh-**NOM**-icks)
- ☐ **exercise physiologist** (**fiz**-ee-**OL**-oh-jist)
- ☐ **fasciitis** (**fas**-ee-**EYE**-tis)
- ☐ **fibromyalgia syndrome** (**figh**-broh-my-**AL**-jee-ah)
- ☐ **ganglion cyst** (**GANG**-glee-on **SIST**)
- ☐ **heel spur**
- ☐ **hemiparesis** (**hem**-ee-pah-**REE**-sis)
- ☐ **hemiplegia** (**hem**-ee-**PLEE**-jee-ah)
- ☐ **hernia** (**HER**-nee-ah)
- ☐ **hyperkinesia** (**high**-per-kye-**NEE**-zee-a)
- ☐ **hypotonia** (**high**-poh-**TOH**-nee-ah)
- ☐ **impingement syndrome** (im-**PINJ**-ment **SIN**-drohm)
- ☐ **insertion**
- ☐ **intermittent claudication** (**klaw**-dih-**KAY**-shun)
- ☐ **muscular dystrophy** (**DIS**-troh-fee)
- ☐ **myasthenia gravis** (**my**-as-**THEE**-nee-ah **GRAH**-vis)
- ☐ **myocele** (**MY**-oh-seel)
- ☐ **myoclonus** (**my**-oh-**KLOH**-nus)
- ☐ **myofascial release** (**my**-oh-**FASH**-ee-ahl)
- ☐ **myolysis** (my-**OL**-ih-sis)
- ☐ **myoparesis** (**my**-oh-**PAR**-eh-sis)
- ☐ **myorrhaphy** (my-**OR**-ah-fee)
- ☐ **neuromuscular** (**new**-roh-**MUS**-kyou-lar)
- ☐ **nocturnal myoclonus** (nock-**TER**-nal **my**-oh-**KLOH**-nus)
- ☐ **oblique** (oh-**BLEEK**)
- ☐ **paralysis** (pah-**RAL**-ih-sis)
- ☐ **paraplegia** (**par**-ah-**PLEE**-jee-ah)
- ☐ **physiatrist** (**fiz**-ee-**AT**-rist)
- ☐ **plantar fasciitis** (**PLAN**-tar **fas**-ee-**EYE**-tis)
- ☐ **polymyositis** (**pol**-ee-**my**-oh-**SIGH**-tis)
- ☐ **pronation** (proh-**NAY**-shun)
- ☐ **quadriplegia** (**kwad**-rih-**PLEE**-jee-ah)
- ☐ **range of motion testing**
- ☐ **sarcopenia** (**sar**-koh-**PEE**-nee-ah)
- ☐ **shin splint**
- ☐ **singultus** (sing-**GUL**-tus)
- ☐ **spasmodic torticollis** (spaz-**MOD**-ick **tor**-tih-**KOL**-is)
- ☐ **sphincter** (**SFINK**-ter)
- ☐ **sprain**
- ☐ **tenodesis** (ten-**ODD**-eh-sis)
- ☐ **tenosynovitis** (**ten**-oh-sin-oh-**VYE**-tis)
- ☐ **tenolysis** (ten-**OL**-ih-sis)
- ☐ **tenorrhaphy** (ten-**OR**-ah-fee)
- ☐ **transverse** (trans-**VERSE**)

LEARNING GOALS

On completion of this chapter, you should be able to:

1. Describe the functions and structures of the muscular system, including muscle fibers, fascia, tendons, and the three types of muscle.
2. Recognize, define, pronounce, and spell the primary terms related to muscle movements, and explain how the muscles are named.
3. Recognize, define, pronounce, and spell the primary terms related to the pathology and the diagnostic and treatment procedures of the muscular system.

FUNCTIONS OF THE MUSCULAR SYSTEM

- Muscles hold the body erect and make movement possible.
- Muscle movement generates nearly 85% of the heat that keeps the body warm.
- Muscles move food through the digestive system.
- Muscle movements, such as walking, aid the flow of blood through veins as it returns to the heart.
- Muscle action moves fluids through the ducts and tubes associated with other body systems.

STRUCTURES OF THE MUSCULAR SYSTEM

The muscular and skeletal systems are sometimes referred to jointly as the *musculoskeletal* system. Because of the interactions of these two systems, they provide the body with form, support, stability, and the ability to move.

The body has more than 600 muscles, which make up about 40–45% of the body's weight. Skeletal muscles are made up of fibers that are covered with fascia and are attached to bones by tendons.

Muscle Fibers

Muscle fibers are the long, slender cells that make up muscles. Each muscle consists of a group of fibers that are bound together by connective tissue.

Fascia

Fascia (**FASH**-ee-ah) is a band of connective tissue that envelops, separates, or binds together muscles or groups of muscles (plural, *fasciae* or *fascias*). Fascia is flexible to allow muscle movements.

The term **myofascial** (**my**-oh-**FASH**-ee-ahl) means pertaining to muscle tissue and fascia (**my/o** means muscle, **fasci** means fascia, and **-al** means pertaining to).

Tendons

- A **tendon** is a narrow band of nonelastic, dense, fibrous connective tissue that attaches a muscle to a bone. Do not confuse tendons with *ligaments*, which are bands of fibrous tissue that form joints by connecting one bone to another bone (Figure 4.1). See Chapter 3 for more information on ligaments.
- For example, the ***patellar tendon*** attaches muscles to the bottom of the patella (kneecap), and the ***Achilles tendon*** attaches the gastrocnemius muscle (the major muscle of the calf of the leg) to the heel bone (Figure 4.10).
- An ***aponeurosis*** is a sheet-like fibrous connective tissue, which resembles a flattened tendon that serves as a fascia to bind muscles together or as a means of connecting muscle to bone (plural, *aponeuroses*). As an example, the abdominal aponeurosis can be seen in Figure 4.9.

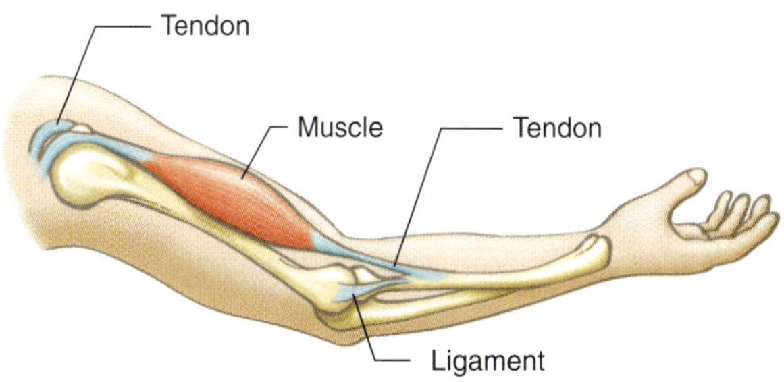

FIGURE 4.1 *Tendons* attach muscle to bone. *Ligaments* join bone to bone.

TYPES OF MUSCLE TISSUE

The three types of muscle tissue are *skeletal, smooth,* and *myocardial* (Figure 4.2). These muscle types are described according to their appearance and function.

Skeletal Muscles

- **Skeletal muscles** are attached to the bones of the skeleton and make body motions possible (Figure 4.2A).

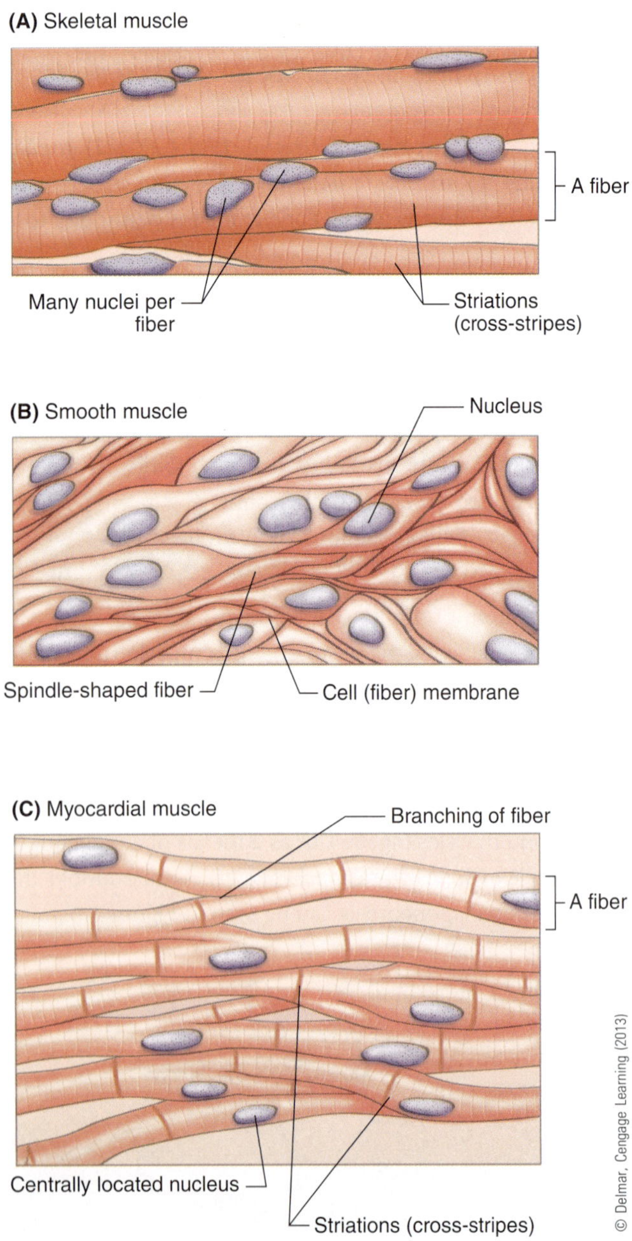

FIGURE 4.2 Types of muscle tissue. (A) Skeletal muscle. (B) Smooth muscle. (C) Myocardial muscle.

- Skeletal muscles are also known as ***voluntary muscles*** because we have conscious (voluntary) control over these muscles.
- Skeletal muscles are also known as ***striated muscles*** because under a microscope, the dark and light bands in the muscle fibers create a striped appearance. ***Striated*** means striped.

Smooth Muscles

Smooth muscles are located in the walls of internal organs such as the digestive tract, blood vessels, and ducts leading from glands (Figure 4.2B). Their function is to move and control the flow of fluids through these structures.

- Smooth muscles are also known as ***involuntary muscles*** because they are under the control of the autonomic nervous system and are *not* under voluntary control. The autonomic nervous system is discussed in Chapter 10.
- Smooth muscles are also known as ***unstriated muscles***. This is because they do *not* have the dark and light bands that produce the striped appearance seen in striated muscles.
- Smooth muscles are also known as ***visceral muscles*** because they are found in hollow structures such as those of the digestive and urinary systems. *Visceral* means relating to the internal organs. These muscles are found in large internal organs, with the exception of the heart.

Myocardial Muscle

Myocardial muscles (**my**-oh-**KAR**-dee-al), also known as ***myocardium*** or ***cardiac muscle***, form the muscular walls of the heart (**my/o** means muscle, **cardi** means heart, and **-al** means pertaining to) (Figure 4.2C).

Myocardial muscle is like striated skeletal muscle in appearance, but is similar to smooth muscle in that its action is involuntary. It is the constant contraction and relaxation of the myocardial muscle that causes the heartbeat. This topic is discussed in Chapter 5.

StudyWARE CONNECTION

Watch the **Types of Muscle** animation in the StudyWARE™.

MUSCLE CONTRACTION AND RELAXATION

A wide range of muscle movements are made possible by the combination of specialized muscle types, muscle innervation, and the organization of muscles into antagonistic muscle pairs.

Muscle Innervation

Muscle innervation (**in**-err-**VAY**-shun) is the stimulation of a muscle by an impulse transmitted by a motor nerve. Motor nerves enable the brain to stimulate a muscle to contract. When the stimulation stops, the muscle relaxes. This information controls the body's voluntary muscular contractions. (Nerves are further described in Chapter 10.)

If the nerve impulse is disrupted due to an injury or disease, the muscle is unable to function properly. For example, it can be paralyzed or unable to contract properly. These conditions are described later in this chapter.

Neuromuscular (**new**-roh-**MUS**-kyou-lar) means pertaining to the relationship between a nerve and muscle (**neur/o** means nerve, **muscul** means muscle, and **-ar** means pertaining to).

Antagonistic Muscle Pairs

All muscles are arranged in antagonistic pairs. The term ***antagonistic*** refers to working in opposition to each other. Muscles within each pair are made up of specialized cells that can change length or shape by contracting and relaxing. When one muscle of the pair contracts, the opposite muscle of the pair relaxes. It is these contrasting motions that make contraction and relaxation possible.

- **Contraction** is the tightening of a muscle. As the muscle contracts, it becomes shorter and thicker, causing the ***belly*** (center) of the muscle to enlarge.
- **Relaxation** occurs when a muscle returns to its original form. As the muscle relaxes, it becomes longer and thinner, and the belly is no longer enlarged.

As an example, the triceps and biceps work as a pair to make movement of the arm possible (Figure 4.3).

CONTRASTING MUSCLE MOTION

These muscle motions, which occur as pairs of opposites, are described in the following text and illustrated in Figures 4.4 through 4.8.

Abduction and Adduction

Abduction (ab-**DUCK**-shun) is the movement of a limb (arm or leg) *away from* the midline of the body (**ab-** means away from, **duct** means to lead, and **-ion** means action). During abduction, the arm moves outward away from the side of the body. An ***abductor*** is a muscle that moves a body part away from the midline.

In contrast, **adduction** (ah-**DUCK**-shun) is the movement of a limb (arm or leg) *toward* the midline of the body (**ad-** means toward, **duct** means to lead, and **-ion** means action). During adduction, the arm moves inward toward the side of the body. An ***adductor*** is a muscle that moves a body part toward the midline (Figure 4.4).

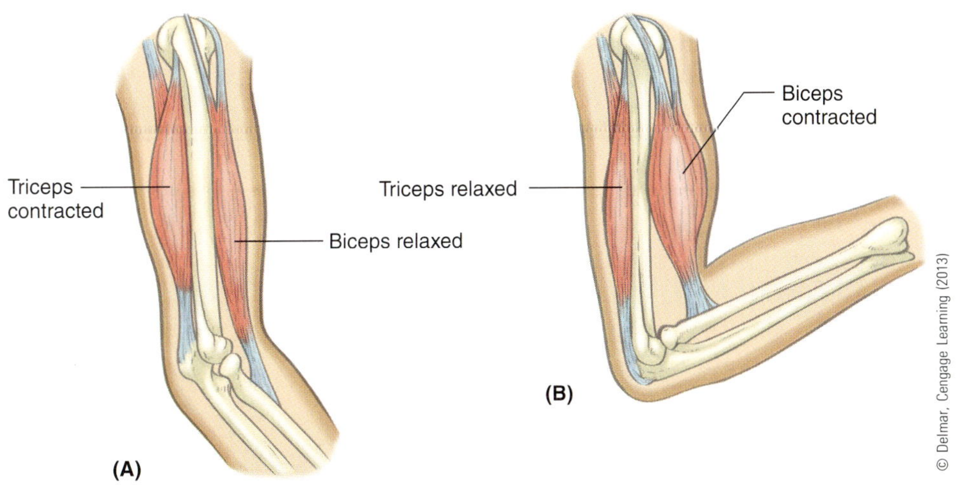

FIGURE 4.3 An antagonistic muscle pair of the upper arm. (A) During *extension*, the *triceps* is contracted and the biceps is *relaxed*. (B) During *flexion*, the *triceps* is relaxed and the *biceps* is contracted.

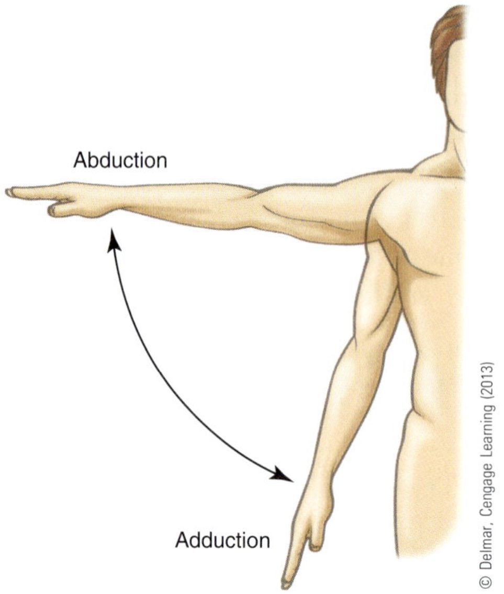

FIGURE 4.4 *Abduction* moves the arm away from the body. *Adduction* moves the arm toward the body.

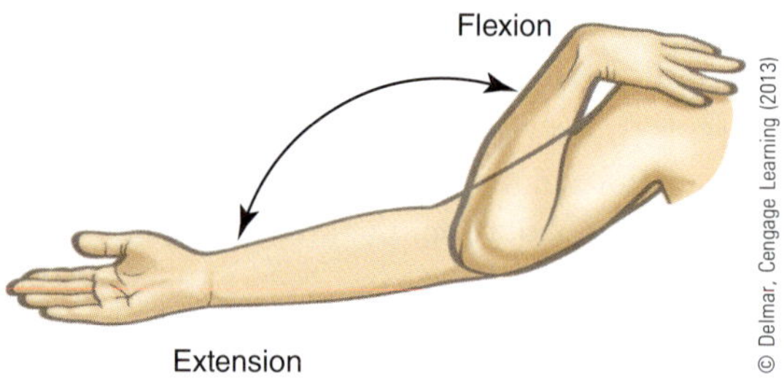

FIGURE 4.5 *Extension* increases the angle of the elbow and moves the hand away from the body. *Flexion* decreases the angle of the elbow and moves the hand toward the body.

Flexion and Extension

Flexion (**FLECK**-shun) means decreasing the angle between two bones by bending a limb at a joint (**flex** means to bend, and **-ion** means action). During flexion, the knee or elbow is bent. A *flexor muscle* bends a limb at a joint.

In contrast, **extension** means increasing the angle between two bones or the straightening out of a limb (**ex-** means away from, **tens** means to stretch out, and **-ion** means action). During extension, the knee or elbow is straightened. An *extensor muscle* straightens a limb at a joint (Figure 4.5).

- **Hyperextension** is the extreme or overextension of a limb or body part beyond its normal limit. For example, movement of the head far backward or far forward beyond the normal range of motion causes hyperextension of the muscles of the neck.

Elevation and Depression

Elevation is the act of raising or lifting a body part. For example, the elevation of the *levator anguli oris* muscles of the face raises the corners of the mouth into a smile. A *levator* is a muscle that raises a body part.

In contrast, **depression** is the act of lowering a body part. The *depressor anguli oris*, for example, lowers the corner of the mouth into a frown. A *depressor* muscle lowers a body part. See Figure 4.9 for illustrations of some of the muscles of the face.

Rotation and Circumduction

Rotation is a circular movement around an axis such as the shoulder joint. An *axis* is an imaginary line that runs lengthwise through the center of the body, and rotation turns a bone on its own axis.

In contrast, **circumduction** (**ser**-kum-**DUCK**-shun) is the circular movement at the far end of a limb. An example of circumduction is the swinging motion of the far end of the arm (Figure 4.6).

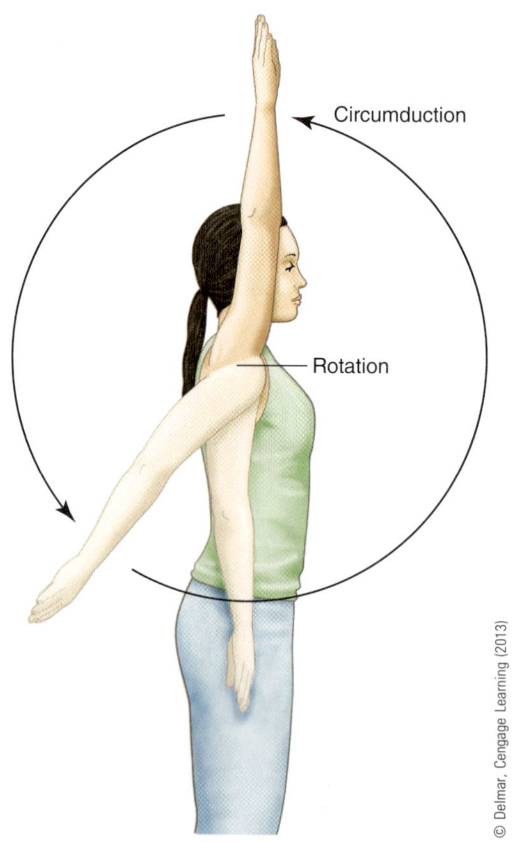

FIGURE 4.6 *Rotation* is a circular movement around an axis such as the shoulder joint. *Circumduction* is the circular movement at the far end of a limb.

- A *rotator muscle* turns a body part on its axis. For example, the head of the **humerus** (**HYUM**-er-us), which is the bone of the upper arm, rotates within the shoulder joint.
- The *rotator cuff* is the group of muscles and their tendons that hold the head of the humerus securely in place as it rotates within the shoulder joint (Figure 4.13).

Supination and Pronation

Supination (**soo**-pih-**NAY**-shun) is the act of rotating the arm or the leg so that the palm of the hand or sole of the foot is turned forward or upward. An easy way to remember this is to think of carrying a bowl of soup.

In contrast, **pronation** (proh-**NAY**-shun) is the act of rotating the arm or leg so that the palm of the hand or sole of the foot is turned downward or backward (Figure 4.7).

Dorsiflexion and Plantar Flexion

Dorsiflexion (**dor**-sih-**FLECK**-shun) is the movement that bends the foot *upward* at the ankle. Pointing the toes and foot upward decreases the angle between the top of the foot and the front of the leg (Figure 4.8).

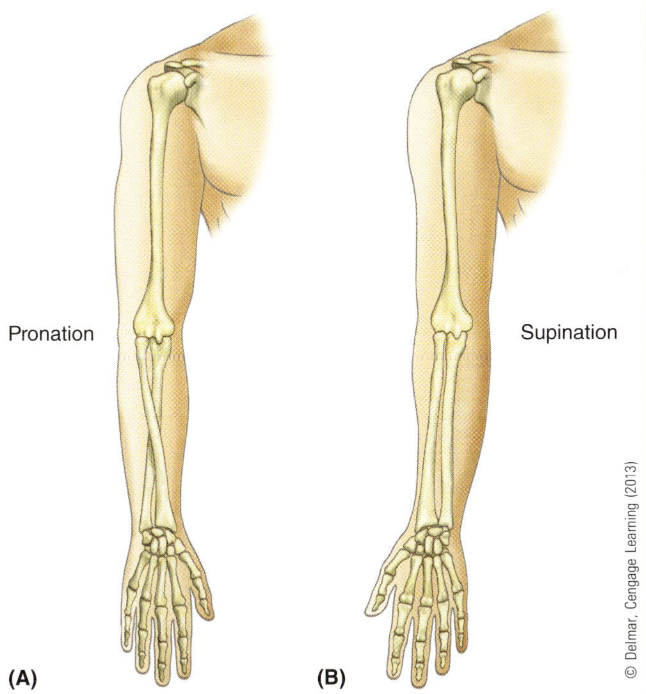

FIGURE 4.7 (A) *Pronation* is turning the arm so the palm of the hand is turned downward. (B) *Supination* is turning the arm so that the palm of the hand is turned upward.

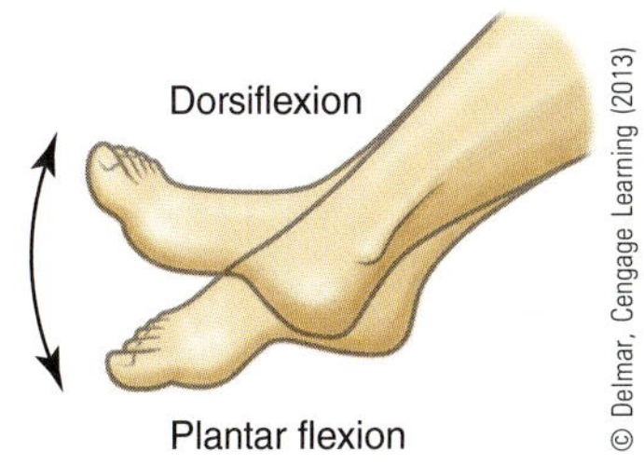

FIGURE 4.8 *Dorsiflexion* bends the foot upward at the ankle. *Plantar flexion* bends the foot downward at the ankle.

In contrast, **plantar flexion** (**PLAN**-tar **FLECK**-shun) is the movement that bends the foot *downward* at the ankle. *Plantar* means pertaining to the sole of the foot. Pointing the toes and foot downward increases the angle between the top of the foot and the front of the leg (Figure 4.8).

HOW MUSCLES ARE NAMED

As you study this section, refer to Figures 4.9 through 4.12.

In Figures 4.9 and 4.10, many of the *superficial* muscles are labeled. These muscles are so called because they are located near the surface, just under the skin.

Muscles Named for Their Origin and Insertion

The movements of skeletal muscles are made possible by two points of attachment. These are known as the origin and insertion, and some muscles are also named for these points.

- The **origin** is where the muscle begins, and it is located nearest the midline of the body or on a less movable part of the skeleton. The origin is the less moveable attachment.
- The **insertion** is where the muscle ends by attaching to a bone or tendon. In contrast to the origin, the insertion is the more movable attachment, and it is the farthest point from the midline of the body.
- The *sternocleidomastoid muscle*, for example, helps bend the neck and rotate the head (Figures 4.9 and 4.11). This muscle is named for its two points of origin, which are **stern/o** meaning breastbone and **cleid/o** meaning collar bone. The **mastoid** muscle inserts at one point of insertion into the mastoid process. (This is part of the temporal bone that is located just behind the ear).

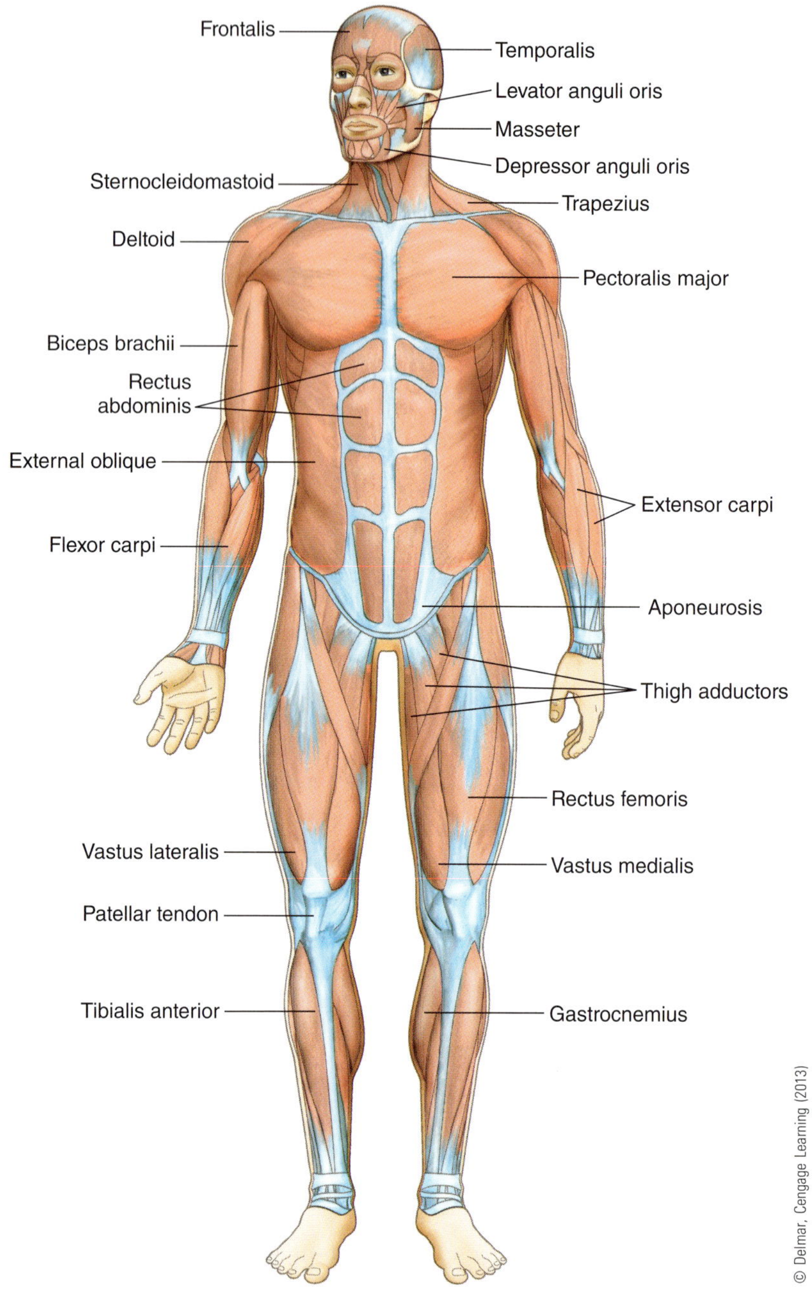

FIGURE 4.9 Superficial muscles of the body (anterior view).

Muscles Named for Their Action

Some muscles are named for their action, such as flexion or extension.

- For example, the ***flexor carpi muscles*** and the ***extensor carpi muscles*** are the pair of muscles that make flexion (bending) and extension (straightening) of the wrist possible (Figure 4.9). ***Carpi*** means wrist or wrist bones.

Muscles Named for Their Location

Some muscles are named for their location on the body or the organ they are near.

- The **pectoralis major** (**peck**-toh-**RAY**-lis), for example, is a thick, fan-shaped muscle situated on the anterior chest wall (Figure 4.9). ***Pectoral*** means relating to the chest.

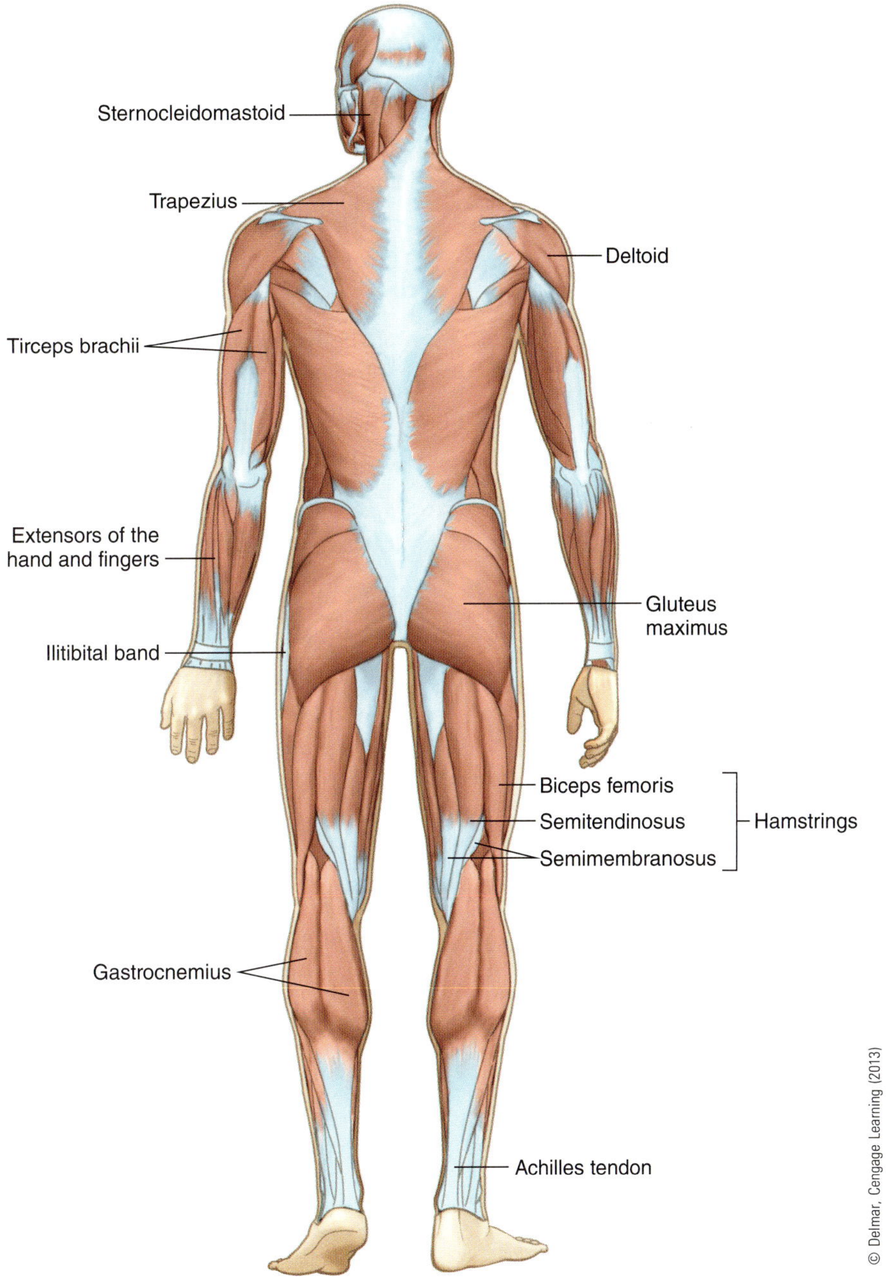

FIGURE 4.10 Superficial muscles of the body (posterior view).

- **Lateralis** means toward the side. For example: the **vastus lateralis** (lat-er-**AY**-lis) is a muscle toward the outer side of the leg.
- **Medialis** means toward the midline. The **vastus medialis** (mee-dee-**AY**-lis) is a muscle toward the midline of the leg. These muscles are part of the quadriceps that flex and extend the leg at the knee. (These muscles can be located on Figure 4.9.)

Muscles Named for Fiber Direction

Some muscles are named for the direction in which their fibers run (Figure 4.12).

- **Oblique** (oh-**BLEEK**) means slanted or at an angle. As an example, the ***external oblique*** and ***internal oblique*** muscles have a slanted alignment.

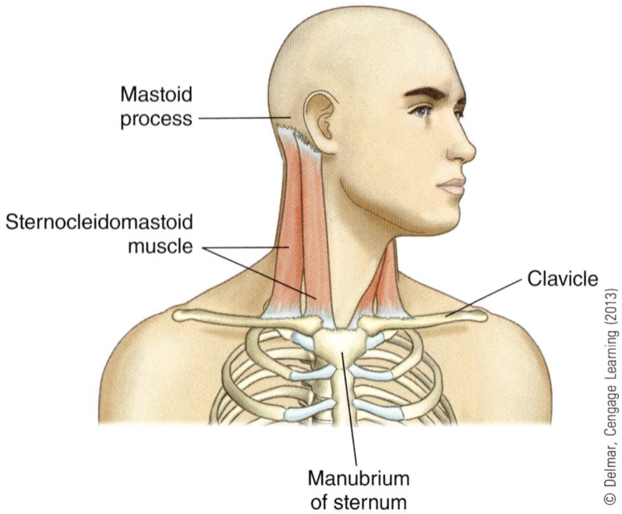

FIGURE 4.11 The *sternocleidomastoid muscle* is named for its *origins* and *insertion.*

- **Rectus** (**RECK**-tus) means in straight alignment with the vertical axis of the body. As an example, the *rectus abdominis* and *rectus femorus* (below, under "Select Muscles and Their Functions") have straight alignment.
- A **sphincter** (**SFINK**-ter) is a ring-like muscle that tightly constricts the opening of a passageway. A sphincter is named for the passage involved. As an example, the *anal sphincter* closes the anus.
- **Transverse** (trans-**VERSE**) means in a crosswise direction. An example is the *transverse abdominis* muscle in the abdomen, which has a crosswise alignment.

Muscles Named for Number of Divisions

Muscles may be named according to the number of divisions forming them. See the muscles of the arm in Figure 4.3 as examples of this.

- The **biceps brachii** (**BYE**-seps **BRAY**-kee-eye), also known as the ***biceps***, is formed from two divisions (**bi-** means two, and **-ceps** means head).
- The **triceps brachii** (**TRY**-seps **BRAY**-kee-eye), also known as the ***triceps***, is formed from three divisions (**tri-** means three, and **-ceps** means head).
- These muscles flex and extend the upper arm.

Muscles Named for Their Size or Shape

Some muscles are named because they are broad or narrow, or large or small.

- The **gluteus maximus** (**GLOO**-tee-us **MAX**-ih-mus) is the largest muscle of the buttock (Figure 4.10). *Maximus* means great or large.
- Other muscles are named because they are shaped like a familiar object. For example, the **deltoid muscle** (**DEL**-toyd), located on the shoulder, is shaped like an inverted triangle, which is the Greek letter *delta.*

Muscles Named for Strange Reasons

Some muscles, such as the hamstrings, have seemingly strange names. The reason this group of muscles is so named is because these are the muscles by which a butcher hangs a slaughtered pig.

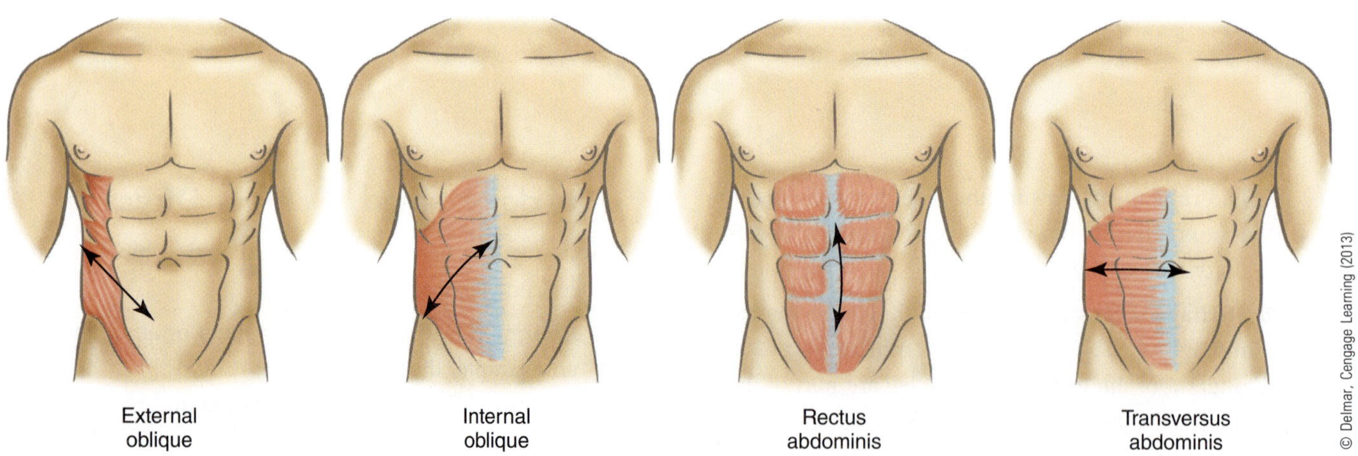

FIGURE 4.12 Many of the muscles of the trunk are named for their direction.

- The **hamstring group**, located at the back of the upper leg, consists of three separate muscles: the *biceps femoris, semitendinosus*, and *semimembranosus* muscles. The primary functions of the hamstrings are knee flexion and hip extension (Figure 4.10).

SELECT MUSCLES AND THEIR FUNCTIONS

Each of the body's 600 muscles has a specific role. Here are just a few listed with their function.

Muscles of the Head

- The **frontalis** (fron-**TAY**-lis), or *occipitofrontalis*, muscle is in the forehead. It raises and lowers the eyebrows.
- The **temporalis** (**tem**-poh-**RAY**-lis) muscle moves the lower jaw up and back to close the mouth.
- The **masseter** (mah-**SEE**-ter) muscle, which is one of the strongest in the body, moves the lower jaw up to close the mouth when chewing.

Muscles of the Trunk

- In the male, the **pectoralis major** makes up the bulk of the chest muscles. In the female, this muscle lies under the breast.
- The **external oblique** and **internal oblique muscles** are found in the abdomen. The external oblique muscles flex and rotate the vertebral column. They also flex the torso and compress the abdomen. The internal oblique muscles flex the spine, support the abdominal contents, help breathe, and rotate the spine.
- The **rectus abdominis** (ab-**DOM**-ih-nus) helps flex the trunk, assists in breathing, and supports the spine.
- The **transverse abdominis** is located on the side of the abdomen. This *core* muscle is engaged when a person laughs or coughs.

Muscles of the Shoulders and Arms

- The **deltoid** forms the muscular cap of the shoulder (Figures 4.9 and 4.10).
- The **trapezius** (trah-**PEE**-zee-us) muscle moves the head and shoulder blade.
- The **biceps brachii**, located in the anterior upper arm, flexes the elbow.
- The **triceps brachii**, located in the posterior upper arm, extends the elbow.

Muscles of the Legs

- The **rectus femoris** (**FEM**-or-iss) extends the leg at the knee.
- The **quadriceps femoris** is made up of four muscles, including the vastus lateralis and vastus medialis, which flex and extend the leg at the knee.
- The **hamstring group** is involved in knee flexion and hip extension.
- The **gastrocnemius** (**gas**-trok-**NEE**-mee-uhs) is the calf muscle that flexes the knee and bends the foot downward. The name comes from the Latin for "stomach of the leg," because of the way this muscle bulges out.

MEDICAL SPECIALTIES RELATED TO THE MUSCULAR SYSTEM

- An **exercise physiologist** (**fiz**-ee-**OL**-oh-jist) is a specialist who works under the supervision of a physician to develop, implement, and coordinate exercise programs, and administer medical tests to promote physical fitness.
- A **neurologist** (new-**ROL**-oh-jist) is a physician who specializes in treating the causes of paralysis and similar muscular disorders in which there is a loss of function.
- A **physiatrist** (**fiz**-ee-**AT**-rist) is a physician who specializes in physical medicine and rehabilitation with the focus on restoring function. *Rehabilitation* is restoration, following disease, illness, or injury, of the ability to function in a normal or near-normal manner.
- A **sports medicine physician** specializes in treating sports-related injuries of the bones, joints, and muscles.

PATHOLOGY OF THE MUSCULAR SYSTEM

Fibers, Fascia, and Tendons

- **Fasciitis** (**fas**-ee-**EYE**-tis), which is also spelled *fascitis*, is inflammation of a fascia (**fasci** means fascia, and **-itis** means inflammation).
- **Fibromyalgia syndrome** (**figh**-broh-my-**AL**-jee-ah) is a debilitating chronic condition characterized by fatigue; diffuse or specific muscle, joint, or bone pain;

and a wide range of other symptoms (**fibr/o** means fibrous tissue, **my** means muscle, and **-algia** means pain). ***Debilitating*** means a condition causing weakness. Contrast fibromyalgia syndrome with *chronic fatigue syndrome.*

- **Tenosynovitis** (**ten**-oh-**sin**-oh-**VYE**-tis) is an inflammation of the sheath surrounding a tendon. (**ten/o** means tendon, **synov** means synovial membrane, and **-itis** means inflammation).
- **Tendinitis** (**ten**-dih-**NIGH**-tis), sometimes spelled ***tendonitis***, is an inflammation of the tendons caused by excessive or unusual use of the joint (**tendin** means tendon, and **-itis** means inflammation). The terms ***tenonitis*** and ***tenontitis*** also mean tendinitis.

Chronic Fatigue Syndrome

Chronic fatigue syndrome (CFS) is a disorder of unknown cause that affects many body systems. It is discussed in this chapter because many of the symptoms are similar to those of the fibromyalgia syndrome.

- CFS is a debilitating and complex disorder characterized by profound fatigue that is not improved by bed rest and may be made worse by physical or mental activity.

Muscle Disorders

- An **adhesion** (ad-**HEE**-zhun) is a band of fibrous tissue that holds structures together abnormally. Adhesions can form in muscles or in internal organs, as the result of an injury or surgery. The term ***frozen shoulder*** refers to adhesions forming in the capsule of connective tissue in the shoulder, tightening around the shoulder joint.
- **Atrophy** (**AT**-roh-fee) means weakness or wearing away of body tissues and structures. Atrophy of a muscle or muscles can be caused by pathology or by disuse of the muscle over a long period of time.
- **Myalgia** (my-**AL**-jee-ah) is tenderness or pain in the muscles (**my** means muscle, and **-algia** means pain).
- A **myocele** (**MY**-oh-seel) is the herniation (protrusion) of muscle substance through a tear in the fascia surrounding it (**my/o** means muscle, and **-cele** means a hernia). A **hernia** (**HER**-nee-ah) is the protrusion of a part of a structure through the tissues normally containing it.
- **Myolysis** (my-**OL**-ih-sis) is the degeneration of muscle tissue (**my/o** means muscle, and **-lysis** means destruction or breaking down in disease). ***Degeneration*** means deterioration or breaking down. ***Deterioration*** means the process of becoming worse.
- **Myorrhexis** (**my**-oh-**RECK**-sis) is the rupture or tearing of a muscle (**my/o** means muscle, and **-rrhexis** means rupture).
- **Polymyositis** (**pol**-ee-**my**-oh-**SIGH**-tis) is a muscle disease characterized by the simultaneous inflammation and weakening of voluntary muscles in many parts of the body (**poly-** means many, **myos** means muscle, and **-itis** means inflammation). The affected muscles are typically those closest to the trunk or torso, and the resulting weakness can be severe.
- **Sarcopenia** (**sar**-koh-**PEE**-nee-ah) is the loss of muscle mass, strength, and function that come with aging (**sarc/o** means flesh, and **-penia** means deficiency). A weight or resistance training program can significantly improve muscle mass and slow, but not stop, this process.

Muscle Tone

Muscle tone is the state of balanced muscle tension (contraction and relaxation) that makes normal posture, coordination, and movement possible.

- **Atonic** (ah-**TON**-ick) means lacking normal muscle tone or strength (**a-** means without, **ton** means tone, and **-ic** means pertaining to).
- **Dystonia** (dis-**TOH**-nee-ah) is a condition of abnormal muscle tone that causes the impairment of voluntary muscle movement (**dys-** means bad, **ton** means tone, and **-ia** means condition).
- **Hypotonia** (**high**-poh-**TOH**-nee-ah) is a condition in which there is diminished tone of the skeletal muscles (**hypo-** means deficient, **ton** means tone, and **-ia** means condition).

Muscle Movement

- **Ataxia** (ah-**TACK**-see-ah) is the lack of muscle coordination during voluntary movement (**a-** means without, **tax** means coordination, and **-ia** means condition). These movements, which are often shaky and unsteady, are most frequently caused by abnormal activity in the cerebellum (see Chapter 10).
- A **contracture** (kon-**TRACK**-chur) is the permanent tightening of fascia, muscles, tendons, ligaments, or skin that occurs when normally elastic connective tissues are replaced with nonelastic fibrous tissues. The most common causes of contractures are scarring or the lack of use due to immobilization or inactivity.

- **Intermittent claudication** (**klaw**-dih-**KAY**-shun) is pain in the leg muscles that occurs during exercise and is relieved by rest. ***Intermittent*** means coming and going at intervals, and ***claudication*** means limping. This condition, which is due to poor circulation, is associated with peripheral vascular disease (see Chapter 5).
- A **spasm** is a sudden, involuntary contraction of one or more muscles. Also known as a ***charley horse***, especially when occurring in the leg.
- A **cramp** is a painful localized muscle spasm often named for its cause, such as menstrual cramps or writer's cramp.
- **Spasmodic torticollis** (spaz-**MOD**-ick **tor**-tih-**KOL**-is), also known as ***wryneck***, is a stiff neck due to spasmodic contraction of the neck muscles that pull the head toward the affected side. ***Spasmodic*** means relating to a spasm, and ***torticollis*** means a contraction, or shortening, of the muscles of the neck.

Muscle Function

- **Bradykinesia** (**brad**-ee-kih-**NEE**-zee-ah) is extreme slowness in movement (**brady-** means slow, **kines** means movement, and **-ia** means condition). This is one of the symptoms of Parkinson's disease, which is discussed in Chapter 10.
- **Dyskinesia** (**dis**-kih-**NEE**-zee-ah) is the distortion or impairment of voluntary movement such as a tic or spasm (**dys-** means bad, **kines** means movement, and **-ia** means condition). A ***tic*** is a spasmodic muscular contraction that often involves parts of the face. Although these movements appear purposeful, they are not under voluntary control.
- **Hyperkinesia** (**high**-per-kye-**NEE**-zee-ah), also known as ***hyperactivity***, is abnormally increased muscle function or activity (**hyper-** means excessive, **kines** means movement, and **-ia** means condition).

Myoclonus

Myoclonus (**my**-oh-**KLOH**-nus) is the sudden, involuntary jerking of a muscle or group of muscles (**my/o** means muscle, **clon** mean violent action, and **-us** is a singular noun ending).

- **Nocturnal myoclonus** (nock-**TER**-nal **my**-oh-**KLOH**-nus) is jerking of the limbs that can occur normally as a person is falling asleep. ***Nocturnal*** means pertaining to night.
- **Singultus** (sing-**GUL**-tus), also known as ***hiccups***, is myoclonus of the diaphragm that causes the characteristic hiccup sound with each spasm.

Myasthenia Gravis

Myasthenia gravis (MG) (**my**-as-**THEE**-nee-ah **GRAH**-vis) is a chronic autoimmune disease that affects the neuromuscular junction (where the neuron activates muscle to contract) and produces serious weakness of voluntary muscles. Muscles that control eye movement, facial expression, chewing, talking, and swallowing are often affected by this condition. ***Myasthenia*** means muscle weakness (**my** means muscle, and **-asthenia** means weakness or lack of strength). ***Gravis*** comes from the Latin word meaning grave or serious.

Muscular Dystrophy

The condition commonly known as **muscular dystrophy** (**DIS**-troh-fee) is properly referred to in the plural, which is *muscular dystrophies.* This general term describes a group of more than 30 genetic diseases that are characterized by progressive weakness and degeneration of the skeletal muscles that control movement, without affecting the nervous system. There is no specific treatment to stop or reverse any form of muscular dystrophy. Two of the most common forms are:

- ***Duchenne muscular dystrophy*** (DMD) is the most common form of muscular dystrophy in children. This condition affects primarily boys with onset between the ages of 3 and 5 years. The disorder progresses rapidly so that most of these boys are unable to walk by age 12 and later need a respirator to breathe.
- ***Becker muscular dystrophy*** (BMD) is very similar to, but less severe than, Duchenne muscular dystrophy.

Repetitive Stress Disorders

Repetitive stress disorders, also known as ***repetitive motion disorders***, are a variety of muscular conditions that result from repeated motions performed in the course of normal work, daily activities, or recreation such as sports. The symptoms caused by these frequently repeated motions involve muscles, tendons, nerves, and joints.

- **Compartment syndrome** involves the compression of nerves and blood vessels due to swelling within the enclosed space created by the fascia that separates groups of muscles. This syndrome can be caused by trauma, tight bandages or casts, or by repetitive activities such as running.
- **Overuse injuries** are minor tissue injuries that have not been given time to heal. These injuries can be caused by spending hours at the computer keyboard or by lengthy sports training sessions.

- **Overuse tendinitis** (**ten**-dih-**NIGH**-tis), also known as ***overuse tendinosis***, is an inflammation of tendons caused by excessive or unusual use of a joint (**tendin-** means tendon, and **-itis** means inflammation).
- **Stress fractures**, which are also overuse injuries, are discussed in Chapter 3.

Myofascial Pain Syndrome

Myofascial pain syndrome (**my**-oh-**FASH**-ee-ahl) is a chronic pain disorder that affects muscles and fascia throughout the body. This condition, which is caused by the development of trigger points, produces local and referred muscle pain. ***Trigger points*** are tender areas that most commonly develop where the fascia comes into contact with a muscle. ***Referred pain*** describes pain that originates in one area of the body, but is felt in another.

Rotator Cuff Injuries

- **Impingement syndrome** (im-**PINJ**-ment) occurs when inflamed and swollen tendons are caught in the narrow space between the bones within the shoulder joint. A common sign of impingement syndrome is discomfort when raising your arm above your head.
- **Rotator cuff tendinitis** (**ten**-dih-**NIGH**-tis) is an inflammation of the tendons of the rotator cuff (Figure 4.13). This condition is often named for the cause, such as ***tennis shoulder*** or ***pitcher's shoulder***.
- A **ruptured rotator cuff** develops when rotator cuff tendinitis is left untreated or if the overuse continues. This occurs as the irritated tendon weakens and tears (Figure 4.13).

Carpal Tunnel Syndrome

Carpal tunnel syndrome symptoms occur when the tendons that pass through the carpal tunnel are chronically overused and become inflamed and swollen. The carpal tunnel is a narrow, bony passage under the carpal ligament that is located one-fourth of an inch below the inner surface of the wrist. The median nerve and the tendons that bend the fingers pass through this tunnel (Figure 4.14). ***Carpal*** means pertaining to the wrist.

- This swelling of carpal tunnel syndrome creates pressure on the median nerve as it passes through the tunnel.
- **Carpal tunnel release** is the surgical enlargement of the carpal tunnel or cutting of the carpal ligament to relieve the pressure on tendons and nerves.

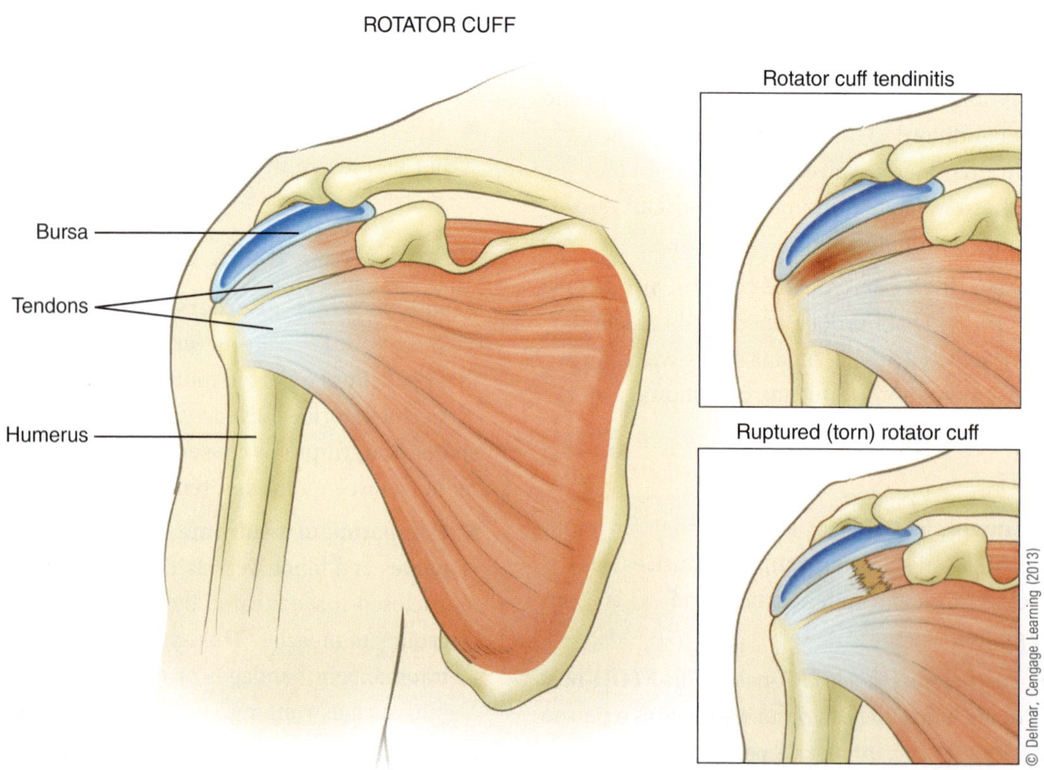

FIGURE 4.13 Diagrammatic views of the *rotator cuff* in health (left) and with injuries (right).

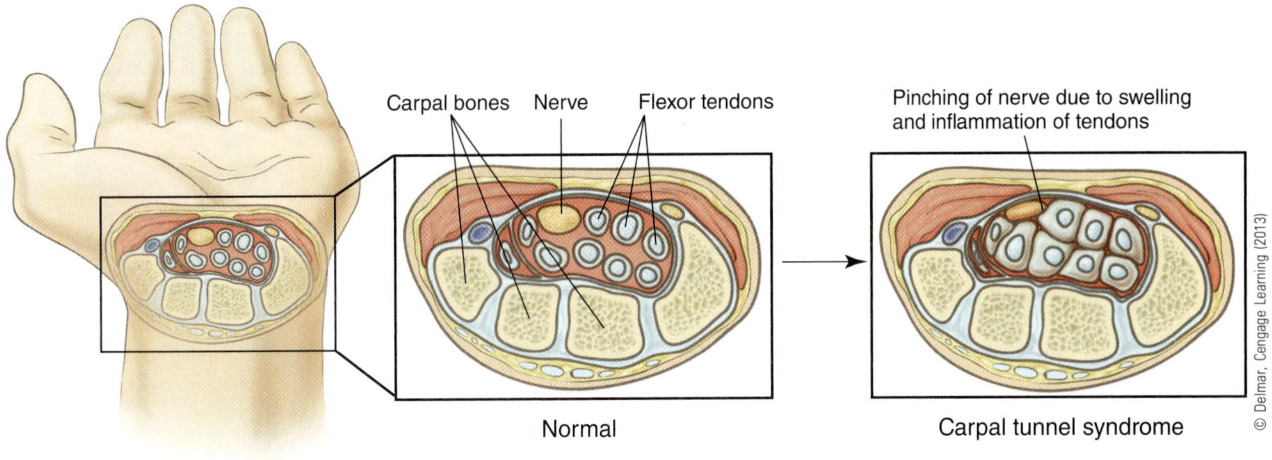

FIGURE 4.14 When the tendons that pass through the carpal tunnel become inflamed and swollen, they pinch the nerve and cause *carpal tunnel syndrome*.

Ganglion Cyst

A **ganglion cyst** (**GANG**-glee-on **SIST**) is a harmless fluid-filled swelling that occurs most commonly on the outer surface of the wrist. This condition, which can be caused by repeated minor injuries, is usually painless and does not require treatment. (Do not confuse this use of the term *ganglion* here with the nerve ganglions described in Chapter 10.)

Epicondylitis

Epicondylitis (**ep**-ih-**kon**-dih-**LYE**-tis) is inflammation of the tissues surrounding the elbow (**epi-** means on, **condyl** means condyle, and **-itis** means inflammation). *Condyle* refers to the round prominence at the end of a bone.

- *Lateral epicondylitis*, also known as *tennis elbow*, is characterized by pain on the outer side of the forearm.
- *Medial epicondylitis*, also known as *golfer's elbow*, is characterized by pain on the palm-side of the forearm.

Ankle and Foot Problems

- A **heel spur** is a calcium deposit in the plantar fascia near its attachment to the calcaneus (heel) bone that can be one of the causes of *plantar fasciitis*.
- **Plantar fasciitis** (**PLAN**-tar **fas**-ee-**EYE**-tis) is an inflammation of the plantar fascia on the sole of the foot. This condition causes foot or heel pain when walking or running (Figure 4.15).

Sports Injuries

The following injuries are frequently associated with sports overuse; however, some may also be caused by other forms of trauma.

- A **sprain** is an injury to a joint, such as an ankle, knee, or wrist, which usually occurs when a ligament is wrenched or torn (Figure 4.16).
- A **strain** is an injury to the body of the muscle or to the attachment of a tendon. Strains usually are associated with overuse injuries that involve a stretched or torn muscle or tendon attachment.
- A **shin splint** is a painful condition caused by the *tibialis anterior* muscle tearing away from the tibia (shin bone). Shin splints can develop in the anterolateral (front and

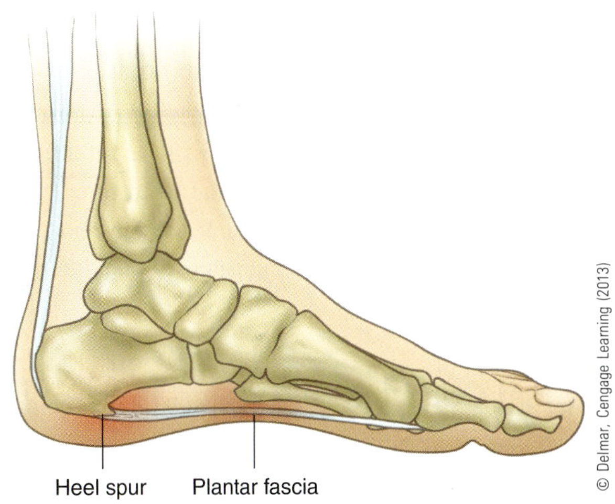

FIGURE 4.15 A *heel spur* and *plantar fasciitis*.

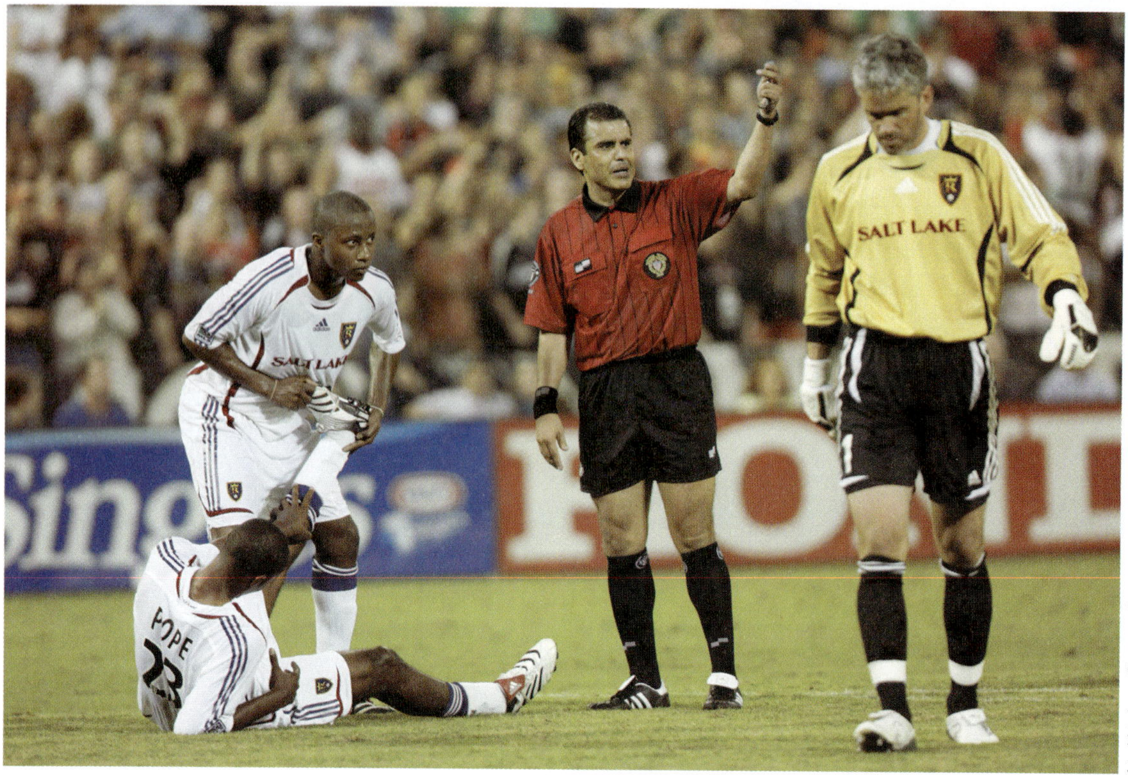

fstockfoto/www.Shutterstock.com

FIGURE 4.16 A *sprained ankle* involving one or more wrenched or torn ligaments is a common sports injury.

side) muscles or in the posteromedial (back and middle) muscles of the lower leg (Figures 4.10 and 4.11). This type of injury is usually caused by repeated stress to the lower leg, such as running on hard surfaces.

- A **hamstring injury** can be a strain or tear on any of the three hamstring muscles that straighten the hip and bend the knee. When these muscles contract too quickly, an injury can occur that is characterized by sudden and severe pain in the back of the thigh.
- **Achilles tendinitis** (**ten**-dih-**NIGH**-tis) is a painful inflammation of the Achilles tendon caused by excessive stress being placed on that tendon.
- **Iliotibial band syndrome** (ITBS) (**ill**-ee-oh-**TIB**-ee-al) is an overuse injury. The iliotibial band runs from the hip bone, diagonally across the leg to the tibia. ITBS is caused by this band rubbing against bone, often in the area of the knee.

Spinal Cord Injuries

As described in Chapter 3, the spinal cord is surrounded and protected by the bony vertebrae. This protection is essential because the spinal cord is soft, with the consistency of toothpaste.

- The type of paralysis caused by a **spinal cord injury** (SCI) is determined by the level of the vertebra closest to the injury. The higher on the spinal cord the injury occurs, the greater the area of the body that may be affected.
- An injury occurs when a vertebra is broken and a piece of the broken bone is pressing into the spinal cord. The cord can also be injured if the vertebrae are pushed or pulled out of alignment.
- When the spinal cord is injured, the ability of the brain to communicate with the body below the level of the injury may be reduced or lost altogether. When that happens, the affected parts of the body will not function normally.
- An ***incomplete injury*** means that the person has some function below the level of the injury, even though that function isn't normal.
- A ***complete injury*** means that there is complete loss of sensation and muscle control below the level of the injury; however, a complete injury does not mean that there is no hope of any improvement.

Types of Paralysis

Paralysis (pah-**RAL**-ih-sis) is the loss of sensation and voluntary muscle movements in a muscle through disease or injury to its nerve supply. Damage can be either temporary or permanent (plural, *paralyses*).

- **Myoparesis** (**my**-oh-**PAR**-eh-sis) is a weakness or slight muscular paralysis (**my/o** means muscle, and **-paresis** means partial or incomplete paralysis).
- **Hemiparesis** (**hem**-ee-pah-**REE**-sis) is slight paralysis or weakness affecting one side of the body (**hemi-** means half, and **-paresis** means partial or incomplete paralysis). Contrast hemiparesis with *hemiplegia*.
- **Hemiplegia** (**hem**-ee-**PLEE**-jee-ah) is total paralysis affecting only one side of the body (**hemi-** means half, and **-plegia** means paralysis). This form of paralysis is usually associated with a stroke or brain damage. Damage to one side of the brain causes paralysis on the opposite side of the body. An individual affected with hemiplegia is known as a ***hemiplegic***. Contrast with *hemiparesis*.
- **Paraplegia** (**par**-ah-**PLEE**-jee-ah) is the paralysis of both legs and the lower part of the body. An individual affected with paraplegia is known as a ***paraplegic***.
- **Quadriplegia** (**kwad**-rih-**PLEE**-jee-ah) is paralysis of all four extremities (**quadr/i** means four, and **-plegia** means paralysis). An individual affected with quadriplegia is known as a ***quadriplegic***.
- **Cardioplegia** (**kar**-dee-oh-**PLEE**-jee-ah) is paralysis of heart muscle (**cardi/o** means heart, and **-plegia** means paralysis). Although this can be caused by a direct blow or trauma, it is more commonly induced intentionally to perform complicated surgery.

StudyWARE CONNECTION

Watch the **Spinal Cord Injuries** animation in the StudyWARE™.

DIAGNOSTIC PROCEDURES OF THE MUSCULAR SYSTEM

- **Deep tendon reflexes** (DTR) are tested with a reflex hammer that is used to strike a tendon (Figure 4.17). A ***reflex*** is an involuntary response to a stimulus. No response or an abnormal response can indicate a disruption of the nerve supply to the involved muscles. Reflexes also are lost in deep coma or because of medication such as heavy sedation.

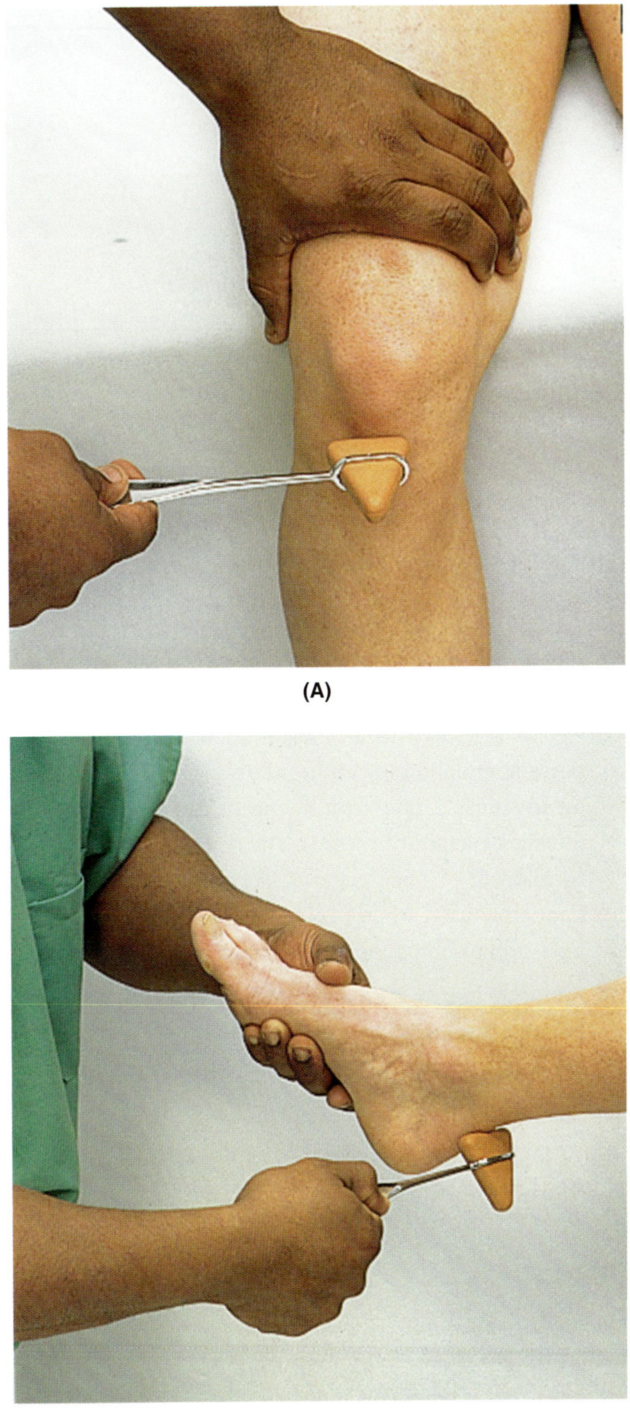

FIGURE 4.17 Assessment of *deep tendon reflexes*. (A) Testing the *patellar reflex*. (B) Testing the *Achilles tendon reflex*.

- **Range-of-motion testing** (ROM) is a diagnostic procedure to evaluate joint mobility and muscle strength (Figure 4.18). Range-of-motion exercises are used to increase strength, flexibility, and mobility.

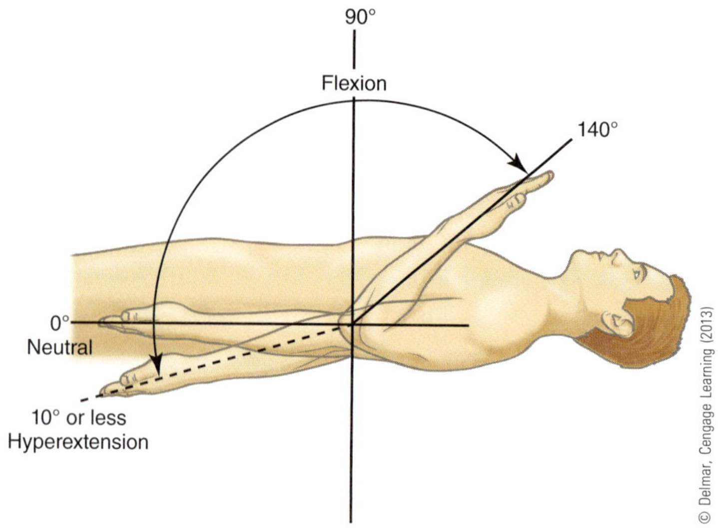

FIGURE 4.18 *Range-of-motion testing* is used to evaluate joint mobility. The results are expressed in degrees.

- **Electromyography** (EMG) (ee-**leck**-troh-my-**OG**-rah-fee) is a diagnostic test that measures the electrical activity within muscle fibers in response to nerve stimulation (**electr/o** means electricity, **my/o** means muscle, and **-graphy** means the process of producing a picture or record). The resulting record is called an *electromyogram*. Electromyography is most frequently used when people have symptoms of weakness, and examination shows impaired muscle strength.
- A **muscle biopsy** involves removal of a plug of tissue for examination. A biopsy needle is commonly used to obtain this specimen, which is later used for examination.

TREATMENT PROCEDURES OF THE MUSCULAR SYSTEM

Medications

- An **antispasmodic**, also known as an *anticholinergic*, is administered to suppress smooth muscle contractions of the stomach, intestine, or bladder. For example, *atropine* is an antispasmodic that can be administered preoperatively to relax smooth muscles during surgery.
- A **skeletal muscle relaxant** is administered to relax certain muscles and to relieve the stiffness, pain, and discomfort caused by strains, sprains, or other muscle injuries. These medications act on the central nervous system and may have a negative interaction with alcohol and some antidepressants (see Chapter 10).
- A **neuromuscular blocker**, also known as a *neuromuscular blocking agent*, is a drug that causes temporary paralysis by blocking the transmission of nerve stimuli to the muscles. These drugs are used as an adjunct to anesthesia during surgery to cause skeletal muscles to relax. As used here, *adjunct* means in addition to.

Ergonomics

Ergonomics (er-goh-**NOM**-icks) is the study of the human factors that affect the design and operation of tools and the work environment. This term is usually applied to the design of equipment and workspaces, with the goal of reducing injuries, strain, and stress.

Treatment Techniques

- **Myofascial release** (**my**-oh-**FASH**-ee-ahl) is a specialized soft-tissue manipulation technique used to ease the pain of conditions such as fibromyalgia syndrome, myofascial pain syndrome, movement restrictions, temporomandibular joint disorders (TMJ), and carpal tunnel syndrome.
- **Occupational therapy** (OT) consists of activities to promote recovery and rehabilitation to assist patients in performing the **activities of daily living** (ADL), which include grooming, eating, and dressing.
- **Physical therapy** (PT) is treatment to prevent disability or restore function through the use of exercise, heat, massage, or other techniques.

- **Therapeutic ultrasound** uses high-frequency sound waves to treat muscle injuries by generating heat deep within muscle tissue. This heat eases pain, reduces muscle spasms, and accelerates healing by increasing the flow of blood into the target tissues.
- **Transcutaneous electrical nerve stimulation** (TENS) uses a device that delivers electrical impulses through the skin, which cause changes in muscles. This is discussed further in Chapter 15.

Rice

The most common first aid treatment of muscular injuries is known by the acronym ***RICE***. These letters stand for ***R****est,* ***I****ce,* ***C****ompression,* and ***E****levation.* Rest and ice are recommended for the first few days after the injury to ease pain. Compression, such as wrapping with a stretch bandage, and elevation help minimize swelling.

After the first few days, as the pain decreases, using heat, accompanied by stretching and light exercises, helps bring blood to the injured area to speed healing.

Fascia

- A **fasciotomy** (**fash**-ee-**OT**-oh-mee) is a surgical incision through the fascia to relieve tension or pressure (**fasci** means fascia, and **-otomy** means a surgical incision). Without this procedure, which is commonly used to treat compartment syndrome, the pressure causes a loss of circulation that damages the affected tissues.
- **Fascioplasty** (**FASH**-ee-oh-**plas**-tee) is the surgical repair of a fascia (**fasci/o** means fascia, and **-plasty** means surgical repair).

Tendons

- **Tenodesis** (ten-**ODD**-eh-sis) is the surgical suturing of the end of a tendon to a bone (**ten/o** means tendon, and **-desis** means to bind or tie together). *Tenodesis* is the opposite of *tenolysis.*
- **Tenolysis** (ten-**OL**-ih-sis), also known as ***tendolysis***, is the release of a tendon from adhesions (**ten/o** means tendon, and **-lysis** means to set free). *Tenolysis* is the opposite of *tenodesis.*
- **Tenorrhaphy** (ten-**OR**-ah-fee) is the surgical suturing together of the divided ends of a tendon (**ten/o** means tendon, and **-rrhaphy** means surgical suturing).

Muscles

- **Myorrhaphy** (my-**OR**-ah-fee) is the surgical suturing a muscle (**my/o** means muscle, and **-rrhaphy** means surgical suturing).
- A **myotomy** (my-**OT**-oh-mee) is a surgical incision into a muscle (**my** means muscle, and **-otomy** means surgical incision).

ABBREVIATIONS RELATED TO THE MUSCULAR SYSTEM

Table 4.1 presents an overview of the abbreviations related to the terms introduced in this chapter. Note: To avoid errors or confusion, always be cautious when using abbreviations.

TABLE 4.1
Abbreviations Related to the Muscular System

activities of daily living = ADL	**ADL** = activities of daily living
carpal tunnel syndrome = CTS	**CTS** = carpal tunnel syndrome
electromyography = EMG	**EMG** = electromyography
fibromyalgia syndrome = FMS	**FMS** = fibromyalgia syndrome
hemiplegia = hemi	**hemi** = hemiplegia
intermittent claudication = IC	**IC** = intermittent claudication
muscular dystrophy = MD	**MD** = muscular dystrophy
myasthenia gravis = MG	**MG** = myasthenia gravis
occupational therapy = OT	**OT** = occupational therapist
polymyositis = PM	**PM** = polymyositis
quadriplegia, quadriplegic = quad	**quad** = quadriplegia, quadriplegic
repetitive stress disorder = RSD	**RSD** = repetitive stress disorder

StudyWARE™ CONNECTION

For more practice and to test your mastery of this material, go to the StudyWARE™ to play interactive games and complete the quiz for this chapter.

DELMAR MOBILE MEDIA

Downloadable audio is available for selected medical terms in this chapter to enhance your learning of medical terminology.

Workbook Practice

Go to your workbook and complete the exercises for this chapter.

CHAPTER 4 LEARNING EXERCISES

MATCHING WORD PARTS 1

Write the correct answer in the middle column.

	Definition	Correct Answer	Possible Answers
4.1.	abnormal condition	______________	**-cele**
4.2.	fascia	______________	**fasci/o**
4.3.	fibrous tissue	______________	**fibr/o**
4.4.	hernia, swelling	______________	**-ia**
4.5.	movement	______________	**kines/o, kinesi/o**

MATCHING WORD PARTS 2

Write the correct answer in the middle column.

	Definition	Correct Answer	Possible Answers
4.6.	coordination	______________	**my/o**
4.7.	muscle	______________	**-rrhexis**
4.8.	rupture	______________	**tax/o**
4.9.	tendon	______________	**tend/o**
4.10.	tone	______________	**ton/o**

MATCHING MUSCLE DIRECTIONS AND POSITIONS

Write the correct answer in the middle column.

	Definition	Correct Answer	Possible Answers
4.11.	crosswise	______________	lateralis
4.12.	ringlike	______________	oblique

4.13. slanted at an angle ______________________ rectus

4.14. straight ______________________ sphincter

4.15. toward the side ______________________ transverse

DEFINITIONS

Select the correct answer, and write it on the line provided.

4.16. The ________________ muscles are under voluntary control.

involuntary nonstriated skeletal visceral

4.17. A/An ________________ is a calcium deposit in the plantar fascia near its attachment to the calcaneus bone.

heel spur impingement syndrome overuse injury shin splint

4.18. Turning the hand so the palm is upward is called ________________.

extension flexion pronation supination

4.19. One of the symptoms of Parkinson's disease is ________________, which is extreme slowness of movement.

bradykinesia dyskinesia hypotonia hyperactivity

4.20. A/An ________________ is a physician who specializes in physical medicine and rehabilitation with the focus on restoring function.

exercise physiologist physiatrist physiologist rheumatologist

4.21. The term ________________ means pertaining to muscle tissue and fascia.

aponeurosis fibrous sheath myocardium myofascial

4.22. A/An ________________ is a narrow band of nonelastic, fibrous connective tissue that attaches a muscle to a bone.

aponeurosis fascia ligament tendon

4.23. A band of fibers that holds structures together abnormally is a/an ________________. These bands can form as the result of an injury or surgery.

adhesion aponeurosis atrophy contracture

4.24. The paralysis of both legs and the lower part of the body is known as ________________.

hemiparesis hemiplegia paraplegia quadriplegia

4.25. The surgical suturing of the end of a tendon to a bone is known as ________________.

tenodesis tenorrhaphy tendinosis tenolysis

MATCHING STRUCTURES

Write the correct answer in the middle column.

	Definition	Correct Answer	Possible Answers
4.26.	heart muscle	________________	gluteus maximus
4.27.	buttock muscle	________________	myocardial
4.28.	fibrous connective tissue	________________	sphincter
4.29.	muscular cap of shoulder	________________	tendon
4.30.	ring-like muscle	________________	deltoid

WHICH WORD?

Select the correct answer, and write it on the line provided.

4.31. An injury to the body of the muscle or the attachment of a tendon is known as a/an ________________. These are usually associated with overuse injuries that involve a wrenched or torn muscle or tendon attachment.

sprain strain

4.32. A ________________ is a drug that causes temporary paralysis by blocking the transmission of nerve stimuli to the muscles.

neuromuscular blocker skeletal muscle relaxant

4.33. The condition of abnormal muscle tone that causes the impairment of voluntary muscle movement is known as ________________.

ataxia dystonia

4.34. Inflamed and swollen tendons caught in the narrow space between the bones within the shoulder joint cause the condition known as ______________________.

impingement syndrome intermittent claudication

4.35. The ______________________ forms the muscular cap of the shoulder.

triceps brachii deltoid

SPELLING COUNTS

Find the misspelled word in each sentence. Then write that word, spelled correctly, on the line provided.

4.36. An antispasmydic is administered to suppress smooth muscle contractions of the stomach, intestine, or bladder. ______________________

4.37. The medical term for hiccups is singulutas. ______________________

4.38. Myasthenia gravus is a chronic autoimmune disease that affects the neuromuscular junction and produces serious weakness of voluntary muscles. ______________________

4.39. A ganglian cyst is a harmless fluid-filled swelling that occurs most commonly on the outer surface of the wrist. ______________________

4.40. Pronetion is the movement that turns the palm of the hand downward or backward. ______________________

ABBREVIATION IDENTIFICATION

Write the correct answer on the line provided.

4.41. **CTS** ______________________

4.42. **DTR** ______________________

4.43. **ROM** ______________________

4.44. **RSD** ______________________

4.45. **SCI** ______________________

TERM SELECTION

Select the correct answer, and write it on the line provided.

4.46. The term ______________________ means the rupture or tearing of a muscle.

myocele myorrhaphy myorrhexis myotomy

4.47. The term meaning the degeneration of muscle tissue is ____________.

myoclonus | myolysis | myocele | myoparesis

4.48. The term ____________ means abnormally increased muscle function or activity.

hyperkinesia | hypertonia | dyskinesia | hypotonia

4.49. A/An ____________ injury can be a strain or tear on any of the three muscles that straighten the hip and bend the knee.

Achilles tendon | hamstring | myofascial | shin splint

4.50. The specialized soft-tissue manipulation technique used to ease the pain of conditions such as fibromyalgia syndrome, movement restrictions, and temporomandibular joint disorders is known as ____________.

myofascial release | occupational therapy | RICE | therapeutic ultrasound

SENTENCE COMPLETION

Write the correct term or terms on the lines provided.

4.51. An inflammation of the tissues surrounding the elbow is known as ____________.

4.52. The movement during which the knees or elbows are bent to decrease the angle of the joints is known as ____________.

4.53. Pain in the leg muscles that occurs during exercise and is relieved by rest is known as ____________. This condition is due to poor circulation and is associated with peripheral vascular disease.

4.54. A weakness or slight muscular paralysis is known as ____________.

4.55. A stiff neck due to spasmodic contraction of the neck muscles that pull the head toward the affected side is known as ____________ or wryneck.

WORD SURGERY

Divide each term into its component word parts. Write these word parts, in sequence, on the lines provided. When necessary, use a slash (/) to indicate a combining vowel. (You may not need all of the lines provided.)

4.56. **Electromyography** is a diagnostic test that measures the electrical activity within muscle fibers.

________ ________ ________ ________

4.57. **Hyperkinesia** means abnormally increased muscle function or activity.

__________ __________ __________ __________

4.58. **Myoclonus** is the sudden, involuntary jerking of a muscle or group of muscles.

__________ __________ __________ __________

4.59. **Polymyositis** is a muscle disease characterized by the simultaneous inflammation and weakening of voluntary muscles in many parts of the body.

__________ __________ __________ __________

4.60. **Sarcopenia** is the loss of muscle mass, strength, and function that comes with aging.

__________ __________ __________ __________

TRUE/FALSE

If the statement is true, write **True** on the line. If the statement is false, write **False** on the line.

4.61. ________________ Overuse tendinitis is inflammation of tendons caused by excessive or unusual use of a joint.

4.62. ________________ Hemiplegia is the total paralysis of the lower half of the body.

4.63. ________________ A spasm is a sudden, involuntary contraction of one or more muscles.

4.64. ________________ Ataxia is the distortion of voluntary movement such as in a tic or spasm.

4.65. ________________ Striated muscles are located in the walls of internal organs such as the digestive tract, blood vessels, and ducts leading from glands.

CLINICAL CONDITIONS

Write the correct answer on the line provided.

4.66. George Quinton developed a swelling on the outer surface of his wrist. His doctor diagnosed this as being a/an ________________ and explained that this was a harmless fluid-filled swelling.

4.67. Raul Valladares has a protrusion of a muscle substance through a tear in the fascia surrounding it. This condition is known as a/an ________________.

4.68. Louisa Ferraro experienced ________________ of her leg muscles due to the disuse of these muscles over a long period of time.

4.69. Jasmine Franklin has ________________________. This is a condition in which there is diminished tone of the skeletal muscles.

4.70. Carolyn Goodwin complained of profound fatigue that is not improved by bed rest and was made worse by physical or mental activity. After ruling out other causes, her physician diagnosed her condition as being ________________________ syndrome.

4.71. Chuan Lee, who is a runner, required treatment for ________________________ ________________________. This condition is a painful inflammation of the Achilles tendon caused by excessive stress being placed on that tendon.

4.72. For the first several days after his fall, Bob Hill suffered severe muscle pain. This condition is known as ________________________.

4.73. Jorge Guendulay could not play for his team because of a/an ________________________. This is a painful condition caused by the muscle tearing away from the tibia.

4.74. Due to a spinal cord injury, Marissa Giannati suffers from ________________________, which is paralysis of all four limbs.

4.75. Duncan McDougle has slight paralysis on one side of his body. This condition, which was caused by a stroke, is known as ________________________.

WHICH IS THE CORRECT MEDICAL TERM?

Select the correct answer, and write it on the line provided.

4.76. The term *muscular* ________________________ describes a group of genetic diseases characterized by progressive weakness and degeneration of the skeletal muscles.

atonic ataxia dystonia dystrophy

4.77. The surgical enlargement of the carpal tunnel or cutting of the carpal ligament to relieve nerve pressure is called ________________________.

carpal tunnel syndrome compartment syndrome carpal tunnel release myofascial pain syndrome

4.78. During ________________________, the arm moves inward and toward the side of the body.

abduction adduction circumduction rotation

4.79. A surgical incision into a muscle is known as ______________________.

myocele myorrhaphy myotomy fascioplasty

4.80. The term ______________________ means bending the foot upward at the ankle.

abduction dorsiflexion elevation plantar flexion

CHALLENGE WORD BUILDING

These terms are *not* found in this chapter; however, they are made up of the following familiar word parts. If you need help in creating the term, refer to your medical dictionary.

poly-	**card/o**	**-desis**
	fasci/o	**-ectomy**
	herni/o	**-itis**
	my/o	**-necrosis**
	sphincter/o	**-otomy**
	-algia	**-pathy**
		-rrhaphy

4.81. Any abnormal condition of skeletal muscles is known as ______________________.

4.82. Pain in several muscle groups is known as ______________________.

4.83. The death of individual muscle fibers is known as ______________________.

4.84. Surgical suturing of torn fascia is known as ______________________.

4.85. Based on word parts, the removal of multiple muscles is known as ______________________.

4.86. The surgical attachment of a fascia to another fascia or to a tendon is known as ______________________.

4.87. Inflammation of the muscle of the heart is known as ______________________.

4.88. The surgical removal of fascia is a/an ______________________.

4.89. The surgical suturing of a defect in a muscular wall, such as the repair of a hernia, is a/an ______________________.

4.90. An incision into a sphincter muscle is a/an ______________________.

LABELING EXERCISES

Identify the movements in the accompanying figures by writing the correct term on the line provided.

4.91. ______________________

4.92. ______________________

4.93. ______________________

4.94. ______________________

4.95. ______________________

4.96. ______________________

4.97. ______________________

4.98. ______________________

4.99. ______________________

4.100. ______________________

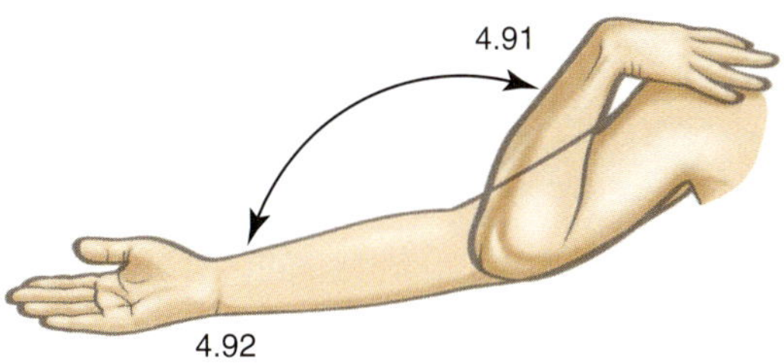

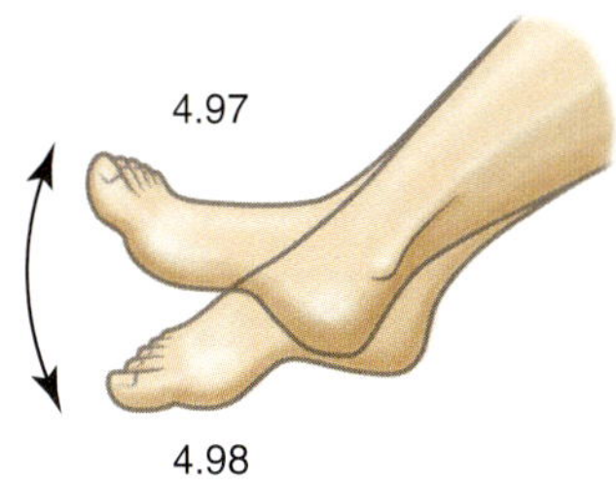

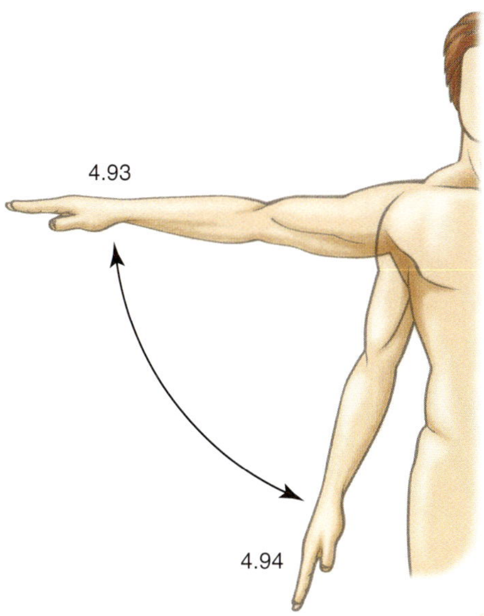

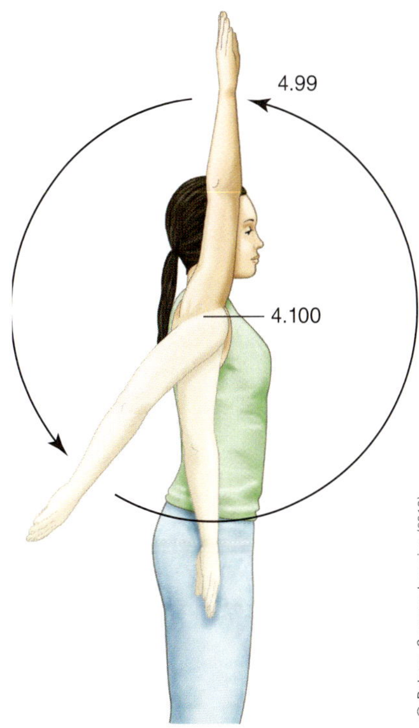

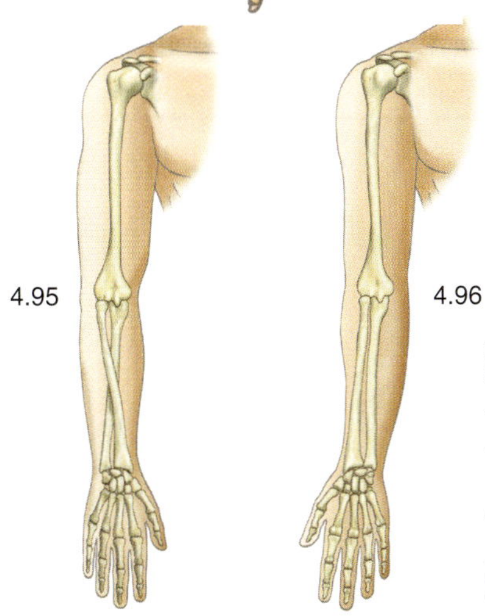

CHAPTER 5

The Cardiovascular System

Overview of STRUCTURES, COMBINING FORMS, AND FUNCTIONS OF THE CARDIOVASCULAR SYSTEM

Major Structures	Related Combining Forms	Primary Functions
Heart	**card/o**, **cardi/o**	Receives blood from the veins and pumps blood into the arteries.
Blood Vessels	**angi/o**, **vas/o**	Transport blood to and from all areas of the body.
Arteries	**arteri/o**	Transport blood away from the heart to all parts of the body.
Capillaries	**capill/o**	Permit the exchange of nutrients and waste products between the blood and the cells.
Veins	**phleb/o**, **ven/o**	Return blood from all body parts to the heart.
Blood	**hem/o**, **hemat/o**	Brings oxygen and nutrients to the cells and carries away waste.

Vocabulary Related to **THE CARDIOVASCULAR SYSTEM**

This list contains essential word parts and medical terms for this chapter. These terms are pronounced in the StudyWARE™ and Audio CDs that are available for use with this text. These and the other important **primary terms** are shown in boldface throughout the chapter. *Secondary terms*, which appear in *orange* italics, clarify the meaning of primary terms.

Word Parts

- ☐ **angi/o** blood or lymph vessel
- ☐ **aort/o** aorta
- ☐ **arteri/o** artery
- ☐ **ather/o** plaque, fatty substance
- ☐ **brady-** slow
- ☐ **cardi/o** heart
- ☐ **-crasia** a mixture or blending
- ☐ **-emia** blood, blood condition
- ☐ **erythr/o** red
- ☐ **hem/o, hemat/o** blood, relating to the blood
- ☐ **leuk/o** white
- ☐ **phleb/o** vein
- ☐ **tachy-** fast, rapid
- ☐ **thromb/o** clot
- ☐ **ven/o** vein

Medical Terms

- ☐ **ACE inhibitor**
- ☐ **anemia** (ah-**NEE**-mee-ah)
- ☐ **aneurysm** (**AN**-you-rizm)
- ☐ **angina** (an-**JIH**-nuh)
- ☐ **angioplasty** (**AN**-jee-oh-**plas**-tee)
- ☐ **anticoagulant** (**an**-tih-koh-**AG**-you-lant)
- ☐ **aplastic anemia** (ay-**PLAS**-tick ah-**NEE**-mee-ah)
- ☐ **arrhythmia** (ah-**RITH**-mee-ah)
- ☐ **atherectomy** (**ath**-er-**ECK**-toh-mee)
- ☐ **atheroma** (**ath**-er-**OH**-mah)
- ☐ **atherosclerosis** (**ath**-er-**oh**-skleh-**ROH**-sis)
- ☐ **atrial fibrillation** (**AY**-tree-al **fih**-brih-**LAY**-shun)
- ☐ **automated external defibrillator** (dee-**fih**-brih-**LAY**-ter)
- ☐ **beta-blocker**
- ☐ **blood dyscrasia** (dis-**KRAY**-zee-ah)
- ☐ **bradycardia** (**brad**-ee-**KAR**-dee-ah)
- ☐ **cardiac arrest**
- ☐ **cardiac catheterization** (**KAR**-dee-ack **kath**-eh-ter-eye-**ZAY**-shun)
- ☐ **cardiomyopathy** (**kar**-dee-oh-my-**OP**-pah-thee)
- ☐ **carotid endarterectomy** (kah-**ROT**-id **end**-ar-ter-**ECK**-toh-mee)
- ☐ **cholesterol** (koh-**LES**-ter-ol)
- ☐ **chronic venous insufficiency**
- ☐ **coronary thrombosis** (**KOR**-uh-**nerr**-ee throm-**BOH**-sis)
- ☐ **defibrillation** (dee-**fih**-brih-**LAY**-shun)
- ☐ **diuretic** (**dye**-you-**RET**-ick)
- ☐ **electrocardiogram** (ee-**leck**-troh-**KAR**-dee-oh-**gram**)
- ☐ **embolism** (**EM**-boh-lizm)
- ☐ **embolus** (**EM**-boh-lus)
- ☐ **endocarditis** (**en**-doh-kar-**DYE**-tis)
- ☐ **erythrocytes** (eh-**RITH**-roh-sights)
- ☐ **hemoglobin** (**hee**-moh-**GLOH**-bin)
- ☐ **hemolytic anemia** (**hee**-moh-**LIT**-ick ah-**NEE**-mee-ah)
- ☐ **hemostasis** (**hee**-moh-**STAY**-sis)
- ☐ **ischemic heart disease** (iss-**KEE**-mick)
- ☐ **leukemia** (loo-**KEE**-mee-ah)
- ☐ **leukocytes** (**LOO**-koh-sites)
- ☐ **leukopenia** (**loo**-koh-**PEE**-nee-ah)
- ☐ **megaloblastic anemia** (**MEG**-ah-loh-**blas**-tick ah-**NEE**-mee-ah)
- ☐ **myelodysplastic syndrome** (**my**-eh-loh-dis-**PLAS**-tick **SIN**-drohm)
- ☐ **myocardial infarction** (**my**-oh-**KAR**-dee-al in-**FARK**-shun)
- ☐ **orthostatic hypotension** (**or**-thoh-**STAT**-ick **high**-poh-**TEN**-shun)
- ☐ **pericardium** (pehr-ih-**KAR**-dee-um)
- ☐ **pernicious anemia** (per-**NISH**-us ah-**NEE**-mee-ah)
- ☐ **phlebitis** (fleh-**BYE**-tis)
- ☐ **Raynaud's disease** (ray-**NOHZ**)
- ☐ **septicemia** (**sep**-tih-**SEE**-mee-ah)
- ☐ **sickle cell anemia**
- ☐ **tachycardia** (**tack**-ee-**KAR**-dee-ah)
- ☐ **temporal arteritis** (**TEM**-poh-**ral ar**-teh-**RYE**-tis)
- ☐ **thallium stress test** (**THAL**-ee-um)
- ☐ **thrombocytopenia** (**throm**-boh-**sigh**-toh-**PEE**-nee-ah)
- ☐ **thrombolytic** (**throm**-boh-**LIT**-ick)
- ☐ **thrombosis** (throm-**BOH**-sis)
- ☐ **thrombotic occlusion** (throm-**BOT**-ick ah-**KLOO**-zhun)
- ☐ **thrombus** (**THROM**-bus)
- ☐ **transfusion reaction**
- ☐ **valvulitis** (**val**-view-**LYE**-tis)
- ☐ **varicose veins** (**VAR**-ih-kohs **VAYNS**)
- ☐ **ventricular fibrillation** (ven-**TRICK**-you-lar **fih**-brih-**LAY**-shun)
- ☐ **ventricular tachycardia** (ven-**TRICK**-you-lar **tack**-ee-**KAR**-dee-ah)

LEARNING GOALS

On completion of this chapter, you should be able to:

1. Describe the heart in terms of chambers, valves, blood flow, heartbeat, and blood supply.
2. Differentiate among the three different types of blood vessels, and describe the major function of each.
3. Identify the major components of blood and the major functions of each component.
4. State the difference between the pulmonary and systemic circulation.
5. Recognize, define, spell, and pronounce the primary terms related to the pathology and the diagnostic and treatment procedures of the cardiovascular system.

FUNCTIONS OF THE CARDIOVASCULAR SYSTEM

The cardiovascular system consists of the heart, blood vessels, and blood. **Cardiovascular** (**kar**-dee-oh-**VAS**-kyou-lar) means pertaining to the heart and blood vessels (**cardi/o** means heart, **vascul** means blood vessels, and **-ar** means pertaining to).

These structures work together to efficiently pump blood to all body tissues.

- Blood is a fluid tissue that transports oxygen and nutrients to the body tissues.
- Blood returns some waste products from these tissues to the kidneys and carries carbon dioxide back to the lungs.
- Blood cells also play important roles in the immune system (see Chapter 6), and in the endocrine system (see Chapter 13).

STRUCTURES OF THE CARDIOVASCULAR SYSTEM

The major structures of the cardiovascular system are the heart, blood vessels, and blood.

The Heart

The **heart** is a hollow, muscular organ located in the thoracic cavity, between the lungs (Figure 5.1). It is a very effective pump that furnishes the power to maintain the blood flow needed throughout the entire body (Figures 5.2 and 5.3). The ***apex*** is the lower tip of the heart.

The Pericardium

The **pericardium** (pehr-ih-**KAR**-dee-um), also known as the ***pericardial sac***, is the double-walled membranous sac that encloses the heart (**peri-** means surrounding, **cardi** means heart, and **-um** is a singular noun ending). ***Membranous*** means pertaining to membrane, which is a thin layer of pliable tissue that covers or encloses a body part.

- The ***parietal pericardium*** is a fibrous sac that surrounds and protects the heart.
- ***Pericardial fluid*** is found between these two layers, where it acts as a lubricant to prevent friction as the heart beats.
- The ***visceral pericardium*** is the inner layer of the pericardium that also forms the outer layer of the heart. When referred to as the outer layer of the heart, it is known as the *epicardium* (Figure 5.4).

The Walls of the Heart

The walls of the heart are made up of these three layers: the epicardium, myocardium, and endocardium (Figure 5.4).

- The **epicardium** (**ep**-ih-**KAR**-dee-um) is the external layer of the heart and the inner layer of the pericardium (**epi-** means upon, **cardi** means heart, and **-um** is a singular noun ending).
- The **myocardium** (my-oh-**KAR**-dee-um) is the middle and thickest of the heart's three layers (**my/o** means muscle, **cardi** means heart, and **-um** is a singular noun ending). Also known as ***myocardial muscle***, this consists of specialized cardiac muscle tissue that is capable of the constant contraction and relaxation of this muscle that creates the pumping movement that is necessary to maintain the flow of blood throughout the body. Myocardial muscle is discussed in Chapter 4.

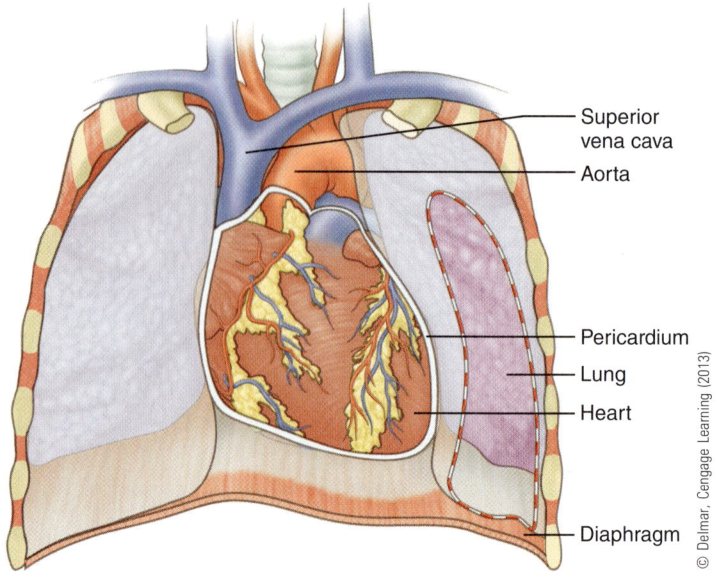

FIGURE 5.1 The heart is located in the thoracic cavity between the lungs.

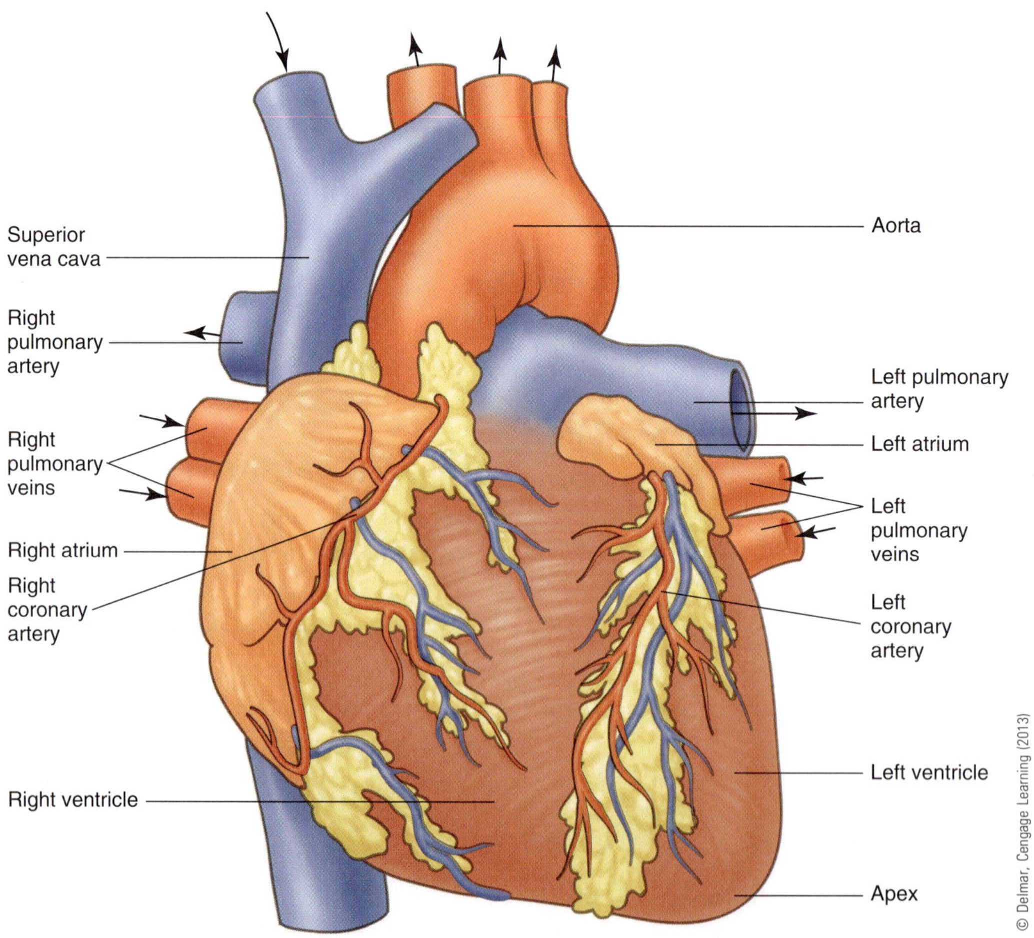

FIGURE 5.2 Anterior external view of the heart.

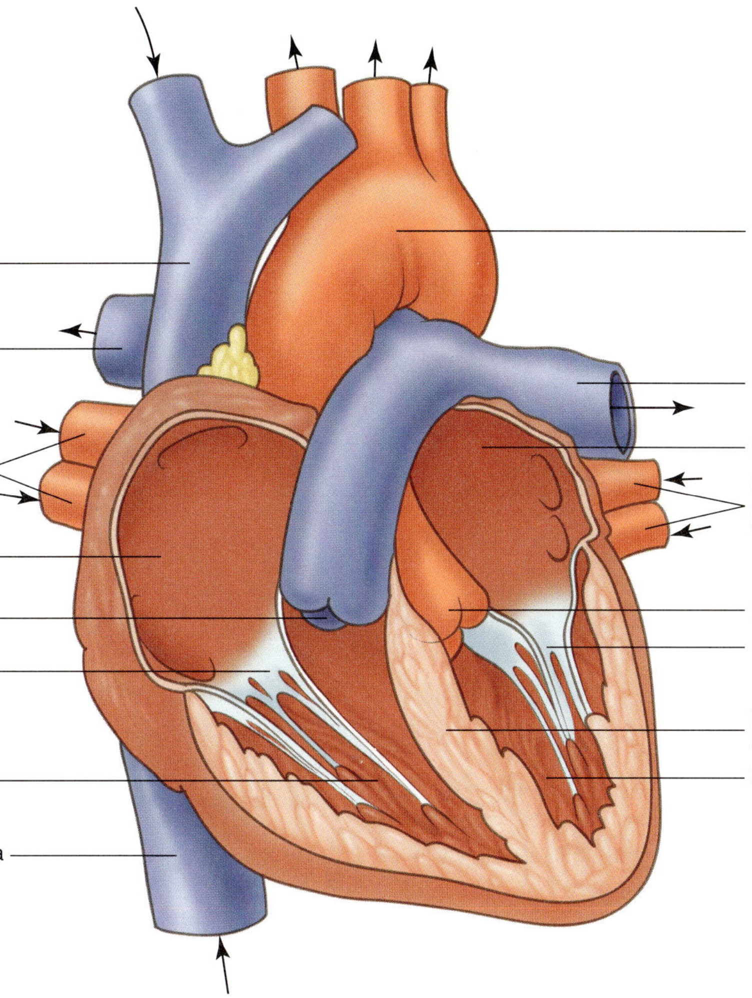

FIGURE 5.3 Anterior cross-section view of the heart.

- The **endocardium** (**en**-doh-**KAR**-dee-um), which consists of epithelial tissue, is the inner lining of the heart (**endo-** means within, **cardi** means heart, and **-um** is a singular noun ending). This is the surface that comes into direct contact with the blood as it is being pumped through the heart.

Blood Supply to the Myocardium

The myocardium, which beats constantly, must have a continuous supply of oxygen and nutrients plus prompt waste removal to survive. If for any reason this blood supply is disrupted, the myocardium of the affected area dies.

The **coronary arteries** (**KOR**-uh-**nerr**-ee), which supply oxygen-rich blood to the myocardium, are shown in red in Figure 5.6. The veins, which are shown in blue, remove waste products from the myocardium.

The Chambers of the Heart

The heart is divided into four chambers, each of which has a specialized function (Figure 5.3):

- The **atria** (**AY**-tree-ah) are the two upper chambers of the heart, and these chambers are divided by ***interatrial septum***. (A *septum* is a wall that separates two chambers.)
- The atria are the receiving chambers, and all blood enters the heart through these chambers. The singular form of *atria* is *atrium*.
- The **ventricles** (**VEN**-trih-kuhls) are the two lower chambers of the heart, and these chambers are divided by the ***interventricular septum***.
- The walls of the ventricles are thicker than those of the atria because the ventricles must pump blood throughout the entire body.
- The term ***ventricle*** is also defined as a normal hollow chamber of the brain (see Chapter 10).

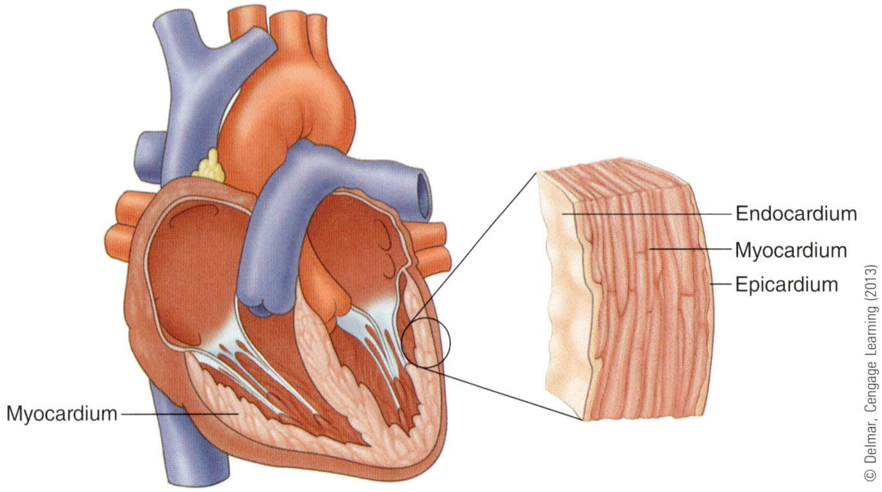

FIGURE 5.4 A simplified view of the tissues of the heart walls.

The Valves of the Heart

The flow of blood through the heart is controlled by four valves as described in this section. If any of these valves is not working correctly, blood cannot flow properly through the heart and cannot be pumped effectively to all parts of the body (Figures 5.3 and 5.5).

- The **tricuspid valve** (try-**KUS**-pid) controls the opening between the right atrium and the right ventricle. The term ***tricuspid*** means having three cusps (points), and this describes the shape of this valve.

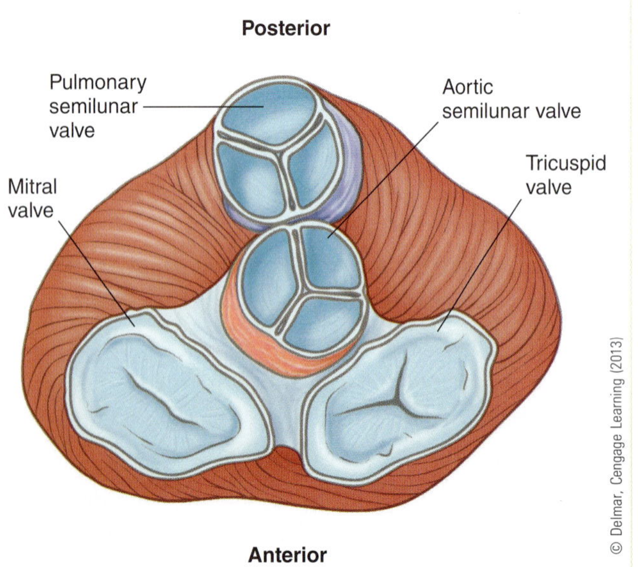

FIGURE 5.5 The valves of the heart viewed from above with the atria removed.

- The **pulmonary semilunar valve** (**PULL**-mah-**nair**-ee **sem**-ee-**LOO**-nar) is located between the right ventricle and the pulmonary artery. ***Pulmonary*** means pertaining to the lungs, and ***semilunar*** means half-moon. This valve is shaped like a half-moon.
- The **mitral valve** (**MY**-tral) is located between the left atrium and left ventricle. ***Mitral*** means shaped like a bishop's miter (hat). This valve is also known as the ***bicuspid valve*** because ***bicuspid*** means having two cusps (points), which describes the shape of this valve.
- The **aortic semilunar valve** (ay-**OR**-tick **sem**-ee-**LOO**-nar) is located between the left ventricle and the aorta. ***Aortic*** means pertaining to the aorta. ***Semilunar*** means half-moon, which describes the shape of this valve.
- The flow of blood through the heart is summarized in Table 5.1. The red arrows indicate oxygenated blood, and blue arrows indicate deoxygenated blood. ***Oxygenated*** means oxygen rich, or containing an adequate supply of oxygen. ***Deoxygenated*** means oxygen poor, or not yet containing an adequate supply of oxygen.

StudyWARE CONNECTION

Watch the **Blood Flow Through the Heart** animation in the StudyWARE™.

TABLE 5.1
Blood Flow Through the Heart

↓	The **right atrium** (RA) receives oxygen-poor blood from all tissues, except the lungs, through the superior and inferior venae cavae. Blood flows out of the RA through the tricuspid valve into the right ventricle.
↓	The **right ventricle** (RV) pumps the oxygen-poor blood through the pulmonary semilunar valve and into the pulmonary artery, which carries it to the lungs.
↓	The **left atrium** (LA) receives oxygen-rich blood from the lungs through the four pulmonary veins. The blood flows out of the LA, through the mitral valve, and into the left ventricle.
↓	The **left ventricle** (LV) receives oxygen-rich blood from the left atrium. Blood flows out of the LV through the aortic semilunar valve and into the aorta, which carries it to all parts of the body, except the lungs.
↓	Oxygen-poor blood is returned by the venae cavae to the right atrium, and the cycle continues.

Systemic and Pulmonary Circulation

Blood is pumped through the systemic and pulmonary circulation systems. Together the blood in these systems brings oxygen to the cells and removes waste products from the cells (Figure 5.6).

Pulmonary circulation is the flow of blood only between the heart and lungs.

- The **pulmonary arteries** carry deoxygenated blood out of the right ventricle and into the lungs. This is the only place in the body where deoxygenated blood is carried by arteries instead of veins.
- In the lungs, carbon dioxide from the body is exchanged for oxygen from the inhaled air.
- The **pulmonary veins** carry the oxygenated blood from the lungs into the left atrium of the heart. This is the only place in the body where veins carry oxygenated blood.

Systemic circulation includes the flow of blood to all parts of the body *except* the lungs.

- Oxygenated blood flows out of the left ventricle and into arterial circulation.
- The veins carry deoxygenated blood into the right atrium.
- From here, the blood flows into the pulmonary circulation before being pumped out of the heart into the arteries again.

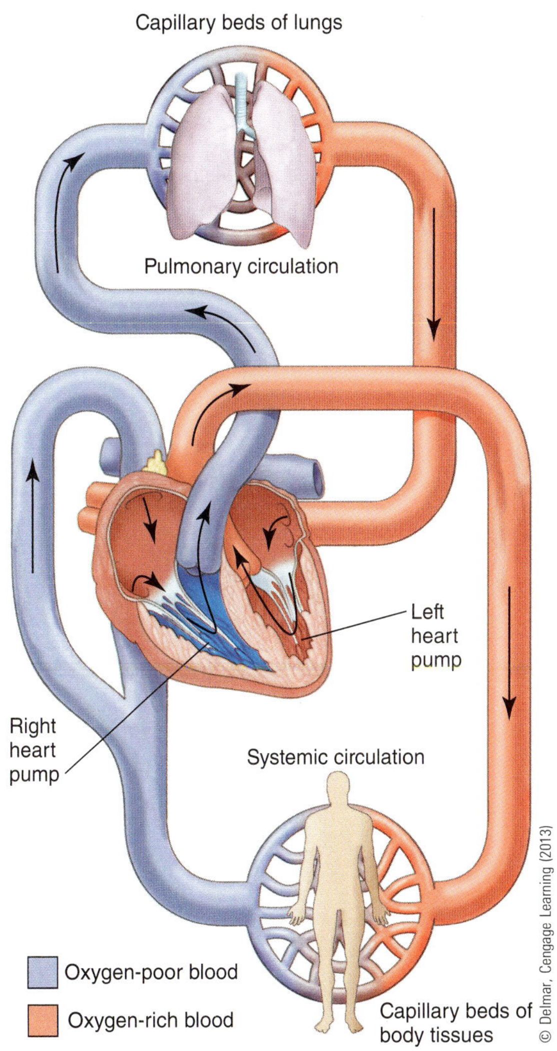

FIGURE 5.6 Systemic and pulmonary blood circulation.

The Heartbeat

The **heartbeat** is the ability to pump blood effectively throughout the body; the contraction and relaxation (beating) of the heart must occur in exactly the correct sequence.

- The rate and regularity of the heartbeat is determined by ***electrical impulses*** from nerves that stimulate the myocardium of the chambers of the heart. (The specialized myocardial muscles that make this pumping action possible are described in Chapter 4.)
- Also known as the ***conduction system***, these electrical impulses are controlled by the sinoatrial (SA) node, atrioventricular (AV) node, and the bundle of His (Figure 5.7).

The Sinoatrial Node

- The **sinoatrial node** (**sigh**-noh-**AY**-tree-ahl), which is often referred to as the ***SA node***, is located in the posterior wall of the right atrium near the entrance of the superior vena cava (Figure 5.7).
- The SA node establishes the basic rhythm and rate of the heartbeat. For this reason, it is known as the ***natural pacemaker*** of the heart.
- Electrical impulses from the SA node start each wave of muscle contraction in the heart.
- The impulse in the right atrium spreads over the muscles of both atria, causing them to contract simultaneously. This contraction forces blood into the ventricles.

The Atrioventricular Node

- The impulses from the SA node also travel to the **atrioventricular node** (**ay**-tree-oh-ven-**TRICK**-you-lar), which is also known as the ***AV node***.
- The AV node is located on the floor of the right atrium near the interatrial septum (Figure 5.7). From here, it transmits the electrical impulses onward to the bundle of His.

The Bundle of His

- The **bundle of His** (**HISS**) is a group of fibers located within the interventricular septum. These fibers carry an electrical impulse to ensure the sequence of the heart contractions (Figure 5.7). These electrical impulses travel onward to the right and left ventricles and the Purkinje fibers.
- **Purkinje fibers** (per-**KIN**-jee) are specialized conductive fibers located within the walls of the ventricles. These fibers relay the electrical impulses to the cells of the ventricles, and it is this stimulation that causes the ventricles to contract. This contraction

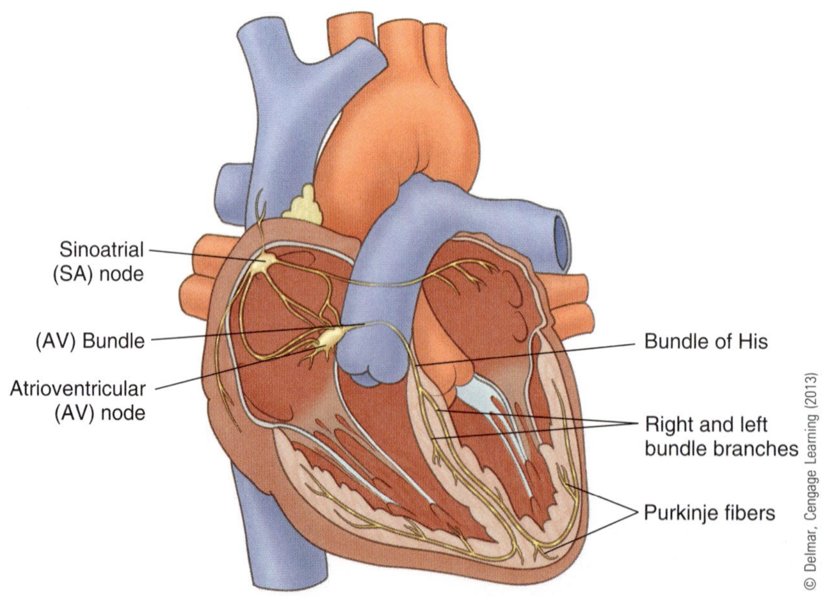

FIGURE 5.7 An electrical impulse from the SA node travels to the AV node and causes the ventricle to contract.

of the ventricles forces blood out of the heart and into the aorta and pulmonary arteries (Figure 5.7).

StudyWARE CONNECTION

Watch the **Electrical Stimulation of the Heart** animation in the StudyWARE™.

Electrical Waves

The activities of the electrical conduction system of the heart can be visualized as wave movements on a monitor or an electrocardiogram. The term ***sinus rhythm*** refers to the normal beating of the heart (Figures 5.8 and 5.16A).

- The ***P wave*** is due to the stimulation (contraction) of the atria.
- The ***QRS complex*** shows the stimulation (contraction) of the ventricles. The atria relax as the ventricles contract.
- The ***T wave*** is the recovery (relaxation) of the ventricles.

THE BLOOD VESSELS

There are three types of blood vessels: arteries, capillaries, and veins. These vessels form the arterial and venous circulatory systems (Figures 5.9 and 5.10).

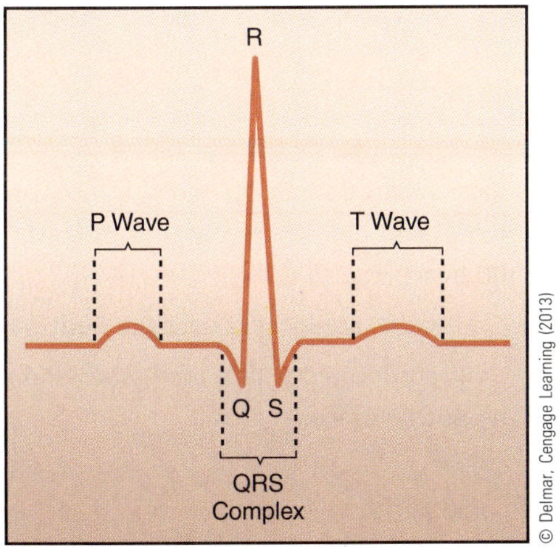

FIGURE 5.8 The waves of contraction and relaxation of the heart can be visualized on a monitor or as an electrocardiogram (EKG or ECG).

Arteries

- The **arteries** are large blood vessels that carry blood away from the heart to all regions of the body.
- The walls of the arteries are composed of three layers. This structure makes the arteries muscular and elastic so they can expand and contract with the pumping beat of the heart. The term ***endarterial*** means within an artery or pertaining to the inner portion of an artery.
- ***Arterial blood*** is bright red in color because it is oxygen rich. The pumping action of the heart causes blood to spurt out when an artery is cut.
- The **aorta** (ay-**OR**-tah) is the largest blood vessel in the body. It begins from the left ventricle of the heart and forms the main trunk of the arterial system (Figures 5.2 and 5.9).
- The **carotid arteries** (kah-**ROT**-id) are the major arteries that carry blood upward to the head.
- The ***common carotid artery*** is located on each side of the neck.
- It divides into the ***internal carotid artery***, which brings oxygen-rich blood to the brain.
- The ***external carotid artery*** brings blood to the face.
- Any disruption in this blood flow can result in a stroke or other brain damage.
- The **arterioles** (ar-**TEE**-ree-ohlz) are the smaller, thinner branches of arteries that deliver blood to the capillaries. As it enters one end of the capillary bed, it is here that the rate of flow of arterial blood slows.

Capillaries

Capillaries (**KAP**-uh-**ler**-eez), which are only one epithelial cell in thickness, are the smallest blood vessels in the body. The capillaries form networks of expanded vascular beds that have the important role of delivering oxygen and nutrients to the cells of the tissues (Figure 5.11).

- The capillaries further slow the flow of blood to allow plasma to flow into the tissues. It is here that the exchange of oxygen, nutrients, and waste materials occur within the surrounding cells.
- After leaving the cells, 90% of this fluid, which is now oxygen poor and contains some waste products, enter the opposite end of the capillary bed through the venules.
- The 10% of this fluid that is left behind in the tissues becomes lymph. This is explained in Chapter 6.

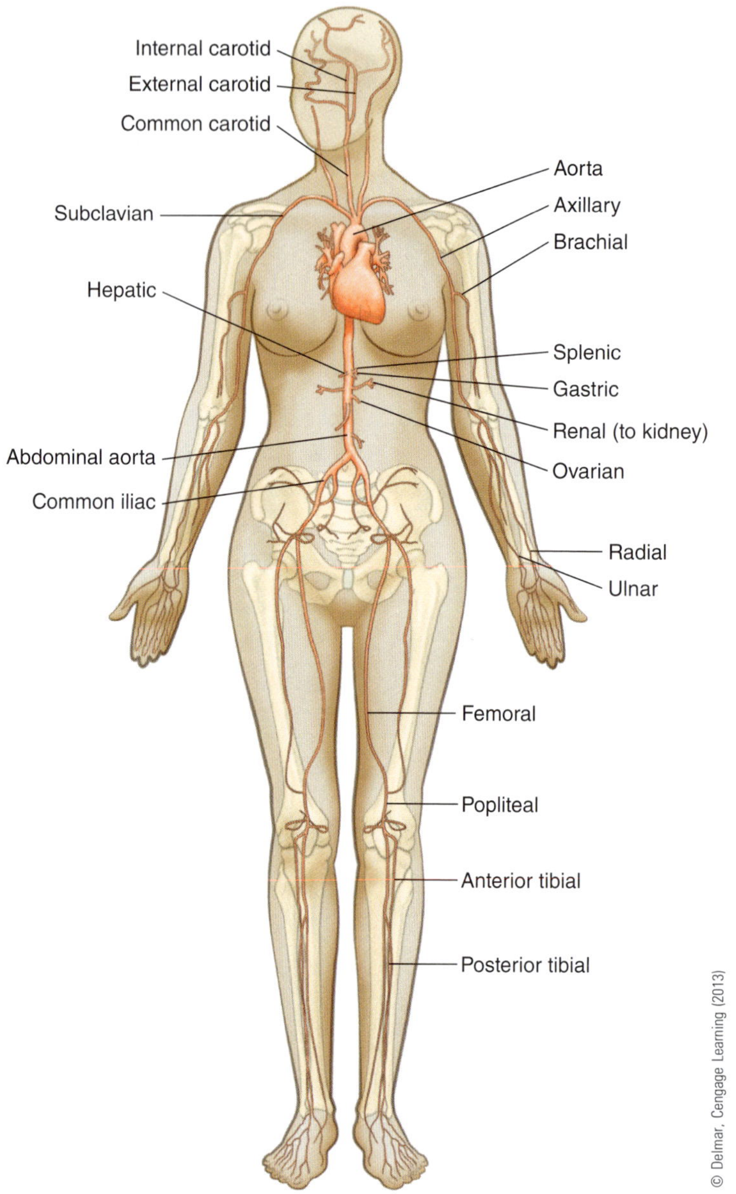

FIGURE 5.9 Anterior view of arterial circulation.

Veins

Veins form a low-pressure collecting system to return oxygen-poor blood to the heart (Figures 5.10 through 5.12).

- **Venules** (**VEN**-youls) are the smallest veins that join to form the larger veins.
- The walls of the veins are thinner and less elastic than those of the arteries.
- The venous blood continues its flow at an increased speed as it continues its return journey to the heart. ***Venous*** means relating to, or contained in, the veins.
- Veins have valves that enable blood to flow only toward the heart and to prevent it from flowing away from the heart (Figure 5.12).
- ***Superficial veins*** are located near the body surface.
- ***Deep veins*** are located within the tissues and away from the body surface.

The Venae Cavae

- The **venae cavae** (**VEE**-nee **KAY**-vee) are the two largest veins in the body. These are the veins that return blood into the heart (singular, *vena cava*).

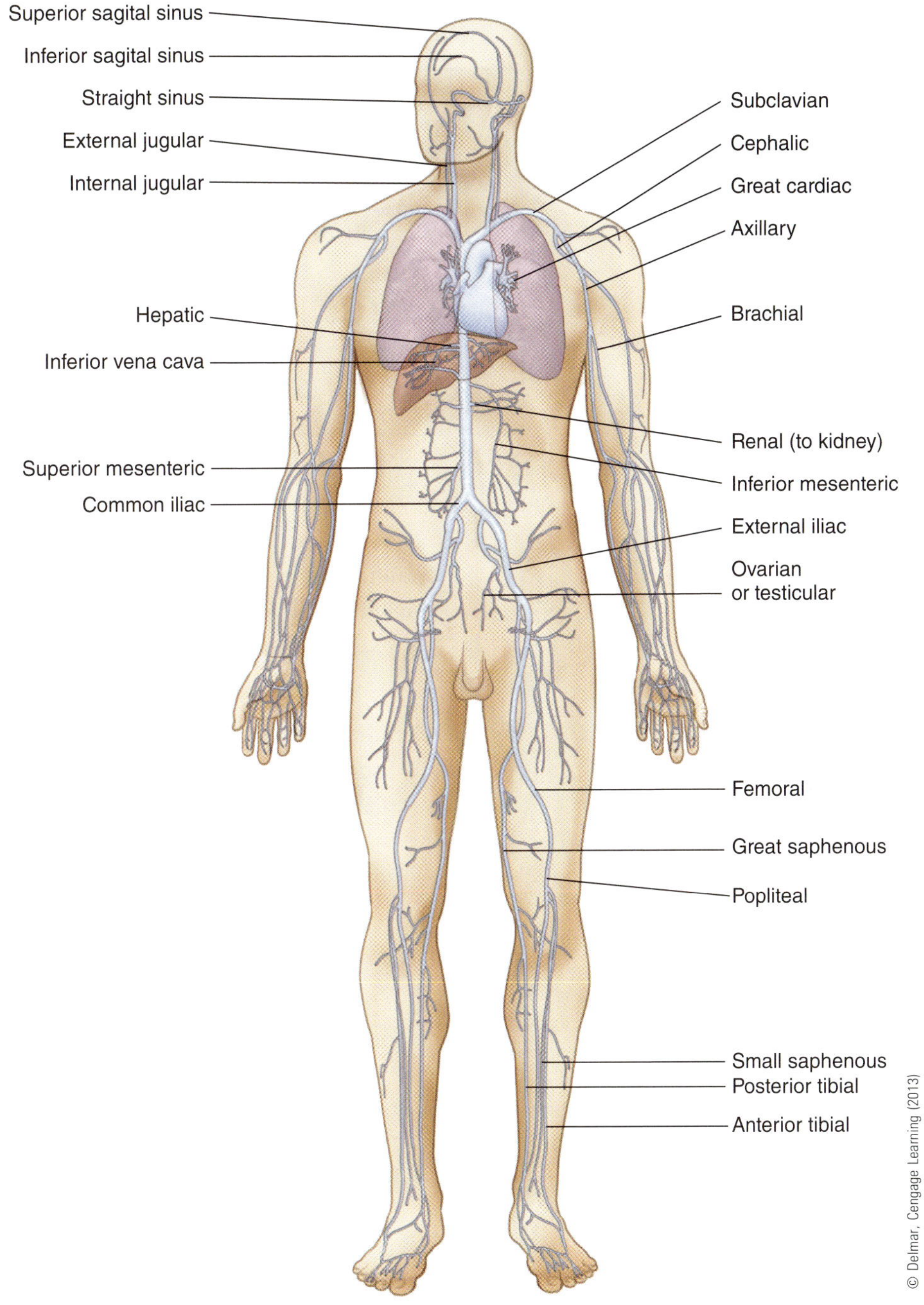

FIGURE 5.10 Anterior view of venous circulation.

- The *superior vena cava* transports blood from the upper portion of the body to the heart (Figures 5.2 and 5.3).
- The *inferior vena cava* transports blood from the lower portion of the body to the heart (Figure 5.3).

Pulse and Blood Pressure

- The **pulse** is the rhythmic pressure against the walls of an artery caused by the contraction of the heart. The *pulse rate* is discussed in Chapter 15.
- **Blood pressure** is the measurement of the amount of systolic and diastolic pressure exerted against the walls of the arteries. How to record blood pressure is discussed in Chapter 15. See Table 5.3 for blood pressure classifications.
- **Systolic pressure** (sis-**TOL**-ick), which occurs when the ventricles contract, is the highest pressure against the walls of an artery. The term *systole* means contraction of the heart, and *systolic* means pertaining to this contraction phase.

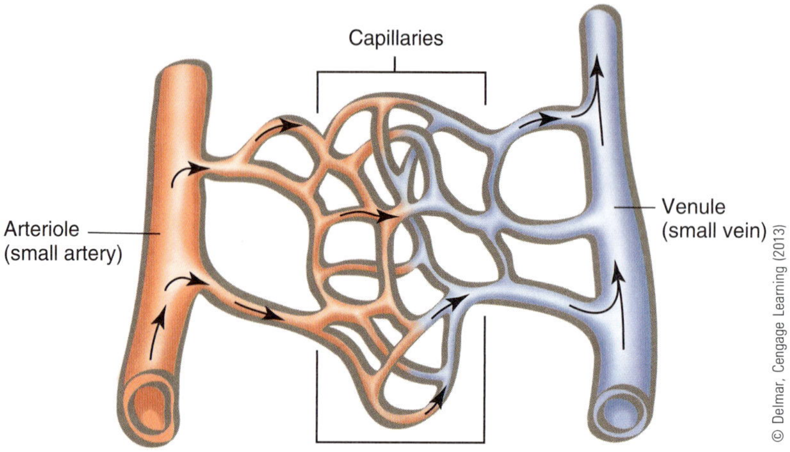

FIGURE 5.11 Oxygen-rich arterial blood is delivered by arterioles to the capillaries. After the oxygen has been extracted, the oxygen-poor blood is returned to circulation as venous blood.

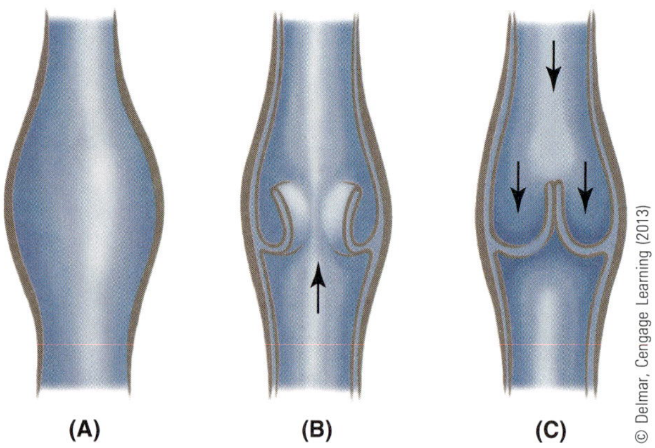

FIGURE 5.12 Veins contain valves to prevent the backward flow of blood. (A) External view of the vein shows wider area of valve. (B) Internal view with the valve open as blood flows through it toward the heart. (C) Internal view with the valve closed to prevent the backflow of blood.

- **Diastolic pressure** (dye-ah-**STOL**-ick), which occurs when the ventricles are relaxed, is the lowest pressure against the walls of an artery. The term *diastole* means relaxation of the heart, and *diastolic* means pertaining to this relaxation phase.

BLOOD

Blood is the fluid tissue in the body. It is composed of 55% liquid plasma and 45% formed elements. As you study these elements, refer to Figure 5.13.

Plasma

Plasma (**PLAZ**-mah) is a straw-colored fluid that contains nutrients, hormones, and waste products. Plasma is 91% water. The remaining 9% consists mainly of proteins, including the clotting proteins.

- **Serum** (**SEER**-um) is plasma fluid after the blood cells and the clotting proteins have been removed.
- **Fibrinogen** (figh-**BRIN**-oh-jen) and **prothrombin** (proh-**THROM**-bin) are the clotting proteins found in plasma. They have an important role in clot formation to control bleeding.

Formed Elements of the Blood

The formed elements of blood include erythrocytes, leukocytes, and thrombocytes.

Erythrocytes

Erythrocytes (eh-**RITH**-roh-sights), also known as *red blood cells* (RBC), are mature red blood cells produced by the red bone marrow (**erythr/o** means red, and **-cytes** means cells). The primary role of these cells is to transport oxygen to the tissues.

This oxygen is transported by **hemoglobin** (**hee**-moh-**GLOH**-bin), which is the oxygen-carrying blood protein pigment of the erythrocytes (**hem/o** means blood, and **-globin** means protein).

Leukocytes

Leukocytes (**LOO**-koh-sites), also known as *white blood cells* (WBC), are the blood cells involved in defending the body against infective organisms and foreign substances (**leuk/o** means white, and **-cytes** means cells). The following are the major groups of leukocytes:

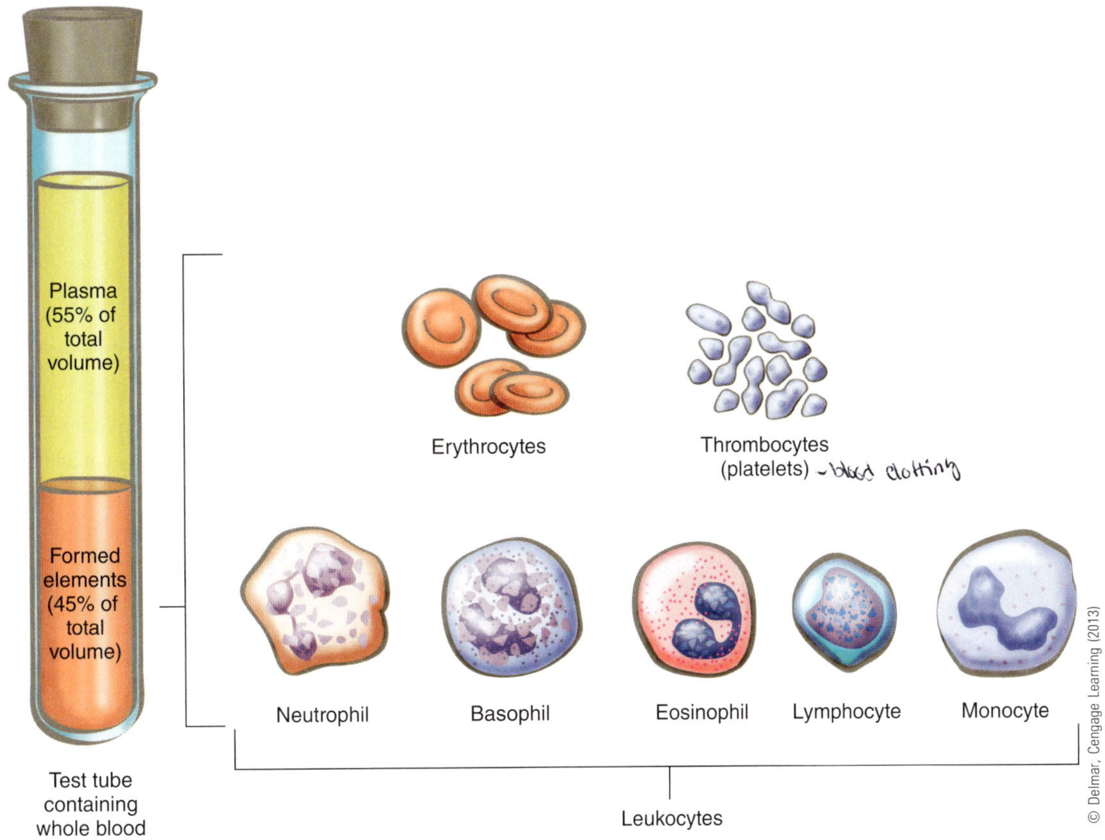

FIGURE 5.13 The major fluid and formed components of blood. The formed elements include erythrocytes, thrombocytes, and leukocytes.

- **Neutrophils** (**NEW**-troh-fills), which are formed in red bone marrow, are the most common type of WBC. Through phagocytosis, neutrophils play a major role in the immune system's defense against pathogens, including bacteria, viruses, and fungi. ***Phagocytosis*** is the process of destroying pathogens by surrounding and swallowing them. (Neutrophils are discussed further in Chapter 6.)
- **Basophils** (**BAY**-soh-fills), which are also formed in red bone marrow, are the least common type of WBC. Basophils are responsible for causing the symptoms of allergies.
- **Eosinophils** (**ee**-oh-**SIN**-oh-fills) are formed in red bone marrow and then migrate to tissues throughout the body. Here these cells destroy parasitic organisms and play a major role in allergic reactions.
- **Lymphocytes** (**LIM**-foh-sights) are formed in red bone marrow, in lymph nodes, and in the spleen. Lymphocytes identify foreign substances and germs (bacteria or viruses) in the body and produce antibodies that specifically target them. (Lymphocytes are discussed further in Chapter 6.)
- **Monocytes** (**MON**-oh-sights) are formed in red bone marrow, lymph nodes, and the spleen. Through phagocytosis, monocytes provide immunological defenses against many infectious organisms.

Thrombocytes

Thrombocytes (**THROM**-boh-sights), which are also known as ***platelets***, are the smallest formed elements of the blood. They play an important role in the clotting of blood (**thromb/o** means clot, and **-cytes** means cells).

- When a blood vessel is damaged, the thrombocytes are activated and become sticky.
- This action causes the thrombocytes to clump together to form a clot to stop the bleeding.

Blood Types

Blood types are classified according to the presence or absence of certain antigens. (An ***antigen*** is any substance that the body regards as being foreign.)

The four major blood types are **A**, **AB**, **B**, and **O**. The A, AB, and B groups are based on the presence of the A or

B antigens or both on the red blood cells. In contrast, in type O blood both the A and B antigens are absent.

The Rh Factor

The **Rh factor** defines the presence or absence of the Rh antigen on red blood cells. The Rh factor was so named because this antigen was first found in rhesus monkeys.

- About 85% of Americans have the Rh antigen, and these individuals are described as being ***Rh positive*** (Rh+).
- The remaining 15% of Americans *do not have* the Rh antigen, and these individuals are described as being ***Rh negative*** (Rh–).
- The Rh factor is an important consideration in cross-matching blood for transfusions (see Chapter 15).
- The Rh factor can cause difficulties when an Rh-positive infant is born to an Rh-negative mother (see Chapter 14).

Blood Gases

Blood gases are gases that are normally dissolved in the liquid portion of blood. The major blood gases are *oxygen* (O_2), *carbon dioxide* (CO_2), and *nitrogen* (N_2).

MEDICAL SPECIALTIES RELATED TO THE CARDIOVASCULAR SYSTEM

- A **cardiologist** (**kar**-dee-**OL**-oh-jist) is a physician who specializes in diagnosing and treating abnormalities, diseases, and disorders of the heart (**cardi** means heart, and **-ologist** means specialist).
- A **hematologist** (**hee**-mah-**TOL**-oh-jist) is a physician who specializes in diagnosing and treating abnormalities, diseases, and disorders of the blood and blood-forming tissues (**hemat** means blood, and **-ologist** means specialist).
- A **vascular surgeon** is a physician who specializes in the diagnosis, medical management, and surgical treatment of disorders of the blood vessels.

PATHOLOGY OF THE CARDIOVASCULAR SYSTEM

Disorders of the heart can be congenital (present from or before birth) or can develop at any time throughout life.

Congenital Heart Defects

Congenital heart defects are structural abnormalities caused by the failure of the heart to develop normally before birth. ***Congenital*** means present at birth. Some congenital heart defects are apparent at birth, whereas others may not be detected until later in life.

Coronary Artery Disease (CAD)

Coronary artery disease (CAD) is atherosclerosis of the coronary arteries that reduces the blood supply to the heart muscle. This creates an insufficient supply of oxygen that can cause angina (pain), a myocardial infarction (heart attack), or death. ***End-stage coronary artery disease*** is characterized by unrelenting angina pain and a severely limited lifestyle.

Atherosclerosis

Atherosclerosis (**ath**-er-**oh**-skleh-**ROH**-sis) is hardening and narrowing of the arteries caused by a buildup of cholesterol plaque on the interior walls of the arteries (**ather/o** means plaque or fatty substance, and **-sclerosis** means abnormal hardening) (Figures 5.14 and 5.15).

- This type of **plaque** (**PLACK**), which is found within the lumen of an artery, is a fatty deposit that is similar to the buildup of rust inside a pipe. (This substance is not the same as *dental plaque*, which is discussed in Chapter 8.) The ***lumen*** is the opening within these vessels through which the blood flows.
- The plaque can protrude outward into the lumen from the wall of the blood vessel or protrude inward into the wall of the vessel.
- An **atheroma** (**ath**-er-**OH**-mah), which is a characteristic of atherosclerosis, is a deposit of plaque on or within the arterial wall (**ather** means plaque, and **-oma** means tumor).

Ischemic Heart Disease

Ischemic heart disease (iss-**KEE**-mick) is a group of cardiac disabilities resulting from an insufficient supply of oxygenated blood to the heart. These diseases are usually associated with coronary artery disease. ***Ischemic*** means pertaining to the disruption of the blood supply. (See also *ischemic stroke* in Chapter 10.)

- **Ischemia** (iss-**KEE**-mee-ah) is a condition in which there is an insufficient supply of oxygen in the tissues due to a restricted blood flow to a part of the body

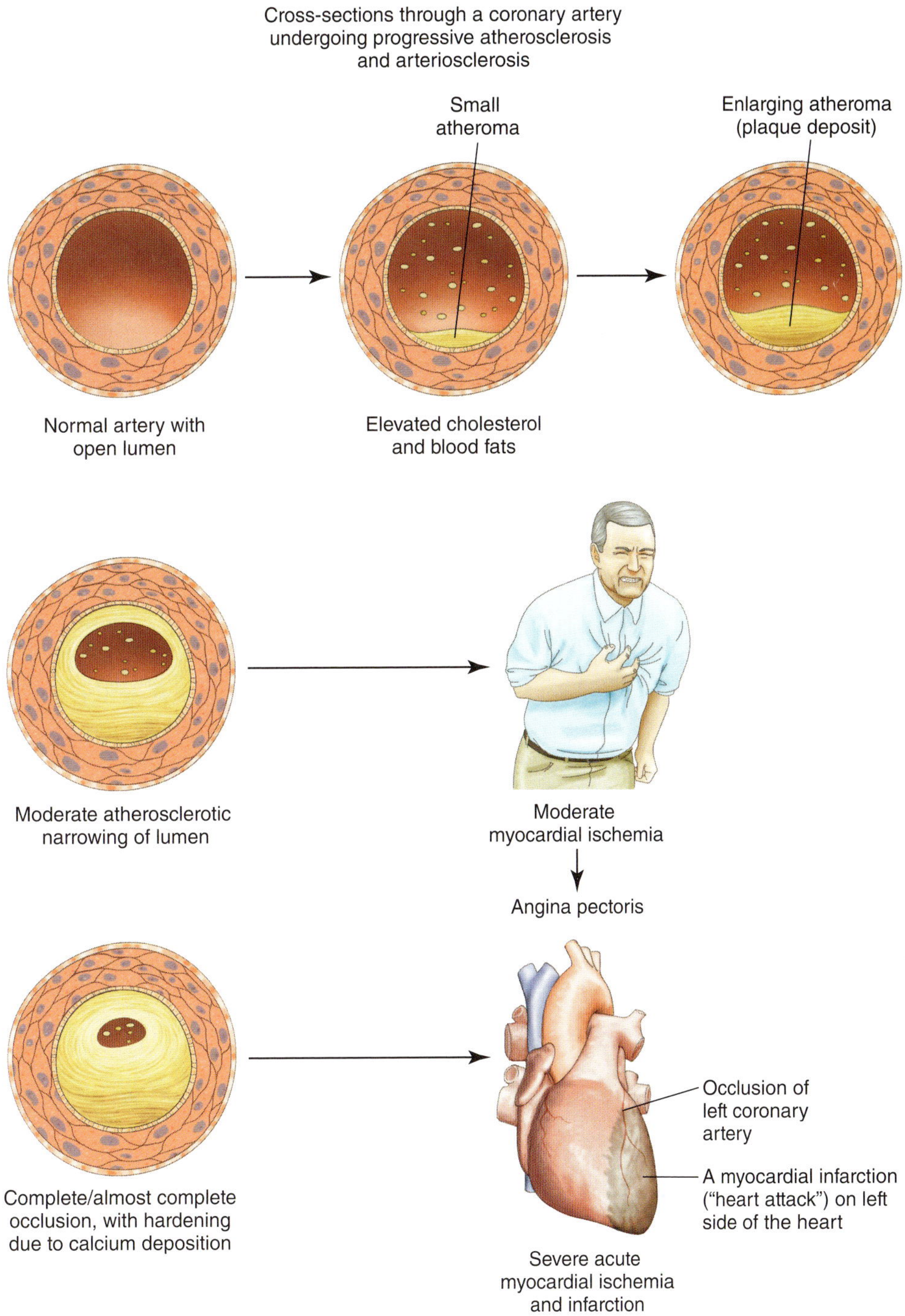

FIGURE 5.14 The progression of coronary heart disease resulting in a myocardial infarction.

(**isch** means to hold back, and **-emia** means blood). For example, ***cardiac ischemia*** is the lack of blood flow and oxygen to the heart muscle.

Angina

Angina (an-**JIH**-nuh), also known as ***angina pectoris***, is a condition in which severe episodes of chest pain occur due to an inadequate blood flow to the myocardium. These episodes are due to ischemia of the heart muscle and often progressively worsen as the blood flow continues to be compromised, until a myocardial infarction occurs.

- ***Stable angina*** occurs during exertion (exercise) and resolves with rest.
- ***Unstable angina*** may occur either during exertion or rest, and is a precursor to a myocardial infarction.

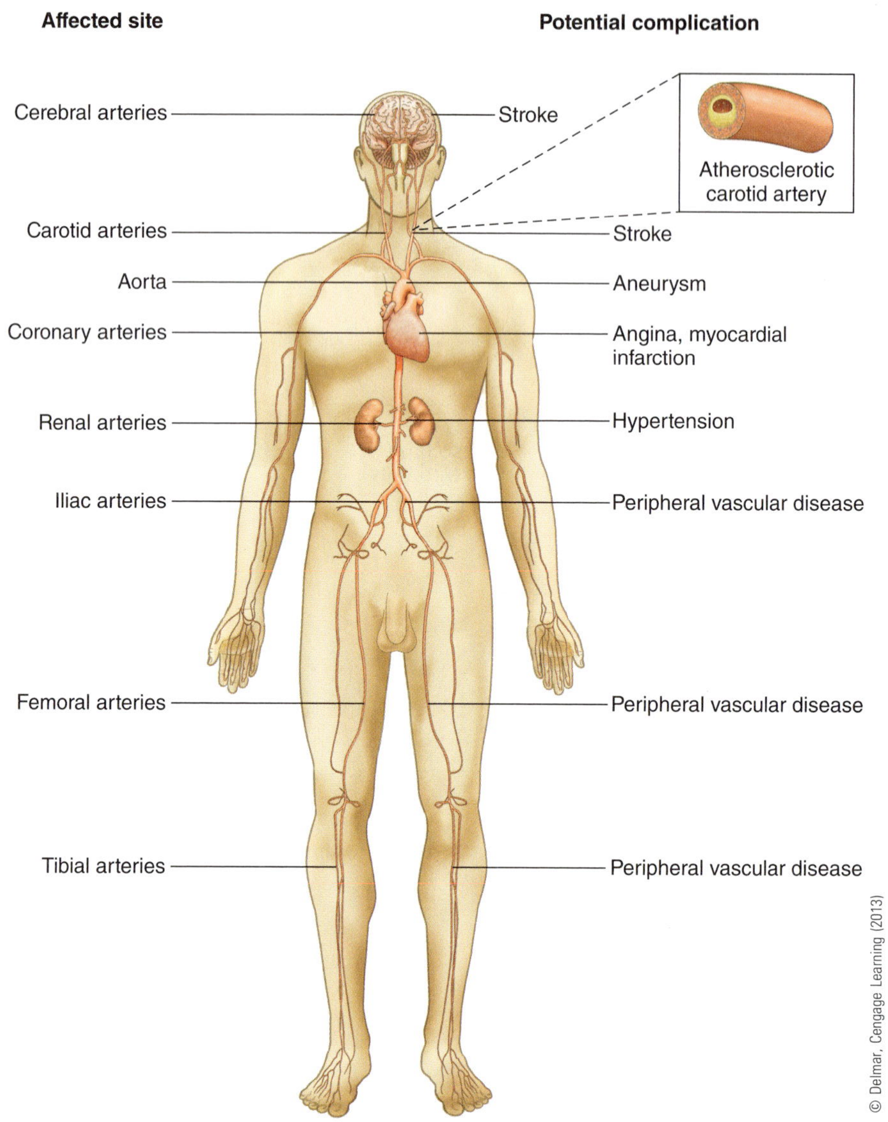

FIGURE 5.15 The sites affected by atherosclerosis (left column) and the potential complications of this condition (right column).

Myocardial Infarction

A **myocardial infarction** (**my**-oh-**KAR**-dee-al in-**FARK**-shun), commonly known as a ***heart attack***, is the occlusion (blockage) of one or more coronary arteries caused by plaque buildup. As used here, ***occlusion*** means total blockage.

- The term ***infarction*** means a sudden insufficiency of blood.
- An ***infarct*** is a localized area of dead tissue caused by a lack of blood.
- This damage to the myocardium impairs the heart's ability to pump blood throughout the body (Figure 5.14).
- The most frequently recognized symptoms of a myocardial infarction include pain or pressure in the middle of the chest that may spread to the back, jaw, or left arm. Many individuals having a heart attack have mild symptoms or none at all.
- Women are more likely to have atypical symptoms, including weakness and fatigue.

Heart Failure

Heart failure, which is also referred to as ***congestive heart failure (CHF)***, occurs most commonly in the elderly. In this chronic condition the heart is unable to pump out all of the blood that it receives. The decreased pumping action causes the congestion. The term ***congestion*** describes a fluid buildup.

- ***Left-sided heart failure*** causes an accumulation of fluid in the lungs also known as ***pulmonary edema***. This occurs because the left side of the heart is unable to efficiently pump oxygen-rich blood from the lungs to the rest of the body (see Chapter 7). The increase in pressure in the veins of the lungs results in localized fluid accumulation.
- ***Right-sided heart failure*** causes fluid buildup throughout the rest of the body. This occurs because the right side of the heart is unable to efficiently pump blood throughout the rest of the body. Due to the pressure of gravity, this edema, or swelling, is first noticeable in the feet and legs. As this swelling worsens, it can also affect the liver, gastrointestinal tract, or the arms.
- **Cardiomegaly** (**kar**-dee-oh-**MEG**-ah-lee) is the abnormal enlargement of the heart that is frequently associated with heart failure as the heart enlarges in an effort to compensate for its decreased pumping ability (**cardi/o** means heart, and **-megaly** means enlargement).

Carditis

Carditis (kar-**DYE**-tis) is an inflammation of the heart (**card** means heart, and **-itis** means inflammation). Note the spelling of *carditis*: In this term, the word root (combining form) **card/o** is used to avoid having a double *i* when it is joined with the suffix **-itis**.

- **Endocarditis** (**en**-doh-kar-**DYE**-tis) is an inflammation of the inner lining of the heart (**endo-** means within, **card** means heart, and **-itis** means inflammation).
- **Bacterial endocarditis** is an inflammation of the lining or valves of the heart caused by the presence of bacteria in the bloodstream. One cause of this condition is bleeding during dental surgery because it allows bacteria from the mouth to enter the bloodstream.
- **Pericarditis** (**pehr**-ih-kar-**DYE**-tis) is an inflammation of the pericardium (**peri-** means surrounding, **card** means heart, and **-itis** means inflammation). This inflammation causes an accumulation of fluid within the pericardial sac, and this excess fluid restricts the beating of the heart, thereby reducing the ability of the heart to pump blood throughout the body.
- **Myocarditis** (**my**-oh-kar-**DYE**-tis) is an uncommon condition that is an inflammation of the myocardium (heart muscle) that develops as a complication of a viral infection (**my/o** means muscle, **card** means heart, and **-itis** means inflammation).

Diseases of the Myocardium

- **Cardiomyopathy** (**kar**-dee-oh-my-**OP**-pah-thee) is the term used to describe all diseases of the heart muscle (**cardi/o** means heart, **my/o** means muscle, and **-pathy** means disease).
- ***Dilated cardiomyopathy*** is a disease of the heart muscle that causes the heart to become enlarged and to pump less strongly. The progression of this condition is usually slow and only presents with symptoms when quite advanced. ***Dilated*** means the expansion of a hollow structure.

Heart Valves

- A **heart murmur** is an abnormal blowing or clicking sound heard when listening to the heart or a neighboring large blood vessels. Heart murmurs are most often caused by defective heart valves, but do not usually require surgery unless they affect the patient's quality of life.
- **Valvulitis** (**val**-view-**LYE**-tis) is an inflammation of a heart valve (**valvul** means valve, and **-itis** means inflammation).
- **Valvular prolapse** (**VAL**-voo-lar proh-**LAPS**) is the abnormal protrusion of a heart valve that results in the inability of the valve to close completely (**valvul** means valve, and **-ar** means pertaining to). ***Prolapse*** means the falling or dropping down of an organ or internal part. This condition is named for the affected valve, such as a ***mitral valve prolapse***.
- **Valvular stenosis** (steh-**NOH**-sis) is a condition in which there is narrowing, stiffening, thickening, or blockage of one or more valves of the heart. ***Stenosis*** is the abnormal narrowing of an opening. These conditions are named for the affected valve, such as ***aortic valve stenosis***.

Cardiac Arrest and Arrhythmia

An **arrhythmia** (ah-**RITH**-mee-ah) is the loss of the normal rhythm of the heartbeat. This can be a minor, temporary episode, or it can be a fatal event. The severity of this episode depends on how much the heart's ability to pump blood is compromised. Rather than being an abnormality in the heart muscle, arrhythmias are usually caused by an abnormality in the electrical conduction system of the heart.

- **Asystole** (ay-**SIS**-toh-lee), known as a *flat line* (**a-** means without, and **systole** means contraction), is the complete lack of electrical activity in the heart. The resulting lack of heart contractions, with no blood pumping from the heart and no blood flow through the body, is one of the conditions required for a medical practitioner to certify death.
- **Cardiac arrest** is an event in which the heart abruptly stops beating or develops an arrhythmia that prevents it from pumping blood effectively.
- **Sudden cardiac death** results when treatment of cardiac arrest is not provided within a few minutes.
- **Bradycardia** (**brad**-ee-**KAR**-dee-ah) is an abnormally slow resting heart rate (**brady-** means slow, **card** means heart, and **-ia** means abnormal condition). The term *bradycardia* is usually applied to a *heartbeat rate* of less than 60 beats per minute. This condition is the opposite of *tachycardia.*
- **Tachycardia** (**tack**-ee-**KAR**-dee-ah) is an abnormally rapid resting heart rate (**tachy-** means rapid, **card** means heart, and **-ia** means abnormal condition). The term *tachycardia* is usually applied to a heartbeat rate of greater than 100 beats per minute. This condition is the opposite of *bradycardia.*
- **Palpitation** (**pal**-pih-**TAY**-shun) is a pounding or racing heartbeat with or without irregularity in rhythm. This condition is associated with certain heart disorders; however, it can also occur during a panic attack (see Chapter 10).

Atrial and Ventricular Fibrillations

The term **fibrillation** (**fih**-brih-**LAY**-shun) describes a rapid and uncontrolled heartbeat. The addition of the term *atrial* or *ventricular* identifies which heart chambers are affected.

- **Atrial fibrillation** (**AY**-tree-al **fih**-brih-**LAY**-shun), also known as *A-fib*, occurs when the normal rhythmic contractions of the atria are replaced by rapid, irregular twitching of the muscular heart wall. This causes an irregular and quivering action of the atria (Figure 5.16B).

Some of the increased electrical impulses reach the ventricles, and this makes them contract more rapidly and less efficiently than normal, causing an irregular rate of 80–180 beats per minute or more.

- **Paroxysmal supraventricular tachycardia** (**par**-ock-**SIZ**-mal **soo**-prah-ven-**TRICK**-you-lar **tack**-ee-**KAR**-dee-ah), also known as *PSVT*, is an episode that begins and ends abruptly during which there are very rapid and regular heartbeats that originate in the atrium or in the AV node (Figure 5.16C). ***Paroxysmal*** means pertaining to sudden occurrence. Compare *PSVT* with *ventricular tachycardia.*
- **Ventricular fibrillation** (ven-**TRICK**-you-lar **fih**-brih-**LAY**-shun), also known as *V-fib*, consists of rapid, irregular, and useless contractions of the ventricles. Instead of pumping strongly, the heart muscle quivers ineffectively. This condition is the cause of many sudden cardiac deaths (Figure 5.16D).
- **Ventricular tachycardia** (ven-**TRICK**-you-lar **tack**-ee-**KAR**-dee-ah), also known as *V-tach*, is a very rapid heartbeat that begins within the ventricles. This condition is potentially fatal because the heart is beating so rapidly that it is unable to adequately pump blood through the body. For some patients, this condition can be controlled with an automated implantable cardioverter-defibrillator. Compare *V-tach* with *paroxysmal supraventricular tachycardia.*

Blood Vessel Abnormalities

- **Vasculitis** (**vas**-kyou-**LYE**-tis) is the inflammation of a blood vessel (**vascul** means blood vessels, and **-itis** means inflammation). There are many types of vasculitis, including phlebitis (under "Veins") and *angiitis* or *arteritis* (inflammation of the arteries).
  - **Polyarteritis** (**pol**-ee-**ar**-teh-**RYE**-tis) is a form of vasculitis involving several medium and small arteries at the same time (**poly-** means many, **arter** means artery, and **-itis** mean inflammation). Polyarteritis is a rare but serious blood vessel disease that occurs when certain immune cells attack the affected arteries.
  - **Temporal arteritis** (**TEM**-poh-**ral ar**-teh-**RYE**-tis), also known as *giant cell arteritis*, is a form of vasculitis that can cause headaches, visual impairment, jaw pain, and other symptoms. It is diagnosed when a biopsy shows the presence of abnormally large cells. Temporal arteritis can cause unilateral or bilateral blindness, and more rarely, a stroke.
- **Angiostenosis** (**AN**-jee-oh-steh-**NOH**-sis) is the abnormal narrowing of a blood vessel (**angi/o** means vessel, and **-stenosis** means abnormal narrowing).
- A **hemangioma** (hee-**man**-jee-**OH**-mah) is a benign tumor made up of newly formed blood vessels (**hem** means blood, **angi** means blood or lymph vessel, and **-oma** means tumor) (see birthmarks in Chapter 12).

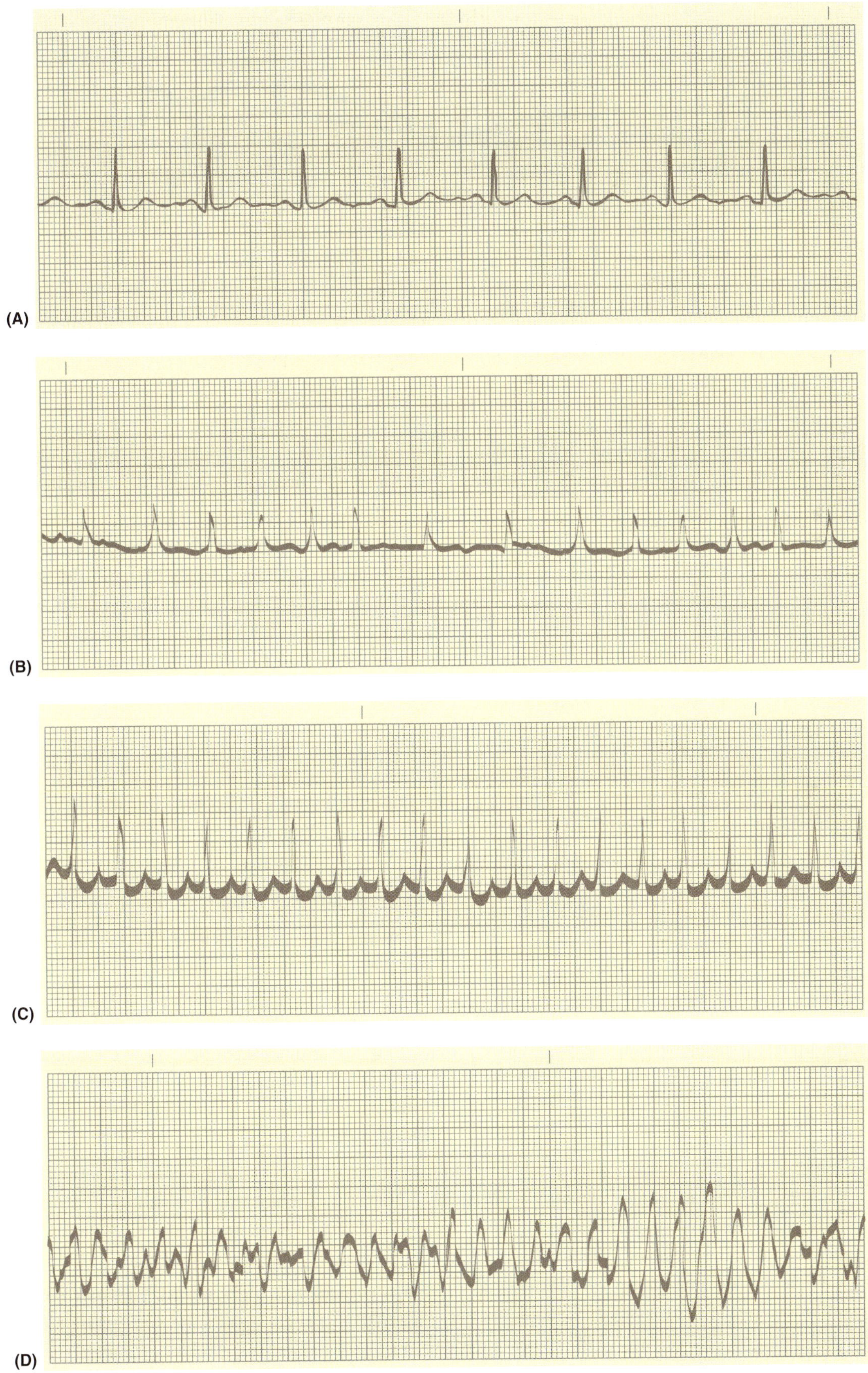

FIGURE 5.16 Electrocardiograms showing disruptions of heart rhythms. (A) Normal sinus rhythm. (B) Atrial fibrillation. (C) Paroxysmal supraventricular tachycardia. (D) Ventricular fibrillation.

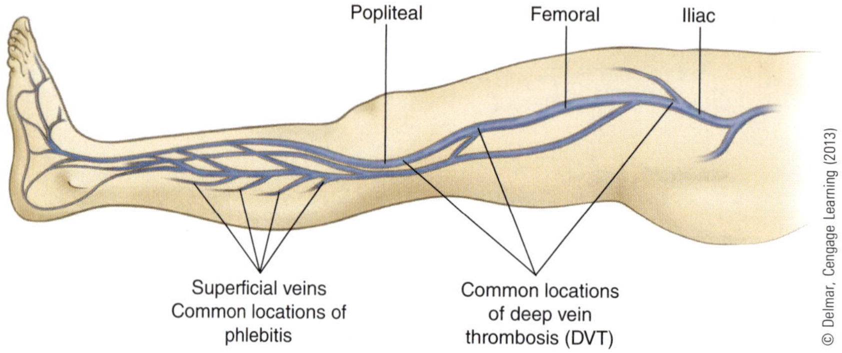

FIGURE 5.17 Common sites for the development of phlebitis and deep vein thrombosis.

- **Hypoperfusion** (**high**-poh-per-**FYOU**-zhun) is a deficiency of blood passing through an organ or body part. ***Perfusion*** is the flow of blood through the vessels of an organ.

Arteries

- An **aneurysm** (**AN**-you-rizm) is a localized weak spot or balloon-like enlargement of the wall of an artery. The rupture of an aneurysm can be fatal because of the rapid loss of blood. Aneurysms are named for the artery involved such as ***aortic aneurysm***, ***abdominal aortic aneurysm***, and ***popliteal aneurysm***.
- **Arteriosclerosis** (ar-**tee**-ree-oh-skleh-**ROH**-sis), also known as ***hardening of the arteries***, is any of a group of diseases characterized by thickening and the loss of elasticity of arterial walls (**arteri/o** means artery, and **-sclerosis** mean abnormal hardening).
- **Arteriostenosis** (ar-**tee**-ree-oh-steh-**NOH**-sis) is the abnormal narrowing of an artery or arteries (**arteri/o** means artery, and **-stenosis** means abnormal narrowing).

Veins

- **Chronic venous insufficiency**, also known as ***venous insufficiency***, is a condition in which venous circulation is inadequate due to partial vein blockage or to the leakage of venous valves. This condition primarily affects the feet and ankles, and the leakage of venous blood into the tissues causes discoloration of the skin.
- **Phlebitis** (fleh-**BYE**-tis) is the inflammation of a vein (**phleb** means vein, and **-itis** means inflammation). It is also known as ***thrombophlebitis***, because the walls of the vein are often infiltrated and a clot (thrombus) formed. This condition usually occurs in a superficial vein (Figure 5.17).
- **Varicose veins** (**VAR**-ih-kohs **VAYNS**) are abnormally swollen veins that usually occur in the superficial veins of the legs. This condition occurs when the valves in these veins do not function properly, so blood pools in the veins, causing them to enlarge.

Thromboses and Embolisms

Thromboses and embolisms are serious conditions that can result in the blockage of a blood vessel.

Thrombosis

A **thrombosis** (throm-**BOH**-sis) is the abnormal condition of having a thrombus (**thromb** means clot, and **-osis** means abnormal condition or disease) (Figure 5.18). The plural form is *thromboses.*

A **thrombus** (**THROM**-bus) is a blood clot attached to the interior wall of an artery or vein (**thromb** means clot, and **-us** is a singular noun ending) (plural, *thrombi*).

- A **thrombotic occlusion** (throm-**BOT**-ick ah-**KLOO**-zhun) is the blocking of an artery by a thrombus. ***Thrombotic*** means caused by a thrombus. As used here, ***occlusion*** means blockage.
- A **coronary thrombosis** (**KOR**-uh-**nerr**-ee throm-**BOH**-sis) is damage to the heart muscle caused by a thrombus blocking a coronary artery (**coron** means crown, and **-ary** means pertaining to, and **thromb** means clot, and **-osis** means abnormal condition).

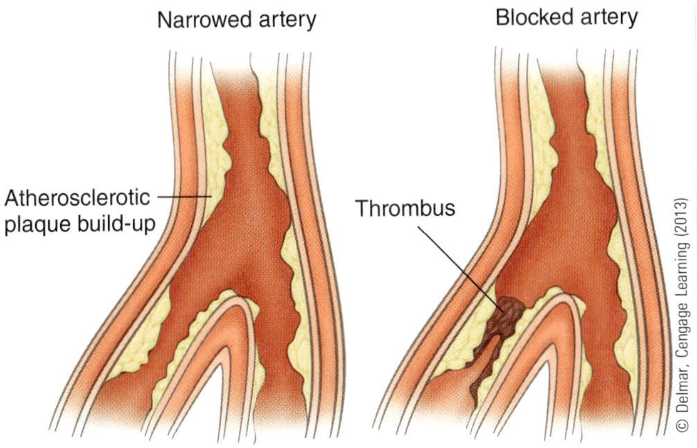

FIGURE 5.18 A thrombus is a blood clot attached to the interior wall of an artery or vein.

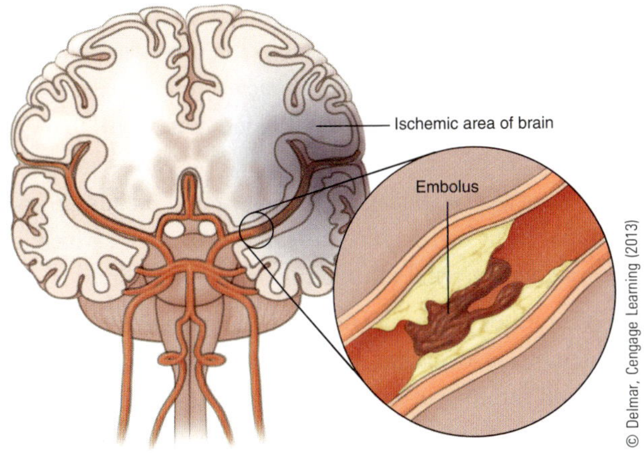

FIGURE 5.19 An embolus is a foreign object circulating in the blood.

- A **deep vein thrombosis** (DVT), also known as a ***deep venous thrombosis***, is the condition of having a thrombus attached to the interior wall of a deep vein. Sometimes such a blockage forms in the legs of a bedridden patient or in someone who has remained seated too long in an airplane or car. The danger is that the thrombus (clot) will break loose and travel to a lung where it can be fatal by causing a blockage (Figure 5.17).

Embolism

An **embolism** (**EM**-boh-lizm) is the sudden blockage of a blood vessel by an embolus (**embol** means something inserted, and **-ism** means condition). The embolism is often named for the causative factor, such as an ***air embolism*** or a ***fat embolism*** (Figure 5.19), or its location, such as ***pulmonary embolism***.

- An **embolus** (**EM**-boh-lus) is a foreign object, such as a blood clot, a quantity of air or gas, or a bit of tissue or tumor that is circulating in the blood (**embol** means something inserted, and **-us** is a singular noun ending) (plural, *emboli*).

Peripheral Vascular Diseases

Peripheral vascular diseases are disorders of blood vessels that are located outside of the heart and brain. These conditions usually involve narrowing of the vessels that carry blood to the legs, arms, stomach, or kidneys.

- **Peripheral arterial occlusive disease** (per-**IH**-feh-**ral** ar-**TEE**-ree-al oh-**KLOO**-siv), also known as ***peripheral artery disease***, is an example of a peripheral vascular disease that is caused by atherosclerosis. This condition is a common and serious problem affecting more than 20% of all patients over 70 years of age. Impaired circulation to the extremities and vital organs can cause changes in the skin color and temperature. It is also involved with *intermittent claudication*, which is discussed in Chapter 4.
- **Raynaud's disease** (ray-**NOHZ**) is a peripheral arterial occlusive disease in which intermittent attacks are triggered by cold or stress. The symptoms, which are due to constricted circulation, include pallor (paleness), cyanosis (blue color), and redness of the fingers and toes.

Blood Disorders

- **Blood dyscrasia** (dis-**KRAY**-zee-ah) is any pathologic condition of the cellular elements of the blood (**dys-** means bad, and **-crasia** means a mixture or blending).
- **Hemochromatosis** (**hee**-moh-**kroh**-mah-**TOH**-sis), also known as ***iron overload disease***, is a genetic disorder in which the intestines absorb too much iron (**hem/o** means blood, **chromat** means color, and **-osis** means abnormal condition or disease). The excess iron that is absorbed enters the bloodstream and accumulates in organs where it causes damage.
- **Leukopenia** (**loo**-koh-**PEE**-nee-ah) is a decrease in the number of disease-fighting white blood cells circulating in the blood (**leuk/o** means white, and **-penia** means deficiency). This condition, which is also known as a ***low white blood cell count***, places the patient at an increased of risk of developing or having difficulty fighting infections.
- **Polycythemia** (**pol**-ee-sy-**THEE**-mee-ah) is an abnormal increase in the number of red cells in the blood due to excess production of these cells by the bone marrow.

- **Septicemia** (**sep**-tih-**SEE**-mee-ah) is often associated with severe infections caused by the presence of bacteria in the blood. Also known as **bacteremia** (**bacter** means bacteria, and **-emia** means a blood condition), this condition can begin with a sudden onset of symptoms that include a spiking fever, chills, rapid breathing, and rapid heart rate. Septicemia can lead to *sepsis*, which is a systemic bacterial infection in the bloodstream.
- **Thrombocytopenia** (**throm**-boh-**sigh**-toh-**PEE**-nee-ah) is a condition in which there is an abnormally small number of platelets circulating in the blood (**thromb/o** means clot, **cyt/o** means cell, and **-penia** means deficiency). Because these cells help the blood to clot, this condition is sometimes associated with abnormal bleeding.
- **Thromocytosis** (**throm**-boh-sigh-**TOH**-sis) is an abnormal increase in the number of platelets in the circulating blood (**thromb/o** means clot, **cyt** means cell, and **-osis** means abnormal condition).
- A **hemorrhage** (**HEM**-or-idj) is the loss of a large amount of blood in a short time (**hem/o** means blood, and **-rrhage** means bleeding). This term also means *to bleed.*
- A **transfusion reaction** is a serious and potentially fatal complication of a blood transfusion in which a severe immune response occurs because the patient's blood and the donated blood do not match.

Cholesterol

- **Cholesterol** (koh-**LES**-ter-ol) is a fatty substance that travels through the blood and is found in all parts of the body. It aids in the production of cell membranes, some hormones, and vitamin D. Some cholesterol comes from dietary sources, and some is created by the liver. Excessively high levels of certain types of cholesterol can lead to heart disease (Table 5.2).
- **Hyperlipidemia** (**high**-per-**lip**-ih-**DEE**-mee-ah) is the general term used to describe elevated levels of cholesterol and other fatty substances in the blood (**hyper-** means excessive, **lipid** means fat, and **-emia** means blood condition).

TABLE 5.2
Interpreting Cholesterol Levels

Total cholesterol is measured in terms of milligrams (mg) per deciliter (dL) of blood. A *milligram* is equal to one-thousandth of a gram.A *deciliter* is equal to one-tenth of a liter	*Desirable levels* are below 200 mg/dL. *Borderline high levels* are 200–239 mg/dL. *High levels* are 240 mg/dL and above.
Low-density lipoprotein cholesterol (LDL) is referred to as *bad cholesterol* because excess quantities of LDL contribute to plaque buildup in the arteries.	*Optimal levels* are below 100 mg/dL. *Near optimal* levels are 100–129 mg/dL. *Borderline high* levels are 130–159 mg/dL. *High levels* are 160–189 mg/dL. *Very high levels* are 190 mg/dL and above.
High-density lipoprotein cholesterol (HDL) is referred to as *good cholesterol* because it carries unneeded cholesterol back to the liver for processing and does not contribute to plaque buildup.	*Bad levels* are below 40 mg/dL. *Better levels* are between 40 and 59 mg/dL. *Best levels* are 60 mg/dL and above.
Triglycerides (try-**GLIS**-er-eyeds) are combinations of *fatty acids* attached to glycerol that are also found normally in the blood in limited quantities.	*Desirable levels* are below 150 mg/dL. *Borderline high levels* are 150–199 mg/dL. *High levels* are 200–499 mg/dL. *Very high levels* are 500 mg/dL and above.

Source: National Heart, Lung, and Blood Institute, 2010.

Leukemia

- **Myelodysplastic syndrome** (**my**-eh-loh-dis-**PLAS**-tick) is a group of bone marrow disorders that are characterized by the insufficient production of one or more types of blood cells due to dysfunction of the bone marrow.
- **Leukemia** (loo-**KEE**-mee-ah) is a type of cancer characterized by a progressive increase in the number of abnormal leukocytes (white blood cells) found in blood-forming tissues, other organs, and in the circulating blood (**leuk** means white, and **-emia** means blood condition).

Anemias

Anemia (ah-**NEE**-mee-ah) is a lower-than-normal number of erythrocytes (red blood cells) in the blood (**an-** means without or less than, and **-emia** means blood condition). The severity of this condition is usually measured by a decrease in the amount of hemoglobin in the blood. When inadequate hemoglobin is present, all parts of the body receive less oxygen and have less energy than is needed to function properly.

- **Aplastic anemia** (ay-**PLAS**-tick ah-**NEE**-mee-ah) is characterized by an absence of *all* formed blood elements caused by the failure of blood cell production in the bone marrow (**a-** means without, **plast** means growth, and **-ic** means pertaining to). Anemia, a low red blood cell count, leads to fatigue and weakness. Leukopenia, a low white blood cell count, causes an increased risk of infection. Thrombocytopenia, a low platelet count, results in bleeding especially from mucous membranes and skin.
- **Hemolytic anemia** (**hee**-moh-**LIT**-ick ah-**NEE**-mee-ah) is characterized by an inadequate number of circulating red blood cells due to the premature destruction of red blood cells by the spleen (**hem/o** means relating to blood, and **-lytic** means to destroy). ***Hemolytic*** means pertaining to breaking down of red blood cells.
- **Iron-deficiency anemia** is the most common form of anemia. Iron, an essential component of hemoglobin, is normally obtained through food intake and by recycling iron from old red blood cells. Without sufficient iron to help create hemoglobin, blood cannot carry oxygen effectively.
- **Megaloblastic anemia** (**MEG**-ah-loh-**blas**-tick ah-**NEE**-mee-ah) is a blood disorder characterized by anemia in which the red blood cells are larger than normal (**mega-** means large, **blast** means immature, and **-tic** means pertaining to). This condition usually results from a deficiency of folic acid or of vitamin B_{12}.
- **Pernicious anemia** (per-**NISH**-us ah-**NEE**-mee-ah) is caused by a lack of the protein ***intrinsic factor*** (IF) that helps the body absorb vitamin B_{12} from the gastrointestinal tract. Vitamin B_{12} is necessary for the formation of red blood cells.
- **Sickle cell anemia** is a genetic disorder that causes abnormal hemoglobin, resulting in some red blood cells assuming an abnormal sickle shape. This sickle shape interferes with normal blood flow, resulting in damage to most of the body systems. The genetic transmission of sickle cell anemia is discussed in Chapter 2.
- **Thalassemia** (thal-ah-**SEE**-mee-ah) is an inherited blood disorder that causes mild or severe anemia due to reduced hemoglobin and fewer red blood cells than normal. ***Cooley's anemia*** is the name that is sometimes used to refer to any type of thalassemia that requires treatment with regular blood transfusions.

Hypertension

Hypertension (HTN), commonly known as ***high blood pressure***, is the elevation of arterial blood pressure to a level that is likely to cause damage to the cardiovascular system. Hypertension is the opposite of *hypotension*.

- ***Essential hypertension***, also known as ***primary hypertension*** or ***idiopathic hypertension***, is consistently elevated blood pressure of unknown cause. ***Idiopathic*** means a disease of unknown cause. The classifications of blood pressure for adults with this condition are summarized in Table 5.3.
- ***Secondary hypertension*** is caused by a different medical problem, such as a kidney disorder or a tumor on the adrenal glands. When the other problem is cured, the secondary hypertension is usually resolved.
- ***Malignant hypertension*** is characterized by very high blood pressure. This condition, which can be fatal, is usually accompanied by damage to the organs, the brain, and optic nerves, or failure of the heart and kidneys.

Hypotension

Hypotension (**high**-poh-**TEN**-shun) is lower-than-normal arterial blood pressure. Symptoms can include dizziness, light-headedness, or fainting. *Hypotension* is the opposite of *hypertension*.

TABLE 5.3
Blood Pressure Classifications for Adults

Category	Systolic (mm Hg) Top Number	Diastolic (mm Hg) Bottom Number
Normal blood pressure	less than 120	less than 80
Pre-hypertension	between 120 and 139	between 80 and 89
Stage 1 Hypertension	between 140 and 159	between 90 and 99
Stage 2 Hypertension	160 or higher	100 or higher

- **Orthostatic hypotension** (**or**-thoh-**STAT**-ick **high**-poh-**TEN**-shun), also known as ***postural hypotension***, is low blood pressure that occurs upon standing up. ***Orthostatic*** means relating to an upright or standing position.

DIAGNOSTIC PROCEDURES OF THE CARDIOVASCULAR SYSTEM

- **Blood tests** and **ultrasonic diagnostic procedures** are discussed in Chapter 15.
- **Angiography** (**an**-jee-**OG**-rah-fee) is a radiographic (x-ray) study of the blood vessels after the injection of a contrast medium (**angi/o** means blood vessel, and **-graphy** means the process of recording). The resulting film is an ***angiogram*** (Figure 5.20).

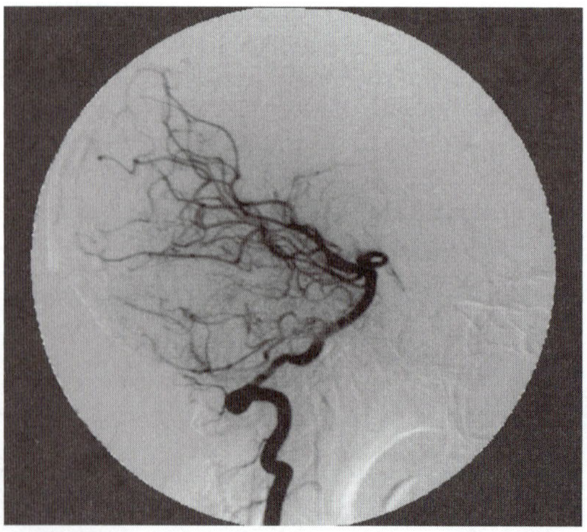

FIGURE 5.20 In angiography, the blood vessels (in black) are made visible through the use of a contrast medium.

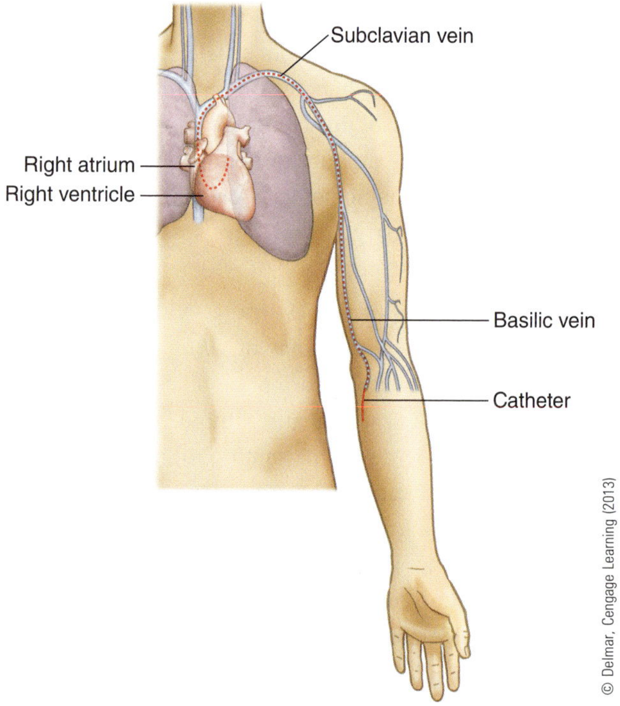

FIGURE 5.21 In *cardiac catheterization* is a catheter is passed into a vein or artery and then guided into the heart.

- **Cardiac catheterization** (**KAR**-dee-ack **kath**-eh-ter-eye-**ZAY**-shun) is a diagnostic procedure in which a catheter is passed into a vein or artery and then guided into the heart (Figure 5.21). When the catheter is in place, a contrast medium is introduced to produce an angiogram to determine how well the heart is working. This procedure is also used during treatment. See the section on clearing blocked arteries later in this chapter.
- **Digital subtraction angiography** (DSA) combines angiography with computerized components to clarify the view of the area of interest by removing the soft tissue and bones from the images.

- **Duplex ultrasound** is a diagnostic procedure to image the structures of the blood vessels and the flow of blood through these vessels. This is a combination of ***diagnostic ultrasound*** to show the structure of the blood vessels and ***Doppler ultrasound*** to show the movement of the red blood cells through these vessels. Diagnostic and Doppler ultrasounds are discussed in Chapter 15.
- **Phlebography** (fleh-**BOG**-rah-fee), also known as ***venography***, is a radiographic test that provides an image of the leg veins after a contrast dye is injected into a vein in the patient's foot (**phleb/o** means vein, and **-graphy** means the process of recording). The resulting film is a ***phlebogram***. This is a very accurate test for detecting deep vein thrombosis.

Electrocardiography

Electrocardiography (ee-**leck**-troh-kar-dee-**OG**-rah-fee) is the noninvasive process of recording the electrical activity of the myocardium (**electr/o** means electric, **cardi/o** means heart, and **graphy** means the process of recording a picture or record) (Figure 5.22). A ***noninvasive*** procedure does not require the insertion of an instrument or device through the skin or a body opening for diagnosis or treatment.

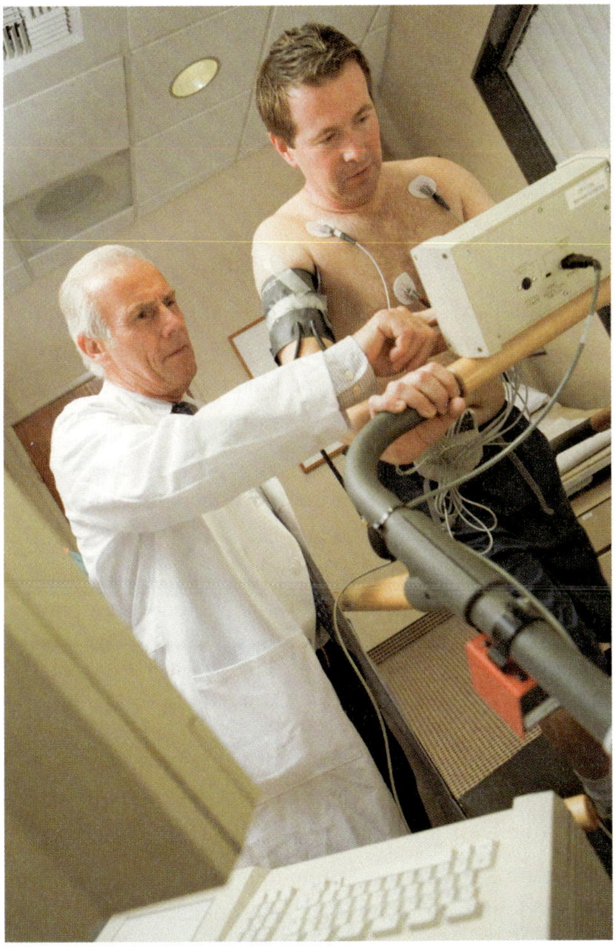

iStockphoto/Catherine Yeulet

FIGURE 5.22 In *electrocardiography*, the electrical activity of the myocardium is captured and externally recorded by electrodes placed on the skin.

- An **electrocardiogram** (ee-**leck**-troh-**KAR**-dee-oh-**gram**) (EKG or ECG) is a record of the electrical activity of the myocardium (**electr/o** means electric, **cardi/o** means heart, and **-gram** means picture or record) (Figure 5.16).
- A **Holter monitor** is a portable electrocardiograph that is worn by an ambulatory patient to continuously monitor the heart rates and rhythms over a 24- or 48-hour period.
- A **stress test** is performed to assess cardiovascular health and function during and after stress. This involves monitoring with an electrocardiogram while the patient exercises on a treadmill, or is injected with a chemical to increase the patient's heart rate if he or she is unable to use a treadmill. The test can also be performed in conjunction with an echocardiogram (see Chapter 15).
- A **thallium stress test** (**THAL**-ee-um) is performed to evaluate how well blood flows through the coronary arteries of the heart muscle during exercise by injecting a small amount of thallium into the bloodstream. If it is not taken up equally by all heart muscle cells, it shows a decrease in blood flow to part of the heart.

TREATMENT PROCEDURES OF THE CARDIOVASCULAR SYSTEM

Medications

Many heart conditions are controlled with medications; however, successful treatment depends on patient compliance. ***Compliance*** is the accuracy and consistency with which the patient follows the physician's instructions.

Antihypertensives

An **antihypertensive** (**an**-tih-**high**-per-**TEN**-siv) is a medication administered to lower blood pressure. Some of these drugs are also used to treat other heart conditions.

- An **ACE inhibitor** (***angiotensin-converting enzyme***) blocks the action of the enzyme that causes the blood vessels to contract, resulting in hypertension.

When this enzyme is blocked, the blood vessels are able to dilate (enlarge), and this reduces the blood pressure. These medications are used primarily to treat hypertension and heart failure. ***Angiotensin II receptor blockers (ARBs)*** have a similar action and effect.

- A **beta-blocker** reduces the workload of the heart by slowing the rate of the heartbeat. They are commonly prescribed to lower blood pressure, relieve angina, or to treat heart failure.
- **Calcium channel blocker agents** cause the heart and blood vessels to relax by decreasing the movement of calcium into the cells of these structures. This relaxation reduces the workload of the heart by increasing the supply of blood and oxygen. Some calcium channel blocking agents are used to treat hypertension or to relieve and control angina.
- A **diuretic** (**dye**-you-**RET**-ick) is administered to stimulate the kidneys to increase the secretion of urine to rid the body of excess sodium and water. These medications are administered to treat hypertension and heart failure by reducing the amount of fluid circulating in the blood.

Additional Medications

- An **antiarrhythmic** (**an**-tih-ah-**RITH**-mick) is a medication administered to control irregularities of the heartbeat.
- An **anticoagulant** (**an**-tih-koh-**AG**-you-lant) slows coagulation and prevents new clots from forming. ***Coagulation*** is the process of clotting blood (see Coumadin).
- **Aspirin** taken in a very small daily dose, such as 81 mg, which is commonly known as ***baby aspirin***, may be recommended to reduce the risk of a heart attack or stroke by reducing the ability of the blood to clot.
- **Cholesterol-lowering drugs**, such as ***statins***, are used to combat hyperlipidemia by reducing the undesirable cholesterol levels in the blood.
- **Coumadin**, which is a brand name for ***warfarin***, is an anticoagulant administered to prevent blood clots from forming or growing larger. This medication is often prescribed for patients with clotting difficulties, certain types of heartbeat irregularities, or after a heart attack or heart valve replacement surgery.
- **Digitalis** (**dij**-ih-**TAL**-is), also known as ***digoxin***, strengthens the contraction of the heart muscle, slows the heart rate, and helps eliminate fluid from body tissues. It is often used to treat heart failure or certain types of arrhythmias.
- A **thrombolytic** (**throm**-boh-**LIT**-ick), also known as a ***clot-busting drug***, dissolves or causes a thrombus to break up (**thromb/o** means clot, and **-lytic** means to destroy).
- **Tissue plasminogen activator** (TPA) (plaz-**MIN**-oh-jen) is a thrombolytic that is administered to some patients having a heart attack or stroke. If administered within a few hours after symptoms begin, this medication can dissolve the damaging blood clots.
- A **vasoconstrictor** (**vas**-oh-kon-**STRICK**-tor) causes blood vessels to narrow. Examples of these medications include antihistamines and decongestants. A vasoconstrictor is the opposite of a *vasodilator*.
- A **vasodilator** (**vas**-oh-dye-**LAYT**-or) causes blood vessels to expand. A vasodilator is the opposite of a *vasoconstrictor*.
- **Nitroglycerin** (**nye**-troh-**GLIH**-sih-rin) is a vasodilator that is prescribed to prevent or relieve the pain of angina by dilating the blood vessels to the heart. This increases the blood flow and oxygen supply to the heart. Nitroglycerin can be administered sublingually (under the tongue), transdermally (through the skin), or orally as a spray.

Clearing Blocked Arteries

- **Angioplasty** (**AN**-jee-oh-**plas**-tee) is the technique of mechanically widening a narrowed or obstructed blood vessel (**angi/o** means blood vessel, and **-plasty** means surgical repair). The narrowing is typically caused by atherosclerosis.
- **Percutaneous transluminal coronary angioplasty** (PTCA) is also known as a ***balloon angioplasty***. This is a procedure in which a small balloon on the end of a catheter is used to open a partially blocked coronary artery by flattening the plaque deposit and stretching the lumen (Figure 5.23).
- **Laser angioplasty** (**AN**-jee-oh-**plas**-tee) involves a laser on the end of a catheter, which uses beams of light to remove the plaque deposit. It can be used separately or in conjunction with PTCA.
- A **stent** is a wire-mesh tube that is commonly placed after the artery has been opened. This provides support to the arterial wall, keeps the plaque from expanding again, and prevents restenosis (Figure 5.24).

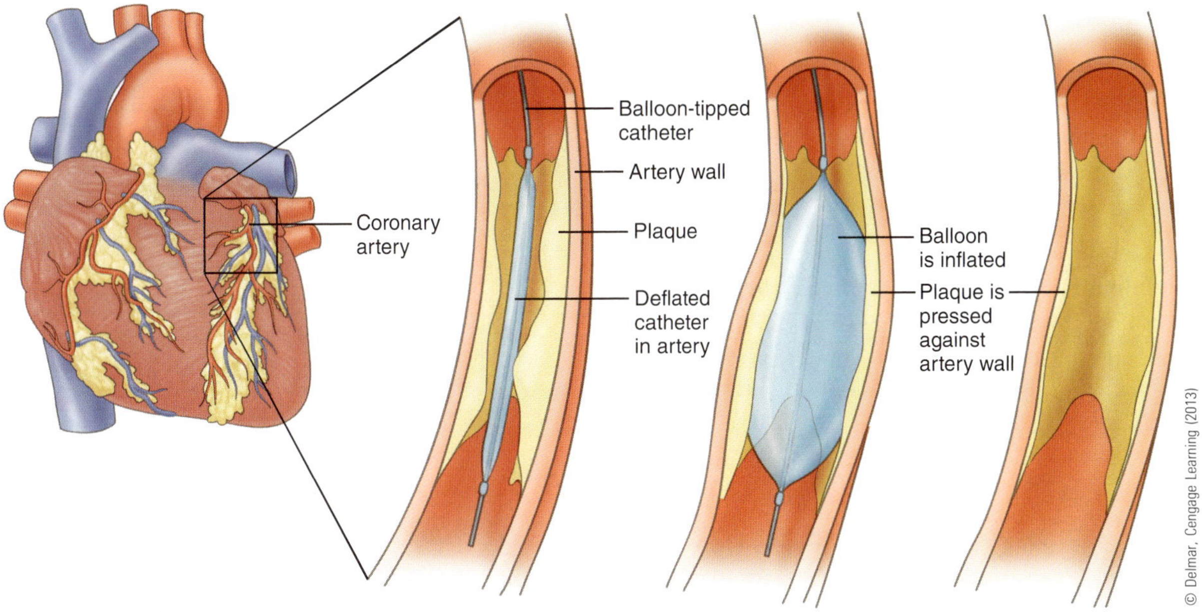

FIGURE 5.23 *Balloon angioplasty* is performed to reopen a blocked coronary artery.

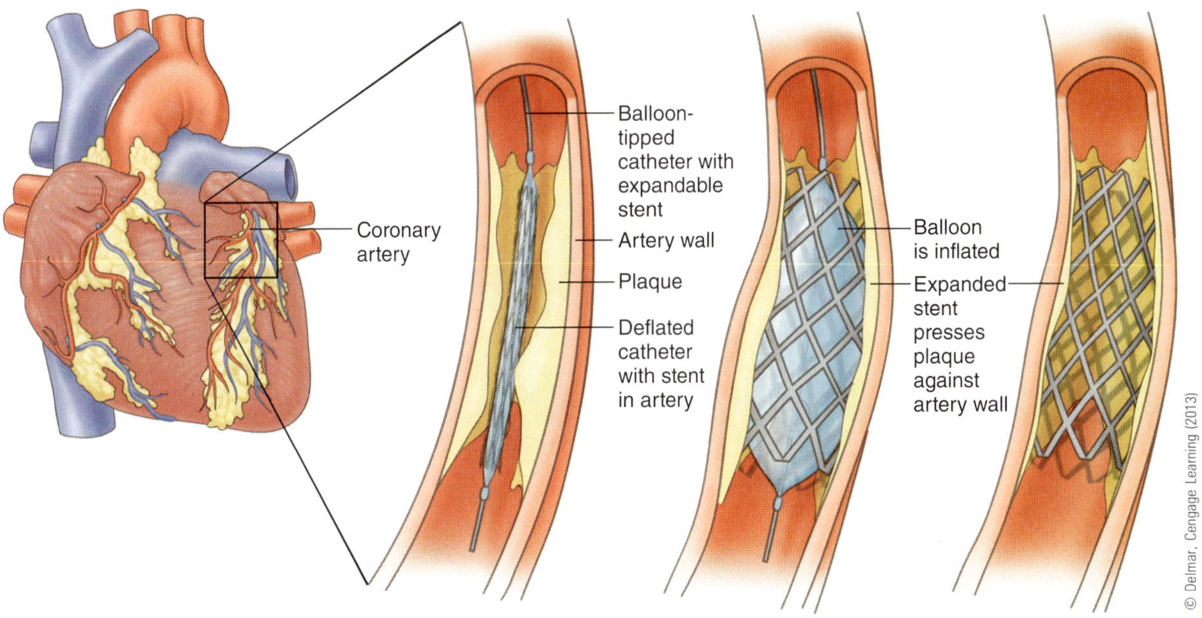

FIGURE 5.24 A *stent* is put in place to prevent *restenosis* of a treated artery.

- **Restenosis** describes the condition when an artery that has been opened by angioplasty closes again (**re-** means again, and **-stenosis** means narrowing).
- An **atherectomy** (**ath**-er-**ECK**-toh-mee) is the surgical removal of plaque buildup from the interior of an artery (**ather** means plaque, and **-ectomy** means surgical removal). A stent may be put in place after the atherectomy to prevent the artery from becoming blocked again.
- A **carotid endarterectomy** (kah-**ROT**-id **end**-ar-ter-**ECK**-toh-mee) is the surgical removal of the lining of a portion of a clogged carotid artery leading to the brain. This procedure is performed to reduce the risk of a stroke caused by a disruption of the blood flow to the brain. Strokes are discussed in Chapter 10.

Coronary Artery Bypass Graft

Coronary artery bypass graft (CABG) is also known as *bypass surgery* (Figure 5.25). In this operation, which requires opening the chest, a piece of vein from the leg or chest is implanted on the heart to replace a blocked coronary artery and to improve the flow of blood to the heart.

- A **minimally invasive coronary artery bypass**, also known as a *keyhole bypass* or a *buttonhole bypass*, is an alternative technique for some bypass patients. This procedure is performed with the aid of a fiberoptic camera through small openings between the ribs.

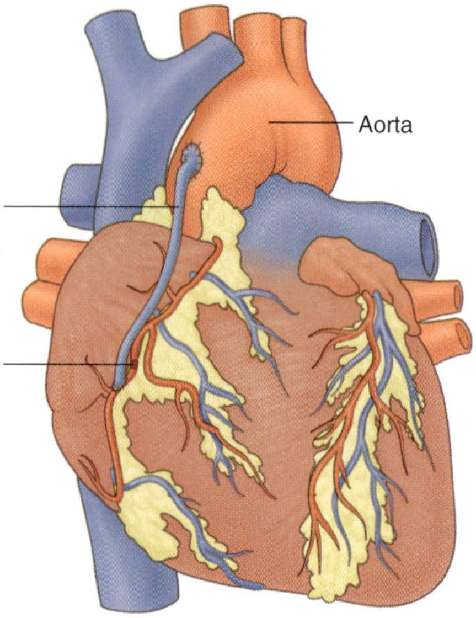

FIGURE 5.25 *Coronary artery bypass surgery* is performed to allow the flow of blood by placing vein grafts to bypass blocked arteries.

Treatment of Cardiac Arrhythmias

- **Defibrillation** (dee-**fih**-brih-**LAY**-shun), also known as *cardioversion*, is the use of electrical shock to restore the heart's normal rhythm. This shock is provided by a device known as a *defibrillator* (Figure 5.26).
- An **automated external defibrillator** (AED) is designed for use by nonprofessionals in emergency situations when defibrillation is required. This piece of equipment automatically samples the electrical rhythms of the heart and if necessary, externally shocks the heart to restore a normal cardiac rhythm.
- An **artificial pacemaker** is used primarily as treatment for bradycardia or atrial fibrillation. This electronic device can be attached externally or implanted under the skin with connections leading into the heart to regulate the heartbeat.

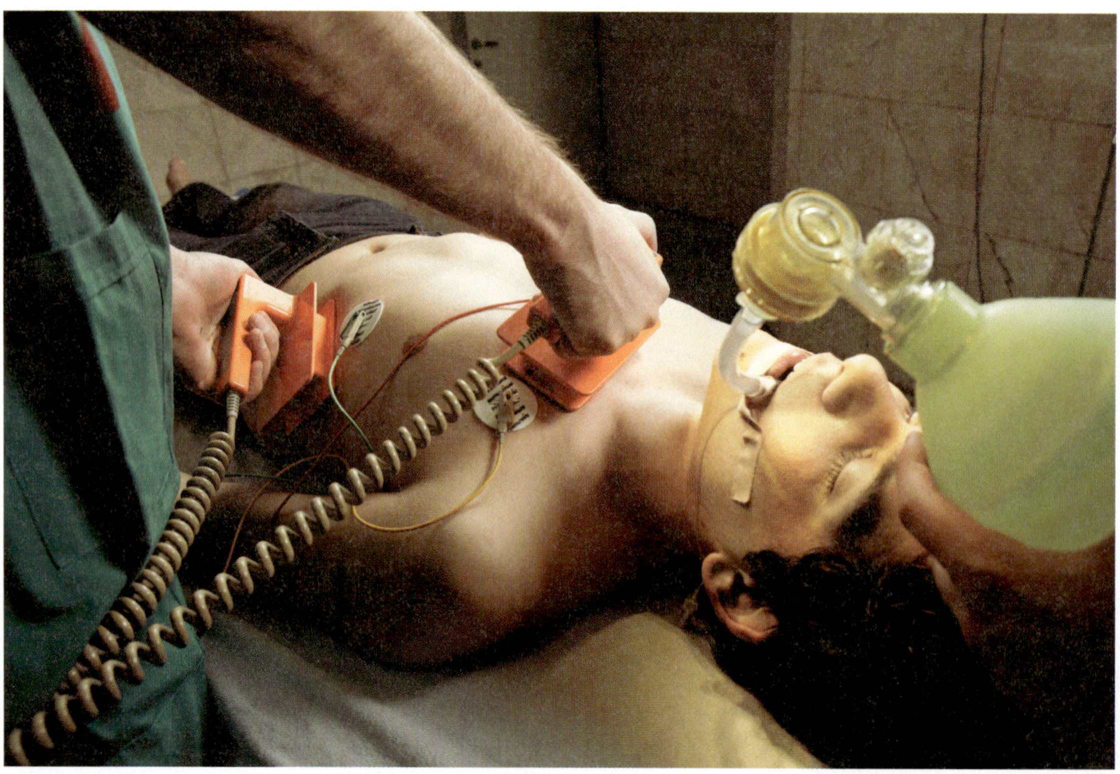

FIGURE 5.26 *Defibrillation* uses electrical shock to attempt to restore the heart to its usual rhythm.

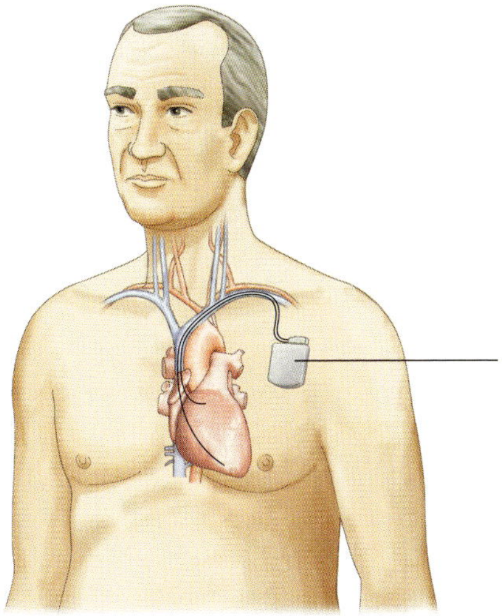

FIGURE 5.27 An *automated implantable cardioverter-defibrillator* constantly regulates the heartbeat and if necessary, acts as an automatic defibrillator.

- An **automated implantable cardioverter-defibrillator** (**KAR**-dee-oh-**ver**-ter dee-**fib**-rih-**LAY**-ter) (AICD) is a double-action pacemaker. (1) It constantly regulates the heartbeat to ensure that the heart does not beat too slowly. (2) If a dangerous disruption of the heart's rhythm occurs, it acts as an automatic defibrillator (Figure 5.27).
- **Valvoplasty** (**VAL**-voh-**plas**-tee), also known as ***valvuloplasty***, is the surgical repair or replacement of a heart valve (**valv/o** means valve, and **-plasty** means surgical repair).
- **Cardiopulmonary resuscitation**, commonly known as ***CPR***, is an emergency procedure for life support consisting of artificial respiration and manual external cardiac compression. ***Cardiopulmonary*** means pertaining to the heart and lungs.
- ***Compression-only resuscitation*** can be effective in keeping a patient suffering from cardiac arrest alive until professional responders arrive, although artificial respiration is still recommended for children, drowning victims, and drug overdoses.

Blood Vessels, Blood, and Bleeding

- An **aneurysmectomy** (**an**-you-riz-**MECK**-toh-mee) is the surgical removal of an aneurysm (**aneurysm** means aneurysm, and **-ectomy** means surgical removal).
- An **aneurysmorrhaphy** (**an**-you-riz-**MOR**-ah-fee), also known as ***aneurysmoplasty***, is the surgical suturing of an aneurysm (**aneurysm/o** means aneurysm, and **-rrhaphy** means surgical suturing).
- An **arteriectomy** (**ar**-teh-ree-**ECK**-toh-mee) is the surgical removal of part of an artery (**arteri** means artery, and **-ectomy** means surgical removal).
- **Hemostasis** (**hee**-moh-**STAY**-sis) means to stop or control bleeding (**hem/o** means blood, and **-stasis** means stopping or controlling). This could be accomplished by the formation of a blood clot by the body or through the external application of pressure to block the flow of blood.
- **Plasmapheresis** (**plaz**-mah-feh-**REE**-sis), also known as ***plasma exchange***, is the removal of whole blood from the body and separation of the blood's cellular elements. The red blood cells and platelets are suspended in saline or a plasma substitute and returned to the circulatory system. For blood donors, this makes more frequent donations possible. Patients with certain autoimmune disorders receive their own red blood cells and platelets back cleansed of antibodies.

ABBREVIATIONS RELATED TO THE CARDIOVASCULAR SYSTEM

Table 5.4 presents an overview of the abbreviations related to the terms introduced in this chapter. Note: To avoid errors or confusion, always be cautious when using abbreviations.

TABLE 5.4

Abbreviations Related to the Cardiovascular System

atrial fibrillation = A-fib	**A-fib** = atrial fibrillation
automated external defibrillator = AED	**AED** = automated external defibrillator
automated implantable cardioverter-defibrillator = AICD	**AICD** = automated implantable cardioverter-defibrillator
cardiac catheterization = card cath, CC	**card cath, CC** = cardiac catheterization
chronic venous insufficiency = CVI	**CVI** = chronic venous insufficiency
coronary artery bypass graft = CABG	**CABG** = coronary artery bypass graft
coronary artery disease = CAD	**CAD** = coronary artery disease
electrocardiogram = EKG, ECG	**EKG, ECG** = electrocardiogram
hypertension = HTN	**HTN** = hypertension
myocardial infarction = MI	**MI** = myocardial infarction
peripheral artery disease = PAD	**PAD** = peripheral artery disease
peripheral vascular disease = PVD	**PVD** = peripheral vascular disease
thallium stress test = TST	**TST** = thallium stress test
tissue plasminogen activator = tPA	**tPA** = tissue plasminogen activator
ventricular fibrillation = V-fib	**V-fib** = ventricular fibrillation

StudyWARE CONNECTION

For more practice and to test your mastery of this material, go to the StudyWARE™ to play interactive games and complete the quiz for this chapter.

Workbook Practice

Go to your workbook and complete the exercises for this chapter.

DELMAR MOBILE MEDIA

Downloadable audio is available for selected medical terms in this chapter to enhance your learning of medical terminology.

CHAPTER 5

LEARNING EXERCISES

MATCHING WORD PARTS 1

Write the correct answer in the middle column.

	Definition	Correct Answer	Possible Answers
5.1.	aorta	________	angi/o
5.2.	artery	________	aort/o
5.3.	plaque, fatty substance	________	arteri/o
5.4.	relating to blood or lymph vessels	________	ather/o
5.5.	slow	________	brady-

MATCHING WORD PARTS 2

Write the correct answer in the middle column.

	Definition	Correct Answer	Possible Answers
5.6.	blood or blood condition	________	cardi/o
5.7.	heart	________	-crasia
5.8.	mixture or blending	________	ven/o
5.9.	red	________	-emia
5.10.	vein	________	erythr/o

MATCHING WORD PARTS 3

Write the correct answer in the middle column.

	Definition	Correct Answer	Possible Answers
5.11.	white	____________	**hem/o**
5.12.	vein	____________	**leuk/o**
5.13.	fast, rapid	____________	**phleb/o**
5.14.	clot	____________	**tachy-**
5.15.	blood, relating to blood	____________	**thromb/o**

DEFINITIONS

Select the correct answer, and write it on the line provided.

5.16. The term meaning white blood cells is ____________.

erythrocytes leukocytes platelets thrombocytes

5.17. Commonly known as the natural pacemaker, the medical name of the structure is the ____________.

atrioventricular node bundle of His Purkinje fiber sinoatrial node

5.18. The myocardium receives its blood supply from the ____________ arteries.

aorta coronary arteries inferior vena cava superior vena cava

5.19. The ____________ are formed in red bone marrow and then migrate to tissues throughout the body. These blood cells destroy parasitic organisms and play a major role in allergic reactions.

basophils eosinophils erythrocytes monocytes

5.20. The bicuspid valve is also known as the ____________ valve.

aortic mitral pulmonary tricuspid

5.21. The ____________ pumps blood into the pulmonary artery, which carries it to the lungs.

left atrium left ventricle right atrium right ventricle

5.22. The ______________ are the smallest formed elements in the blood, and they play an important role in blood clotting.

erythrocytes leukocytes monocytes thrombocytes

5.23. A foreign object, such as a bit of tissue or air, circulating in the blood is known as a/an ______________.

embolism embolus thrombosis thrombus

5.24. The ______________ carries blood to all parts of the body except the lungs.

left atrium left ventricle right atrium right ventricle

5.25. The ______________ are the most common type of white blood cell.

erythrocytes leukocytes neutrophils thrombocytes

MATCHING STRUCTURES

Write the correct answer in the middle column.

	Definition	Correct Answer	Possible Answers
5.26.	a hollow, muscular organ	______________	endocardium
5.27.	cardiac muscle	______________	epicardium
5.28.	external layer of the heart	______________	heart
5.29.	inner lining of the heart	______________	myocardium
5.30.	sac enclosing the heart	______________	pericardium

WHICH WORD?

Select the correct answer, and write it on the line provided.

5.31. High-density ______________ is also known as good cholesterol.

lipoprotein cholesterol total cholesterol

5.32. An abnormally slow resting heart rate is described as ______________.

bradycardia tachycardia

5.33. In ________________ fibrillation, instead of pumping strongly, the heart muscle quivers ineffectively.

atrial ventricular

5.34. The highest pressure against the blood vessels is ________________ pressure, and it occurs when the ventricles contract.

diastolic systolic

5.35. The diagnostic procedure that images the structures of the blood vessels and the flow of blood through these vessels is known as ________________.

digital angiography duplex ultrasound

SPELLING COUNTS

Find the misspelled word in each sentence. Then write that word, spelled correctly, on the line provided.

5.36. The autopsy indicated that the cause of death was a ruptured aneuryism. ________________

5.37. A deficiency of blood passing through an organ or body part is known as hypoprefusion. ________________

5.38. An arrhythemia is an abnormal heart rhythm in which the heartbeat is faster or slower than normal. ________________

5.39. Reynaud's disease is a condition with symptoms that include of intermittent attacks of pallor, cyanosis, and redness of the fingers and toes. ________________

5.40. An automated implantable cardioverter-defibrilator is a double-action pacemaker. ________________

ABBREVIATION IDENTIFICATION

In the space provided, write the words that each abbreviation stands for.

5.41. **CAD** ________________

5.42. **EKG, ECG** ________________

5.43. **A-fib** ________________

5.44. **MI** ________________

5.45. **VF** ________________

TERM SELECTION

Select the correct answer, and write it on the line provided.

5.46. The systemic condition often associated with severe infections caused by the presence of bacteria in the blood is known as ________________________.

dyscrasia endocarditis pericarditis septicemia

5.47. A/An ________________________ reduces the workload of the heart by slowing the rate of the heartbeat.

ACE inhibitor beta-blocker calcium blocker statin inhibitor

5.48. The blood disorder characterized by anemia in which the red blood cells are larger than normal is known as ________________________ anemia.

aplastic hemolytic megaloblastic pernicious

5.49. A/An ________________________ is administered to lower high blood pressure.

antiarrhythmic antihypertensive aspirin diuretic

5.50. A bacterial infection of the lining or valves of the heart is known as bacterial ________________________.

endocarditis myocarditis pericarditis valvulitis

SENTENCE COMPLETION

Write the correct term or terms on the lines provided.

5.51. Plasma with the clotting proteins removed is known as ________________________.

5.52. Having an abnormally small number of platelets in the circulating blood is known as ________________________.

5.53. The surgical removal of the lining of a portion of a clogged carotid artery leading to the brain is known as a/an ________________________.

5.54. The abnormal protrusion of a heart valve that results in the inability of the valve to close completely is known as a/an ________________________ ________________________.

5.55. The medication ________________________ is prescribed to prevent or relieve the pain of angina by dilating the blood vessels to the heart.

WORD SURGERY

Divide each term into its component word parts. Write these word parts, in sequence, on the lines provided. When necessary, use a slash (/) to indicate a combining vowel. (You may not need all of the lines provided.)

5.56. **Aneurysmorrhaphy** means the surgical suturing a ruptured aneurysm.

__________ __________ __________ __________

5.57. **Aplastic** anemia is characterized by an absence of *all* formed blood elements.

__________ __________ __________ __________

5.58. **Electrocardiography** is the process of recording the electrical activity of the myocardium.

__________ __________ __________ __________

5.59. **Polyarteritis** is a form of vasculitis involving several medium and small arteries at the same time.

__________ __________ __________ __________

5.60. **Valvoplasty** is the surgical repair or replacement of a heart valve.

__________ __________ __________ __________

TRUE/FALSE

If the statement is true, write **True** on the line. If the statement is false, write **False** on the line.

5.61. ________________ A thrombus is a clot or piece of tissue circulating in the blood.

5.62. ________________ Hemochromatosis is also known as iron overload disease.

5.63. ________________ Plasmapheresis is the removal of whole blood from the body, separation of its cellular elements, and reinfusion of these cellular elements suspended in saline or a plasma substitute.

5.64. ________________ A vasoconstrictor is a drug that enlarges the blood vessels.

5.65. ________________ Peripheral vascular disease is a disorder of the blood vessels located outside the heart and brain.

CLINICAL CONDITIONS

Write the correct answer on the line provided.

5.66. Alberta Fleetwood has a/an ________________. This condition is a benign tumor made up of newly formed blood vessels.

5.67. After his surgery, Ramon Martinez developed a deep vein ________________ in his leg.

5.68. During her pregnancy, Polly Olson suffered from abnormally swollen veins in her legs. The medical term for this condition is ______________________ veins.

5.69. Thomas Wilkerson suffers from episodes of severe chest pain due to inadequate blood flow to the myocardium. This is a condition is known as ______________________.

5.70. When Mr. Klein stands up too quickly, his blood pressure drops. His physician describes this as postural or ______________________.

5.71. Juanita Gomez was diagnosed as having ______________________. This bone marrow disorder is characterized by the insufficient production of one or more types of blood cells.

5.72. Dr. Lawson read her patient's ______________________. This diagnostic record is also known as an ECG or EKG.

5.73. Jason Turner suffered from cardiac arrest. The paramedics arrived promptly and saved his life by using ______________________ (CPR).

5.74. Darlene Nolan was diagnosed as having a deep vein thrombosis. Her doctor immediately prescribed a/an ______________________ to cause the thrombus to dissolve.

5.75. Hamilton Edwards Sr. suffers from ______________________ (IHD). This is a group of cardiac disabilities resulting from an insufficient supply of oxygenated blood to the heart.

WHICH IS THE CORRECT MEDICAL TERM?

Select the correct answer, and write it on the line provided.

5.76. A/An ______________________, which is a characteristic of atherosclerosis, is a deposit of plaque on or within the arterial wall.

vasculitis | angiostenosis | arteriosclerosis | atheroma

5.77. The term ______________________ means to stop or control bleeding.

hemochromatosis | hemostasis | plasmapheresis | transfusion reaction

5.78. Inflammation of a vein is known as ______________________.

arteriostenosis | endocarditis | phlebitis | carditis

5.79. Blood ________________ is any pathologic condition of the cellular elements of the blood.

anemia dyscrasia hemochromatosis septicemia

5.80. The surgical removal of an aneurysm is a/an ________________.

aneurysmectomy aneurysmoplasty aneurysmorrhaphy aneurysmotomy

CHALLENGE WORD BUILDING

These terms are *not* found in this chapter; however, they are made up of the following familiar word parts. If you need help in creating the term, refer to your medical dictionary.

peri-	**angi/o**	**-itis**
	arter/o	**-necrosis**
	cardi/o	**-rrhaphy**
	phleb/o	**-rrhexis**
	-ectomy	**-stenosis**

5.81. Inflammation of an artery or arteries is known as ________________.

5.82. The surgical removal of a portion of a blood vessel is a/an ________________.

5.83. The abnormal narrowing of the lumen of a vein is known as ________________.

5.84. The surgical removal of a portion of the tissue surrounding the heart is a/an ________________.

5.85. To surgically suture the wall of the heart is a/an ________________.

5.86. Rupture of a vein is known as ________________.

5.87. The suture repair of any vessel, especially a blood vessel, is a/an ________________.

5.88. Rupture of the heart is known as ________________.

5.89. To suture the tissue surrounding the heart is a/an ________________.

5.90. The tissue death of the walls of the blood vessels is known as ________________.

LABELING EXERCISES

Identify the numbered items in the accompanying figures.

5.91. superior ____________________

5.92. right ____________________

5.93. right ____________________

5.94. left pulmonary ____________________

5.95. left pulmonary ____________________

5.96. pulmonary ____________________ valve

5.97. ____________________ valve

5.98. ____________________

5.99. ____________________ semilunar valve

5.100. ____________________ valve

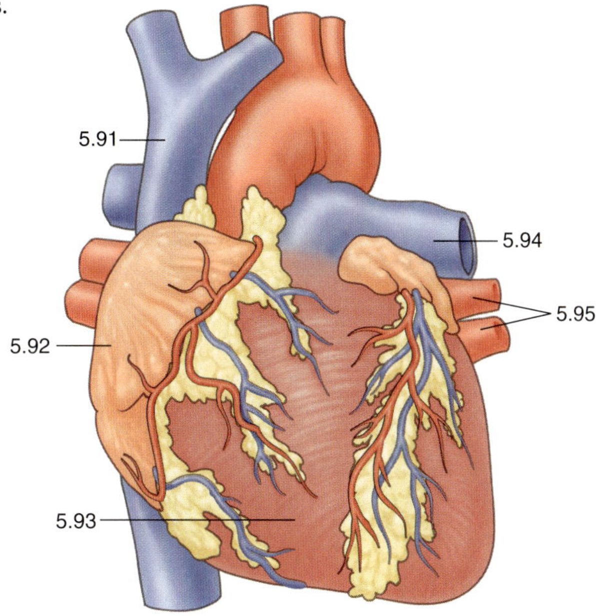

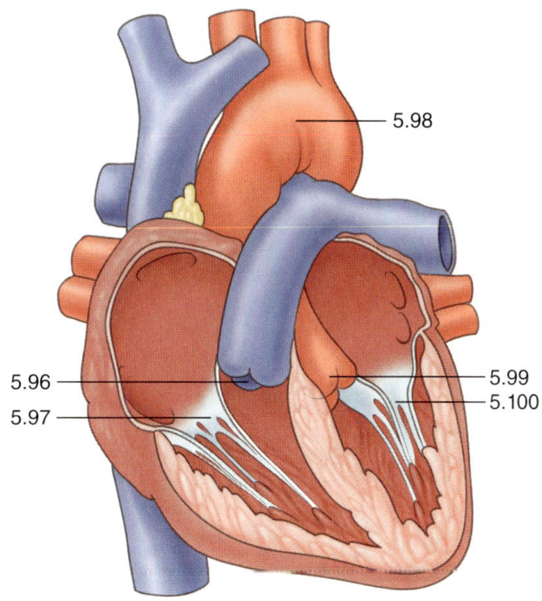

CHAPTER 6

The Lymphatic and Immune Systems

Overview of STRUCTURES, COMBINING FORMS, AND FUNCTIONS OF THE LYMPHATIC AND IMMUNE SYSTEMS

Major Structures	Related Combining Forms	Primary Functions
Lymph	**lymph/o**	The fluid that removes cellular waste products, pathogens, and dead blood cells from the tissues.
Lymphatic Vessels and Ducts	**lymphangi/o**	The capillaries, vessels, and ducts that return lymph from the tissues to the venous bloodstream.
Lymph Nodes	**lymphaden/o**	Bean-shaped structures of the lymphatic system where pathogens and other harmful substances are filtered from the lymph by specialized cells of the immune system.
Tonsils and Adenoids	**tonsill/o**, **adenoid/o**	Lymphoid structures of the lymphatic system that protect the entry to the respiratory system.
Spleen	**splen/o** (Note: this combining form is spelled with only one *e*.)	A sac-like mass of lymphoid tissue with protective roles in both the immune and lymphatic systems.
Bone Marrow	**myel/o**	Produces lymphocytes, which are specialized leukocytes (white blood cells). **Myel/o** also means spinal cord (see Chapter 10).
Lymphocytes	**lymphocyt/o**	Specialized leukocytes that play important roles in the immune reactions.
Thymus	**thym/o**	A gland located in the upper chest with specialized roles in both the lymphatic and immune systems.

Vocabulary Related to **THE LYMPHATIC AND IMMUNE SYSTEMS**

This list contains essential word parts and medical terms for this chapter. These terms are pronounced in the StudyWARE™ and Audio CDs that are available for use with this text. These and the other important **primary terms** are shown in boldface throughout the chapter. *Secondary terms*, which appear in *orange* italics, clarify the meaning of primary terms.

Word Parts

- ☐ **anti-** against
- ☐ **carcin/o** cancerous
- ☐ **immun/o** immune, protection, safe
- ☐ **lymph/o** lymph, lymphatic tissue
- ☐ **lymphaden/o** lymph node or gland
- ☐ **lymphangi/o** lymph vessel
- ☐ **neo-, ne/o** new, strange
- ☐ **-oma** tumor, neoplasm
- ☐ **onc/o** tumor
- ☐ **phag/o** eat, swallow
- ☐ **-plasm** formative material of cells
- ☐ **sarc/o** flesh, connective tissue
- ☐ **splen/o** spleen
- ☐ **-tic** pertaining to
- ☐ **tox/o** poison, poisonous

Medical Terms

- ☐ **acquired immunodeficiency syndrome** (**im**-you-noh-deh-**FISH**-en-see)
- ☐ **allergen** (**AL**-er-jen)
- ☐ **anaphylaxis** (**an**-ah-fih-**LACK**-sis)
- ☐ **antibiotics**
- ☐ **antibody** (**AN**-tih-**bod**-ee)
- ☐ **antifungal** (**an**-tih-**FUNG**-gul)
- ☐ **antigen** (**AN**-tih-jen)
- ☐ **antigen-antibody reaction**
- ☐ **autoimmune disorder** (**aw**-toh-ih-**MYOUN**)
- ☐ **bacilli** (bah-**SILL**-eye)
- ☐ **bacteria** (back-**TEER**-ree-ah)
- ☐ **candidiasis** (kan-dih-**DYE**-ah-sis)
- ☐ **carcinoma** (**kar**-sih-**NOH**-mah)
- ☐ **carcinoma in situ** (**kar**-sih-**NOH**-mah in **SIGH**-too)
- ☐ **complement system** (**KOM**-pleh-ment)
- ☐ **cytokines** (**SIGH**-toh-kyens)
- ☐ **cytomegalovirus** (**sigh**-toh-**meg**-ah-loh-**VYE**-rus)
- ☐ **cytotoxic drug** (**sigh**-toh-**TOK**-sick)
- ☐ **ductal carcinoma in situ** (**DUCK**-tal kar-sih-**NOH**-mah in **SIGH**-too)
- ☐ **hemolytic** (**hee**-moh-**LIT**-ick)
- ☐ **herpes zoster** (**HER**-peez **ZOS**-ter)
- ☐ **Hodgkin's lymphoma** (**HODJ**-kinz lim-**FOH**-mah)
- ☐ **human immunodeficiency virus** (**im**-you-noh-deh-**FISH**-en-see)
- ☐ **immunodeficiency disorder** (**im**-you-noh-deh-**FISH**-en-see)
- ☐ **immunoglobulins** (**im**-you-noh-**GLOB**-you-lins)
- ☐ **immunosuppressant** (**im**-you-noh-soo-**PRES**-ant)
- ☐ **immunotherapy** (ih-**myou**-noh-**THER**-ah-pee)
- ☐ **infectious mononucleosis** (**mon**-oh-**new**-klee-**OH**-sis)
- ☐ **infiltrating ductal carcinoma** (in-**FILL**-trate-ing **DUK**-tal kar-sih-**NOH**-mah)
- ☐ **interferons** (**in**-ter-**FEAR**-onz)
- ☐ **lymphadenitis** (lim-**fad**-eh-**NIGH**-tis)
- ☐ **lymphadenopathy** (lim-**fad**-eh-**NOP**-ah-thee)
- ☐ **lymphangioma** (lim-**fan**-jee-**OH**-mah)
- ☐ **lymphedema** (**lim**-feh-**DEE**-mah)
- ☐ **lymphocytes** (**LIM**-foh-sights)
- ☐ **lymphoma** (lim-**FOH**-mah)
- ☐ **lymphoscintigraphy** (**lim**-foh-sin-**TIH**-grah-fee)
- ☐ **macrophage** (**MACK**-roh-fayj)
- ☐ **malaria** (mah-**LAY**-ree-ah)
- ☐ **mammography** (mam-**OG**-rah-fee)
- ☐ **metastasis** (meh-**TAS**-tah-sis)
- ☐ **metastasize** (meh-**TAS**-tah-sighz)
- ☐ **myoma** (my-**OH**-mah)
- ☐ **myosarcoma** (**my**-oh-sahr-**KOH**-mah)
- ☐ **non-Hodgkin's lymphoma** (non-**HODJ**-kinz lim-**FOH**-mah)
- ☐ **opportunistic infection** (**op**-ur-too-**NIHS**-tick)
- ☐ **osteosarcoma** (**oss**-tee-oh-sar-**KOH**-mah)
- ☐ **parasite** (**PAR**-ah-sight)
- ☐ **rabies** (**RAY**-beez)
- ☐ **rickettsia** (rih-**KET**-see-ah)
- ☐ **rubella** (roo-**BELL**-ah)
- ☐ **sarcoma** (sar-**KOH**-mah)
- ☐ **spirochetes** (**SPY**-roh-keets)
- ☐ **splenomegaly** (**splee**-noh-**MEG**-ah-lee)
- ☐ **staphylococci** (**staf**-ih-loh-**KOCK**-sigh)
- ☐ **streptococci** (**strep**-toh-**KOCK**-sigh)
- ☐ **systemic reaction**
- ☐ **teletherapy** (**tel**-eh-**THER**-ah-pee)
- ☐ **toxoplasmosis** (**tock**-soh-plaz-**MOH**-sis)
- ☐ **varicella** (**var**-ih-**SEL**-ah)

LEARNING GOALS

On completion of this chapter, you should be able to:

1. Describe the major functions and structures of the lymphatic and immune systems.
2. Identify the medical specialists who treat disorders of the lymphatic and immune systems.
3. Recognize, define, spell, and pronounce the primary terms related to the structures, functions, pathology, and the diagnostic and treatment procedures of the lymphatic and immune systems.
4. Recognize, define, spell, and pronounce the primary terms related to oncology.

FUNCTIONS OF THE LYMPHATIC SYSTEM

The three main functions of the lymphatic system are to:

1. Absorb fats and fat-soluble vitamins through the lacteals of the small intestine.
2. Remove waste products from the tissues, and cooperate with the immune system in destroying invading pathogens.
3. Return filtered lymph to the veins at the base of the neck.

Absorption of Fats and Fat-Soluble Vitamins

Food is digested in the small intestine, which is lined with small fingerlike projections known as *villi*. Each *villus* (singular) contains lacteals and blood vessels.

- **Lacteals** (**LACK**-tee-ahlz) are specialized structures of the lymphatic system that absorb those fats that cannot be transported by the bloodstream. These dietary fats are transformed in the cells of the lacteals. The lymphatic vessels then return them to the venous circulation so they can be used throughout the body as nutrients.
- The blood vessels absorb the nutrients, fats, and fat-soluble vitamins from the digested food directly into the bloodstream for use throughout the body. This is discussed further in Chapter 8.

Interstitial Fluid and Lymph Creation

Interstitial fluid (**in**-ter-**STISH**-al), which is also known as *intercellular* or *tissue fluid*, is plasma from arterial blood that flows out of the arterioles and into the capillaries, and then flows into the spaces between the cells of the tissues.

- This fluid delivers nutrients, oxygen, and hormones to the cells.
- When interstitial fluid leaves the cells, it brings with it waste products and protein molecules that were created within the cells. About 90% of this fluid returns to the bloodstream.

Lymph (**limf**) is made up of the remaining 10% of the returning interstitial fluid. Lymph is a clear, watery fluid containing electrolytes and proteins. It plays essential roles in the lymphatic system as it works in close cooperation with the immune system.

- Lymph collects the protein molecules created within the cells as it leaves. Lymph also removes dead cells, debris, and pathogens (including cancer cells) that were still left in the intercellular spaces.
- The lymph enters very small capillaries within the tissues and then flows into progressively larger vessels and ducts as it travels in a one-way trip upward toward the neck.
- At this stage, the lymph begins to play an active role in cooperation with the immune system to protect the body against invading microorganisms and diseases. These functions are described in the discussion of the immune system.

STRUCTURES OF THE LYMPHATIC SYSTEM

Many of the structures of the lymphatic system cooperate and also perform roles in other body systems.

Lymphatic Circulation

The **lymphatic circulatory system** and blood circulatory system work closely together, and because of these similarities the lymphatic circulatory system is often referred to as the ***secondary circulatory system***. However, it is also very important to understand the differences in these two systems. While studying this section, compare Figure 6.1 with Figures 5.9 and 5.10 in Chapter 5.

- Blood circulates throughout the entire body in a loop, pumped by the heart. The bloodstream flows in an open system in which it leaves and reenters the blood vessels through the capillaries
- Since the lymphatic system does not have a pump-like organ, it must depend on the pumping motion of muscles to move the fluid upward.
- Lymph flows in only one direction. From its point of origin, lymph can move only upward until it returns to the circulatory system at the base of the neck. Once lymph enters a lymphatic capillary, it must continue this upward flow.
- Blood is filtered by the kidneys, and waste products are excreted by the urinary system. Lymph is filtered by lymph nodes, which are located along lymphatic vessels. These nodes contain specialized cells of the immune system.
- The color of blood makes the arteries and veins readily visible. Since lymph is a clear fluid, the lymphatic vessels are not readily visible.

Lymphatic Capillaries

Lymphatic capillaries are microscopic, blind-ended tubes located near the surface of the body with capillary walls that are only one cell in thickness. These cells separate briefly to allow the lymph to enter the capillary. Then the action of the cells as they close forces the lymph to flow upward and forward (Figure 6.2).

Lymphatic Vessels and Ducts

Lymph flows from the lymphatic capillaries into the progressively larger **lymphatic vessels**, which are located deeper within the tissues. Like veins, lymphatic vessels have valves to prevent the backward flow of lymph.

The larger lymphatic vessels eventually join together to form two ducts. Each duct drains a specific part of the body and returns the lymph to the venous circulation (Figure 6.1).

- The **right lymphatic duct** collects lymph from the right side of the head and neck, the upper right quadrant of the body, and the right arm. The right lymphatic duct empties into the right subclavian vein. The ***subclavian*** vein is the proximal part of the main vein of the arm.
- The **thoracic duct**, which is the largest lymphatic vessel in the body, collects lymph from the left side of the head and neck, the upper left quadrant of the trunk, the left arm, the entire lower portion of the trunk, and both legs. The thoracic duct empties into the left subclavian vein.

Lymph Nodes

Each small, bean-shaped **lymph node** contains specialized lymphocytes that are capable of destroying pathogens. Unfiltered lymph flows into the nodes, and here the lymphocytes destroy harmful substances such as bacteria, viruses, and malignant cells. Additional structures within the node filter the lymph to remove other impurities. After these processes are complete, the lymph leaves the node and continues its journey to become part of the venous circulation again.

There are between 400 and 700 lymph nodes located along the larger lymphatic vessels, and approximately half of these nodes are in the abdomen. Most of the other nodes are positioned on the branches of the larger lymphatic vessels throughout the body. The exceptions are the three major groups of lymph nodes that are named for their locations (Figure 6.1).

- **Cervical lymph nodes** (**SER**-vih-kal) are located along the sides of the neck (**cervic** means neck, and **-al** means pertaining to).
- **Axillary lymph nodes** (**AK**-sih-**lar**-ee) are located under the arms in the area known as the armpits (**axill** means armpit, and **-ary** means pertaining to).
- **Inguinal lymph nodes** (**ING**-gwih-nal) are located in the inguinal (groin) area of the lower abdomen (**inguin** means groin, and **-al** means pertaining to).

StudyWARE CONNECTION

Watch the **Lymph Nodes** animation in the StudyWARE™.

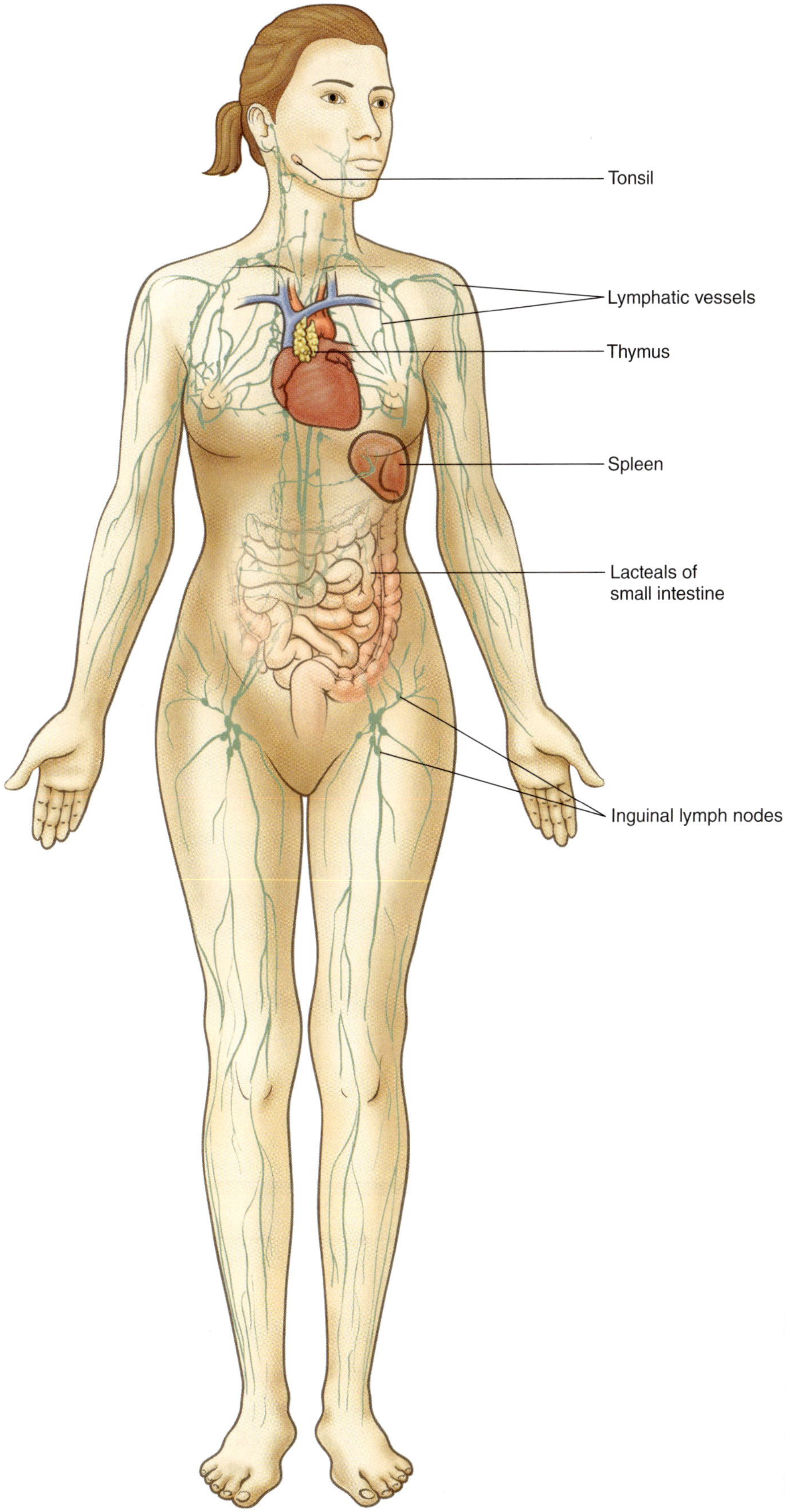

FIGURE 6.1 The vessels and organs of the lymphatic system; only inguinal lymph nodes are labeled.

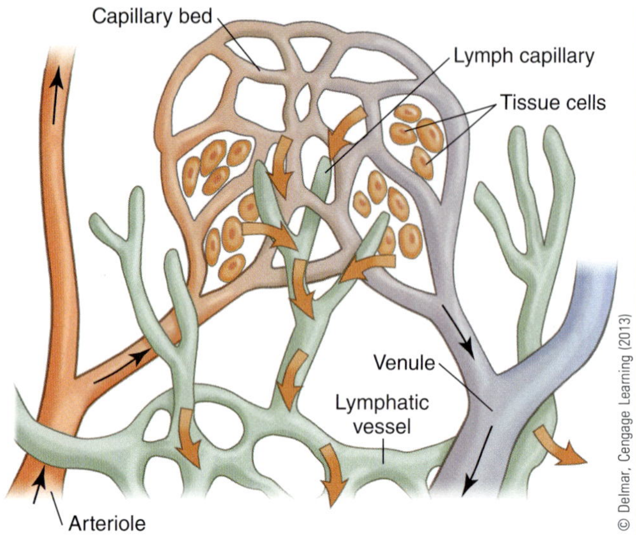

FIGURE 6.2 *Lymph capillaries* begin as blind-ended tubes. Lymph enters between the cells of the capillary wall and flows into progressively larger lymphatic vessels.

Lymphocytes

Lymphocytes (**LIM**-foh-sights), also known as ***lymphoid cells***, are leukocytes that are formed in bone marrow as stem cells (**lymph/o** means lymph, and **-cytes** means cells). There are three types of lymphocytes: natural killer cells, B cells, and T cells.

- Lymphocytes undergo further maturation and differentiation in lymphoid tissues throughout the body. These changes enable these lymphocytes to act as specialized antibodies that are capable of attacking specific antigens. ***Maturation*** means the process of becoming mature. ***Differentiation*** means to be modified to perform a specific function.
- **Natural killer cells** (NK cells) play an important role in the killing of cancer cells and cells infected by viruses.

B Cells

- **B cells**, also known as ***B lymphocytes***, are specialized lymphocytes that produce antibodies. Each lymphocyte makes a specific antibody that is capable of destroying a specific antigen.
- B cells are most effective against viruses and bacteria that are circulating in the blood. When a B cell is confronted with the antigen that it is coded to destroy, that B cell is transformed into a plasma cell.
- **Plasma cells** develop from B cells and secrete a large volume of antibodies coded to destroy specific antigens.

T Cells

- **T cells**, also known as ***T lymphocytes***, belong to a group of leukocytes known as lymphocytes. These cells, which get the 'T' in their name from their origin in the thymus, play a central role in cell-mediated immunity.
- **Cytokines** (**SIGH**-toh-kyens) are a group of proteins such as interferons and interleukins released primarily by the T cells. These cells act as intracellular signals to begin the immune response.
- **Interferons** (**in**-ter-**FEAR**-onz) (IFNs) are produced in response to the presence of antigens, particularly viruses or tumor cells. Interferons activate the immune system, fight viruses by slowing or stopping their multiplication, and signal other cells to increase their defenses.
- **Interleukins** (**in**-ter-**LOO**-kinz) play multiple roles in the immune system, including directing B and T cells to divide and proliferate.

ADDITIONAL STRUCTURES OF THE LYMPHATIC SYSTEM

The remaining structures of this body system are made up of lymphoid tissue. The term ***lymphoid*** means pertaining to the lymphatic system or resembling lymph or lymphatic tissue. Although these structures consist of lymphoid tissue, their primary roles are in conjunction with the immune system (Figure 6.3).

The Tonsils

The **tonsils** (**TON**-sils) are three masses of lymphoid tissue that form a protective ring around the back of the nose and upper throat (Figure 6.4). The tonsils play an important role in the immune system by preventing pathogens from entering the respiratory system when breathing through the nose and mouth.

- The **adenoids** (**AD**-eh-noids), also known as the ***nasopharyngeal tonsils***, are located in the nasopharynx, which is the upper part of the pharynx and is described in Chapter 7.
- The **palatine tonsils** (**PAL**-ah-tine) are located on the left and right sides of the throat in the area that is visible at the back of the mouth. ***Palatine*** describes the hard and soft palates that form the roof of the mouth.
- The **lingual tonsils** (**LING**-gwal) are located at the base of the tongue; however, they are not readily visible. ***Lingual*** means pertaining to the tongue.

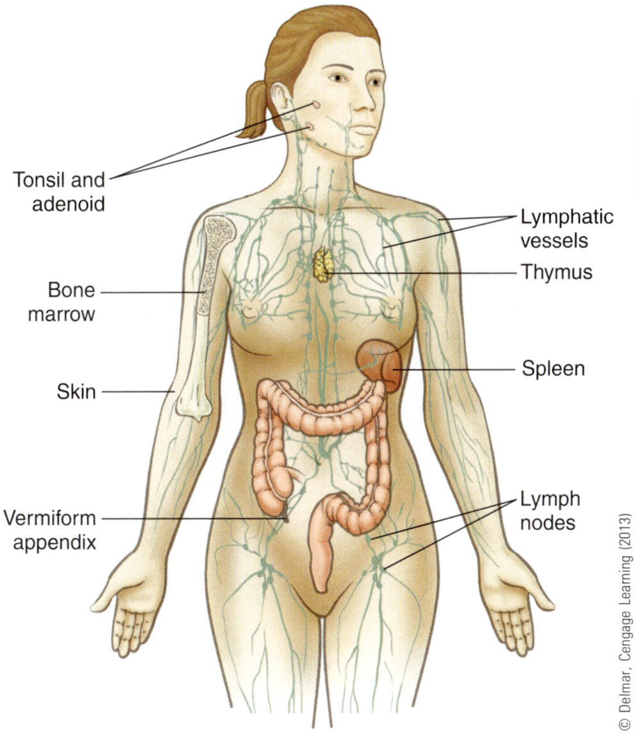

FIGURE 6.3 Structures consisting of lymphoid tissues play many important roles in the immune system.

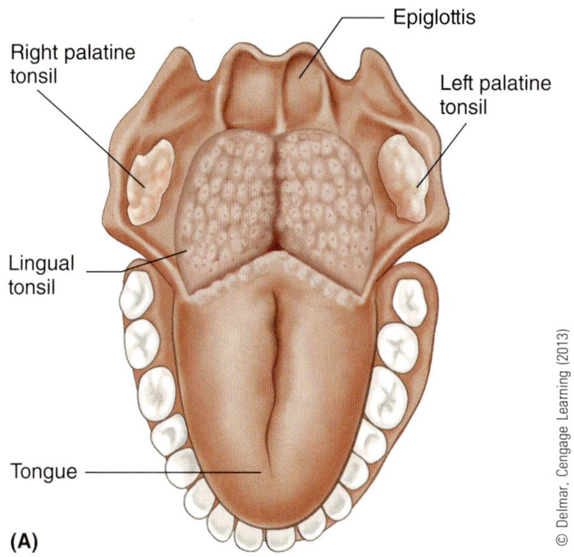

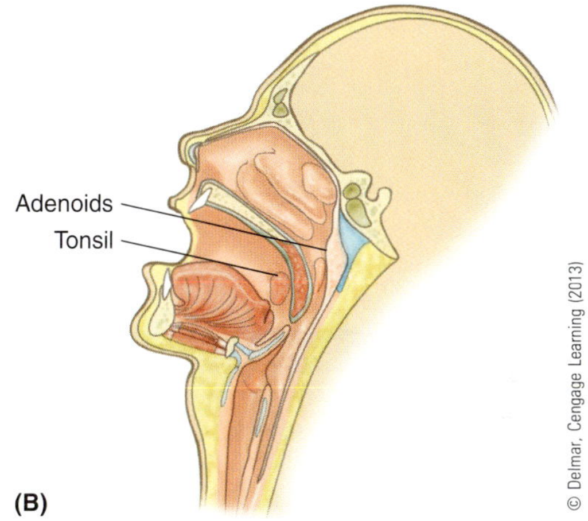

FIGURE 6.4 The *tonsils* form a protective ring around the entrance to the respiratory system.

The Thymus Gland

The **thymus** (**THIGH**-mus), which is a mass of lymphoid tissue located above the heart, reaches its greatest size at puberty and becomes smaller with age.

- As part of the endocrine system, the thymus secretes a hormone that stimulates the maturation of lymphocytes into T cells (see Chapter 13).
- These T cells, which are essential to the immune system, leave the thymus through the bloodstream and the lymphatic system.

The Vermiform Appendix

The **vermiform appendix**, commonly referred to as the *appendix*, hangs from the lower portion of the cecum, which is the first section of the large intestine. Although its purpose was unknown for many years, recent research indicates that the appendix may play an important role in the immune system.

The Spleen

The **spleen** is a sac-like mass of lymphoid tissue located in the left upper quadrant of the abdomen, just inferior to (below) the diaphragm and posterior to (behind) the stomach (Figure 6.5).

- The spleen filters microorganisms and other foreign material from the blood.
- The spleen forms *lymphocytes* and *monocytes*, which are specialized leukocytes (white blood cells) with roles to play in the immune system.
- The spleen has the **hemolytic** (**hee**-moh-**LIT**-ick) function of destroying worn-out erythrocytes (red blood cells) and releasing their hemoglobin for reuse (**hem/o** means blood, and **-lytic** means to destroy).
- The spleen also stores extra erythrocytes (red blood cells) and maintains the appropriate balance between these cells and the plasma of the blood.

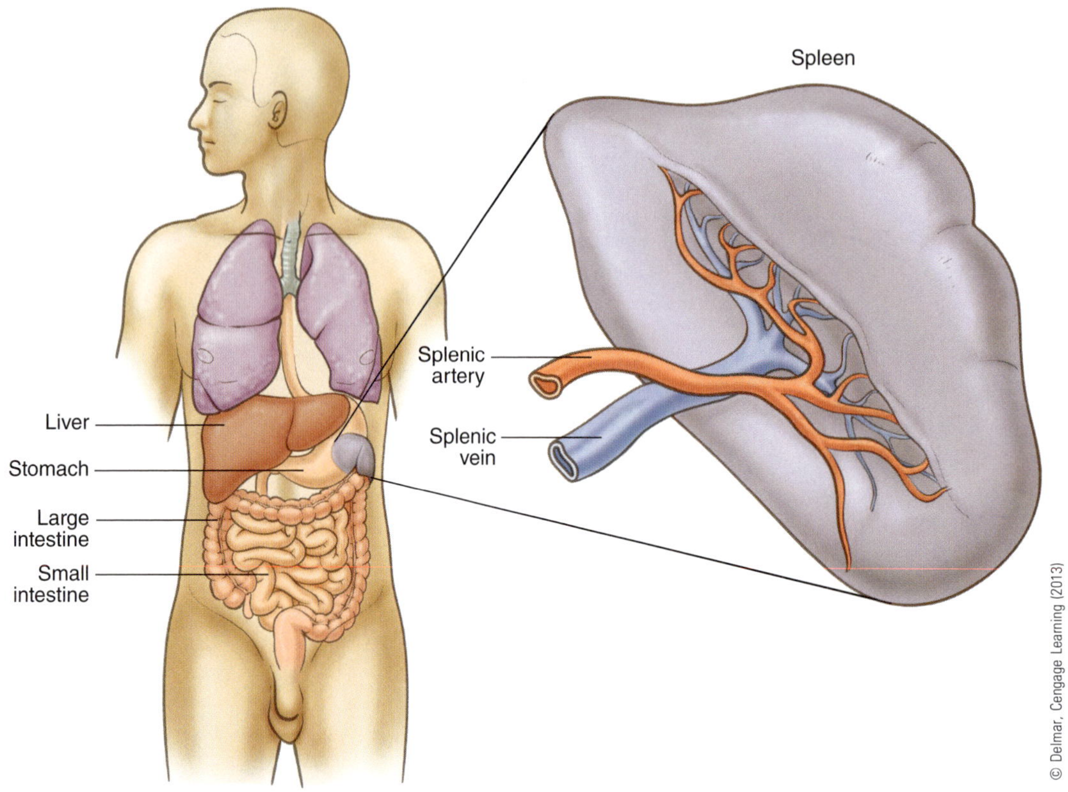

FIGURE 6.5 The spleen performs important functions related to both the immune and cardiovascular systems.

StudyWARE CONNECTION

Watch **The Lymphatic System** animation in the StudyWARE™.

FUNCTIONS AND STRUCTURES OF THE IMMUNE SYSTEM

The primary function of the immune system is to maintain good health and to protect the body from harmful substances such as:

- ***Pathogens***, which are disease-producing microorganisms.
- ***Allergens***, which are substances that produce allergic reactions.
- ***Toxins***, which are poisonous or harmful substances.
- ***Malignant cells***, which are potentially life-threatening cancer cells.

The immune system first attempts to prevent the entry of these harmful substances into the body. If harmful substances do gain entry into the body, the immune system immediately begins working to destroy them.

- The immune system uses a complex system of chemical signaling between specialized cells to identify, attack, and remember antigens.
- This is accomplished by coordinating a highly specific response based on the type of antigen and differentiating it from the body's own tissues to avoid attacking itself.
- After encountering an antigen once, the immune system's "memory" of the invader enables the body to mount a more efficient future defense against that antigen.

The Immune System's First Line of Defense

Unlike other body systems, the immune system is not contained within a single set of organs or vessels. Instead, its functions use structures from several other body systems. The first line of defense includes:

- **Intact skin** that wraps the body in a physical barrier to prevent invading organisms from entering the body. ***Intact*** means that there are no cuts, scrapes, open sores, or breaks in the skin. The skin is also covered with an ***acid mantle*** that makes it an inhospitable environment for most bacteria.

- The **respiratory system** traps breathed-in foreign matter with nose hairs and the moist mucous membrane lining of the respiratory system. The tonsils form a protective ring around the entrance to the throat. If foreign matter gets past these barriers, coughing and sneezing help expel it from the respiratory system.
- The **digestive system** uses the acids and enzymes produced by the stomach to destroy invaders that are swallowed or consumed with food.
- The structures of the **lymphatic system** and specialized leukocytes (white blood cells) work together in specific ways to attack and destroy pathogens that have succeeded in entering the body.

The Antigen-Antibody Reaction

An **antigen-antibody reaction**, also known as the *immune reaction*, involves binding antigens to antibodies. This reaction labels a potentially dangerous antigen so it can be recognized and destroyed by other cells of the immune system.

- An **antigen** (**AN**-tih-jen) is any substance that the body regards as being foreign. This includes viruses, bacteria, toxins, and transplanted tissues. The immune system immediately responds to the presence of any antigen. (Figure 6.6).
- **Tolerance** refers to an acquired unresponsiveness to a specific antigen. The term is also used to describe a decline in the effective response to a drug, usually due to repeated use.

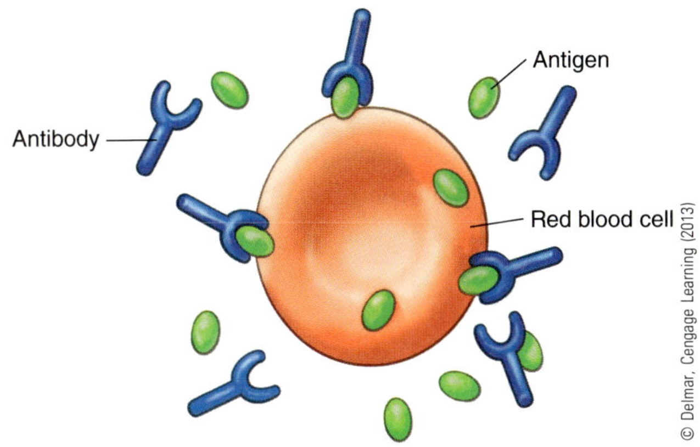

FIGURE 6.6 Antibodies bind together foreign antigens to neutralize them and to flag them for destruction by the microphages.

- An **antibody** (**AN**-tih-**bod**-ee) is a disease-fighting protein created by the immune system in response to the presence of a specific antigen (the prefix **anti-** means against). The terms *antibody* and *immunoglobulin* are often used interchangeably.

Immunoglobulins

- **Immunoglobulins** (**im**-you-noh-**GLOB**-you-lins) bind with specific antigens in the antigen-antibody response. The five primary types of immunoglobulins, which are secreted by plasma cells, are also known as antibodies (Table 6.1).

TABLE 6.1
Immunoglobulins and Their Roles

Immunoglobulin G (IgG) is the most abundant class of antibodies, and they are found in blood serum and lymph. These antibodies are active against bacteria, fungi, viruses, and foreign particles.
Immunoglobulin A (IgA) is the class of antibodies produced predominantly against ingested antigens. These antibodies are found in body secretions such as saliva, sweat, or tears, and function to prevent the attachment of viruses and bacteria to the epithelial surfaces that line most organs.
Immunoglobulin M (IgM) is the class of antibodies that are found in circulating body fluids. These are the first antibodies to appear in response to an initial exposure to an antigen.
Immunoglobulin D (IgD) is the class of antibodies found only on the surface of B cells. These antibodies are important in B cell activation.
Immunoglobulin E (IgE) is the class of antibodies produced in the lungs, skin, and mucous membranes. These antibodies are responsible for allergic reactions.
Note: Synthetic immunoglobulins, which are used as medications, are discussed later in this chapter.

Phagocytes

Phagocytes (**FAG**-oh-sights) are specialized leukocytes that act as part of the antigen-antibody reaction by destroying substances such as cell debris, dust, pollen, and pathogens by the process of phagocytosis (**phag/o** means to eat or swallow, and **-cyte** means cell). ***Phagocytosis*** is the process of destroying pathogens by surrounding and swallowing them. Phagocytes include monocytes, macrophages, dendritic cells, and mast cells. Mast cells are discussed in Chapter 12.

- **Monocytes** are leukocytes that provide immunological defenses against many infectious organisms. Macrophages derive from monocytes after they leave the bloodstream and enter into the tissue. Monocytes replenish macrophages and dendritic cells.
- A **macrophage** (**MACK**-roh-fayj) is a type of leukocyte that surrounds and kills invading cells (**macro-** means large, and **-phage** means a cell that eats). Macrophages also remove dead cells and stimulate the action of other immune cells.
- **Dendritic cells** (den-**DRIT**-ic) are specialized leukocytes that patrol the body searching for antigens that produce infections. When such a cell is found, the dendritic cell grabs it, swallows, and alerts B and T cells to act against this specific antigen.

The Complement System

The complement system (**KOM**-pleh-ment) is a group of proteins that normally circulate in the blood in an inactive form. When needed, these cells complement the ability of antibodies to ward off pathogens by combining with them to dissolve and remove pathogenic bacteria and other foreign cells. ***Complement*** means to complete or make whole.

Immunity

Immunity is the state of being resistant to a specific disease. This resistance can be present naturally or it can be acquired.

- **Natural immunity**, which is also known as ***passive immunity***, is resistance to a disease present without the administration of an antigen or exposure to a disease. Natural immunity is either present at birth or it is passed from the mother to her child through breast milk.
- **Acquired immunity** is obtained by having had a contagious disease. Being ***vaccinated*** against a contagious disease provides protection against that disease, such as measles or polio, without having been exposed to the risk of actually having the disease.
- A ***vaccine*** is a preparation containing an antigen, consisting of whole or partial disease-causing organisms, which have been killed or weakened. For some diseases, such as tetanus (discussed in Chapter 10), a periodic booster shot is required to maintain the effectiveness of the immunity.
- ***Vaccination*** provides protection against the disease; however, for some conditions a periodic booster is required to maintain the effectiveness of the immunization.

MEDICAL SPECIALTIES RELATED TO THE LYMPHATIC AND IMMUNE SYSTEMS

- The lymphatic and immune systems work in close cooperation to protect and maintain the health of the body. Some functions and structures of these systems are performed by specialized structures or shared structures. Some medical specialists treat disorders that affect both of these body systems.
- An **allergist** (**AL**-er-jist) specializes in diagnosing and treating conditions of altered immunologic reactivity, such as allergic reactions.
- An **immunologist** (**im**-you-**NOL**-oh-jist) specializes in diagnosing and treating disorders of the immune system (**immun** means protected, and **-ologist** means specialist).
- A **lymphologist** (lim-**FOL**-oh-jist) is a physician who specializes in diagnosing and treating disorders of the lymphatic system (**lymph** means lymphatic system, and **-ologist** means specialist).
- An **oncologist** (ong-**KOL**-oh-jist) is a physician specializing in the diagnosing and treatment of malignant disorders such as tumors and cancer (**onc** mean tumor, and **-ologist** means specialist).

PATHOLOGY AND DIAGNOSTIC PROCEDURES OF THE LYMPHATIC SYSTEM

- **Lymphadenitis** (lim-**fad**-eh-**NIGH**-tis), commonly known as ***swollen glands***, is an inflammation of the lymph nodes (**lymphaden** means lymph node, and

-itis means inflammation). The terms *lymph nodes* and *lymph glands* are sometimes used interchangeably. Swelling of the lymph nodes is frequently an indication of an infection.

- **Lymphadenopathy** (lim-**fad**-eh-**NOP**-ah-thee) is any disease process affecting a lymph node or nodes (**lymphaden/o** means lymph node, and **-pathy** means disease).
- A **lymphangioma** (lim-**fan**-jee-**OH**-mah) is a benign tumor formed by an abnormal collection of lymphatic vessels due to a congenital malformation of the lymphatic system (**lymph** means lymph, **angi** means lymph vessel, and **-oma** means tumor).
- **Splenomegaly** (**splee**-noh-**MEG**-ah-lee) is an abnormal enlargement of the spleen (**splen/o** means spleen, and **-megaly** means enlargement). This condition can be due to bleeding caused by an injury, an infectious disease such as mononucleosis, or abnormal functioning of the immune system.
- **Splenorrhagia** (**splee**-noh-**RAY**-jee-ah) is bleeding from the spleen (**splen/o** means spleen, and **-rrhagia** means bleeding).
- **Tonsillitis** and **tonsillectomy** are discussed in Chapter 1.
- **Lymphoscintigraphy** (**lim**-foh-sin-**TIH**-grah-fee) is a diagnostic test that is performed to detect damage or malformations of the lymphatic vessels. A radioactive substance is injected into lymph ducts, and a scanner or probe is used to follow the movement of the substance on a computer screen. This technique is used to find a sentinel node.

Lymphedema

Lymphedema (**lim**-feh-**DEE**-mah) is swelling of the tissues due to an abnormal accumulation of lymph fluid within the tissues (**lymph** means lymph, and **-edema** means swelling). This is not the type of swelling that occurs due to an injury such as a sprained ankle. It is caused by damage to the lymphatic system that prevents lymph from draining properly. Because lymph is rich in protein, which is an environment that pathogens thrive in, lymphedema is often associated with infections.

- **Primary lymphedema** is a hereditary condition of the lymphatic system that develops with swelling beginning in the feet and progressing into the ankles and in an upward direction along the legs. The disorder occurs most frequently in females when the symptoms begin to appear during puberty.
- **Secondary lymphedema** is caused by damage to lymphatic vessels that is most frequently due to cancer treatment, surgery, trauma, or burns.
- Primary and secondary lymphedema are most commonly treated with compression and exercise to control the swelling and to minimize the infections. Although this treatment helps, at this time it is not possible to cure lymphedema.
- **Bioimpedance spectroscopy** (**BYE**-oh-im-**pee**-dens) is a noninvasive method of diagnosing lymphedema. It measures the resistance to an electrical current passed through the affected limb, with abnormally low results showing a buildup of lymph. If this condition can be diagnosed with this technique at an early stage, there is hope that it will not develop any further.

PATHOLOGY AND DIAGNOSTIC PROCEDURES OF THE IMMUNE SYSTEM

The effectiveness of the immune system depends upon the individual's:

- *General health.* If the immune system is compromised by poor health, it cannot be fully effective.
- *Age.* Older individuals usually have more acquired immunity; however, their immune system tends to respond less quickly or effectively to new challenges.
- *Age.* Babies and very young children do not yet have as much acquired immunity, and their bodies sometimes have difficulty resisting challenges to the immune system.
- *Heredity.* Genes and genetic disorders affect the individual's general health and the functioning of his or her immune system.

Allergic Reactions

- An **allergic reaction** occurs when the body's immune system reacts to a harmless allergen such as pollen, food, or animal dander as if it were a dangerous invader.
- An **allergy**, also known as ***hypersensitivity***, is an overreaction by the body to a particular antigen. For *allergic rhinitis*, an allergic reaction to airborne allergens, see Chapter 7.
- An **allergen** (**AL**-er-jen) is a substance that produces an allergic reaction in an individual.

- A **localized allergic response**, also known as a ***cellular response***, includes redness, itching, and burning where the skin has come into contact with an allergen. For example, contact with poison ivy can cause a localized allergic response in the form of an itchy rash (see Chapter 12). Although the body reacts mildly the first time it is exposed to the allergen, sensitivity is established, and future contacts can cause much more severe symptoms.
- A **systemic reaction**, which is also described as **anaphylaxis** (**an**-ah-fih-**LACK**-sis) or as ***anaphylactic shock***, is a severe response to an allergen. As shown in Figure 6.7, the symptoms of this response develop quickly. Without prompt medical aid, the patient can die within a few minutes.
- A ***scratch test*** is a diagnostic test to identify commonly troublesome allergens such as tree pollen and ragweed. Swelling and itching indicate an allergic reaction (Figure 6.8).
- **Antihistamines** are medications administered to relieve or prevent the symptoms of hay fever, which is a common allergy to wind-borne pollens, and other types of allergies. Antihistamines work by preventing the effects of ***histamine***, which is a substance produced by the body that causes the itching, sneezing, runny nose, and watery eyes of an allergic reaction.

Autoimmune Disorders

An **autoimmune disorder** (**aw**-toh-ih-**MYOUN**), also known as an ***autoimmune disease***, is any of a large group of diseases characterized by a condition in which the immune system produces antibodies against its own tissues, mistaking healthy cells, tissues, or organs for antigens.

- This abnormal functioning of the immune system appears to be genetically transmitted and predominantly occurs in women during the childbearing years.

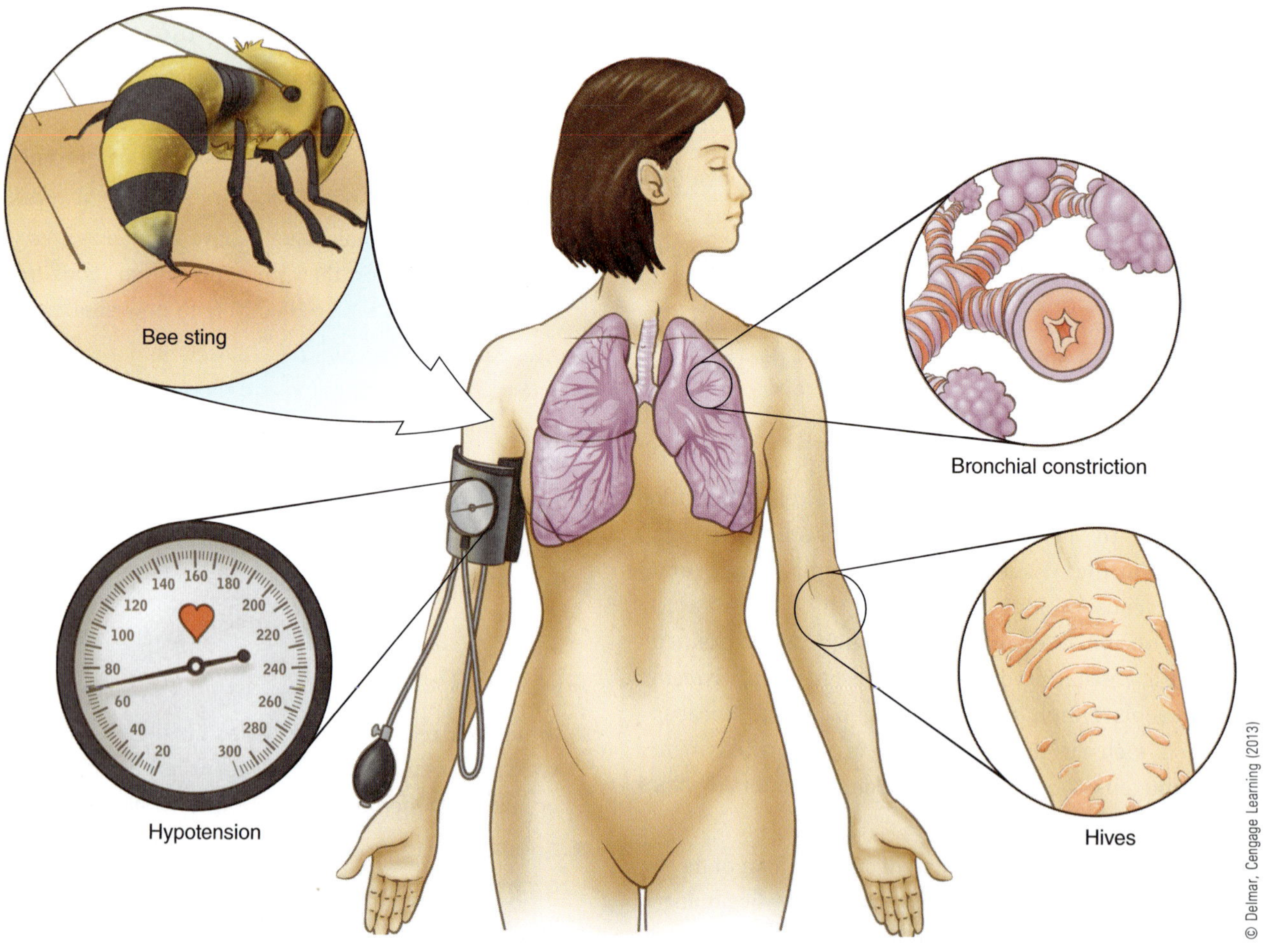

FIGURE 6.7 A severe anaphylactic allergic reaction involves several body systems and requires prompt treatment. Shown here are the many systems that may respond to a bee sting.

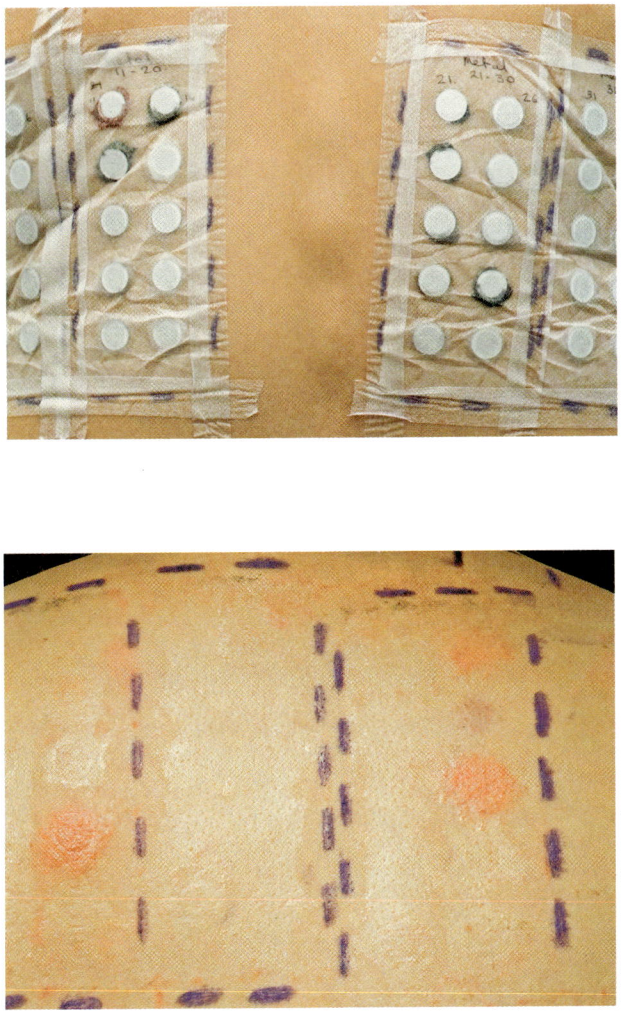

Andy Lidstone/www.Shutterstock.com

Andy Lidstone/www.Shutterstock.com

FIGURE 6.8 In scratch tests, allergens are placed on the skin, the skin is scratched, and the allergen is labeled. Reactions usually begin to occur within 20 minutes.

- It is estimated that 3% of Americans have an autoimmune disorder, with women affected 2.7 times more often than men. Autoimmune disorders affect most body systems. For examples, see Table 6.2.

Immunodeficiency Disorders

An **immunodeficiency disorder** (**im**-you-noh-deh-**FISH**-en-see) occurs when the immune response is compromised. *Compromised* means weakened or not functioning properly.

HIV: Human Immunodeficiency Virus

The **human immunodeficiency virus** (**im**-you-noh-deh-**FISH**-en-see), commonly known as *HIV*, is a bloodborne infection in which the virus damages or kills the T cells of the immune system, causing it to progressively fail, thus leaving the body at risk of developing many life-threatening opportunistic infections (Figure 6.9). Medical intervention including reverse transcriptase (RT), protease, and fusion inhibitors can now prolong the patient's life, especially if administered starting in the early stages of HIV.

- An **opportunistic infection** (**op**-ur-too-**NIHS**-tick) is caused by a pathogen that does not normally produce an illness in healthy humans. However, when the host is debilitated, these pathogens are able to cause an infection. *Debilitated* means weakened by another condition.
- **Acquired immunodeficiency syndrome**, commonly known as *AIDS*, is the most advanced and fatal stage of an HIV infection.

TABLE 6.2
Examples of Autoimmune Disorders and the Affected Body Systems

Body System	Autoimmune Disorder
Skeletal System	*Rheumatoid arthritis* affects joints and connective tissue.
Muscular System	*Myasthenia gravis* affects nerve and muscle synapses.
Cardiovascular System	*Pernicious anemia* affects the red blood cells.
Digestive System	*Crohn's disease* affects the intestines, ileum, or the colon.
Nervous System	*Multiple sclerosis* affects the brain and spinal cord.
Integumentary System	*Scleroderma* affects the skin and connective tissues.
Endocrine System	*Graves' disease* affects the thyroid gland.

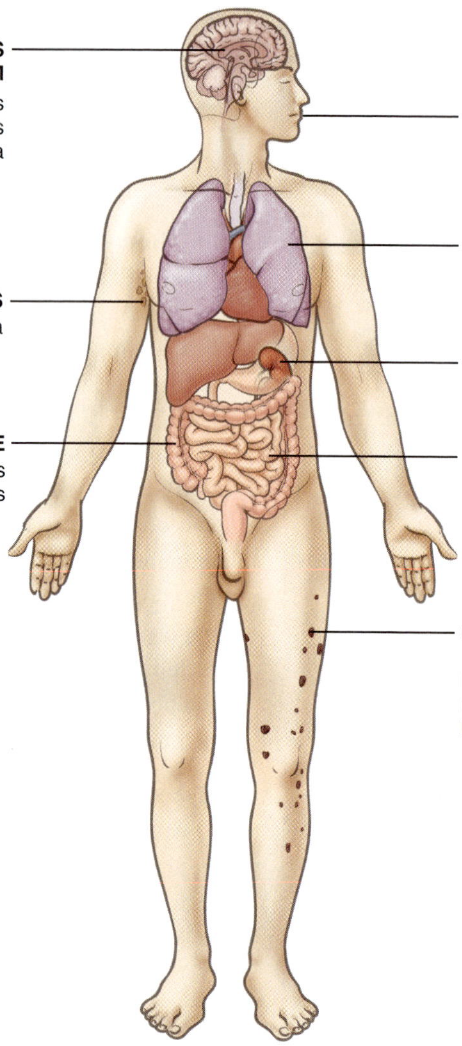

FIGURE 6.9 Pathologies associated with Acquired immunodeficiency syndrome (AIDS). (Each condition is discussed in the appropriate body system chapter.)

- **Kaposi's sarcoma** (**KAP**-oh-seez sar-**KOH**-mah) is an example of an opportunistic infection that is frequently associated with HIV. This cancer causes patches of abnormal tissue to grow under the skin; in the lining of the mouth, nose, and throat; or in other organs.
- **ELISA**, which is the acronym for *enzyme-linked immunosorbent assay*, is a blood test used to screen for the presence of HIV antibodies.
- A **Western blot test** is a blood test that produces more accurate results than the ELISA test. The Western blot test is performed to confirm the diagnosis when the results of the ELISA test are positive. This is necessary because the ELISA test sometimes produces a *false positive* result in which the test erroneously indicates the presence of HIV.

TREATMENT OF THE IMMUNE SYSTEM

A variety of treatment procedures are used to correct or control the symptoms of disorders of the immune system.

Immunotherapy

Immunotherapy (ih-**myou**-noh-**THER**-ah-pee), also called *biological therapy*, is a disease treatment that involves either stimulating or repressing the immune response (**immun/o** means immune, and **-therapy** means treatment).

- In the treatment of cancers, immunotherapy is used to stimulate the immune response to fight the malignancy. *Stimulate* means to cause greater activity.

- In the treatment of allergies, immunotherapy is used to repress the body's sensitivity to a particular allergen. ***Repress*** means to decrease or stop a normal response. This treatment is also known as ***allergy desensitization***.

Antibody Therapy

- **Synthetic immunoglobulins**, also known as ***immune serum***, are used as a postexposure preventive measure against certain viruses, including rabies and some types of hepatitis. ***Postexposure*** means that the patient has been exposed to the virus, for example, by being bitten by an animal with rabies. The goal of this treatment is to prevent the disease from developing by providing temporary immunity.
- **Synthetic interferon** is used in the treatment of multiple sclerosis, hepatitis C, and some cancers.
- **Monoclonal antibodies** are any of a class of antibodies produced in the laboratory by identical offspring of a clone of specific cells. These artificially produced antibodies are used to enhance the patient's immune response to certain malignancies, including some non-Hodgkin's lymphoma, melanoma, breast cancer, and colon cancer. ***Monoclonal*** means pertains to a single clone of cells. As used here, a ***clone*** is an exact replica of a group of bacteria.

Immunosuppression

Immunosuppression (**im**-you-noh-sup-**PRESH**-un) is treatment to repress or interfere with the ability of the immune system to respond to stimulation by antigens.

- An **immunosuppressant** (**im**-you-noh-soo-**PRES**-ant) is a substance that prevents or reduces the body's normal immune response. This medication is administered to prevent the rejection of donor tissue and to depress autoimmune disorders.
- A **corticosteroid drug** (**kor**-tih-koh-**STEHR**-oid) is a hormone-like preparation administered primarily as an anti-inflammatory and as an immunosuppressant. The natural production of corticosteroids by the endocrine system is discussed in Chapter 13.
- A **cytotoxic drug** (**sigh**-toh-**TOK**-sick) is a medication that kills or damages cells (**cyt/o** means cell, **tox** means poison, and **-ic** means pertaining to). These drugs are used as immunosuppressants or as antineoplastics. *Antineoplastics* are discussed under "Chemotherapy" later in this chapter.

PATHOGENIC ORGANISMS

A **pathogen** (**PATH**-oh-jen) is a microorganism that causes a disease in humans. A ***microorganism*** is a living organism that is so small it can be seen only with the aid of a microscope. ***Pathogenic*** means capable of producing disease (Figure 6.10).

Bacteria

Bacteria (back-**TEER**-ree-ah) are one-celled microscopic organisms (singular, *bacterium*). Most bacteria are not harmful to humans. The following bacteria are pathogenic:

- **Bacilli** (bah-**SILL**-eye) are rod-shaped spore-forming bacteria (**bacilli** means rod shaped). (The singular is *bacillus*.)
- **Anthrax** (**AN**-thraks) is a contagious disease that can be transmitted through livestock infected with *bacillus anthracis*. Spores grown in laboratories have been used in biological warfare.
- A **rickettsia** (rih-**KET**-see-ah) is a small bacterium that lives in lice, fleas, ticks, and mites (plural, *rickettsiae*). ***Rocky Mountain spotted fever*** is caused by a rickettsia that is transmitted to humans by the bite of an infected tick.
- **Spirochetes** (**SPY**-roh-keets) are long, slender spiral-shaped bacteria that have flexible walls and are capable of movement.
- **Lyme disease** (**LIME**) is caused by a spirochete belonging to the genus *Borrelia*. Lyme disease, which can affect the joints, heart, and central nervous system, is transmitted by the bite of an infected deer tick. Syphilis is also caused by spirochetes (see Chapter 14).
- **Staphylococci** (**staf**-ih-loh-**KOCK**-sigh) are a group of about 30 species of bacteria that form irregular groups or clusters resembling grapes (**staphyl/o** means clusters or bunches of grapes, and **-cocci** means spherical bacteria). (The singular is *staphylococcus*.) Most staphylococci are harmless and reside normally on the skin and mucous membranes of humans and other organisms; however, others are capable of producing very serious infections.

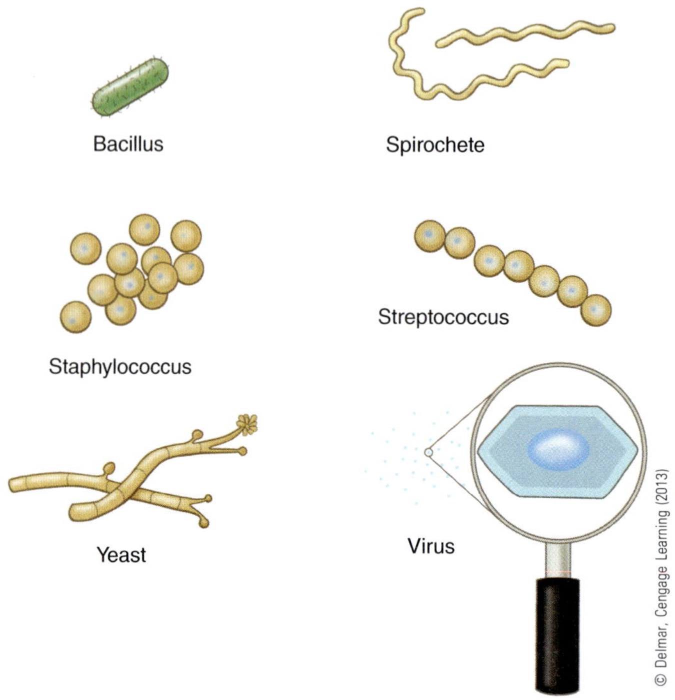

FIGURE 6.10 Shown here are examples of types of pathogens. The single virus shown at the right is magnified to illustrate details of its structure.

- **Staphylococcus aureus** (**staf**-ih-loh-**KOCK**-us **OR**-ee-us), also known as ***staph aureus***, is a form of staphylococci that often infects wounds and causes serious problems such as toxic shock syndrome or food poisoning.
- **Streptococci** (**strep**-toh-**KOCK**-sigh) are bacteria that form a chain (**strept/o** means twisted chain, and **-cocci** means spherical bacteria). (The singular is *streptococcus.*) Many streptococcal species are harmless; however, other members of this group are responsible for serious illnesses such as strep throat, meningitis (see Chapter 10), endocarditis (see Chapter 5), and necrotizing fasciitis (see Chapter 12).

Septic Shock

Septic shock is a serious condition that occurs when an overwhelming bacterial infection affects the body. Toxins that are released by pathogens can produce direct tissue damage, resulting in low blood pressure.

This damage causes vital organs (the brain, heart, kidneys, and liver) not to function properly or to fail completely. Septic shock occurs most frequently in the very old and the very young. It also occurs in those with underlying or debilitating illnesses.

Antibiotic-Resistant Bacteria

Antibiotic-resistant bacteria occur when antibiotics fail to kill all of the bacteria they target. When this occurs, the surviving bacteria become resistant to this particular drug. As more and more bacteria become resistant to first-line antibiotics, the consequences are severe because the illness lasts longer, and the risks of complications and death increase.

Originally these infections were nosocomial (hospital acquired), but now these antibiotic-resistant bacteria are increasingly common in the general population.

Methicillin-resistant *Staphylococcus aureus*, commonly known as ***MRSA***, is one of several types of bacteria that are now resistant to most antibiotics.

- The first symptom of MRSA looks like small, red bumps with a black top. These bumps soon become abscesses that require immediate care.
- MRSA infections are serious, difficult to treat, can be fatal, and often occur repeatedly as breaks in the skin allow the bacteria entry. These infections are becoming increasingly present in the general population.

Fungus and Yeast Infections

A **fungus** (**FUNG**-gus) is a simple parasitic organism (plural, *fungi*). Some of these fungi are harmless to humans; others are pathogenic. **Tinea pedis**, commonly known as *athlete's foot*, is a fungal infection that develops between the toes (see Chapter 12).

Yeast is a type of fungus. An example is **candidiasis** (**kan**-dih-**DYE**-ah-sis), is also known as a *yeast infection*. These infections occur on the skin or mucous membranes in warm, moist areas such as the vagina or mouth and are caused by the pathogenic yeast *Candida albicans*. *Oral thrush* is a yeast infection that occurs in the mouth, whereas *vaginal candidiasis* occurs in the vagina (see Chapter 14).

Parasites

A **parasite** (**PAR**-ah-sight) is a plant or animal that lives on or within another living organism at the expense of that organism.

- **Malaria** (mah-**LAY**-ree-ah) is caused by a parasite that lives in certain mosquitoes and is transferred to humans by the bite of an infected mosquito. Symptoms develop from 7 days to 4 weeks after being infected and include fever, shaking chills, headache, muscle aches, and tiredness.
- **Toxoplasmosis** (**tock**-soh-plaz-**MOH**-sis) is another example of a parasite that is most commonly transmitted from pets to humans by contact with contaminated animal feces. A pregnant woman should avoid such contact because it can transmit diseases in the developing child such as *microcephalus* (an abnormally small head and underdeveloped brain) or *hydrocephalus* (excess cerebrospinal fluid accumulates in the ventricles of the brain).
- **West Nile virus** is also spread to humans by the bite of an infected mosquito. A mild form of this condition has flu-like symptoms. A more severe variety spreads to the spinal cord and brain. West Nile virus is a member of the *Flavivirus* genus, which also includes the viruses that cause dengue fever.
- **Lyme disease** is transmitted to humans by the bite of an infected blacklegged tick. The tick becomes infected by having bitten a deer infected with the bacterium *Borrelia burgdorferi*. The symptoms of Lyme disease include fever, headache, fatigue, and a characteristic skin rash known as *erythema migrans*. If untreated, Lyme disease can spread to the joints, heart, and nervous system.

Viral Infections

Viruses (**VYE**-rus-ez) are very small infectious agents that live only by invading other cells. After invading the cell, the virus reproduces and then breaks the wall of the infected cell to release the newly formed viruses. These viruses spread to other cells and repeat the process.

- **Influenza** (**in**-floo-**EN**-zah), commonly known as the *flu*, is a highly contagious viral respiratory infection that usually occurs in seasonal epidemics. Flu symptoms include fever, sore throat, muscle aches, cough, runny nose, and fatigue. Complications can include pneumonia. A vaccine is available annually to protect against the most common strains of influenza.
- **Measles** are an acute, highly contagious infection that is transmitted by respiratory droplets of the *rubeola virus*. Symptoms include a red, itchy rash over the entire body, a high fever, runny nose, and coughing. Serious complications of measles can include *photophobia*, which is a serious sensitivity to light.
- **Mumps** is an acute viral infection that is characterized by the swelling of the parotid glands, which are the salivary glands located just in front of the ears. In adults, mumps can also cause painful swelling of the ovaries or testicles.
- **Rubella** (roo-**BELL**-ah), also known as *German measles* or *3-day measles*, is a viral infection characterized by a low-grade fever, swollen glands, inflamed eyes, and a fine, pink rash. Although not usually severe or long lasting, rubella is serious in a woman during early pregnancy because it can cause defects in a developing fetus.
- The **measles, mumps, and rubella vaccination** (MMR) immunization can prevent these three viral conditions and should be administered in early childhood.
- **Rabies** (**RAY**-beez) is an acute viral infection that is transmitted to humans through the bite or saliva of an infected animal. An infected animal is said to be *rabid*. If risk is suspected, it is necessary to undergo testing immediately so that postexposure treatment can be started as quickly as possible. Without testing and treatment, the signs and symptoms of rabies usually occur 30 to 90 days after the bite, and once symptoms have developed, rabies is almost always fatal.

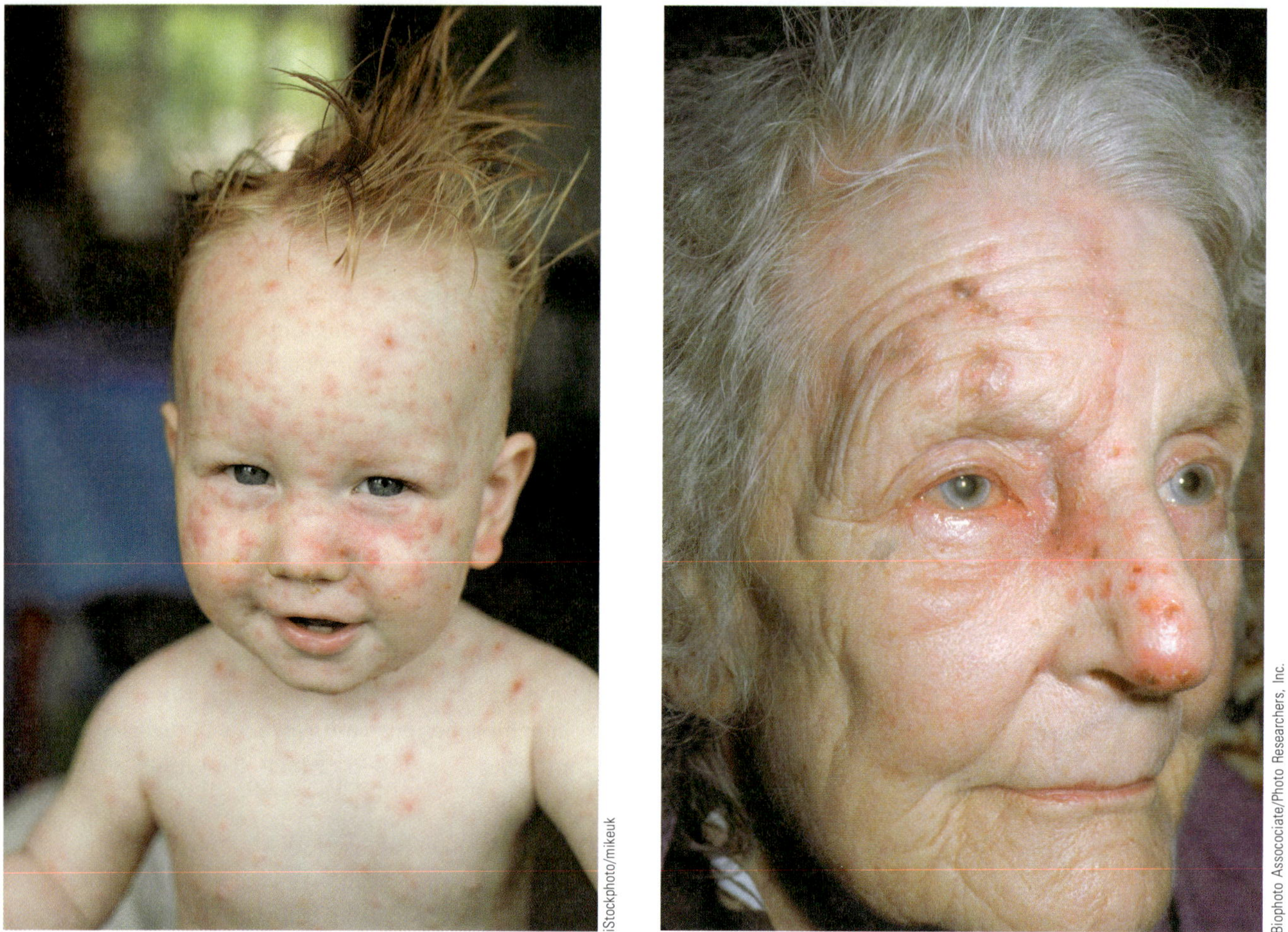

(A) (B)

FIGURE 6.11 Varicella, or chickenpox (A), is caused by the varicella zoster virus, which can remain dormant until later in life when it erupts as herpes zoster, or shingles (B).

Herpesviruses

The group of herpesviruses, which includes *varicella zoster*, *Epstein-Barr*, *cytomegalovirus*, and *herpes simplex*, causes a variety of diseases in humans.

- **Cytomegalovirus** (**sigh**-toh-**meg**-ah-loh-**VYE**-rus) (CMV) is found in most body fluids (**cyt/o** means cell, **megal/o** means large, **vir** means virus, and **-us** is a singular noun ending). It is most often present as a ***silent infection*** in which the individual has no signs or symptoms of the infection, although it can potentially cause a serious illness when the individual has a weakened immune system, or when it is transmitted from the mother to her unborn child. This transmission can cause serious congenital disabilities to the child.
- **Varicella** (**var**-ih-**SEL**-ah), also known as ***chickenpox***, is caused by the herpes virus *Varicella zoster* and is highly contagious. This condition is characterized by a fever and a rash consisting of hundreds of itchy, fluid-filled blisters that burst and form crusts.
- **Herpes zoster** (**HER**-peez **ZOS**-ter), which is also known as ***shingles***, is an acute viral infection characterized by painful skin eruptions that follow the underlying route of an inflamed nerve. This inflammation occurs when the dormant varicella (chickenpox) virus is reactivated later in life. A vaccine is available to prevent shingles; however, this treatment can be effective only if it is administered promptly.

- **Infectious mononucleosis** (**mon**-oh-**new**-klee-**OH**-sis), also known as *mono*, is caused by the Epstein-Barr virus (EBV). This condition is characterized by fever, a sore throat, and enlarged lymph nodes. Swelling of the spleen or liver involvement can also develop.

Medications to Control Infections

- **Antibiotics** are medications capable of inhibiting growth or killing pathogenic bacterial microorganisms (**anti-** means against, **bio** means life, and **-tic** means pertaining to). *Inhibit* means to slow the growth or development. Antibiotics are effective against most bacterial infections; however, they are not effective against viral infections.
- A **bactericide** (back-**TEER**-ih-sighd) is a substance that causes the death of bacteria (**bacteri** means bacteria, and **-cide** means causing death). This group of antibiotics includes penicillins and cephalosporins.
- A *bacteriostatic* agent slows or stops the growth of bacteria (**bacteri** means bacteria, and **-static** means causing control). This group of antibiotics includes tetracycline, sulfonamide, and erythromycin.
- An **antifungal** (**an**-tih-**FUNG**-gul) is an agent that destroys or inhibits the growth of fungi (**anti-** means against, **fung** means fungus, and **-al** means pertaining to). Lotrimin is an example of a topical antifungal that is applied to treat or prevent athlete's foot. This type of medication is also known as an *antimycotic*.
- An **antiviral drug** (**an**-tih-**VYE**-ral), such as acyclovir, is used to treat viral infections or to provide temporary immunity (**anti-** means against, **vir** means virus, and **-al** means pertaining to).

ONCOLOGY

Oncology (ong-**KOL**-oh-jee) is the study of the prevention, causes, and treatment of tumors and cancer (**onc** means tumor, and **-ology** means study of). Most cancers are named for the part of the body where the cancer originated. Cancer can attack all body systems and is the second leading cause of death in the United States after heart conditions.

Tumors

A **tumor**, which is also known as a **neoplasm** (**neo-** means new or strange, and **-plasm** means formation), is an abnormal growth of body tissue. Within this mass, the multiplication of cells is uncontrolled, abnormal, rapid, and progressive.

A *benign tumor* is not a form of cancer, and it is not life-threatening. For example, a **myoma** (my-**OH**-mah) is a benign tumor made up of muscle tissue (**my** means muscle, and **-oma** means tumor). Although this type of tumor is not life threatening, it can cause damage as the tumor grows and places pressure on adjacent structures.

A *malignant tumor* is a form of cancer. It is capable of spreading to distant body sites, including to other body systems, and it is potentially life threatening. For example, a **myosarcoma** (**my**-oh-sahr-**KOH**-mah) is a malignant tumor derived from muscle tissue (**my/o** means muscle, **sarc** means flesh, and **-oma** means tumor).

- **Angiogenesis** (**an**-jee-oh-**JEN**-eh-sis) is the process through which a tumor supports its growth by creating its own blood supply (**angi/o** means vessel, and **-genesis** means reproduction). Angiogenesis is the opposite of *antiangiogenesis*.
- **Antiangiogenesis** (**an**-tih-an-jee-oh-**JEN**-eh-sis) is a form of treatment that disrupts the blood supply to the tumor (**anti-** means against, **angi/o** means vessel, and **-genesis** means reproduction). Antiangiogenesis is the opposite of *angiogenesis*.

Cancer

Cancer is a class of diseases characterized by the uncontrolled division of cells and the ability of these cells to invade other tissues, either by invasion through direct growth into adjacent tissue or by spreading into distant sites by metastasizing.

- To **metastasize** (meh-**TAS**-tah-sighz) is the process by which cancer spreads from one place to another. The cancer moves from the primary site and metastasizes (spreads) to a secondary site.
- A **metastasis** (meh-**TAS**-tah-sis) is the new cancer site that results from the spreading process (**meta-** means beyond, and **-stasis** means stopping). The metastasis can be in the same body system or within another body system at a distance from the primary site (plural, *metastases*).

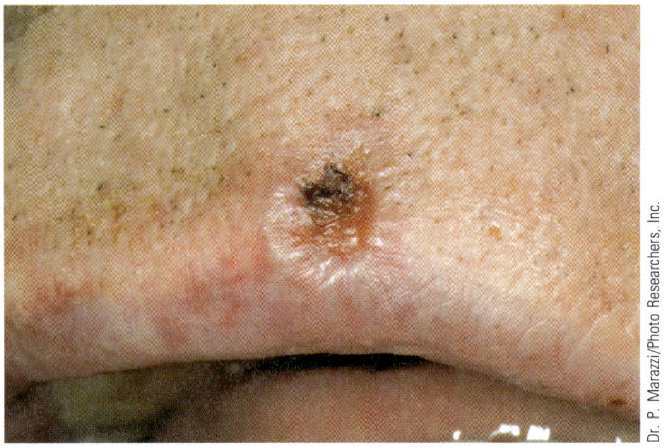

FIGURE 6.12 Basal cell carcinoma of the lip. This type of malignant tumor occurs in the basal cell layer of the epidermis.

Carcinomas

A **carcinoma** (**kar**-sih-**NOH**-mah) is a malignant tumor that occurs in epithelial tissue (**carcin** means cancer, and **-oma** means tumor) (Figure 6.12). Epithelial tissue forms the protective covering for all of the internal and external surfaces of the body.

- Carcinomas tend to infiltrate and produce metastases (new cancer sites) that can affect any organ or part of the body. (*Infiltrate* means to gain access to.)
- A **carcinoma in situ** (**kar**-sih-**NOH**-mah in **SIGH**-too) is a malignant tumor in its original position that has not yet disturbed or invaded the surrounding tissues. *In situ* means in the place where the cancer first occurred.
- For example, an **adenocarcinoma** (**ad**-eh-noh-**kar**-sih-**NOH**-mah) is any one of a large group of carcinomas derived from glandular tissue (**aden/o** means gland, **carcin** means cancer, and **-oma** means tumor).

Sarcomas

A **sarcoma** (sar-**KOH**-mah) is a malignant tumor that arises from connective tissues, including hard, soft, and liquid connective tissues (**sarc** means flesh, and **-oma** means tumor) (plural, *sarcomas* or *sarcomata*).

- *Hard-tissue sarcomas* arise from bone or cartilage (see Chapter 3). For example, an **osteosarcoma** (**oss**-tee-oh-sar-**KOH**-mah) is a hard-tissue sarcoma that usually involves the upper shaft of the long bones, pelvis, or knee (**oste/o** means bone, **sarc** means flesh, and **-oma** means tumor).
- *Soft-tissue sarcomas* are cancers of the muscle, fat, fibrous tissue, blood and lymphatic vessels, or other supporting tissue, including the synovial tissues that line the cavities of joints. For example, a **synovial sarcoma** (sih-**NOH**-vee-al sar-**KOH**-mah) is a tumor of the tissues surrounding a synovial joint such as the knees or elbows.
- *Liquid-tissue sarcomas* arise from blood and lymph. For example, **leukemia** (loo-**KEE**-mee-ah) is a cancer of the white blood-forming cells in the bone marrow (**leuk/o** means white, and **-emia** means pertaining to blood). See Chapter 5 for more about leukemia.

Staging Tumors

Staging is the process of classifying tumors by how far the disease has progressed, the potential for its responding to therapy, and the patient's prognosis. Specific staging systems are used for different types of cancer (Figure 6.13).

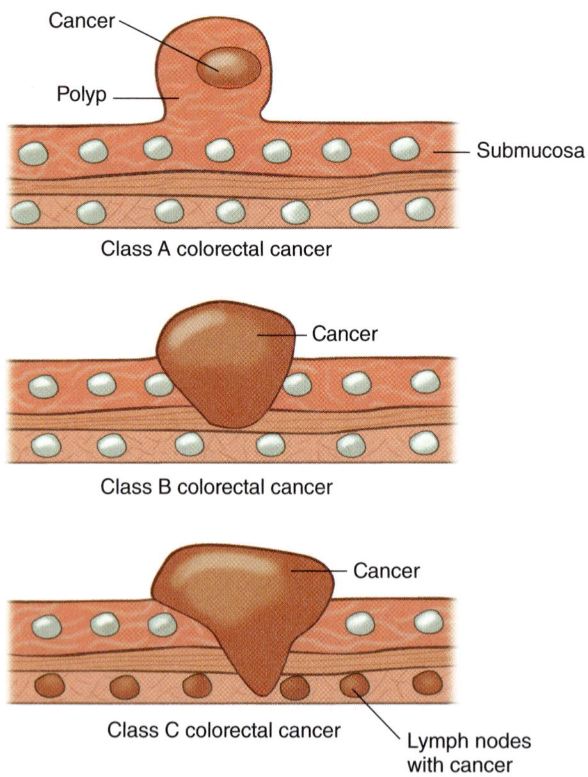

FIGURE 6.13 Stages of colorectal cancer. *Class A*: The cancerous tumor has formed within a polyp inside the colon, but has not yet invaded the surrounding tissue. *Class B*: The cancer has invaded the underlying tissue. *Class C*: The cancer has spread to the underlying tissues and nearby lymph nodes.

Lymphomas

Lymphoma (lim-**FOH**-mah) is a general term applied to malignancies affecting lymphoid tissues (**lymph** means lymph, and **-oma** means tumor). This includes lymph nodes, the spleen, liver, and bone marrow. The two most common types of lymphomas are Hodgkin's lymphoma and non-Hodgkin's lymphoma.

- **Hodgkin's lymphoma** (**HODJ**-kinz lim-**FOH**-mah), also known as ***Hodgkin's disease***, is distinguished from other lymphomas by the presence of large, cancerous lymphocytes known as ***Reed-Sternberg cells***.
- **Non-Hodgkin's lymphoma** is the term used to describe all other lymphomas *other than* Hodgkin's lymphoma. There are many different types of non-Hodgkin's lymphoma, some aggressive (fast growing) and some indolent (slow growing).

Breast Cancer

Breast cancer is a carcinoma that develops from the cells of the breast and can spread to adjacent lymph nodes and other body sites (Figure 6.14). There are several types of breast cancer named for their location or amount of spreading.

- **Ductal carcinoma in situ** is breast cancer at its earliest stage before the cancer has broken through the wall of the milk duct. At this stage, the cure rate is nearly 100%.
- **Infiltrating ductal carcinoma** (in-**FILL**-trate-ing **DUK**-tal kar-sih-**NOH**-mah), also known as ***invasive ductal carcinoma***, starts in the milk duct, breaks through the wall of that duct, and invades the fatty breast tissue. This form of cancer accounts for the majority of all breast cancers. ***Infiltrating*** and ***invasive*** are terms used to describe cancer that has spread beyond the layer of tissue in which it developed and is now growing into surrounding, healthy tissues.
- **Infiltrating lobular carcinoma**, also known as ***invasive lobular carcinoma***, is cancer that starts in the milk glands (lobules), breaks through the wall of the gland, and invades the fatty tissue of the breast. Once this cancer reaches the lymph nodes, it can rapidly spread to distant parts of the body.
- **Inflammatory breast cancer** (IBC) is a rare but aggressive form of breast cancer. IBC grows rapidly, and the symptoms include pain, rapid increase in the breast size, redness or a rash on the breast, and swelling of nearby lymph nodes. Most breast cancers are detected by mammography, ultrasound, or self-examination. In contrast, IBC can be detected only by magnetic resonance imaging (MRI).
- ***Male breast cancer*** can occur in the small amount of breast tissue that is normally present in men. The types of cancers are similar to those occurring in women.

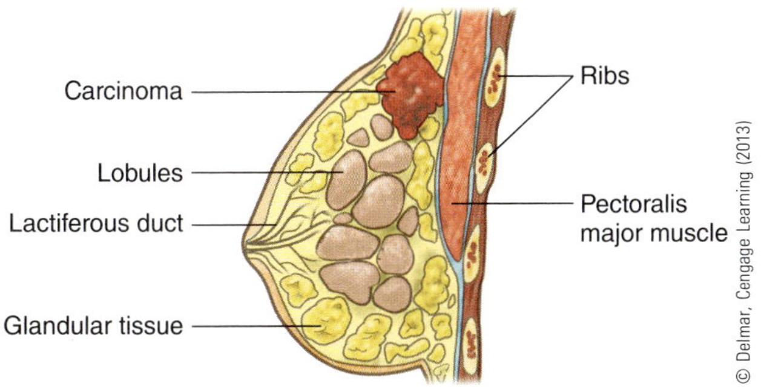

FIGURE 6.14 Most breast cancers are initially detected as a lump. When this lump is malignant, it is a form of carcinoma.

Stages of Breast Cancer

Breast cancer is described as one of the following stages that depend to the size of the cancer, the lymph node involvement, and the presence of metastases (spreading).

Stage 0:	Cancer cells are found only in one location, such as ductal carcinoma in situ.
Stage I:	Cancer cells have moved beyond the duct but have not yet reached the lymph nodes.
Stage II:	Cancer has increased in size, and/or has reached the axillary (armpit) lymph nodes.
Stage III:	Cancer has spread to the cervical (neck) lymph nodes and/or the tissues surrounding the breast, such as the chest wall or skin.
Stage IV:	Cancer has spread to other organs, most commonly the brain, lungs, liver, or bones. This is also known as invasive cancer.

Detection of Breast Cancer

Early detection of breast cancer is important and uses the following techniques.

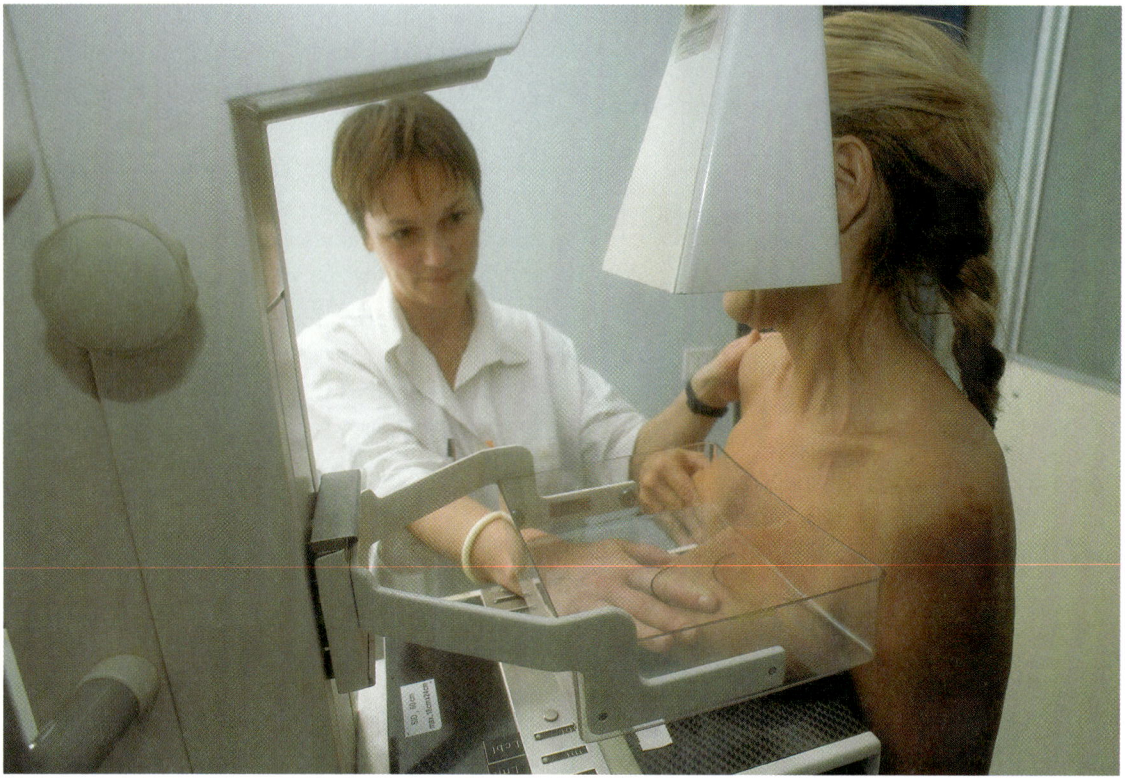

FIGURE 6.15 In mammography, the breast is gently flattened and radiographed from various angles.

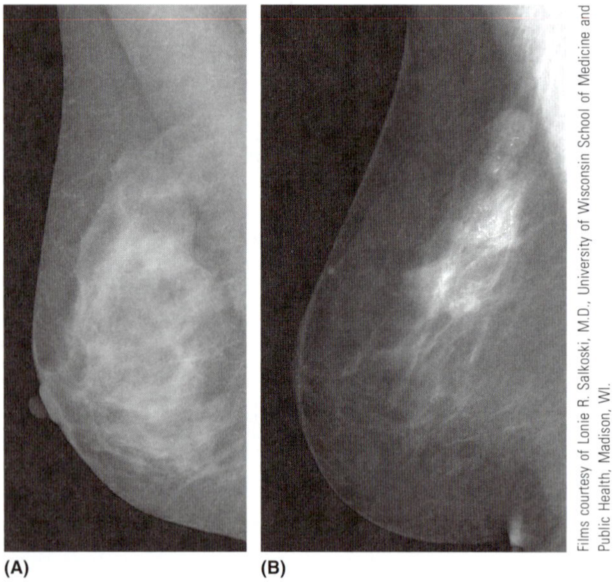

FIGURE 6.16 (A) A normal mammogram in which no abnormal mass is visible. (B) A mammogram in which breast cancer is visible.

- **Breast self-examination** is a self-care procedure for the early detection of breast cancer. The focus of self-examination is checking for a new lump or for changes in an existing lump, shape of the nipple, or the skin covering the breast.
- **Professional palpation of the breast** is performed to feel the texture, size, and consistency of the breast. Palpation is explained in Chapter 15.
- **Mammography** (mam-**OG**-rah-fee) is a radiographic examination of the breasts to detect the presence of tumors or precancerous cells (**mamm/o** means breast, and **-graphy** means the process of producing a picture or record) (Figure 6.15). The resulting record is a ***mammogram*** (Figure 6.16).
- **Ultrasound** is used as an initial follow-up test when an abnormality is found by mammography. (Ultrasound is discussed in Chapter 15.)
- A **needle breast biopsy** is a technique in which an x-ray-guided needle is used to remove small samples of tissue from the breast. It is less painful and disfiguring than a surgical biopsy.
- A **surgical biopsy** (**BYE**-op-see) is the removal of a small piece of tissue for examination to confirm a diagnosis (**bi-** means pertaining to life, and **-opsy** means view of). After a diagnosis has been established, treatment is then planned based on the stage of the cancer.

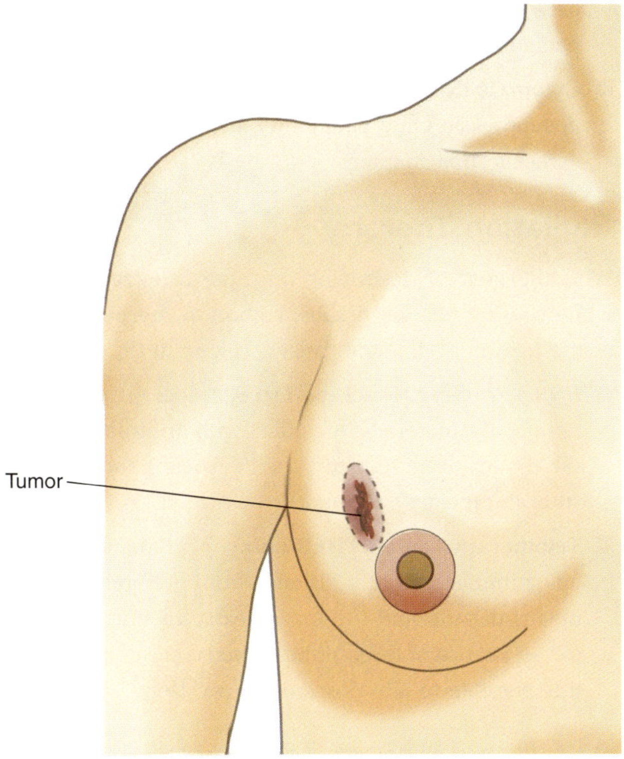

FIGURE 6.17 A lumpectomy is the removal of the cancerous tissue plus a margin of healthy tissue.

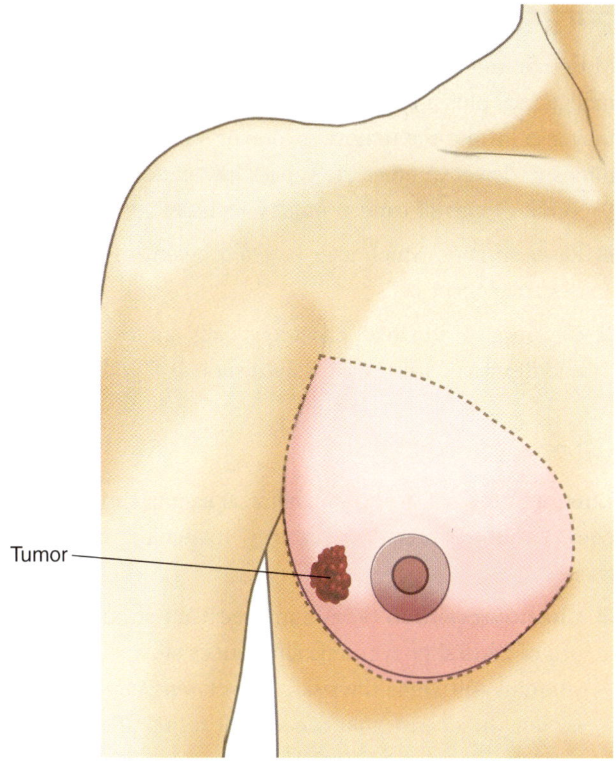

FIGURE 6.18 A modified radical mastectomy is the removal of the entire breast and the adjacent lymph nodes.

- A *sentinel node biopsy* is a biopsy of the first lymph node to come into contact with cancer cells as they leave the organ of origination and start spreading into the rest of the body. After the sentinel lymph node has been identified, only this and the other affected nodes are removed for biopsy.
- **Lymph node dissection** is a surgical procedure in which all of the lymph nodes in a major group are removed to determine or slow the spread of cancer in this area. For example, an *axillary lymph node dissection (ALND)* is sometimes performed as part of the surgical treatment of the breast.

Surgical Treatment of Breast Cancer

- A **lumpectomy** is the surgical removal of only the cancerous tissue with the surrounding margin of normal tissue (Figure 6.17). The remainder of the tissue of the affected breast is not removed.
- A **mastectomy** (mas-**TECK**-toh-mee) is the surgical removal of the entire breast and nipple (**mast** means breast, and **-ectomy** means surgical removal). Although simply described as a mastectomy, this procedure often includes the removal of axillary lymph nodes under the adjacent arm.
- A **radical mastectomy** is the surgical removal of an entire breast and many of the surrounding tissues.
- A **modified radical mastectomy** is the surgical removal of the entire breast and all of the axillary lymph nodes under the adjacent arm (Figure 6.18).

Breast Reconstruction

As an alternative to wearing an external prosthesis, which simulates the shape of the breast within a bra, many women who have undergone a mastectomy elect to have breast reconstruction.

- *Immediate breast reconstruction* begins during the same surgery as the mastectomy when an "expander" is placed to replace the tissue that was removed.
- *Delayed breast reconstruction* may be necessary if the surgery is to be followed by radiation treatment. Several different techniques are used to restore the size and shape of the missing breast.

CANCER TREATMENTS

The most common forms of treatment for all types of cancer are surgery, chemotherapy, and radiation therapy.

Surgery

Most commonly, cancer surgery involves removing the malignancy plus a margin of normal surrounding tissue. It may also involve the removal of one or more nearby lymph nodes to detect whether the cancer has started to spread.

Other types of cancer surgery include:

- Laser surgery, which uses targeted beams of light to destroy cancer cells
- Cryosurgery, in which cancerous cells are frozen and destroyed using a substance such as liquid nitrogen

Chemotherapy

Chemotherapy is the use of chemical agents and drugs in combinations selected to destroy malignant cells and tissues.

- **Chemoprevention** (**kee**-moh-pree-**VEN**-shun) is the use of natural or synthetic substances such as drugs or vitamins to reduce the risk of developing cancer, or to reduce the chance that cancer will recur. Chemoprevention may also be used to reduce the size or slow the development of an existing tumor.
- An **antineoplastic** (**an**-tih-nee-oh-**PLAS**-tick) is a medication that blocks the development, growth, or proliferation of malignant cells (**anti-** means against, **ne/o** means new, **plast** means growth or formation, and **-ic** means pertaining to). *Proliferation* means to increase rapidly.
- **Cytotoxic drugs**, which are also used for both immunosuppression and chemotherapy, are discussed earlier in this chapter.

Radiation Therapy

With the goal of destroying only the cancerous tissues while sparing healthy tissues, **radiation therapy** is used in the treatment of some cancers (Figure 6.19).

- **Brachytherapy** (**brack**-ee-**THER**-ah-pee) is the use of radioactive materials in contact with or implanted into the tissues to be treated (**brachy-** means short, and **-therapy** means treatment).
- **Teletherapy** (**tel**-eh-**THER**-ah-pee) is radiation therapy administered at a distance from the body (**tele-** means distant, and **-therapy** means treatment). With the assistance of three-dimensional computer imaging, it is possible to aim doses more precisely.

Additional Cancer Treatment Therapies

- **Targeted therapy** is a developing form of anti-cancer drug therapy that uses drugs or other substances to identify and attack specific cancer cells without

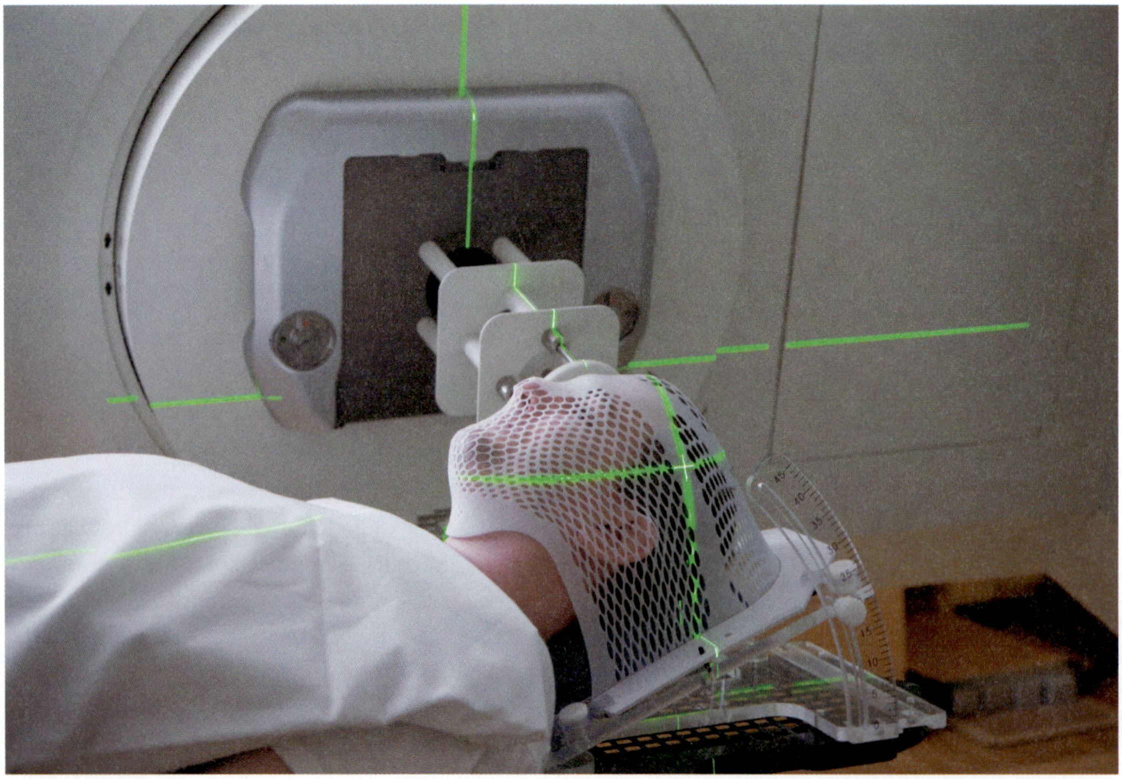

iStockphoto/Mark Kostick

FIGURE 6.19 Radiation therapy destroys cancerous cells while sparing healthy tissues.

harming normal cells. A monoclonal antibody is a type of targeted therapy.

- After the primary cancer treatments have been completed to decrease the chance that a cancer will recur, sometimes **adjuvant therapy** (**AD**-jeh-vant) is used. The term *adjuvant* refers to an agent intended to increase the effectiveness of a drug; however, adjuvant treatments for cancer can also include chemotherapy, hormone therapy, radiation, immunotherapy, or targeted therapy.
- **Clinical trials** involve testing new and promising cancer treatments that have not yet received Food and Drug Administration (FDA) approval on patients who agree to be part of the research.

ABBREVIATIONS RELATED TO THE LYMPHATIC AND IMMUNE SYSTEMS

Table 6.3 presents an overview of the abbreviations related to the terms introduced in this chapter. Note: To avoid errors or confusion, always be cautious when using abbreviations.

StudyWARE CONNECTION

For more practice and to test your mastery of this material, go to the StudyWARE™ to play interactive games and complete the quiz for this chapter.

Workbook Practice

Go to your workbook and complete the exercises for this chapter.

DELMAR MOBILE MEDIA

Downloadable audio is available for selected medical terms in this chapter to enhance your learning of medical terminology.

TABLE 6.3
Abbreviations Related to the Lymphatic and Immune Systems

antibody = A, Ab	**A, Ab** = antibody
antigen = AG, Ag	**AG, Ag** = antigen
carcinoma = CA, Ca	**CA, Ca** = carcinoma
carcinoma in situ = CIS	**CIS** = carcinoma in situ
ductal carcinoma in situ = DCIS	**DCIS** = ductal carcinoma in situ
herpes zoster = HZ	**HZ** = herpes zoster
Hodgkin's lymphoma = HL	**HL** = Hodgkin's lymphoma
immunoglobulin = IG	**IG** = immunoglobulin
lymphedema = LE	**LE** = lymphedema
measles, mumps, and rubella vaccination = MMR	**MMR** = measles, mumps, and rubella vaccination
metastasis = MET	**MET** = metastasis
metastasize = met	**met** = metastasize
non-Hodgkin's lymphoma = NHL	**NHL** = non-Hodgkin's lymphoma
varicella = VSZ	**VSZ** = varicella

CHAPTER 6

LEARNING EXERCISES

MATCHING WORD PARTS 1

Write the correct answer in the middle column.

	Definition	Correct Answer	Possible Answers
6.1.	against	________________	**anti-**
6.2.	eat, swallow	________________	**lymphaden/o**
6.3.	lymph node	________________	**lymphangi/o**
6.4.	lymph vessel	________________	**phag/o**
6.5.	poison	________________	**tox/o**

MATCHING WORD PARTS 2

Write the correct answer in the middle column.

	Definition	Correct Answer	Possible Answers
6.6.	flesh	________________	**immun/o**
6.7.	formative material of cells	________________	**onc/o**
6.8.	protection, safe	________________	**-plasm**
6.9.	spleen	________________	**sarc/o**
6.10.	tumor	________________	**splen/o**

MATCHING TYPES OF PATHOGENS

Write the correct answer in the middle column.

	Definition	Correct Answer	Possible Answers
6.11.	bacteria capable of movement	________________	parasites
6.12.	chain-forming bacteria	________________	spirochetes

6.13. cluster-forming bacteria ______________ staphylococci

6.14. live only by invading cells ______________ streptococci

6.15. live within other organisms ______________ viruses

DEFINITIONS

Select the correct answer, and write it on the line provided.

6.16. The ______________ has/have a hemolytic function.

appendix lymph nodes spleen tonsils

6.17. Inflammation of the lymph nodes is known as ______________.

angiogenesis lymphadenitis lymphedema lymphoma

6.18. The medical term for the condition commonly known as shingles is ______________.

cytomegalovirus herpes zoster rubella varicella

6.19. Proteins who activate the immune system, fight viruses by slowing or stopping their multiplication, and signal other cells to increase their defenses are known as ______________.

T cells immunoglobulins interferons synthetic immunoglobulins

6.20. The ______________ plays specialized roles in both the lymphatic and immune systems.

bone marrow liver spleen thymus

6.21. The protective ring of lymphoid tissue around the back of the nose and upper throat is formed by the ______________.

lacteals lymph nodes tonsils villi

6.22. Secondary ______________ can be caused by cancer treatments, burns, or injuries.

lymphadenitis lymphangioma lymphadenopathy lymphedema

6.23. Fats that cannot be transported by the bloodstream are absorbed by the ______________ that are located in the villi that line the small intestine.

lacteals lymph nodes B cells spleen

6.24. The parasite ______________ is most commonly transmitted from pets to humans by contact with contaminated animal feces.

herpes zoster malaria rabies toxoplasmosis

6.25. A/An ______________ is a type of leukocyte that surrounds and kills invading cells. This type of cell also removes dead cells and stimulates the action of other immune cells.

B lymphocyte macrophage platelet T lymphocyte

MATCHING STRUCTURES

Write the correct answer in the middle column.

	Definition	Correct Answer	Possible Answers
6.26.	filter harmful substances from lymph	______________	complement system cells
6.27.	lymphoid tissue hanging from the lower portion of the cecum	______________	intact skin
6.28.	combine with antibodies to dissolve foreign cells	______________	lymph nodes
6.29.	stores extra erythrocytes	______________	spleen
6.30.	wraps the body in a physical barrier	______________	vermiform appendix

WHICH WORD?

Select the correct answer, and write it on the line provided.

6.31. The ______________ act as intracellular signals to begin the immune response.

cytokines macrophages

6.32. A ______________ drug is a medication that kills or damages cells.

corticosteroid cytotoxic

6.33. The ______________ develop from B cells and secrete large bodies of antibodies coded to destroy specific antigens.

Reed-Sternberg cells plasma cells

6.34. The antibody therapy known as ______________ is used to treat multiple sclerosis, hepatitis C, and some cancers.

monoclonal antibodies synthetic interferon

6.35. Infectious mononucleosis is caused by a ______________.

spirochete virus

SPELLING COUNTS

Find the misspelled word in each sentence. Then write that word, spelled correctly, on the line provided.

6.36. A sarkoma is a malignant tumor that arises from connective tissue. ______________

6.37. The adanoids, which are also known as the nasopharyngeal tonsils, are located in the nasopharynx. ______________

6.38. Lymphiscintigraphy is a diagnostic test that is performed to detect damage or malformations of the lymphatic vessels. ______________

6.39. Antiobiotics are commonly used to combat bacterial infections. ______________

6.40. Varichella is commonly known as chickenpox. ______________

ABBREVIATION IDENTIFICATION

In the space provided, write the words that each abbreviation stands for.

6.41. **CIS** ______________

6.42. **DCIS** ______________

6.43. **LE** ______________

6.44. **MMR** ______________

6.45. **Ag** ______________

TERM SELECTION

Select the correct answer, and write it on the line provided.

6.46. ______________ is the process through which a tumor supports its growth by creating its own blood supply.

metastasis angiogenesis neoplasm malignant tumor

6.47. An opportunistic infection that is frequently associated with HIV is ______________.

Hodgkin's disease Kaposi's sarcoma myasthenia gravis tinea pedis

6.48. Malaria is caused by a ________________ that is transferred to humans by the bite of an infected mosquito.

parasite rickettsiae spirochete virus

6.49. Bacilli, which are rod-shaped, spore-forming bacteria, cause ________________.

Lyme disease measles rubella anthrax

6.50. Swelling of the parotid glands is a symptom of ________________.

measles mumps shingles rubella

SENTENCE COMPLETION

Write the correct term on the line provided.

6.51. A severe systemic reaction to an allergen causing serious symptoms that develop very quickly is known as ________________.

6.52. In ________________, radioactive materials are implanted into the tissues to be treated.

6.53. When testing for HIV, a/an ________________ test produces more accurate results than the ELISA test.

6.54. A/An ________________ is a benign tumor formed by an abnormal collection of lymphatic vessels.

6.55. After primary cancer treatments have been completed, ________________ therapy is used to decrease the chances that the cancer will recur.

WORD SURGERY

Divide each term into its component word parts. Write these word parts, in sequence, on the lines provided. When necessary, use a slash (/) to indicate a combining vowel. (You may not need all of the lines provided.)

6.56. An **antineoplastic** is a medication that blocks the development, growth, or proliferation of malignant cells.

__________ __________ __________ __________

6.57. **Metastasis** is the new cancer site that results from the spreading process.

__________ __________ __________ __________

6.58. **Osteosarcoma** is a hard-tissue sarcoma that usually involves the upper shaft of the long bones, pelvis, or knee.

________ ________ ________ ________

6.59. **Cytomegalovirus** is a member of the *herpesvirus* family that causes a variety of diseases.

________ ________ ________ ________

6.60. **Antiangiogenesis** is a form of cancer treatment that disrupts the blood supply to the tumor.

________ ________ ________ ________

TRUE/FALSE

If the statement is true, write **True** on the line. If the statement is false, write **False** on the line.

6.61. ________ Inflammatory breast cancer is the most aggressive and least common form of breast cancer.

6.62. ________ Lymph carries nutrients and oxygen to the cells.

6.63. ________ A myosarcoma is a benign tumor derived from muscle tissue.

6.64. ________ Reed-Sternberg cells are present in Hodgkin's lymphoma.

6.65. ________ Septic shock is caused by a viral infection.

CLINICAL CONDITIONS

Write the correct answer on the line provided.

6.66. Dr. Wei diagnosed her patient as having an enlarged spleen due to damage caused by his injuries. The medical term for this condition is ____________.

6.67. At the beginning of the treatment of Juanita Phillips' breast cancer, a/an ____________ breast biopsy was performed using an x-ray-guided needle.

6.68. Mr. Grossman described his serious illness as being caused by a "superbug infection." His doctor describes these bacteria as being ____________.

6.69. Dorothy Peterson was diagnosed with breast cancer. She and her doctor agreed upon treating this surgically with a/an ____________. This is a procedure in which the cancerous tissue with a margin of normal tissue are removed.

6.70. Every day since his kidney transplant, Mr. Lanning must take a/an ____________ to prevent rejection of the donor organ.

6.71. Rosita Sanchez is 2 months pregnant, and she and her doctor are worried because her rash was diagnosed as ____________________. They are concerned because this condition can produce defects in Rosita's developing child.

6.72. Tarana Inglis took ____________________ to relieve the symptoms of her allergies.

6.73. The ____________________ virus is spread to humans through the bite of an infected mosquito. The more severe variety spreads to the spinal cord and brain.

6.74. John Fogelman was diagnosed with having a/an ____________________. This is a malignant tumor that arises from connective tissues, including hard, soft, and liquid tissues.

6.75. Jane Doe is infected with HIV. One of her medications is acyclovir, which is a/an ____________________ drug.

WHICH IS THE CORRECT MEDICAL TERM?

Select the correct answer, and write it on the line provided.

6.76. The ____________________ are specialized lymphocytes that produce antibodies. Each lymphocyte makes a specific antibody that is capable of destroying a specific antigen.

B cells bacilli immunoglobulins T cells

6.77. Any of a large group of diseases characterized by a condition in which the immune system produces antibodies against its own tissues is known as a/an ____________________ disorder.

autoimmune allergy rubella immunodeficiency

6.78. The ____________________ lymph nodes are located in the groin.

axillary cervical inguinal subcutaneous

6.79. A/An ____________________ is any one of a large group of carcinomas derived from glandular tissue.

adenocarcinoma lymphoma myosarcoma myoma

6.80. A/An ____________________ drug is used either as an immunosuppressant or as an antineoplastic.

corticosteroid cytotoxic immunoglobulin monoclonal

CHALLENGE WORD BUILDING

These terms are *not* found in this chapter; however, they are made up of the following familiar word parts. If you need help in creating the term, refer to your medical dictionary.

adenoid/o	**-ectomy**
lymphaden/o	**-itis**
lymphang/o	**-ology**
immun/o	**-oma**
splen/o	**-rrhaphy**
tonsill/o	
thym/o	

6.81. The study of the immune system is known as ________________.

6.82. Surgical removal of the spleen is a/an ________________.

6.83. Inflammation of the thymus is known as ________________.

6.84. Inflammation of the lymph vessels is known as ________________.

6.85. The term meaning to suture the spleen is ________________.

6.86. The surgical removal of the adenoids is a/an ________________.

6.87. The surgical removal of a lymph node is a/an ________________.

6.88. A tumor originating in the thymus is known as ________________.

6.89. Inflammation of the tonsils is known as ________________.

6.90. Inflammation of the spleen is known as ________________.

LABELING EXERCISES

Identify the numbered items on the accompanying figures on the next page.

6.91. tonsils and ________________

6.92. Lymphocytes are formed in bone ________________

6.93. large intestine and ________________

6.94. ________________

6.95. ______________________

6.96. ______________________ lymph nodes

6.97. Right ______________________ empties into the right subclavian vein.

6.98. ______________________ duct

6.99. ______________________ lymph nodes

6.100. ______________________ lymph nodes

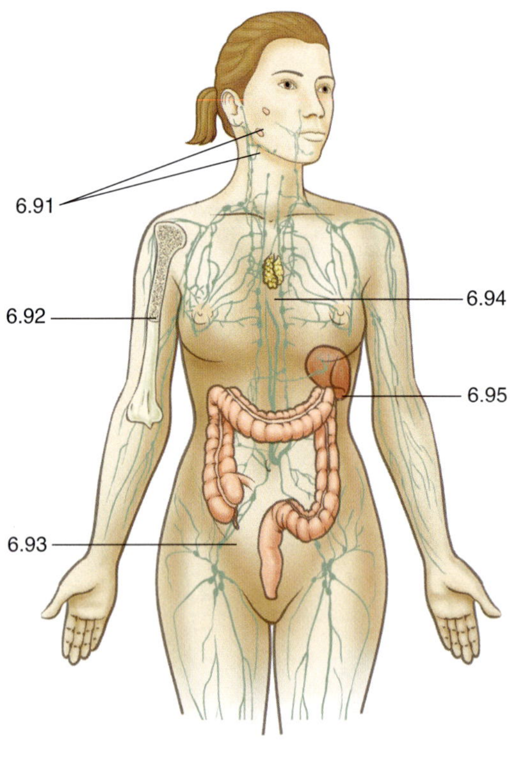

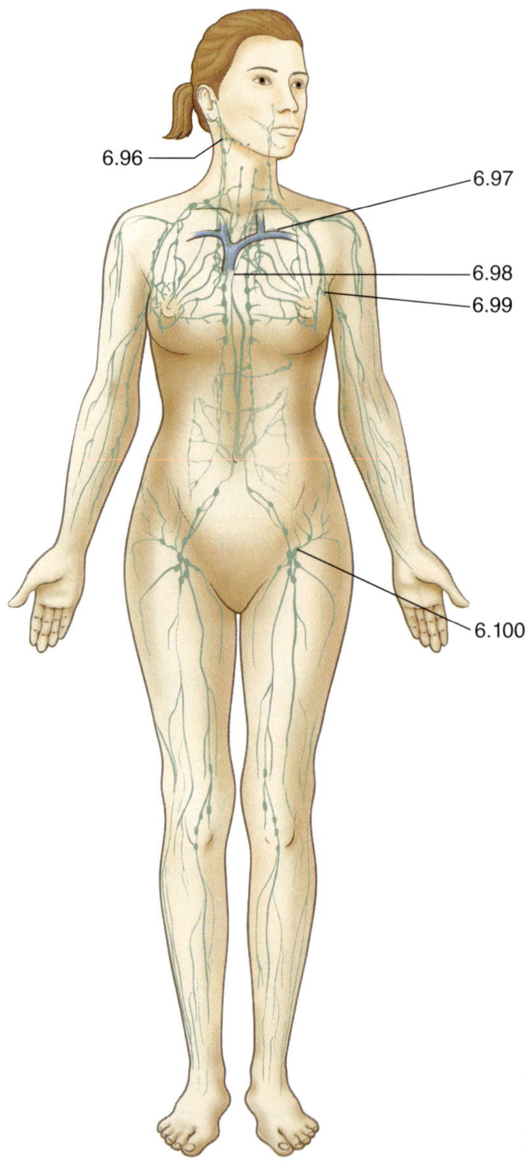

CHAPTER 7

The Respiratory System

Overview of STRUCTURES, COMBINING FORMS, AND FUNCTIONS OF THE RESPIRATORY SYSTEM

Major Structures	Related Combining Forms	Primary Functions
Nose	**nas/o**	Exchanges air during inhaling and exhaling; warms, moisturizes, and filters inhaled air.
Sinuses	**sinus/o**	Produce mucus for the nasal cavities, make bones of the skull lighter, aid in sound production.
Pharynx	**pharyng/o**	Transports air back and forth between the nose and the trachea.
Larynx	**laryng/o**	Makes speech possible.
Epiglottis	**epiglott/o**	Closes off the trachea during swallowing.
Trachea	**trache/o**	Transports air back and forth between the pharynx and the bronchi.
Bronchi	**bronch/o**, **bronchi/o**	Transports air from the trachea into the lungs.
Alveoli	**alveol/o**	Air sacs that exchange gases with the pulmonary capillary blood.
Lungs	**pneum/o**, **pneumon/o**, **pulmon/o**	Bring oxygen into the body, and remove carbon dioxide and some water waste from the body.

Vocabulary Related to **THE RESPIRATORY SYSTEM**

This list contains essential word parts and medical terms for this chapter. These terms are pronounced in the StudyWARE™ and Audio CDs that are available for use with this text. These and the other important **primary terms** are shown in boldface throughout the chapter. *Secondary terms*, which appear in *orange* italics, clarify the meaning of primary terms.

Word Parts

- ☐ **bronch/o**, **bronchi/o** bronchial tube, bronchus
- ☐ **laryng/o** larynx, throat
- ☐ **nas/o** nose
- ☐ **ox/i**, **ox/o**, **ox/y** oxygen
- ☐ **pharyng/o** throat, pharynx
- ☐ **phon/o** sound, voice
- ☐ **pleur/o** pleura, side of the body
- ☐ **-pnea** breathing
- ☐ **pneum/o**, **pneumon/o**, **pneu-** lung, air
- ☐ **pulm/o**, **pulmon/o** lung
- ☐ **sinus/o** sinus
- ☐ **somn/o** sleep
- ☐ **spir/o** to breathe
- ☐ **thorac/o**, **-thorax** chest, pleural cavity
- ☐ **trache/o**, **trachea** windpipe

Medical Terms

- ☐ **alveoli** (al-**VEE**-oh-lye)
- ☐ **anoxia** (ah-**NOCK**-see-ah)
- ☐ **antitussive** (**an**-tih-**TUSS**-iv)
- ☐ **aphonia** (ah-**FOH**-nee-ah)
- ☐ **asbestosis** (**ass**-beh-**STOH**-sis)
- ☐ **asphyxia** (ass-**FICK**-see-ah)
- ☐ **asthma** (**AZ**-mah)
- ☐ **atelectasis** (**at**-ee-**LEK**-tah-sis)
- ☐ **bradypnea** (**brad**-ihp-**NEE**-ah)
- ☐ **bronchodilator** (**brong**-koh-dye-**LAY**-tor)
- ☐ **bronchorrhea** (**brong**-koh-**REE**-ah)
- ☐ **bronchoscopy** (brong-**KOS**-koh-pee)
- ☐ **bronchospasm** (**brong**-koh-spazm)
- ☐ **Cheyne-Stokes respiration** (**CHAYN-STOHKS**)
- ☐ **croup** (**KROOP**)
- ☐ **cyanosis** (**sigh**-ah-**NOH**-sis)
- ☐ **cystic fibrosis** (**SIS**-tick figh-**BROH**-sis)
- ☐ **diphtheria** (dif-**THEE**-ree-ah)
- ☐ **dysphonia** (dis-**FOH**-nee-ah)
- ☐ **dyspnea** (**DISP**-nee-ah)
- ☐ **emphysema** (**em**-fih-**SEE**-mah)
- ☐ **empyema** (**em**-pye-**EE**-mah)
- ☐ **endotracheal intubation** (**en**-doh-**TRAY**-kee-al **in**-too-**BAY**-shun)
- ☐ **epistaxis** (**ep**-ih-**STACK**-sis)
- ☐ **hemoptysis** (hee-**MOP**-tih-sis)
- ☐ **hemothorax** (**hee**-moh-**THOH**-racks)
- ☐ **hypercapnia** (**high**-per-**KAP**-nee-ah)
- ☐ **hyperpnea** (**high**-perp-**NEE**-ah)
- ☐ **hypopnea** (**high**-poh-**NEE**-ah)
- ☐ **hypoxemia** (**high**-pock-**SEE**-mee-ah)
- ☐ **hypoxia** (high-**POCK**-see-ah)
- ☐ **laryngectomy** (**lar**-in-**JECK**-toh-mee)
- ☐ **laryngitis** (**lar**-in-**JIGH**-tis)
- ☐ **laryngoscopy** (**lar**-ing-**GOS**-koh-pee)
- ☐ **laryngospasm** (lah-**RING**-goh-spazm)
- ☐ **mediastinum** (**mee**-dee-as-**TYE**-num)
- ☐ **nebulizer** (**NEB**-you-lye-zer)
- ☐ **otolaryngologist** (**oh**-toh-**lar**-in-**GOL**-oh-jist)
- ☐ **pertussis** (per-**TUS**-is)
- ☐ **pharyngitis** (fah-rin-**JIGH**-tis)
- ☐ **phlegm** (**FLEM**)
- ☐ **pleurisy** (**PLOOR**-ih-see)
- ☐ **pleurodynia** (**ploor**-oh-**DIN**-ee-ah)
- ☐ **pneumoconiosis** (**new**-moh-**koh**-nee-**OH**-sis)
- ☐ **pneumonectomy** (**new**-moh-**NECK**-toh-mee)
- ☐ **pneumonia** (new-**MOH**-nee-ah)
- ☐ **pneumothorax** (**new**-moh-**THOR**-racks)
- ☐ **polysomnography** (**pol**-ee-som-**NOG**-rah-fee)
- ☐ **pulmonologist** (**pull**-mah-**NOL**-oh-jist)
- ☐ **pulse oximeter** (ock-**SIM**-eh-ter)
- ☐ **pyothorax** (**pye**-oh-**THOH**-racks)
- ☐ **sinusitis** (**sigh**-nuh-**SIGH**-tis)
- ☐ **sleep apnea** (**AP**-nee-ah)
- ☐ **spirometer** (spih-**ROM**-eh-ter)
- ☐ **tachypnea** (**tack**-ihp-**NEE**-ah)
- ☐ **thoracentesis** (**thoh**-rah-sen-**TEE**-sis)
- ☐ **thoracotomy** (**thoh**-rah-**KOT**-toh-mee)
- ☐ **tracheostomy** (**tray**-kee-**OS**-toh-mee)
- ☐ **tracheotomy** (**tray**-kee-**OT**-oh-mee)
- ☐ **tuberculosis** (too-**ber**-kew-**LOH**-sis)

LEARNING GOALS

On completion of this chapter, you should be able to:

1. Describe the major functions of the respiratory system.
2. Name and describe the structures of the respiratory system.
3. Recognize, define, spell, and pronounce the primary terms related to the pathology and the diagnostic and treatment procedures of the respiratory system.

FUNCTIONS OF THE RESPIRATORY SYSTEM

The functions of the respiratory system are to:

- Deliver air to the lungs.
- Convey oxygen from the inhaled air to the blood for delivery to the body cells.
- Expel the waste products (carbon dioxide and a small amount of water) returned to the lungs by the blood through exhalation.
- Produce the airflow through the larynx that makes speech possible.

STRUCTURES OF THE RESPIRATORY SYSTEM

The **respiratory system** supplies the blood with oxygen for transportation to the cells in all parts of the body (Figure 7.1). Oxygen is vital to the survival and function of these cells. The respiratory system also removes carbon dioxide and some water waste from the body. For descriptive purposes, the respiratory system is divided into upper and lower respiratory tracts (Figures 7.1 and 7.2).

- The **upper respiratory tract** consists of the nose (nostrils), mouth, pharynx, epiglottis, larynx, and trachea. (Figure 7.2)

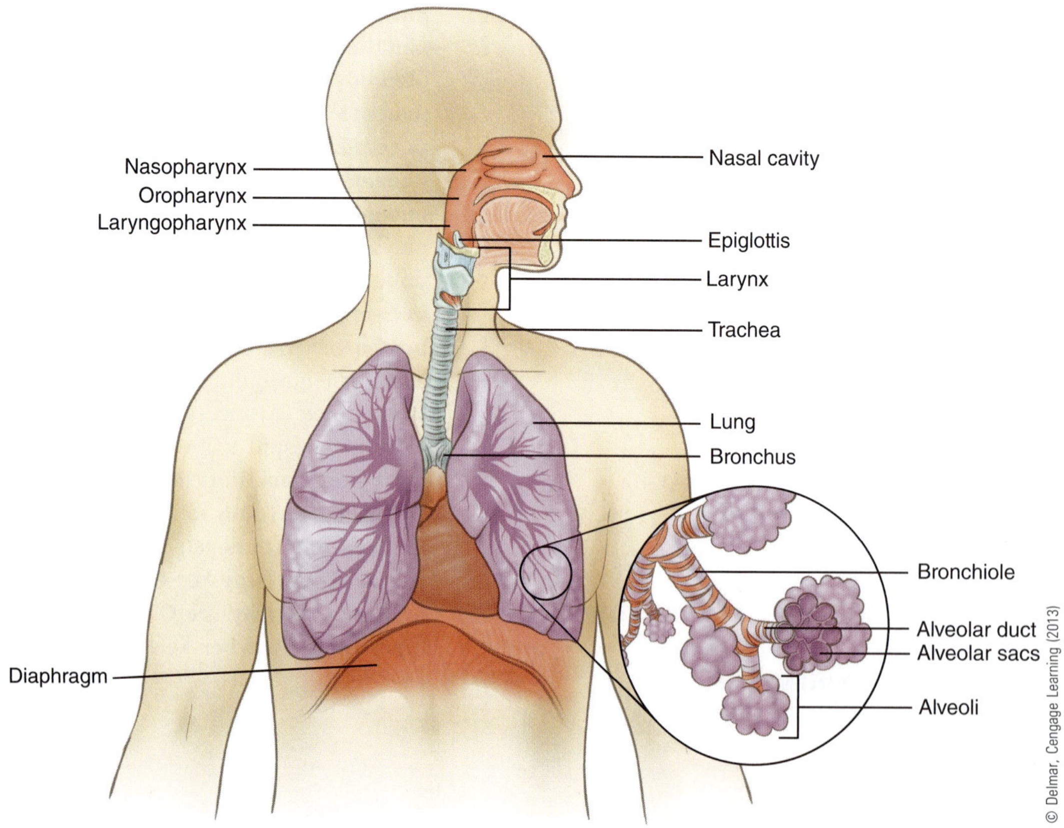

FIGURE 7.1 Structures of the respiratory system.

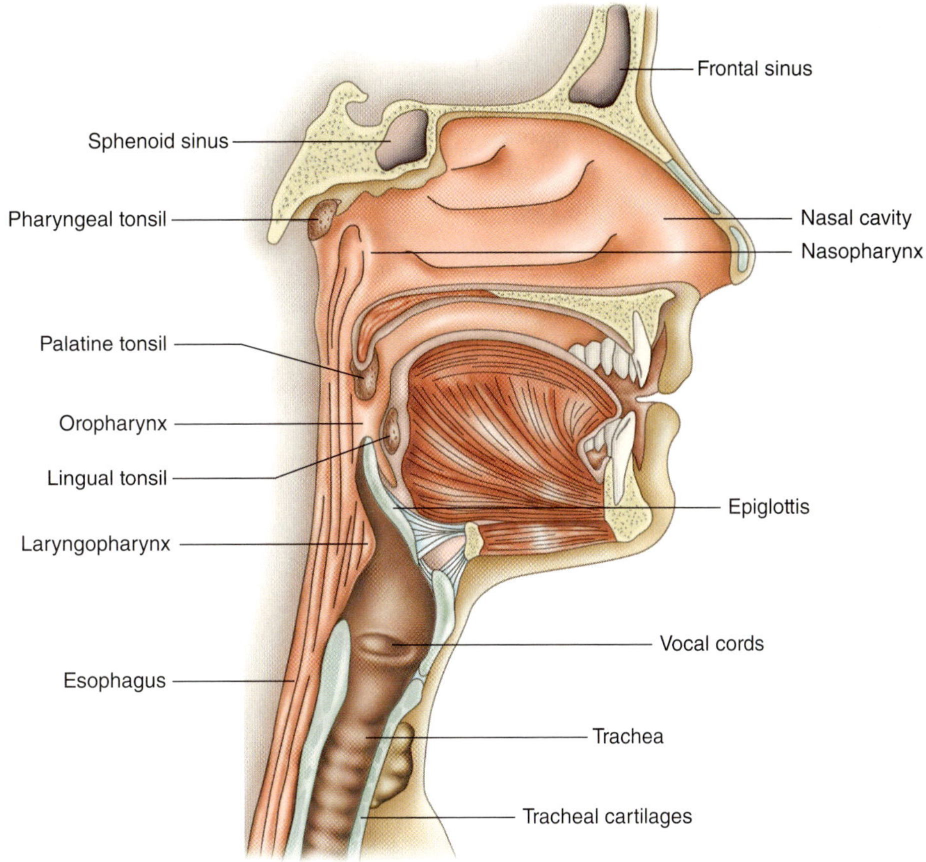

FIGURE 7.2 Structures of the upper respiratory tract.

- The **lower respiratory tract** consists of the bronchial tree and lungs. These structures are located within and protected by the **thoracic cavity** (thoh-**RAS**-ick), or **thorax**, also known as the *rib cage*.
- The upper respiratory tract and the bronchial tree of the lower respiratory tract are sometimes referred to as the *airway*.

The Nose

Air enters the body through the **nose** and passes through the *nasal cavity*, which is the interior portion of the nose.

- The *nostrils* are the external openings of the nose.
- The **nasal septum** (**NAY**-zal **SEP**-tum) is a wall of cartilage that divides the nose into two equal sections. A *septum* is a wall that separates two chambers.
- **Cilia** (**SIL**-ee-ah), the thin hairs located just inside the nostrils, filter incoming air to remove debris. The *nostrils* are the external openings of the nose.
- **Mucous membranes** (**MYOU**-kus) line the nose. These specialized tissues also line the digestive, reproductive, and urinary systems as well as other parts of the respiratory system.
- **Mucus** (**MYOU**-kus) is a slippery secretion produced by the mucous membranes that protects and lubricates these tissues. In the nose, mucus helps moisten, warm, and filter the air as it enters. Notice that mucous and mucus have different spellings; however, they share the same pronunciation. Mucous is the name of the tissue (which comes first, both anatomically and alphabetically); mucus is the secretion that flows from the tissue.
- The **olfactory receptors** (ol-**FACK**-toh-ree) are nerve endings that act as the receptors for the sense of smell. They are also important to the sense of taste. These receptors are located in the mucous membrane in the upper part of the nasal cavity.

The Tonsils

The **tonsils** and **adenoids** are part of the lymphatic system described in Chapter 6. They help protect the body from infection coming through the nose or the mouth. The tonsils, also called the *palatine tonsils*, are located at the back of the mouth. The adenoids, also called the *nasopharyngeal tonsils*, are higher up, behind the nose and the roof of the mouth.

The Paranasal Sinuses

The **paranasal sinuses**, which are air-filled cavities lined with mucous membrane, are located in the bones of the skull (**para-** means near, **nas** means nose, and **-al** means pertaining to). A ***sinus*** can be a sac or cavity in any organ or tissue; however, the term *sinus* most commonly refers to the paranasal sinuses.

The functions of these sinuses are (1) to make the bones of the skull lighter, (2) to help produce sound by giving resonance to the voice, and (3) to produce mucus to provide lubrication for the tissues of the nasal cavity. The sinuses are connected to the nasal cavity via short ducts. The four pairs of paranasal sinuses are located on either side of the nose and are named for the bones in which they are located.

- The **frontal sinuses** are located in the frontal bone just above the eyebrows. An infection here can cause severe pain in this area.
- The **sphenoid sinuses**, which are located in the sphenoid bone behind the eye and under the pituitary gland, are close to the optic nerves, and an infection here can damage vision.
- The **maxillary sinuses**, which are the largest of the paranasal sinuses, are located in the maxillary bones under the eyes. An infection in these sinuses can cause pain in the posterior maxillary teeth.
- The **ethmoid sinuses**, which are located in the ethmoid bones between the nose and the eyes, are irregularly shaped air cells that are separated from the orbital (eye) cavity by only a thin layer of bone.

The Pharynx

The **pharynx** (**FAR**-inks), which is commonly known as the ***throat***, receives the air after it passes through the nose or mouth, as well as food. (Its role in the digestive system is discussed in Chapter 8.)

The pharynx is made up of three divisions (Figure 7.2):

- The **nasopharynx** (**nay**-zoh-**FAR**-inks), which is the first division, is posterior to the nasal cavity and continues downward to behind the mouth (**nas/o** means nose, and **-pharynx** means throat). This portion of the pharynx is used only by the respiratory system for the transport of air and opens into the oropharynx.
- The **oropharynx** (**oh**-roh-**FAR**-inks), which is the second division, is the portion that is visible when looking into the mouth (**or/o** means mouth, and **-pharynx** means throat). The oropharynx is shared by the respiratory and digestive systems and transports air, food, and fluids downward to the laryngopharynx.
- The **laryngopharynx** (lah-**ring**-goh-**FAR**-inks), which is the third division, is also shared by both the respiratory and digestive systems (**laryng/o** means larynx, and **-pharynx** means throat). Air, food, and fluids continue downward to the openings of the esophagus and trachea where air enters the trachea and food and fluids flow into the esophagus. See the later section "Protective Swallowing Mechanisms."

Larynx

The **larynx** (**LAR**-inks), also known as the ***voice box***, is a triangular chamber located between the pharynx and the trachea (Figure 7.3).

- The larynx is protected and supported by a series of nine separate cartilages. The ***thyroid cartilage*** is the largest, and when enlarged it projects from the front of the throat and is commonly known as the ***Adam's apple***.
- The larynx contains the ***vocal cords***. During breathing, the cords are separated to let air pass. During speech, they close together, and sound is produced as air is expelled from the lungs, causing the cords to vibrate against each other.

Protective Swallowing Mechanisms

The respiratory and digestive systems share part of the pharynx. During swallowing, there is the risk of a blocked airway or aspiration pneumonia caused by food or water going into the trachea and entering the lungs, instead of

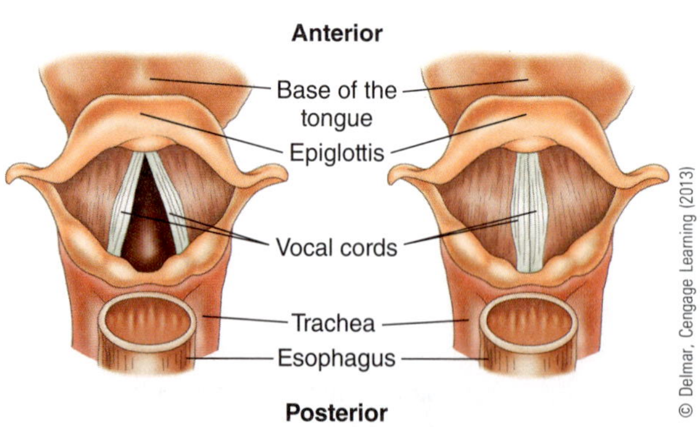

FIGURE 7.3 View of the larynx and vocal cords from above. Shown on the left, the vocal cords are open during breathing. On the right, the vocal cords vibrate together during speech.

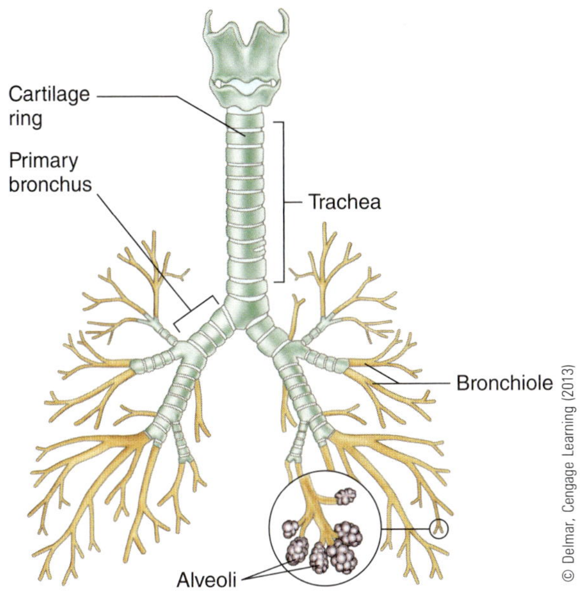

FIGURE 7.4 The trachea, bronchial tree, and alveoli.

going into the esophagus. Two protective mechanisms act automatically during swallowing to ensure that *only* air goes into the lungs:

- The soft palate, which is the muscular posterior portion of the roof of the mouth, moves up and backward during swallowing to close off the nasopharynx. This prevents food or liquid from going up into the nose. Structures of the mouth are discussed further in Chapter 8.
- At the same time, the **epiglottis** (**ep**-ih-**GLOT**-is), which is a lid-like structure located at the base of the tongue, swings downward and closes off the laryngopharynx so that food does not enter the trachea and the lungs.

The Trachea

- The role of the **trachea** (**TRAY**-kee-ah) is to transport air to and from the lungs. This tube, which is commonly known as the *windpipe*, is located directly in front of the esophagus.
- The trachea is held open by a series of flexible C-shaped cartilage rings that make it possible for the trachea to compress so that food can pass down the esophagus (Figure 7.4).

StudyWARE CONNECTION

Watch the **Respiratory Safeguards** animation in the StudyWARE™.

The Bronchi

The **bronchi** (**BRONG**-kee) are two large tubes, also known as *primary bronchi*, which branch out from the trachea and convey air into the two lungs (singular, *bronchus,* pronounced **BRONG**-kus). Because of the similarity of these structures to an inverted tree, this is referred to as the *bronchial tree* (Figures 7.1 and 7.4).

- Within the lung, each primary bronchus divides and subdivides into increasingly smaller **bronchioles** (**BRONG**-kee-ohlz), which are the smallest branches of the bronchi.

The Alveoli

Alveoli (al-**VEE**-oh-lye), also known as *air sacs*, are the very small grapelike clusters found at the end of each bronchiole (singular, *alveolus,* pronounced al-**VEE**-oh-lus). The alveoli are where the exchange of oxygen and carbon dioxide takes place. Each lung contains millions of alveoli (Figures 7.1 and 7.4).

- During respiration, the alveoli are filled with air from the bronchioles.
- A network of microscopic pulmonary capillaries surrounds the alveoli. **Pulmonary** (**PULL**-mah-**nair**-ee) means relating to or affecting the lungs.
- The exchange of oxygen and carbon dioxide between the air inside the alveoli and the blood in the pulmonary capillaries occurs through the thin, elastic walls of the alveoli.
- The alveoli produce a detergent-like substance, known as a *surfactant*, which reduces the surface tension of the fluid in the lungs. This makes the alveoli more stable so they do not collapse when an individual exhales. Premature babies often lack adequate surfactant.

The Lungs

The **lungs**, which are the essential organs of respiration, are divided into lobes (Figure 7.5). A *lobe* is a subdivision or part of an organ.

- The **right lung** is larger and has three lobes: the upper, middle, and lower (or superior, middle, and inferior).
- The **left lung** has only two lobes, the upper and lower, due to space restrictions because the heart is located on that side of the body.

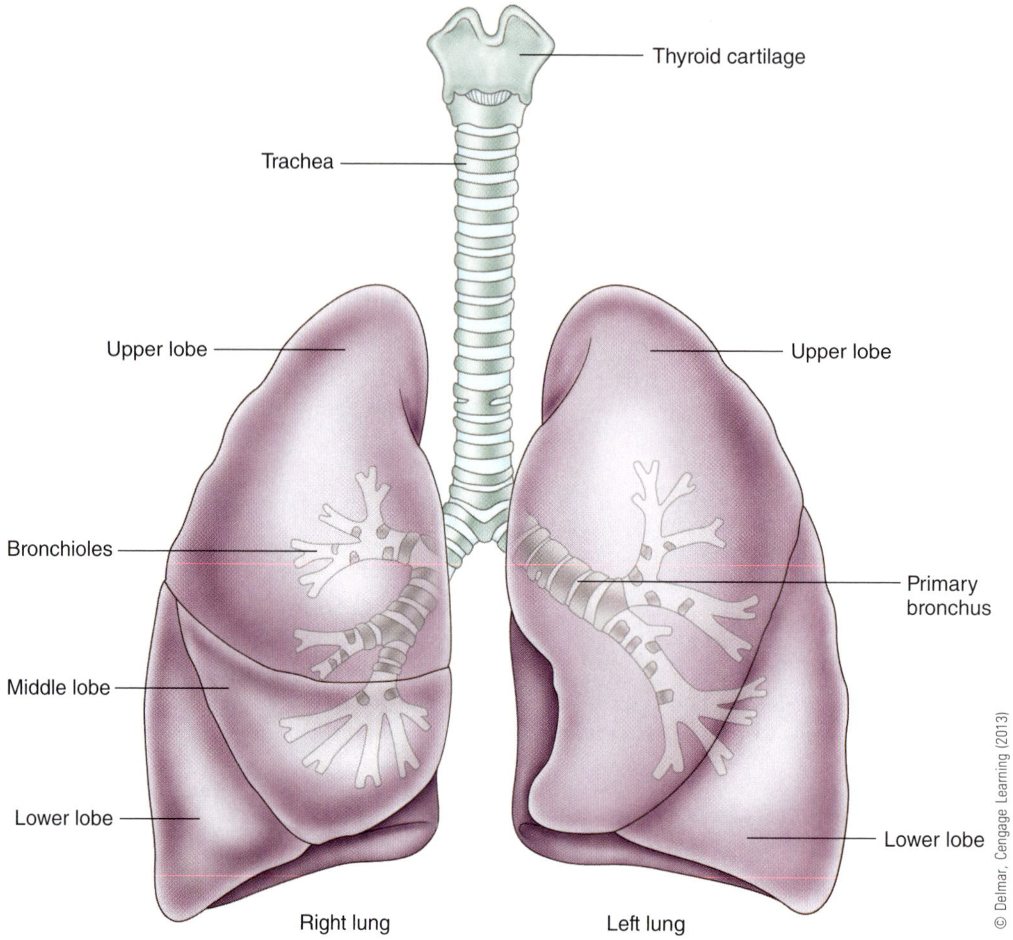

FIGURE 7.5 External view of the lungs. Note the three lobes of the right lung and the two lobes of the left lung.

The Mediastinum

The **mediastinum** (**mee**-dee-as-**TYE**-num) is the middle section of the chest cavity and is located between the lungs. This cavity contains connective tissue and organs, including the heart and its veins and arteries, the esophagus, trachea, bronchi, the thymus gland, and lymph nodes (Figure 7.6).

The Pleura

The **pleura** (**PLOOR**-ah) is a thin, moist, and slippery membrane that covers the outer surface of the lungs and lines the inner surface of the thoracic cavity (Figure 7.6).

- The **parietal pleura** (pah-**RYE**-eh-tal) is the outer layer of the pleura. It lines the walls of the thoracic cavity, covers the diaphragm, and forms the sac containing each lung. The parietal pleura is attached to the chest wall. ***Parietal*** means relating to the walls of a cavity.
- The **visceral pleura** (**VIS**-er-al), which is the inner layer of pleura that covers each lung, is attached directly to the lungs. ***Visceral*** means relating to the internal organs.
- The **pleural cavity**, also known as the ***pleural space***, is the thin fluid-filled space between the parietal and visceral pleural membranes. The fluid acts as a lubricant, allowing the membranes to slide easily over each other during respiration.

The Diaphragm

The **diaphragm** (**DYE**-ah-fram), also known as the ***thoracic diaphragm***, is a dome-shaped sheet of muscle that separates the thoracic cavity from the abdomen. It is the contraction and relaxation of this muscle that makes breathing possible.

- The **phrenic nerves** (**FREN**-ick) stimulate the diaphragm and cause it to contract (Figure 7.7).

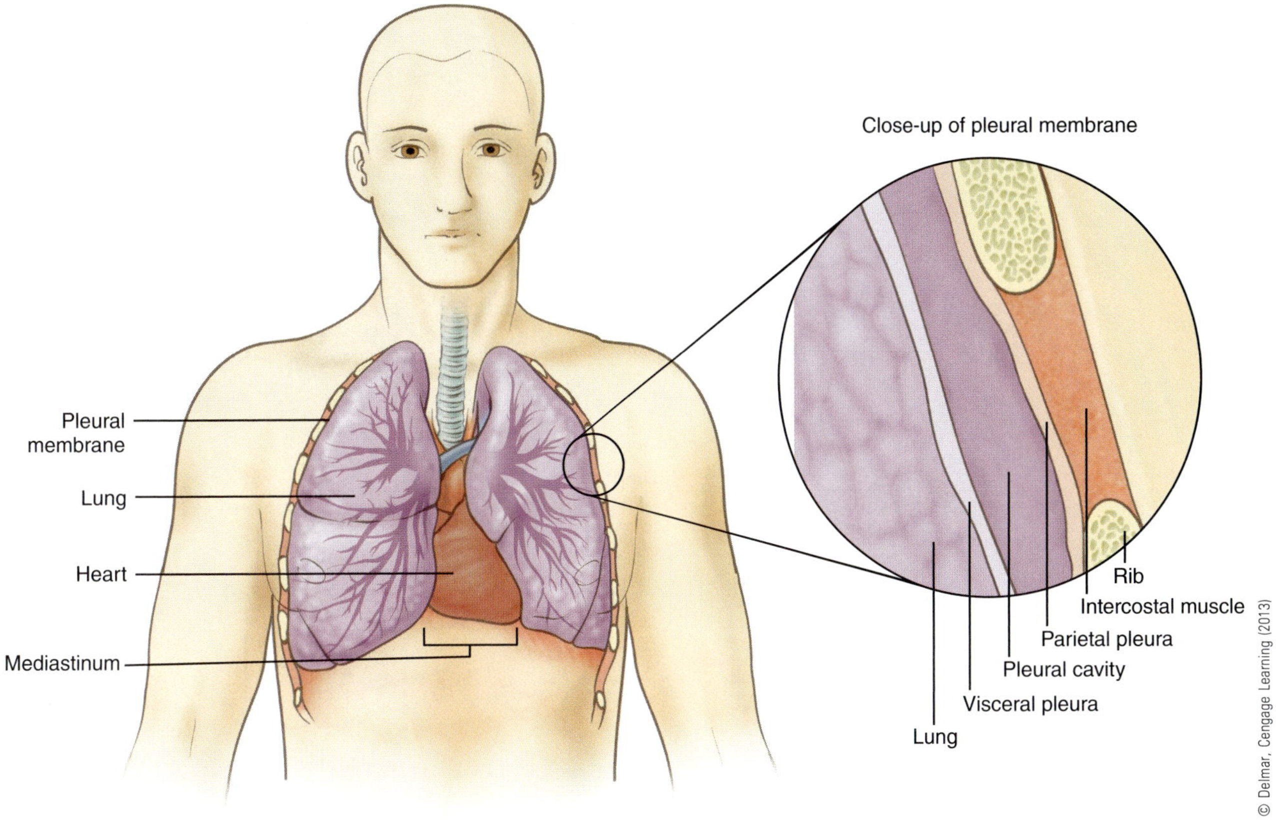

FIGURE 7.6 The pleura allows the lungs to move smoothly within the chest.

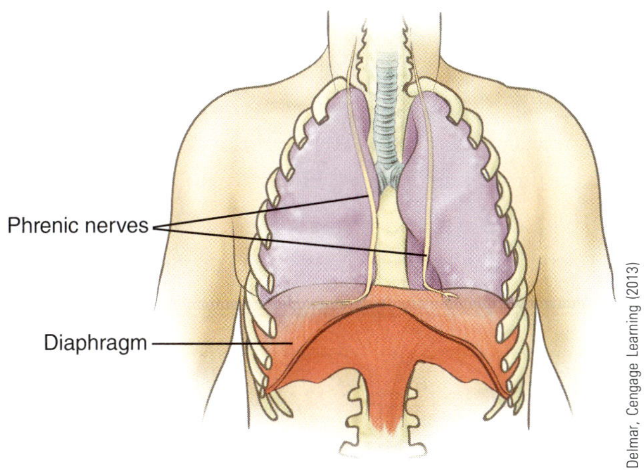

FIGURE 7.7 The diaphragm is controlled by the phrenic nerves.

■ Note: the word *diaphragm* refers to a dividing structure, so the term is also used to describe a contraceptive device that separates the vagina from the cervix.

RESPIRATION

Respiration, or breathing, is the exchange of oxygen for carbon dioxide that is essential to life. A single respiration, or ***breath***, consists of one inhalation and one exhalation (Figure 7.8). ***Ventilation*** is another word for moving air in and out of the lungs.

Inhalation and Exhalation

Inhalation (**in**-hah-**LAY**-shun) is the act of taking in air as the diaphragm contracts and pulls downward (Figure 7.8 left). This action causes the thoracic cavity to expand. This produces a vacuum within the thoracic cavity that draws air into the lungs.

Exhalation (**ecks**-hah-**LAY**-shun) is the act of breathing out. As the diaphragm relaxes, it moves upward, causing the thoracic cavity to become narrower. This action forces air out of the lungs (Figure 7.8 right).

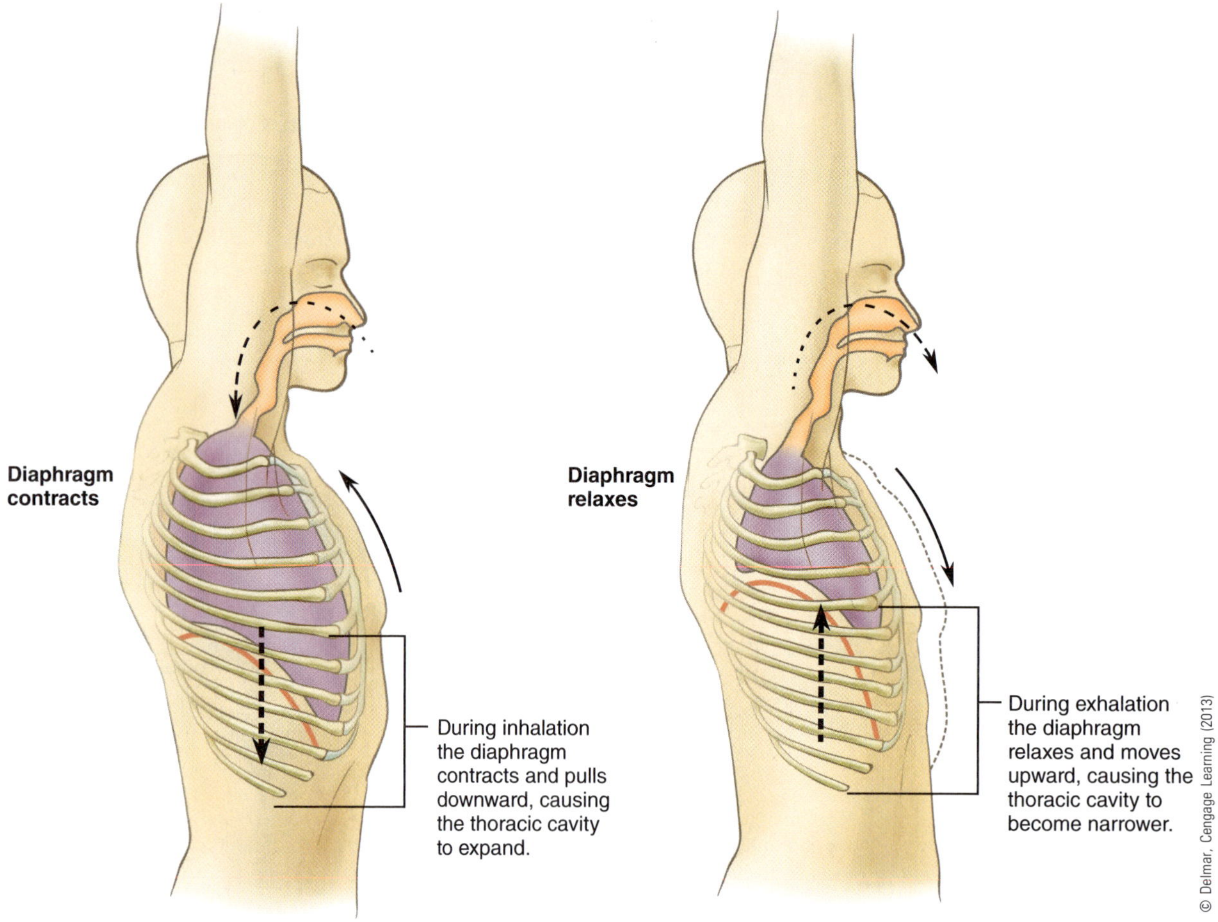

FIGURE 7.8 Movements of the diaphragm and thoracic cavity produce inhalation (left) and exhalation (right).

External Respiration

External respiration is the act of bringing air in and out of the lungs from the outside environment and in the process, exchanging oxygen for carbon dioxide (Figure 7.9).

- As air is ***inhaled*** into the alveoli, oxygen immediately passes into the surrounding capillaries and is carried by the erythrocytes (red blood cells) to all body cells.
- At the same time, the waste product carbon dioxide that has passed into the bloodstream is transported into the air spaces of the lungs to be ***exhaled***.

Internal Respiration

Internal respiration, which is also known as ***cellular respiration***, is the exchange of gases within the cells of the blood and tissues (Figure 7.9).

- In this process, oxygen passes from the bloodstream into the cells.
- The cells give off the waste product carbon dioxide, and this passes into the bloodstream.
- The bloodstream transports the carbon dioxide to the lungs, where it is expelled during exhalation.

MEDICAL SPECIALTIES RELATED TO THE RESPIRATORY SYSTEM

- An **otolaryngologist** (**oh**-toh-**lar**-in-**GOL**-oh-jist), also known as an **ENT** (ear, nose, throat), is a physician with specialized training in the diagnosis and treatment of diseases and disorders of the head and neck (**ot/o** means ear, **laryng/o** means larynx, and **-ologist** means specialist).

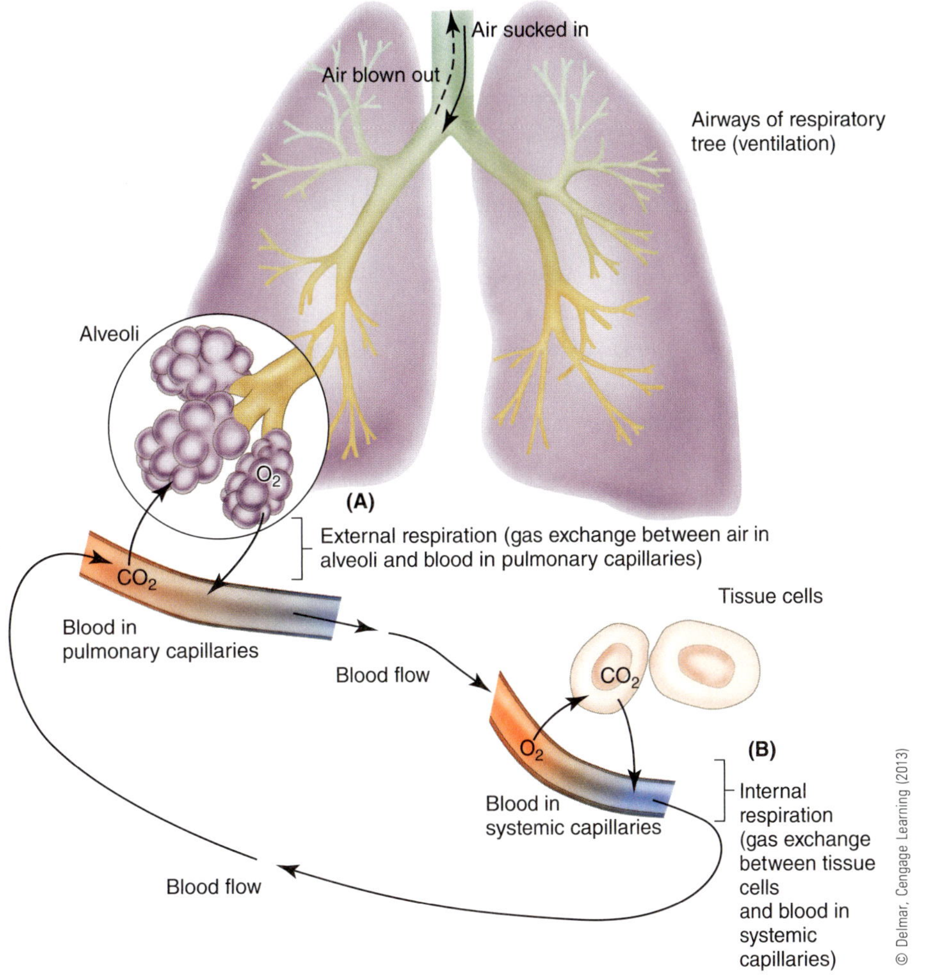

FIGURE 7.9 External and internal respiration compared. (A) External respiration occurs in the lungs. (B) Internal respiration occurs at the cellular level within the blood and tissues.

- A **pulmonologist** (**pull**-mah-**NOL**-oh-jist) is a physician who specializes in diagnosing and treating diseases and disorders of the respiratory system (**pulmon** means lung, and **-ologist** means specialist).
- A **thoracic surgeon** performs operations on the organs inside the thorax, or chest, including the heart, lungs, and esophagus.

PATHOLOGY OF THE RESPIRATORY SYSTEM

Chronic Obstructive Pulmonary Disease

Chronic obstructive pulmonary disease (COPD) is a group of lung diseases in which the bronchial airflow is obstructed, making it hard to breathe. Chronic obstructive pulmonary disease, which is most often caused by long-term smoking, is generally permanent and progressive. Most people with COPD suffer from two related conditions: chronic bronchitis and emphysema.

Chronic Bronchitis

Chronic bronchitis (brong-**KYE**-tis) is a disease in which the airways have become inflamed due to recurrent exposure to an inhaled irritant, usually cigarette smoke (**bronch** means bronchus, and **-itis** means inflammation). An increase in the number and size of mucus-producing cells results in excessive mucus production and a thickening of the walls of the air passages. This causes chronic coughing, difficulty getting air in and out of the lungs, and sometimes also bacterial lung infections.

Emphysema

Emphysema (**em**-fih-**SEE**-mah) is the progressive, long-term loss of lung function, usually due to smoking. Emphysema is characterized by (1) a decrease in the total number of alveoli, (2) the enlargement of the remaining alveoli, and (3) the progressive destruction of the walls of these remaining alveoli.

As the alveoli are destroyed, breathing becomes increasingly rapid, shallow, and difficult. In an effort to compensate for the loss of capacity, the lungs chronically overinflate and the rib cage stays partially expanded all the time, resulting in a slightly rounded shape called a *barrel chest* (Figure 7.10).

Asthma

Asthma (**AZ**-mah) is a chronic inflammatory disease of the bronchial tubes, often triggered by an allergic reaction. Asthma is characterized by episodes of severe breathing difficulty, coughing, and wheezing. These episodes are known as *asthmatic attacks*.

Wheezing is a breathing sound caused by a partially obstructed airway. The frequency and severity of asthmatic attacks is influenced by a variety of factors, including allergens, environmental agents, exercise, and infection.

- Figure 7.11A shows the exterior of the airway before an attack. Figure 7.11B shows the factors within and surrounding the airway that cause breathing difficulty during an attack.
- **Airway inflammation** is the swelling and clogging of the bronchial tubes with mucus. This usually occurs after the airway has been exposed to inhaled allergens.
- A **bronchospasm** (**brong**-koh-spazm) is a contraction of the smooth muscle in the walls of the bronchi and bronchioles, tightening and squeezing the airway shut (**bronch/o** means bronchi, and **-spasm** means involuntary contraction).
- *Exercise-induced asthma* is the narrowing of the airways that develops after 5 to 15 minutes of physical exertion. This also can be due to cold weather or allergies.
- A person who suffers from asthma is known as an *asthmatic*.

StudyWARE CONNECTION

Watch the **Asthma** animation in the StudyWARE™.

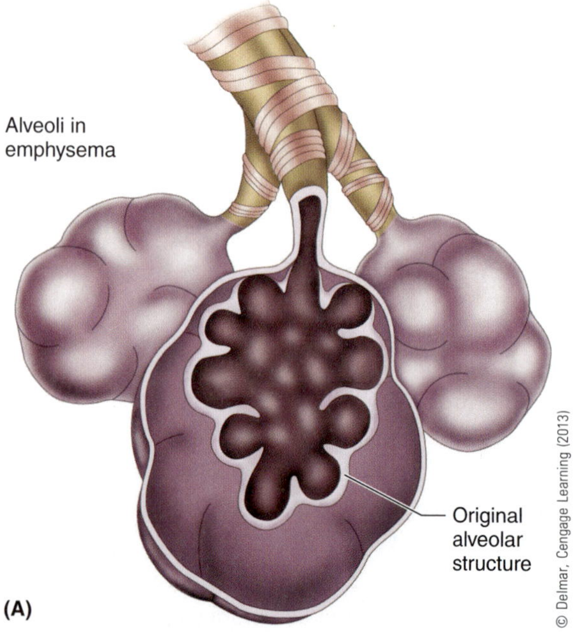

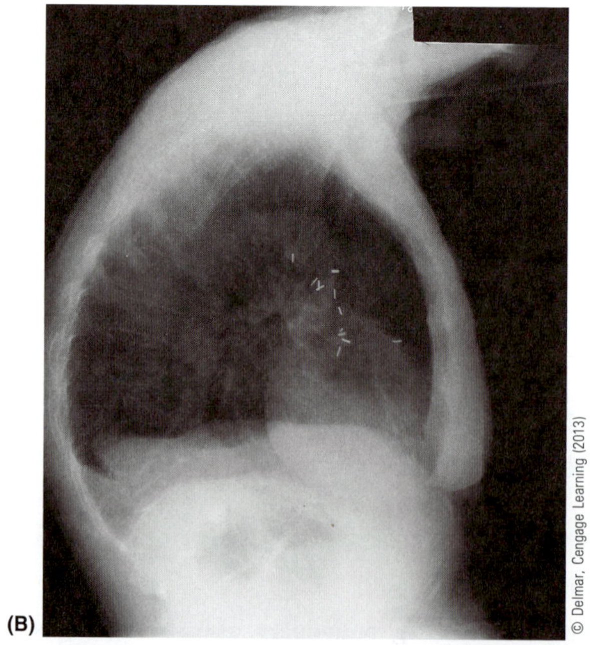

FIGURE 7.10 Emphysema. (A) Changes in the alveoli as the disease progresses. (B) Lateral x-ray showing lung enlargement and abnormal barrel chest in emphysema. (Note: the short white lines shown in the x-ray are surgical clips.)

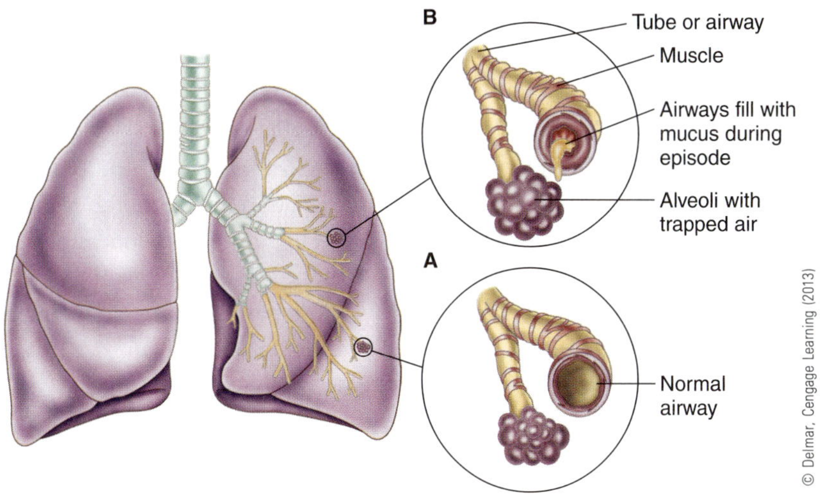

FIGURE 7.11 Changes in the airways during an asthma episode. (A) Before the episode, the muscles are relaxed and the airways are open. (B) During the episode, the muscles tighten and the airways fill with mucus.

UPPER RESPIRATORY DISEASES

- **Upper respiratory infections** (URI) and ***acute nasopharyngitis*** are among the terms used to describe the ***common cold***. An upper respiratory infection can be caused by any one of 200 different viruses, the most common of which is the ***human rhinovirus***.
- **Allergic rhinitis** (rye-**NIGH**-tis), commonly referred to as an ***allergy***, is an allergic reaction to airborne allergens that causes an increased flow of mucus (**rhin** means nose, and **-itis** means inflammation). Allergies are discussed in Chapter 6.
- **Croup** (**KROOP**) is an acute respiratory infection in children and infants characterized by obstruction of the larynx, hoarseness, and swelling around the vocal cords resulting in a barking cough and stridor. ***Stridor*** is a harsh, high-pitched sound caused by a blockage present when breathing in.
- **Diphtheria** (dif-**THEE**-ree-ah) is an acute bacterial infection of the throat and upper respiratory tract. The diphtheria bacteria produce toxins that can damage the heart muscle and peripheral nerves. Through immunization the disease is now largely prevented.
- **Epistaxis** (**ep**-ih-**STACK**-sis), also known as a ***nosebleed***, is bleeding from the nose that may be caused by dry air, an injury, medication to prevent blood clotting, or high blood pressure.
- **Influenza** (**in**-flew-**EN**-zah), also known as the ***flu***, is an acute, highly contagious viral infection characterized by respiratory inflammation, fever, chills, and muscle pain. Influenza is spread by respiratory droplets and occurs most commonly in epidemics during the colder months. There are many strains of the influenza virus. Some strains can be prevented by annual immunization.
- **Pertussis** (per-**TUS**-is), also known as ***whooping cough***, is a contagious bacterial infection of the upper respiratory tract that is characterized by recurrent bouts of a paroxysmal cough, followed by breathlessness and a noisy inspiration. ***Paroxysmal*** means sudden or spasmlike. Childhood immunization against diphtheria, pertussis, and tetanus are given together (DPT); however, the incidence of pertussis is on the rise.
- **Rhinorrhea** (**rye**-noh-**REE**-ah), also known as a ***runny nose***, is the watery flow of mucus from the nose (**rhin/o** means nose, and **-rrhea** means abnormal discharge).
- **Sinusitis** (**sigh**-nuh-**SIGH**-tis) is an inflammation of the sinuses (**sinus** means sinus, and **-itis** means inflammation).

Pharynx and Larynx

- **Pharyngitis** (fah-rin-**JIGH**-tis), also known as a ***sore throat***, is an inflammation of the pharynx (**pharyng** means pharynx, and **-itis** means inflammation). It is often a symptom of a cold, flu, or sinus infection.

■ A **laryngospasm** (lah-**RING**-goh-spazm) is the sudden spasmodic closure of the larynx (**laryng/o** means larynx, and **-spasm** means a sudden involuntary contraction). It is sometimes associated with gastroesophageal reflux disease (GERD), which is discussed in Chapter 8.

Voice Disorders

■ **Aphonia** (ah-**FOH**-nee-ah) is the loss of the ability of the larynx to produce normal speech sounds (**a-** means without, **phon** means sound or voice, and **-ia** means abnormal condition).

■ **Dysphonia** (dis-**FOH**-nee-ah) is difficulty in speaking, which may include any impairment in vocal quality, including hoarseness, weakness, or the cracking of a boy's voice during puberty (**dys-** means bad, **phon** means sound or voice, and **-ia** means abnormal condition).

■ **Laryngitis** (**lar**-in-**JIGH**-tis) is an inflammation of the larynx (**laryng** means larynx, and **-itis** means inflammation). This term is also commonly used to describe voice loss that is caused by this inflammation.

Trachea and Bronchi

■ **Tracheorrhagia** (**tray**-kee-oh-**RAY**-jee-ah) is bleeding from the mucous membranes of the trachea (**trache/o** means trachea, and **-rrhagia** means bleeding).

■ **Bronchiectasis** (**brong**-kee-**ECK**-tah-sis) is the permanent dilation of the bronchi, caused by chronic infection and inflammation (**bronch/i** means bronchus, and **-ectasis** means stretching or enlargement).

■ **Bronchorrhea** (**brong**-koh-**REE**-ah) is an excessive discharge of mucus from the bronchi (**bronch/o** means bronchus, and **-rrhea** means abnormal flow). This is often caused by chronic bronchitis or asthma.

Pleural Cavity

■ **Pleurisy** (**PLOOR**-ih-see), also known as ***pleuritis***, is an inflammation of the pleura, the membranes that cover the lungs and line the pleural cavity. Pleurisy, which causes pleurodynia, may result from trauma, tuberculosis, connective tissue disease, or an infection (**pleur** means pleura, and **-isy** is a noun ending).

■ **Pleurodynia** (**ploor**-oh-**DIN**-ee-ah) is a sharp pain that occurs when the inflamed membranes rub against each other with each inhalation (**pleur/o** means pleura, and **-dynia** means pain).

■ **Pleural effusion** (eh-**FEW**-zhun) is the excess accumulation of fluid in the pleural space. This produces a feeling of breathlessness because it prevents the lung from fully expanding. ***Effusion*** is the escape of fluid from blood or lymphatic vessels into the tissues or into a body cavity (Figure 7.12).

■ **Pyothorax** (**pye**-oh-**THOH**-racks), also known as ***empyema of the pleural cavity***, is the presence of pus in the pleural cavity between the layers of the pleural membrane (**py/o** means pus, and **-thorax** means chest).

■ **Empyema** (**em**-pye-**EE**-mah) refers to a collection of pus in a body cavity.

■ **Hemothorax** (**hee**-moh-**THOH**-racks) is a collection of blood in the pleural cavity (**hem/o** means blood, and **-thorax** means chest). This condition often results from chest trauma, such as a stab wound, or it can be caused by disease or surgery.

■ A **pneumothorax** (**new**-moh-**THOR**-racks) is the accumulation of air in the pleural space resulting in a pressure imbalance that causes the lung to fully or partially collapse (**pneum/o** means lung or air, and **-thorax** means chest). This can have an external cause, such as a stab wound through the chest wall, or can occur when there is a lung-disease-related rupture in the pleura that allows air to leak into the pleural space (Figure 7.13).

Lungs

■ **Acute respiratory distress syndrome** (ARDS) is a lung condition usually caused by trauma, pneumonia, smoke or fumes, inhaled vomit, or sepsis. ***Sepsis*** is a systemic

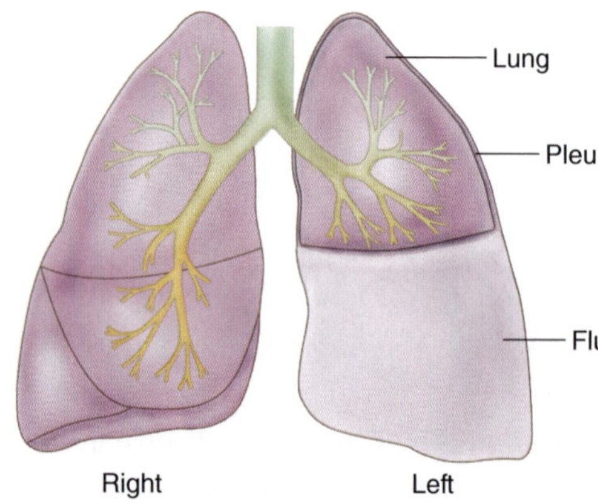

FIGURE 7.12 In pleural effusion, excess fluid in the pleural cavity prevents the lung from fully expanding.

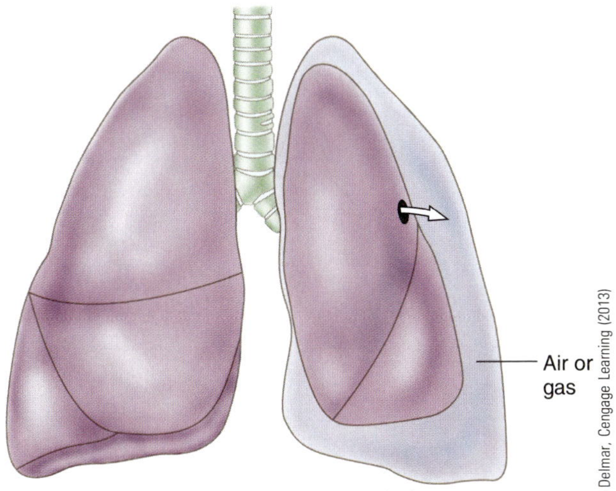

FIGURE 7.13 Pneumothorax is an accumulation of air or gas in the pleural space that causes the lung to collapse. In the left lung, a perforation in the pleura allowed air to escape into the pleural space.

bacterial infection in the bloodstream. ARDS is a life-threatening condition in which inflammation in the lungs and fluid in the alveoli lead to low levels of oxygen in the blood.

- **Atelectasis** (**at**-ee-**LEK**-tah-sis), or ***collapsed lung***, is the incomplete expansion of part or all of a lung due to a blockage of the air passages or pneumothorax (**atel** means incomplete, and **-ectasis** means stretching or enlargement).
- **Pulmonary edema** (eh-**DEE**-mah) is an accumulation of fluid in lung tissues, especially the alveoli. ***Edema*** means swelling. Pulmonary edema is often a symptom of heart failure and is discussed in Chapter 5.
- **Pulmonary embolism** (**EM**-boh-lizm) is the sudden blockage of a pulmonary artery by foreign matter or by an embolus that has formed in the leg or pelvic region.
- **Pneumorrhagia** (**new**-moh-**RAY**-jee-ah) is bleeding from the lungs (**pneum/o** means lungs, and **-rrhagia** means bleeding).

Tuberculosis

Tuberculosis (too-**ber**-kew-**LOH**-sis) (TB), which is an infectious disease caused by *Mycobacterium tuberculosis*, usually attacks the lungs; however, it can also affect other parts of the body. Pleurisy and coughing up blood (hemoptysis) can be symptoms of TB in the lungs.

- TB occurs most commonly in individuals whose immune systems are weakened by another condition such as AIDS. A healthy individual can carry latent TB without showing symptoms of the disease. ***Latent*** means present but not active.
- ***Multidrug-resistant tuberculosis*** is a dangerous form of tuberculosis because the germs have become resistant to the effect of the primary TB drugs.

Pneumonia Named for the Affected Lung Tissue

Pneumonia (new-**MOH**-nee-ah) is a serious inflammation of the lungs in which the alveoli and air passages fill with pus and other fluids (**pneumon** means lung, and **-ia** means abnormal condition). Pneumonia is most commonly caused by an infection and often follows a cold, flu, chronic illness, or other condition that weakens the immune system and its ability to stave off infection.

There are two types of bacterial pneumonia named for the parts of the lungs affected (Figure 7.14). These are:

- **Bronchopneumonia** (**brong**-koh-new-**MOH**-nee-ah) is a localized form of pneumonia that often affects the bronchioles (**bronch/o** means bronchial tubes, **pneumon** means lung, and **-ia** means abnormal condition). Bronchopneumonia often leads to lobar pneumonia.
- **Lobar pneumonia** affects larger areas of the lungs, often including one or more sections, or lobes, of a lung. ***Double pneumonia*** is lobar pneumonia involving both lungs and is usually a form of bacterial pneumonia.

Pneumonia Named for the Causative Agent

As many as 30 causes of pneumonia have been identified; however, the most common causative agents are air pollution, bacteria, fungi, viruses, and inhaled liquid or chemicals.

- **Aspiration pneumonia** (**ass**-pih-**RAY**-shun) can occur when a foreign substance, such as vomit, is inhaled into the lungs. As used here, ***aspiration*** means inhaling or drawing a foreign substance into the upper respiratory tract.
- **Bacterial pneumonia** is most commonly caused by *Streptococcus pneumoniae*. ***Pneumococcal pneumonia*** is the only form of pneumonia that can be prevented through vaccination.
- **Community-acquired pneumonia** is a type of pneumonia that results from contagious infection outside of a hospital or clinic.

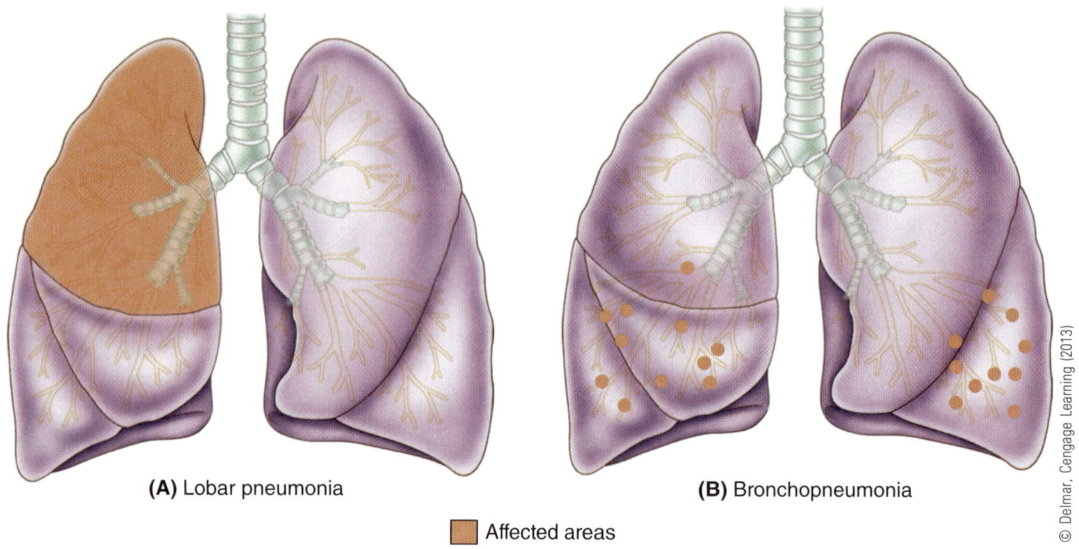

FIGURE 7.14 Types of pneumonia are usually named for the area of the lung that is involved, or for the causative agent. (A) Lobar pneumonia affects larger areas of the lungs. (B) Bronchopneumonia affects the bronchioles and surrounding alveoli.

- **Hospital-acquired pneumonia**, or ***nosocomial pneumonia***, is a type of pneumonia contracted during a stay in the hospital when a patient's defenses are impaired. Patients on a respirator are particularly at risk. *Nosocomial* means hospital-acquired.
- **Walking pneumonia**, also known as ***mycoplasma pneumonia***, is a milder but longer-lasting form of the disease caused by the bacteria *Mycoplasma pneumoniae.* It gets its name from the fact that the patient is often not bedridden.
- **Pneumocystis pneumonia** (**new**-moh-**SIS**-tis new-**MOH**-nee-ah) is an opportunistic infection caused by the yeast-like fungus *Pneumocystis carinii.* Opportunistic infections are discussed in Chapter 6.
- **Viral pneumonia**, which can be caused by several different types of viruses, accounts for approximately a third of all pneumonias.

Interstitial Lung Disease

Interstitial lung disease (**in**-ter-**STISH**-al) refers to a group of almost 200 disorders that cause inflammation and scarring of the alveoli and their supporting structures. ***Interstitial*** means relating to spaces within or around a tissue or an organ. In these lung conditions the tissue around the alveoli becomes scarred or stiff, leading to a reduction of oxygen being transferred to the blood.

- **Pulmonary fibrosis** (figh-**BROH**-sis), or ***interstitial fibrosis***, is the progressive formation of scar tissue in the lung, resulting in decreased lung capacity and increased difficulty in breathing (**fibros** means fibrous connective tissue, and **-is** is the noun ending). ***Fibrosis*** is a condition in which normal tissue is replaced by fibrotic (hardened) tissue.

Many connective tissue diseases such as rheumatoid arthritis, scleroderma, and lupus can cause pulmonary fibrosis, as can environmental toxins such as asbestos and silica. Pulmonary fibrosis can also occur without a known cause.

Environmental and Occupational Interstitial Lung Diseases

- **Pneumoconiosis** (**new**-moh-**koh**-nee-**OH**-sis) is any fibrosis of the lung tissues caused by dust in the lungs after prolonged environmental or occupational contact (**pneum/o** means lung, **coni** means dust, and **-osis** means abnormal condition or disease).
- **Anthracosis** (**an**-thrah-**KOH**-sis), also known as ***coal miner's pneumoconiosis*** or ***black lung disease***, is caused by coal dust in the lungs (**anthrac** means coal dust, and **-osis** means abnormal condition or disease).
- **Asbestosis** (**ass**-beh-**STOH**-sis) is caused by asbestos particles in the lungs and usually occurs after working with asbestos (**asbest** means asbestos, and **-osis** means abnormal condition or disease).
- **Silicosis** (**sill**-ih-**KOH**-sis) is caused by inhaling silica dust in the lungs and usually occurs after working in occupations including foundry work, quarrying, ceramics, glasswork, and sandblasting (**silic** means glass, and **-osis** means abnormal condition or disease).

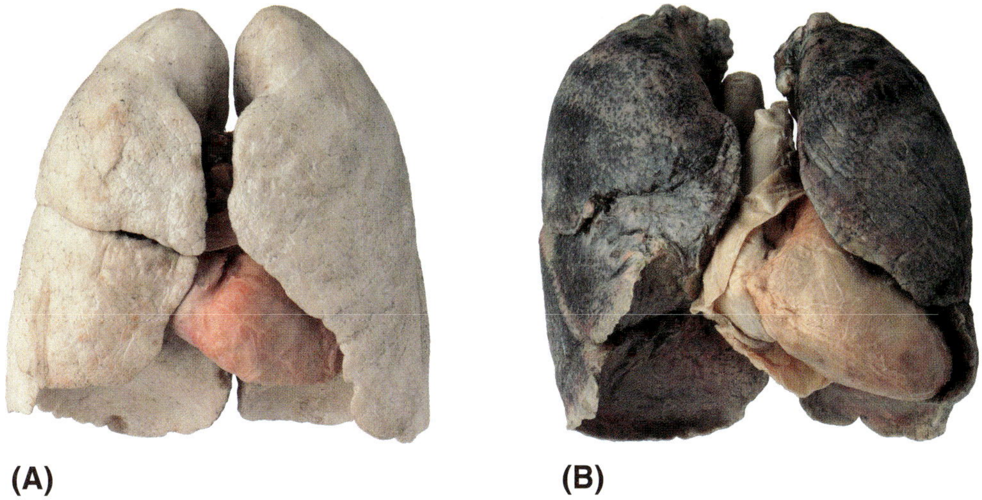

FIGURE 7.15 Photographs of actual lung and heart specimens. (A) Healthy lungs of a nonsmoker. (B) Damaged lungs of a smoker.

Cystic Fibrosis

Cystic fibrosis (**SIS**-tick figh-**BROH**-sis) is a life-threatening genetic disorder in which the lungs and pancreas are clogged with large quantities of abnormally thick mucus. This results in damage to the lungs, poor growth, and nutritional deficiencies. Treatments for cystic fibrosis include:

- *Pancreatic enzymes* to aid the digestive system
- *Antibiotics* to prevent and treat lung infections
- *Bronchodilators* to keep airways open
- *Chest percussion*, which is a therapeutic technique to remove excess mucus from the lungs. This is often performed with the patient positioned at an angle to allow gravity to help drain the secretions. Percussion is described in Chapter 15.

Lung Cancer

Lung cancer, which is the leading cause of cancer death in the United States, is a condition in which cancer cells form in the tissues of the lung. Important risk factors for lung cancer are smoking and inhaling secondhand smoke (Figure 7.15).

Breathing Disorders

The general term *breathing disorders* describes abnormal changes in the rate or depth of breathing. Specific terms describe in greater detail the changes that are occurring (Figure 7.16).

- **Eupnea** (youp-**NEE**-ah) is easy or normal breathing (**eu-** means good, and **-pnea** means breathing). This is the baseline for judging some breathing disorders (Figure 7.16A). Eupnea is the opposite of *apnea.*
- **Apnea** (**AP**-nee-ah) is the temporary absence of spontaneous respiration (**a-** means without, and **-pnea** means breathing) (Figure 7.16D). It is a common respiratory problem in premature infants. Apnea is the opposite of *eupnea.*
- **Bradypnea** (**brad**-ihp-**NEE**-ah) is an abnormally slow rate of respiration, usually of less than 10 breaths per minute (**brady-** means slow, and **-pnea** means breathing) (Figure 7.16C). Bradypnea is the opposite of *tachypnea.*
- **Cheyne-Stokes respiration** (**CHAYN-STOHKS**) is an irregular pattern of breathing characterized by alternating rapid or shallow respiration followed by slower respiration or apnea (Figure 7.16E). This pattern sometimes occurs in comatose patients or those nearing death.
- **Tachypnea** (**tack**-ihp-**NEE**-ah) is an abnormally rapid rate of respiration usually of more than 20 breaths per minute (**tachy-** means rapid, and **-pnea** means breathing) (Figure 7.16B). Tachypnea is the opposite of *bradypnea.*
- **Dyspnea** (**DISP**-nee-ah), also known as *shortness of breath (SOB)*, is difficult or labored breathing (**dys-** means painful, and **-pnea** means breathing). Shortness of breath is frequently one of the first symptoms of heart failure. It can also be caused by strenuous physical exertion or can be due to lung damage that produces dyspnea even at rest.

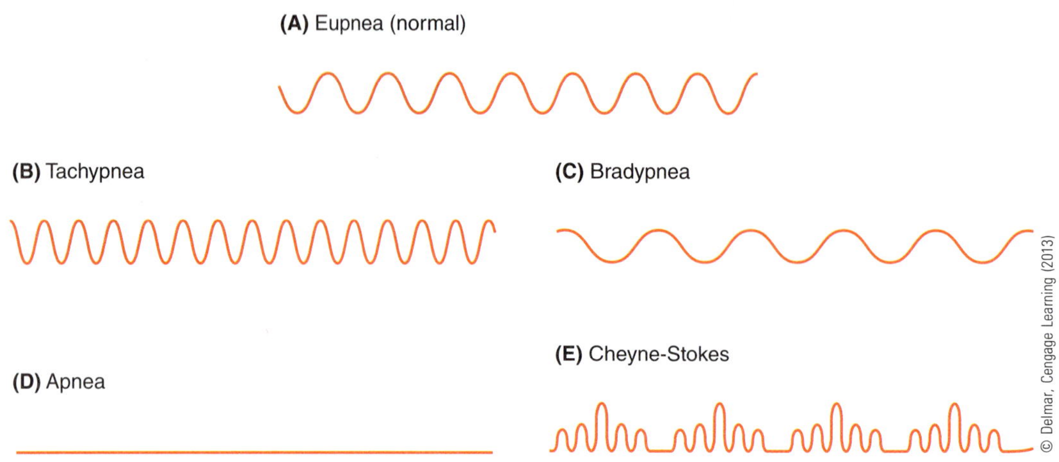

FIGURE 7.16 Respiratory patterns. (A) Eupnea is normal breathing. (B) Tachypnea is abnormally rapid breathing. (C) Bradypnea is abnormally slow breathing. (D) Apnea is the absence of breathing. (E) Cheyne-Stokes is an alternating series of abnormal patterns.

- **Hyperpnea** (**high**-perp-**NEE**-ah), which is commonly associated with exertion, is breathing that is deeper and more rapid than is normal at rest (**hyper-** means excessive, and **-pnea** means breathing). Hyperpnea may also occur at high altitude, or be caused by anemia or sepsis. Hyperpnea is the opposite of *hypopnea*.
- **Hypopnea** (**high**-poh-**NEE**-ah) is shallow or slow respiration (**hypo-** means decreased, and **-pnea** means breathing). Hypopnea is the opposite of *hyperpnea*.
- **Hyperventilation** (**high**-per-**ven**-tih-**LAY**-shun) is an abnormally rapid rate of deep respiration that is usually associated with anxiety (**hyper-** means excessive, and **-ventilation** means breathing). This decreases the level of carbon dioxide in the blood, causing dizziness and tingling in the fingers and toes.

Sleep-Related Breathing Disorders

Sleep related breathing disorders are characterized by disruptions of normal breathing patterns that only occur during sleep and are associated with higher risks of cardiovascular disease and strokes.

- **Sleep apnea** is a potentially serious disorder in which breathing repeatedly stops and starts during sleep for long-enough periods to cause a measurable decrease in blood oxygen levels. ***Obstructive sleep apnea*** is caused by the muscles at the back of the throat relaxing and narrowing the airways.
- ***Snoring***, which can be a symptom of sleep apnea, is noisy breathing caused by vibration of the soft palate.

Coughing

- **Expectoration** (eck-**SPEK**-toh-**rate**) is the act of coughing up and spitting out saliva, mucus, or other body fluid (**expector/o** means to cough up, and **-ation** means state or action).
- **Hemoptysis** (hee-**MOP**-tih-sis) is the expectoration of blood or blood-stained sputum derived from the lungs or bronchial tubes as the result of a pulmonary or bronchial hemorrhage (**hem/o** means blood, and **-ptysis** means spitting).

Lack of Oxygen

- **Airway obstruction**, commonly known as ***choking***, occurs when food or a foreign object partially or completely blocks the airway and prevents air from entering or leaving the lungs. This can be a life-threatening emergency requiring immediate action through the performance of the ***abdominal thrust maneuver***. This is also known as the ***Heimlich maneuver***.
- **Anoxia** (ah-**NOCK**-see-ah) is the absence of oxygen from the body's tissues and organs even though there is an adequate flow of blood (**an-** means without, **ox** means oxygen, and **-ia** means abnormal condition). If anoxia continues for more than 4 to 6 minutes, irreversible brain damage can occur.
- **Hypoxia** (high-**POCK**-see-ah) is the condition of having deficient oxygen levels in the body's tissues and organs; however, it is less severe than anoxia (**hyp-** means deficient, **ox** means oxygen, and **-ia** means abnormal condition). This condition can be caused by

a variety of factors, including head trauma, carbon monoxide poisoning, suffocation, and high altitudes. Compare with *hypoxemia*.

- ***Altitude hypoxia***, also known as ***altitude sickness***, is a condition that can be brought on by the decreased oxygen in the air at higher altitudes, usually above 8,000 feet.
- **Asphyxia** (ass-**FICK**-see-ah) is the loss of consciousness that occurs when the body cannot get the oxygen it needs to function. Asphyxia can be caused by choking, suffocation, drowning, or inhaling gases such as carbon monoxide.
- ***Asphyxiation*** is a state of asphyxia or suffocation. In this life-threatening condition, oxygen levels in the blood drop quickly, carbon dioxide levels rise, and unless the patient's breathing is restored within a few minutes, death or serious brain damage follows.
- **Cyanosis** (**sigh**-ah-**NOH**-sis) is a bluish discoloration of the skin and mucous membranes caused by a lack of adequate oxygen in the blood (**cyan** means blue, and **-osis** means abnormal condition or disease).
- **Hypercapnia** (**high**-per-**KAP**-nee-ah) is the abnormal buildup of carbon dioxide in the blood (**hyper-** means excessive, **capn** means carbon dioxide, and **-ia** means abnormal condition).
- **Hypoxemia** (**high**-pock-**SEE**-mee-ah) is the condition of having low oxygen levels in the blood, usually due to respiratory disorders or heart conditions (**hyp-** means deficient, **ox** means oxygen, and **-emia** means blood). Compare with *hypoxia*.
- **Respiratory failure** (RF), also known as ***respiratory acidosis***, is a condition in which the level of oxygen in the blood becomes dangerously low (hypoxemia) or the level of carbon dioxide becomes dangerously high (hypercapnia). It is a medical emergency that can result from a chronic condition or develop suddenly.
- **Smoke inhalation** is damage to the lungs in which particles from a fire coat the alveoli and prevent the normal exchange of gases.

Sudden Infant Death Syndrome

Sudden infant death syndrome (SIDS) is the sudden and unexplainable death of an apparently healthy sleeping infant between the ages of 2 months and 6 months. Although the cause of SIDS is still unknown, it is suspected to be a heart problem or interruption in breathing. The recommendation that infants sleep on their back or side instead of facedown has reduced the incidence of SIDS.

DIAGNOSTIC PROCEDURES OF THE RESPIRATORY SYSTEM

- The ***respiratory rate***, which is an important vital sign, is discussed in Chapter 15. It is a count of the number of breaths (one inhalation and one exhalation) per minute.
- ***Respiratory sounds*** such as *rale, rhonchi,* and *stridor* provide information about the condition of the lungs and pleura. These are described in Chapter 15.
- **Bronchoscopy** (brong-**KOS**-koh-pee) is the visual examination of the bronchi using a bronchoscope (**bronch/o** means bronchus, and **-scopy** means direct visual examination). A ***bronchoscope*** is a flexible, fiber-optic device that is passed through the nose or mouth and down the airways. It can also be used for operative procedures, such as tissue repair or the removal of a foreign object.
- A **chest x-ray** (CXR), also known as ***chest imaging***, is a valuable tool for diagnosing pneumonia, lung cancer, pneumothorax, pleural effusion, tuberculosis, and emphysema (Figure 7.10B).
- **Laryngoscopy** (**lar**-ing-**GOS**-koh-pee) is the visual examination of the larynx and vocal cords using a flexible or rigid laryngoscope inserted through the mouth (**laryng/o** means larynx, and **-scopy** means a direct visual examination). ***Indirect laryngoscopy*** is a simpler version of this test in which the larynx is viewed by shining a light on an angled mirror held at the back of the soft palate.
- A **peak flow meter** is an inexpensive handheld device used to let patients with asthma measure air flowing out of the lungs, revealing any narrowing of the airways in advance of an asthma attack (Figure 7.17).
- **Polysomnography** (**pol**-ee-som-**NOG**-rah-fee), also known as a ***sleep study***, measures physiological activity during sleep and is often performed to detect nocturnal defects in breathing associated with sleep apnea (**poly-** means many, **somn/o** means sleep, and **-graphy** means the process of recording).
- **Pulmonary function tests** (PFTs) are a group of tests that measure volume and flow of air by using a spirometer. These tests are measured against a norm for the individual's age, height, and sex.

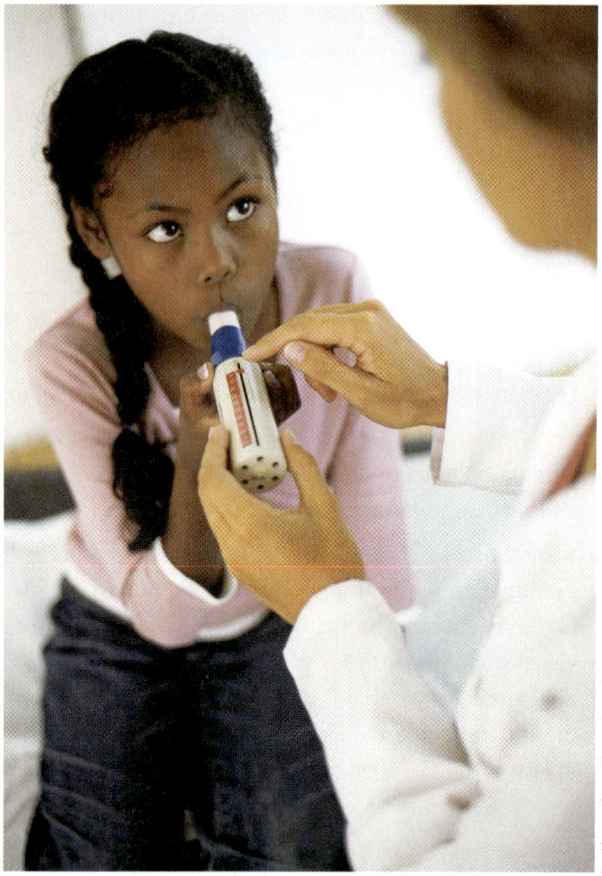

Ian Hooton/Photo Researchers, Inc.

FIGURE 7.17 A peak flow meter is often used to measure how quickly a patient with asthma can expel air.

- A **spirometer** (spih-**ROM**-eh-ter) is a recording device that measures the amount of air inhaled or exhaled (volume) and the length of time required for each breath (**spir/o** means to breathe, and **-meter** means to measure).
- A **pulse oximeter** (ock-**SIM**-eh-ter) is an external monitor placed on the patient's fingertip or earlobe to measure the oxygen saturation level in the blood (**ox/i** means oxygen, and **-meter** means to measure). This is a noninvasive method of assessing basic respiratory function (Figure 7.18).
- **Phlegm** (**FLEM**) is thick mucus secreted by the tissues lining the respiratory passages.
- **Sputum** (**SPYOU**-tum) is phlegm ejected through the mouth that can be examined for diagnostic purposes. ***Sputum cytology*** is a procedure in which a sample of mucus is coughed up from the lungs and then examined under a microscope to detect cancer cells.

Tuberculosis Testing

Two kinds of tests can be used to help detect tuberculosis infection: tuberculin skin testing and blood tests. These tests show whether the patient is infected with TB; however, they do not show whether the infection is latent or active.

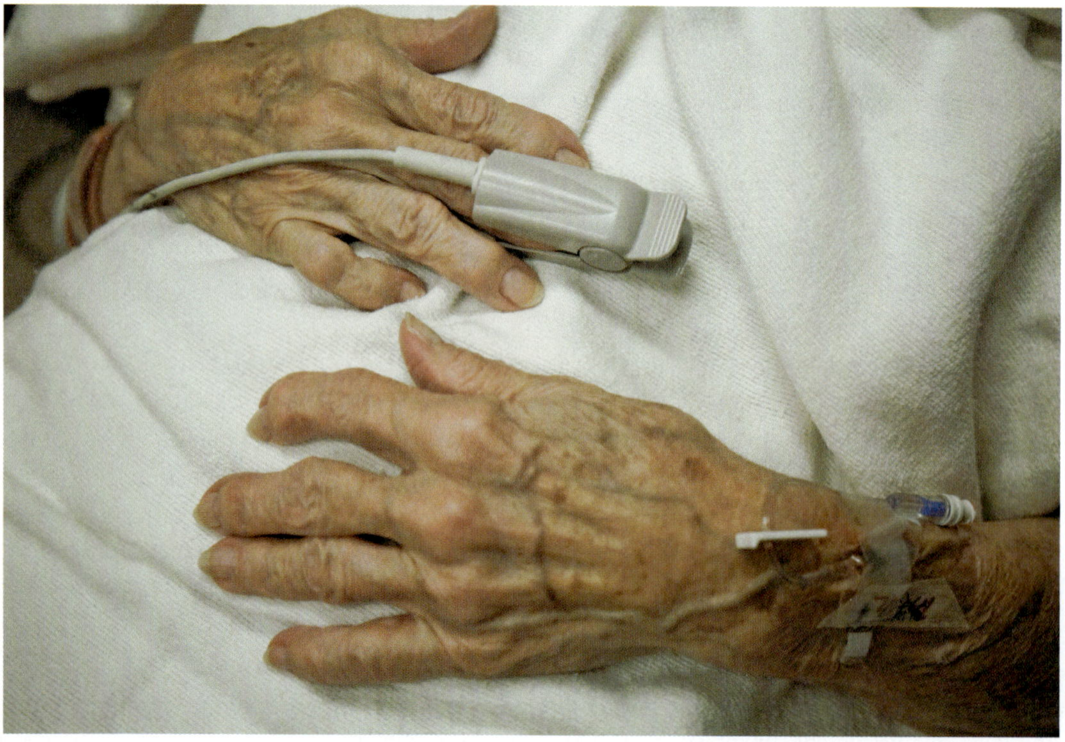

iStockphoto/David Sucsy

FIGURE 7.18 A pulse oximeter is applied to a finger to provide continuous reassessment of the patient's levels of oxygenation.

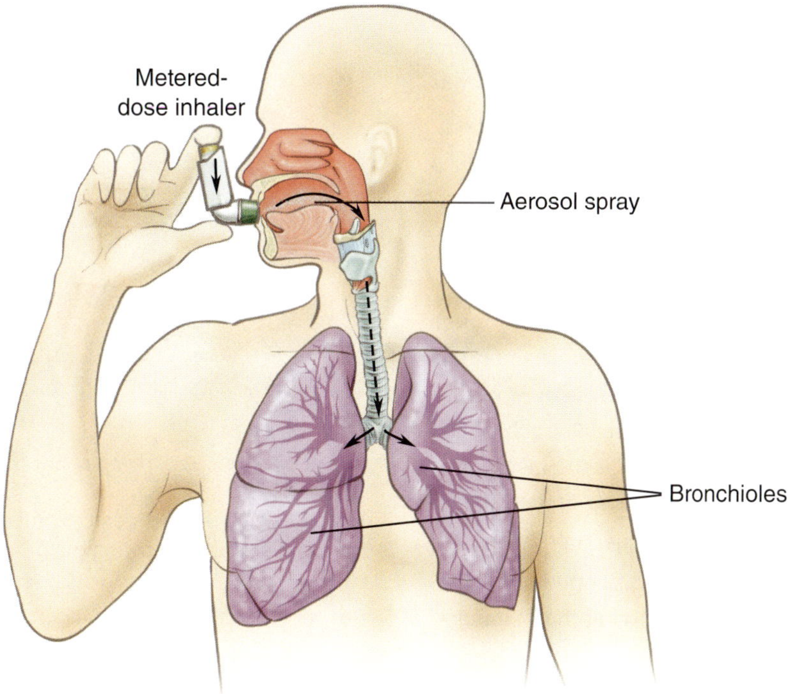

FIGURE 7.19 The metered-dose inhaler delivers medication for inhalation directly into the airways.

- **Tuberculin skin testing** is a screening test for tuberculosis in which the skin of the arm is injected with a harmless antigen extracted from TB bacteria. The ***tuberculin tine test*** is performed using an instrument with several small prongs called tines.
- The **Mantoux PPD skin test** is considered a more accurate skin test for diagnosing tuberculosis. A very small amount of PPD tuberculin (a purified protein derivative) is injected just under the top layer of the skin on the forearm. The site is checked for a reaction 48 to 72 hours later.

A positive result indicates the possibility of exposure to the disease, and this response warrants further testing such as a chest x-ray and sputum cytology.

TREATMENT PROCEDURES OF THE RESPIRATORY SYSTEM

Medications and Their Administration

- An **antitussive** (**an**-tih-**TUSS**-iv), commonly known as ***cough medicine***, is administered to prevent or relieve coughing (**anti-** means against, **tuss** means cough, and **-ive** means performs).
- A **bronchodilator** (**brong**-koh-dye-**LAY**-tor) is a medication that relaxes and expands the bronchial passages into the lungs. Patients with asthma use short-acting bronchodilators as needed as rescue medications, while long-acting bronchodilators are used every day to control the condition.
- A **metered-dose inhaler** (MDI) administers a specific amount of a medication such as a bronchodilator in aerosol form. A gas propellant mixes with the medicine to push it into the lungs (Figure 7.19).
- A **nebulizer** (**NEB**-you-lye-zer) is an electronic device that pumps air or oxygen through a liquid medicine to turn it into a mist, which is then inhaled by the patient via a face mask or mouthpiece.

Asthma Treatment

The goal of asthma treatment is to avoid the substances that trigger symptoms and to control airway inflammation. Most people with asthma take two kinds of medicines.

- ***Controller medicines***, such as inhaled corticosteroids, are long-acting medications taken daily to prevent attacks. These medications help control inflammation and stop the airways from reacting to the factors that trigger the asthma.

- *Quick-relief*, or *rescue*, *medicines*, are taken at the first sign of an attack to dilate the airways and make breathing easier. These medications are known as bronchodilators and are discussed under medications. Corticosteroids may also be given intravenously during a severe attack.

The Nose, Throat, and Larynx

- **Endotracheal intubation** (**en**-doh-**TRAY**-kee-al **in**-too-**BAY**-shun) (ETT) is the passage of a tube through the mouth into the trachea to establish or maintain an open airway, especially when a patient is on a ventilator (**endo-** means within, **trache** means trachea, and **-al** means pertaining to). ***Intubation*** is the insertion of a tube, usually for the passage of air or fluids.
- **Functional endoscopic sinus surgery** (FESS) is a procedure performed using an endoscope in which chronic sinusitis is treated by enlarging the opening between the nose and sinus.
- A **laryngectomy** (**lar**-in-**JECK**-toh-mee) is the surgical removal of the larynx (**laryng** means larynx, and **-ectomy** means surgical removal).
- A **laryngotomy** (**lar**-ing-**OT**-oh-mee) is a surgical incision into the larynx, performed when the upper part of the airway is obstructed (**laryng** means larynx, and **-otomy** means surgical incision).
- **Septoplasty** (**SEP**-toh-**plas**-tee) is the surgical repair or alteration of parts of the nasal septum (**sept/o** means septum, and **-plasty** means surgical repair).

The Trachea

- **Tracheostomy** (**tray**-kee-**OS**-toh-mee) is the surgical creation of a stoma into the trachea to insert a temporary or permanent tube to facilitate breathing (**trache** means trachea, and **-ostomy** means surgically creating an opening). The term *tracheostomy* is used to refer to the surgical procedure and to the stoma itself. As used here, a ***stoma*** means a surgically created opening on a body surface (Figure 7.20).
- An emergency **tracheotomy** (**tray**-kee-**OT**-oh-mee) is a procedure in which an incision is made into the trachea to gain access to the airway below a blockage (**trache** means trachea, and **-otomy** means surgical incision).

The Lungs, Pleura, and Thorax

- A **pneumonectomy** (**new**-moh-**NECK**-toh-mee) is the surgical removal of all or part of a lung (**pneumon** means lung, and **-ectomy** means surgical removal).

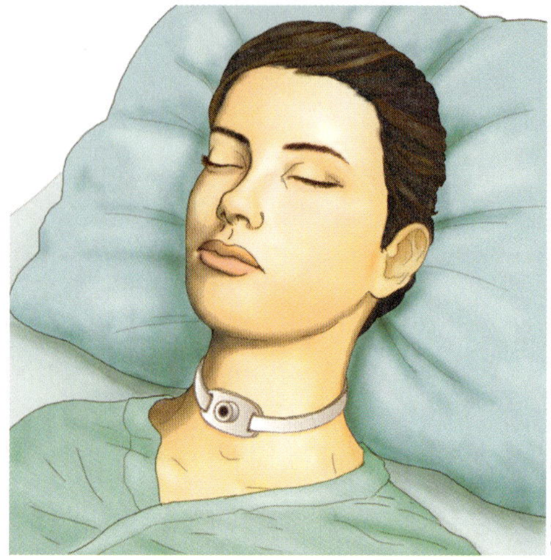

FIGURE 7.20 A tracheostomy tube creates an open airway for a patient unable to maintain his own airway.

- A **lobectomy** (loh-**BECK**-toh-mee) is the surgical removal of a lobe of an organ, usually the lung, brain, or liver (**lob** means lobe, and **-ectomy** means surgical removal).
- **Wedge resection** is a surgery in which a small wedge-shaped piece of cancerous lung tissue is removed, along with a margin of healthy tissue around the cancer.
- **Thoracentesis** (**thoh**-rah-sen-**TEE**-sis) is the surgical puncture of the chest wall with a needle to obtain fluid from the pleural cavity (**thor/a** means thorax or chest, and **-centesis** means surgical puncture to remove fluid). This procedure is performed to remove liquid (pleural effusion) or air (pneumothorax) from the pleural cavity.
- A **thoracotomy** (**thoh**-rah-**KOT**-toh-mee) is a surgical incision into the chest walls to open the pleural cavity for biopsy or treatment (**thorac** means chest, and **-otomy** means surgical incision). A thoracotomy is used to gain access to the lungs, heart, esophagus, diaphragm, and other organs.
- **Video-assisted thoracic surgery** (VATS) is the use of a thoracoscope to view the inside of the pleural cavity through very small incisions. A ***thoracoscope*** is a specialized endoscope used for treating the thorax. This procedure is used to remove small sections of cancerous tissue and to obtain biopsy specimens to diagnose certain types of pneumonia, infections, or tumors of the chest wall. It is also used to treat repeatedly collapsing lungs.

Respiratory Therapy

- **Diaphragmatic breathing**, also known as *abdominal breathing*, is a relaxation technique used to relieve anxiety.
- A **CPAP machine** (continuous positive airway pressure) is a noninvasive ventilation device used in the treatment of sleep apnea. A face mask is connected to a pump that creates constant air pressure in the nasal passages, holding the airway open. Although this does not cure sleep apnea, it does reduce snoring and prevents dangerous apnea disturbances.
- A **BiPAP machine** (bilevel positive airway pressure) is like a CPAP machine; however, it can be set at a higher pressure for inhaling and a lower pressure for exhaling. It is used for sleep apnea in patients with neuromuscular diseases or those who find the CPAP machine uncomfortable.
- An **Ambu bag**, or *bag valve mask*, is an emergency resuscitator used to assist ventilation (Figure 7.21). A flexible air chamber is squeezed to force air through a face mask into the lungs of the patient, a process referred to as "bagging."

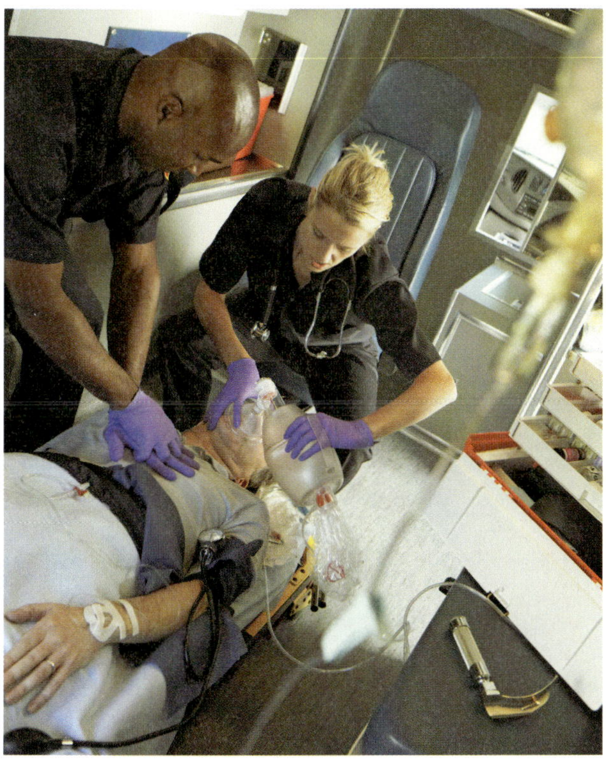

FIGURE 7.21 Emergency medical technicians use an Ambu bag to assist ventilation.

- A **ventilator**, also called a *respirator*, is a mechanical device for artificial respiration that is used to replace or supplement the patient's natural breathing function. The ventilator forces air into the lungs; exhalation takes place passively as the lungs contract.

Supplemental Oxygen Therapy

Supplemental oxygen is administered when the patient is unable to maintain an adequate oxygen saturation level in the blood from breathing normal air. Oxygen is administered by using a compressor either flowing into a hood or tent, or delivered directly to the patient using one of the following devices:

- A *nasal cannula* is a small tube that divides into two nasal prongs (Figure 7.22).
- A *rebreather mask* allows the exhaled breath to be partially reused, delivering up to 60% oxygen.
- A *non-rebreather mask* allows higher levels of oxygen to be added to the air taken in by the patient.

Hyperbaric oxygen therapy (**high**-per-**BARE**-ik) (HBOT) involves breathing pure oxygen in a special chamber that allows air pressure to be raised up to three times higher than normal. The lungs and the bloodstream are thus able to absorb more oxygen, which is delivered throughout the body to promote healing and fight infection.

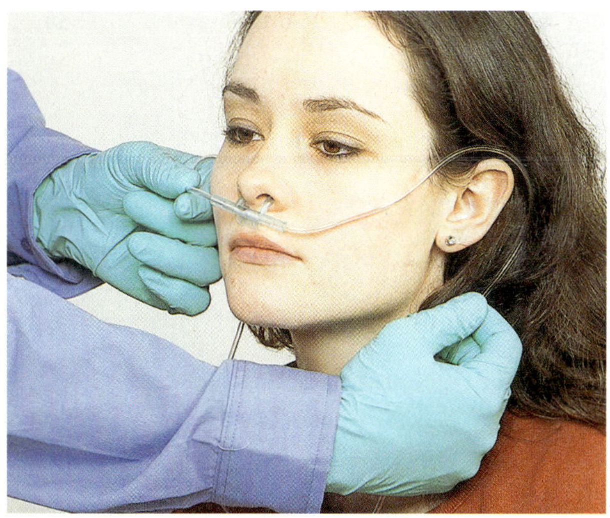

FIGURE 7.22 One method of delivering supplemental oxygen is through a nasal cannula.

ABBREVIATIONS RELATED TO THE RESPIRATORY SYSTEM

Table 7.1 presents an overview of the abbreviations related to the terms introduced in this chapter. Note: To avoid errors or confusion, always be cautious when using abbreviations.

StudyWARE CONNECTION

For more practice and to test your mastery of this material, go to the StudyWARE™ to play interactive games and complete the quiz for this chapter.

Workbook Practice

Go to your workbook, and complete the exercises for this chapter.

DELMAR MOBILE MEDIA

Downloadable audio is available for selected medical terms in this chapter to enhance your learning of medical terminology.

TABLE 7.1
Abbreviations Related to the Respiratory System

acute respiratory distress syndrome = ARDS	**ARDS** = acute respiratory distress syndrome
chronic bronchitis = Br	**Br** = chronic bronchitis
Cheyne-Stokes breathing = CSB	**CSB** = Cheyne-Stokes breathing
chronic obstructive pulmonary disease = COPD	**COPD** = chronic obstructive pulmonary disease
cystic fibrosis = CF	**CF** = cystic fibrosis
endotracheal intubation = ETT	**ETT** = endotracheal intubation
functional endoscopic sinus surgery = FESS	**FESS** = functional endoscopic sinus surgery
hyperbaric oxygen therapy = HBOT	**HBOT** = hyperbaric oxygen therapy
pulmonary function tests = PFT	**PFT** = pulmonary function tests
respiratory failure = RF	**RF** = respiratory failure
sudden infant death syndrome = SIDS	**SIDS** = sudden infant death syndrome
tuberculosis = TB	**TB** = tuberculosis
upper respiratory infection = URI	**URI** = upper respiratory infection

CHAPTER 7

LEARNING EXERCISES

MATCHING WORD PARTS 1

Write the correct answer in the middle column.

	Definition	Correct Answer	Possible Answers
7.1.	nose	____________	nas/o
7.2.	sleep	____________	laryng/o
7.3.	to breathe	____________	pharyng/o
7.4.	throat, pharynx	____________	somn/o
7.5.	larynx, throat	____________	spir/o

MATCHING WORD PARTS 2

Write the correct answer in the middle column.

	Definition	Correct Answer	Possible Answers
7.6.	lung	____________	bronch/o
7.7.	oxygen	____________	ox/o
7.8.	pleura	____________	phon/o
7.9.	bronchus	____________	pleur/o
7.10.	sound or voice	____________	pneum/o

MATCHING WORD PARTS 3

Write the correct answer in the middle column.

	Definition	Correct Answer	Possible Answers
7.11.	windpipe	____________	-pnea
7.12.	sinus	____________	pulmon/o

7.13. lung ______________________ **sinus/o**

7.14. chest ______________________ **-thorax**

7.15. breathing ______________________ **trache/o**

DEFINITIONS

Select the correct answer, and write it on the line provided.

7.16. The heart, aorta, esophagus, and trachea are located in the ______________________.

dorsal cavity manubrium mediastinum pleura

7.17. The ______________________ acts as a lid over the entrance to the laryngopharynx.

Adam's apple epiglottis larynx thyroid cartilage

7.18. The innermost layer of the pleura is known as the ______________________.

parietal pleura pleural space pleural cavity visceral pleura

7.19. The ______________________ sinuses are located just above the eyebrows.

ethmoid frontal maxillary sphenoid

7.20. The smallest divisions of the bronchial tree are the ______________________.

alveoli alveolus bronchioles bronchi

7.21. During respiration, the exchange of oxygen and carbon dioxide takes place through the walls of the ______________________.

alveoli arteries capillaries veins

7.22. The term meaning spitting blood or blood-stained sputum is ______________________.

effusion epistaxis hemoptysis hemothorax

7.23. Black lung disease is the lay term for ______________________.

anthracosis asbestosis pneumoconiosis silicosis

7.24. The term ______________________ means an abnormally rapid rate of respiration.

apnea bradypnea dyspnea tachypnea

7.25. The term meaning any voice impairment is ______________________.

aphonia dysphonia laryngitis laryngospasm

MATCHING STRUCTURES

Write the correct answer in the middle column.

	Definition	Correct Answer	Possible Answers
7.26.	first division of the pharynx	________________	laryngopharynx
7.27.	second division of the pharynx	________________	larynx
7.28.	third division of the pharynx	________________	nasopharynx
7.29.	voice box	________________	oropharynx
7.30.	windpipe	________________	trachea

WHICH WORD?

Select the correct answer, and write it on the line provided.

7.31. The exchange of gases within the cells of the body is known as ________________.

external respiration   internal respiration

7.32. The term that describes the lung disease caused by asbestos particles in the lungs is ________________.

asbestosis   silicosis

7.33. The form of pneumonia that can be prevented through vaccination is ________________.

bacterial pneumonia   viral pneumonia

7.34. The term commonly known as shortness of breath is ________________.

dyspnea   eupnea

7.35. The emergency procedure to gain access below a blocked airway is known as a ________________.

tracheostomy   tracheotomy

SPELLING COUNTS

Find the misspelled word in each sentence. Then write the word, spelled correctly, on the line provided.

7.36. The thick mucus secreted by the tissues that line the respiratory passages is called phlem. ______

7.37. The medical term meaning an accumulation of pus in a body cavity is empiema. ______

7.38. The medical name for the disease commonly known as whooping cough is pertusis. ______

7.39. The frenic nerves stimulate the diaphragm and cause it to contract. ______

7.40. An antitussiff is administered to prevent or relieve coughing. ______

ABBREVIATION IDENTIFICATION

In the space provided, write the words that each abbreviation stands for.

7.41. **ARDS** ______

7.42. **CF** ______

7.43. **FESS** ______

7.44. **SIDS** ______

7.45. **URI** ______

TERM SELECTION

Select the correct answer, and write it on the line provided.

7.46. Inhaling a foreign substance into the upper respiratory tract can cause ______ pneumonia.

aspiration inhalation inspiration respiration

7.47. The term meaning abnormally rapid deep breathing is ______.

dyspnea hyperpnea hypopnea hyperventilation

7.48. The term meaning the surgical creation of a stoma into the trachea to insert a breathing tube is ________________________.

bronchiectasis thoracotomy tracheostomy tracheotomy

7.49. The diaphragm is relaxed during ________________________.

exhalation inhalation internal respiration singultus

7.50. The chronic allergic disorder characterized by episodes of severe breathing difficulty, coughing, and wheezing is known as ________________________.

allergic rhinitis asthma bronchospasm laryngospasm

SENTENCE COMPLETION

Write the correct term on the line provided.

7.51. The term meaning an absence of spontaneous respiration is ________________________.

7.52. The sudden spasmodic closure of the larynx is a/an ________________________.

7.53. The term meaning bleeding from the lungs is ________________________.

7.54. The term meaning pain in the pleura or in the side is ________________________.

7.55. A contraction of the smooth muscle in the walls of the bronchi and bronchioles that tighten and squeeze the airway shut is known as a/an ________________________.

WORD SURGERY

Divide each term into its component word parts. Write these word parts, in sequence, on the lines provided. When necessary, use a slash (/) to indicate a combining vowel. (You may not need all of the lines provided.)

7.56. **Bronchorrhea** means an excessive discharge of mucus from the bronchi.

__________ __________ __________ __________

7.57. The **oropharynx** is visible when looking at the back of the mouth.

__________ __________ __________ __________

7.58. **Polysomnography** measures physiological activity during sleep and is most often performed to detect nocturnal defects in breathing associated with sleep apnea.

__________ __________ __________ __________

7.59. **Pneumorrhagia** is bleeding from the lungs.

__________ __________ __________ __________

7.60. **Rhinorrhea**, also known as a runny nose, is an excessive flow of mucus from the nose.

__________ __________ __________ __________

TRUE/FALSE

If the statement is true, write **True** on the line. If the statement is false, write **False** on the line.

7.61. ________________ A pulse oximeter is a monitor placed inside the ear to measure the oxygen saturation level in the blood.

7.62. ________________ In atelectasis, the lung fails to expand because there is a blockage of the air passages or pneumothorax.

7.63. ________________ Croup is an allergic reaction to airborne allergens.

7.64. ________________ Hypoxemia is the condition of below-normal oxygenation of arterial blood.

7.65. ________________ Emphysema is the progressive loss of lung function in which the chest sometimes assumes an enlarged barrel shape.

CLINICAL CONDITIONS

Write the correct answer on the line provided.

7.66. Baby Jamison was born with ________________ ________________. This is a genetic disorder in which the lungs are clogged with large quantities of abnormally thick mucus.

7.67. Dr. Lee surgically removed a portion of the lung. This procedure is known as a/an ________________.

7.68. Wendy Barlow required the surgical removal of her larynx. This procedure is known as a/an ________________.

7.69. During his asthma attacks, Jamaal Nelson uses an inhaler containing a ________________. This medication expands the opening of the passages into his lungs.

7.70. Each year, Mr. Partin receives a flu shot to prevent ________________.

7.71. When hit during a fight, Marvin Roper's nose started to bleed. The medical term for this condition is ________________.

7.72. The doctor's examination revealed that Juanita Martinez has an accumulation of blood in the pleural cavity. This diagnosis is recorded on her chart as a/an ________________.

7.73. Duncan McClanahan had a/an ________________ performed to correct damage to the septum of his nose.

7.74. Suzanne Holderman is suffering from an inflammation of the bronchial walls. The medical term for Suzanne's condition is chronic ________________.

7.75. Ted Coleman required the permanent placement of a breathing tube. The procedure for the placement of this tube is called a/an ________________.

WHICH IS THE CORRECT MEDICAL TERM?

Select the correct answer, and write it on the line provided.

7.76. An inflammation of the pleura that causes pleurodynia is known as ________________.

atelectasis emphysema pleurodynia pleurisy

7.77. The substance ejected through the mouth and used for diagnostic purposes in respiratory disorders is known as ________________.

phlegm pleural effusion saliva sputum

7.78. The term meaning a bluish discoloration of the skin caused by a lack of adequate oxygen is ________________.

asphyxia cyanosis epistaxis hypoxia

7.79. The medical term meaning sudden spasmodic closure of the larynx is ________________.

aphonia dysphonia laryngitis laryngospasm

7.80. The pattern of alternating periods of rapid breathing, slow breathing, and the absence of breathing is known as ________________.

anoxia Cheyne-Stokes respiration eupnea tachypnea

CHALLENGE WORD BUILDING

These terms are *not* found in this chapter; however, they are made up of the following familiar word parts. If you need help in creating the term, refer to your medical dictionary.

bronch/o	**-itis**
epiglott/o	**-ologist**
laryng/o	**-plasty**
pharyng/o	**-plegia**
pneumon/o	**-rrhagia**
trache/o	**-rrhea**
	-scopy
	-stenosis

7.81. An abnormal discharge from the pharynx is known as ____________________.

7.82. Inflammation of the lungs is known as ____________________.

7.83. A specialist in the study of the larynx is a/an ____________________.

7.84. Bleeding from the larynx is known as ____________________.

7.85. Inflammation of both the pharynx and the larynx is known as ____________________.

7.86. Abnormal narrowing of the lumen of the trachea is known as ____________________.

7.87. The surgical repair of a bronchial defect is a/an ____________________.

7.88. Inflammation of the epiglottis is known as ____________________.

7.89. The inspection of both the trachea and bronchi through a bronchoscope is a/an ____________________.

7.90. Paralysis of the walls of the bronchi is known as ____________________.

LABELING EXERCISES

Identify the parts of numbered items on the accompanying figure.

7.91. ______________________

7.92. ______________________

7.93. ______________________

7.94. ______________________

7.95. ______________________

7.96. ______________________ cavity

7.97. ______________________

7.98. ______________________

7.99. ______________________ lung

7.100. ______________________ sacs

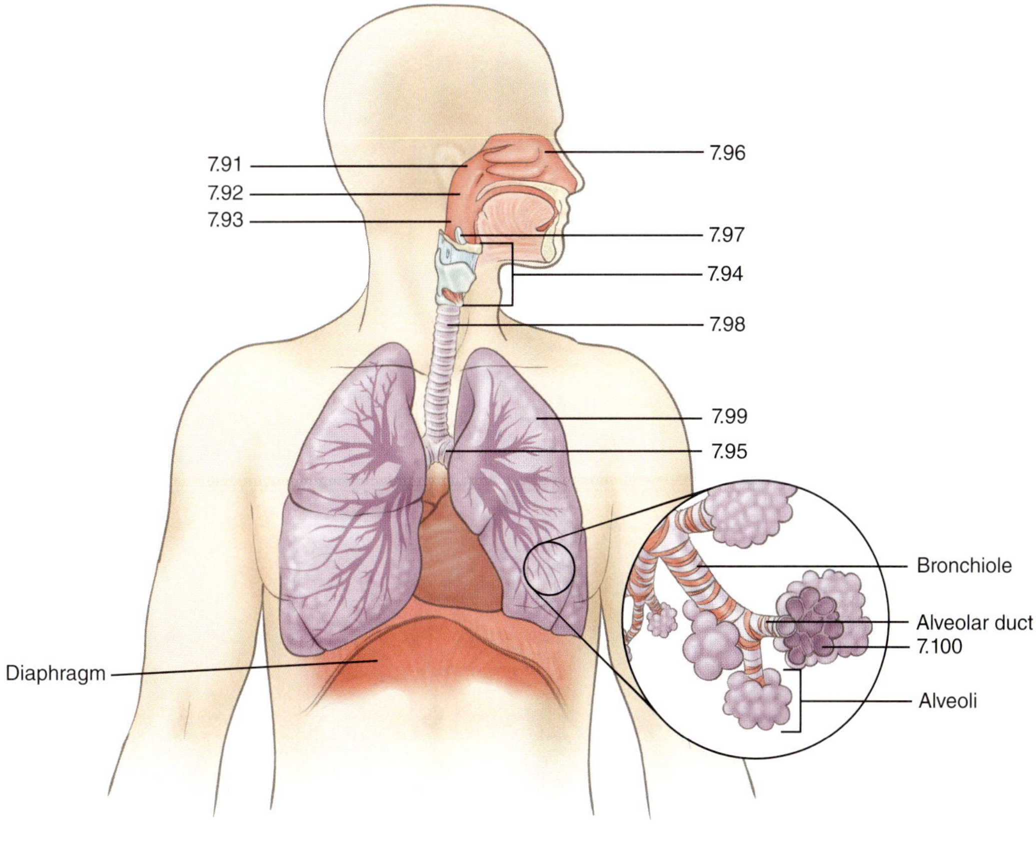

CHAPTER 8

The Digestive System

Overview of STRUCTURES, COMBINING FORMS, AND FUNCTIONS OF THE DIGESTIVE SYSTEM

Major Structures	Related Combining Forms	Primary Functions
Mouth	**or/o**, **stomat/o**	Begins preparation of food for digestion.
Pharynx	**pharyng/o**	Transports food from the mouth to the esophagus.
Esophagus	**esophag/o**	Transports food from the pharynx to the stomach.
Stomach	**gastr/o**	Breaks down food and mixes it with gastric juices.
Small Intestine	**enter/o**	Mixes chyme coming from the stomach with digestive juices to complete the digestion and absorption of most nutrients.
Large Intestine	**col/o**, **colon/o**	Absorbs excess water, and prepares solid waste for elimination.
Rectum and Anus	**an/o**, **proct/o**, **rect/o**	Control the excretion of solid waste.
Liver	**hepat/o**	Secretes bile and enzymes to aid in the digestion of fats.
Gallbladder	**cholecyst/o**	Stores bile, and releases it into the small intestine as needed.
Pancreas	**pancreat/o**	Secretes digestive juices and enzymes into the small intestine as needed.

Vocabulary Related to **THE DIGESTIVE SYSTEM**

This list contains essential word parts and medical terms for this chapter. These terms are pronounced in the student StudyWARE™ and Audio CDs that are available for use with this text. These and the other important **primary terms** are shown in boldface throughout the chapter. *Secondary terms*, which appear in *orange* italics, clarify the meaning of primary terms.

Word Parts

- ☐ **an/o** anus, ring
- ☐ **chol/e** bile, gall
- ☐ **cholecyst/o** gallbladder
- ☐ **col/o**, **colon/o** colon, large intestine
- ☐ **-emesis** vomiting
- ☐ **enter/o** small intestine
- ☐ **esophag/o** esophagus
- ☐ **gastr/o** stomach, belly
- ☐ **hepat/o** liver
- ☐ **-lithiasis** presence of stones
- ☐ **-pepsia** digest, digestion
- ☐ **-phagia** eating, swallowing
- ☐ **proct/o** anus and rectum
- ☐ **rect/o** rectum, straight
- ☐ **sigmoid/o** sigmoid colon

Medical Terms

- ☐ **aerophagia** (**ay**-er-oh-**FAY**-jee-ah)
- ☐ **anastomosis** (ah-**nas**-toh-**MOH**-sis)
- ☐ **anorexia nervosa** (**an**-oh-**RECK**-see-ah ner-**VOH**-sah)
- ☐ **antiemetic** (**an**-tih-ee-**MET**-ick)
- ☐ **aphthous ulcers** (**AF**-thus **UL**-serz)
- ☐ **ascites** (ah-**SIGH**-teez)
- ☐ **bariatrics** (**bayr**-ee-**AT**-ricks)
- ☐ **borborygmus** (**bor**-boh-**RIG**-mus)
- ☐ **bulimia nervosa** (byou-**LIM**-ee-ah ner-**VOH**-sah)
- ☐ **cachexia** (kah-**KEKS**-eeh-ah)
- ☐ **celiac disease** (**SEE**-lee-ak)
- ☐ **cheilosis** (kee-**LOH**-sis)
- ☐ **cholangiography** (koh-**LAN**-jee-**og**-rah-fee)
- ☐ **cholangitis** (**koh**-lan-**JIGH**-tis)
- ☐ **cholecystectomy** (**koh**-luh-sis-**TECK**-toh-mee)
- ☐ **cholecystitis** (**koh**-luh-sis-**TYE**-tis)
- ☐ **choledocholithotomy** (koh-**led**-oh-koh-lih-**THOT**-oh-mee)
- ☐ **cholelithiasis** (**koh**-luh-lih-**THIGH**-ah-sis)
- ☐ **cirrhosis** (sih-**ROH**-sis)
- ☐ **colonoscopy** (**koh**-lun-**OSS**-koh-pee)
- ☐ **colostomy** (koh-**LAHS**-toh-mee)
- ☐ **Crohn's disease**
- ☐ **diverticulitis** (**dye**-ver-tick-you-**LYE**-tis)
- ☐ **diverticulosis** (**dye**-ver-tick-you-**LOH**-sis)
- ☐ **dyspepsia** (dis-**PEP**-see-ah)
- ☐ **dysphagia** (dis-**FAY**-jee-ah)
- ☐ **enteritis** (**en**-ter-**EYE**-tis)
- ☐ **eructation** (eh-ruk-**TAY**-shun)
- ☐ **esophageal varices** (eh-**sof**-ah-**JEE**-al **VAYR**-ih-seez)
- ☐ **esophagogastroduodenoscopy** (eh-**sof**-ah-goh-**gas**-troh-**dew**-oh-deh-**NOS**-koh-pee)
- ☐ **gastroduodenostomy** (**gas**-troh-**dew**-oh-deh-**NOS**-toh-mee)
- ☐ **gastroesophageal reflux disease** (gas-troh-eh-**sof**-ah-**JEE**-al **REE**-flucks)
- ☐ **gastrostomy tube** (gas-**TROS**-toh-mee)
- ☐ **hematemesis** (**hee**-mah-**TEM**-eh-sis)
- ☐ **Hemoccult test** (**HEE**-moh-kult)
- ☐ **hepatitis** (**hep**-ah-**TYE**-tis)
- ☐ **herpes labialis** (**HER**-peez **lay**-bee-**AL**-iss)
- ☐ **hiatal hernia** (high-**AY**-tal **HER**-nee-ah)
- ☐ **hyperemesis** (**high**-per-**EM**-eh-sis)
- ☐ **ileus** (**ILL**-ee-us)
- ☐ **inguinal hernia** (**ING**-gwih-nal **HER**-nee-ah)
- ☐ **jaundice** (**JAWN**-dis)
- ☐ **leukoplakia** (**loo**-koh-**PLAY**-kee-ah)
- ☐ **melena** (meh-**LEE**-nah)
- ☐ **morbid obesity** (**MOR**-bid oh-**BEE**-sih-tee)
- ☐ **nasogastric intubation** (**nay**-zoh-**GAS**-trick **in**-too-**BAY**-shun)
- ☐ **obesity** (oh-**BEE**-sih-tee)
- ☐ **palatoplasty** (**PAL**-ah-toh-**plas**-tee)
- ☐ **peptic ulcers** (**UL**-serz)
- ☐ **peristalsis** (**pehr**-ih-**STAL**-sis)
- ☐ **polyp** (**POL**-up)
- ☐ **proctologist** (prock-**TOL**-oh-jist)
- ☐ **regurgitation** (ree-**gur**-jih-**TAY**-shun)
- ☐ **salmonellosis** (**sal**-moh-nel-**LOH**-sis)
- ☐ **sigmoidoscopy** (**sig**-moi-**DOS**-koh-pee)
- ☐ **stomatitis** (**stoh**-mah-**TYE**-tis)
- ☐ **trismus** (**TRIZ**-mus)
- ☐ **ulcerative colitis** (**UL**-ser-**ay**-tiv koh-**LYE**-tis)
- ☐ **volvulus** (**VOL**-view-lus)
- ☐ **xerostomia** (**zeer**-oh-**STOH**-mee-ah)

LEARNING GOALS

On completion of this chapter, you should be able to:

1. Identify and describe the major structures and functions of the digestive system.
2. Describe the processes of digestion, absorption, and metabolism.
3. Recognize, define, spell, and pronounce the primary terms related to the pathology and the diagnostic and treatment procedures of the digestive system.

STRUCTURES OF THE DIGESTIVE SYSTEM

The digestive system consists primarily of the **gastrointestinal tract** (**gas**-troh-in-**TESS**-tih-nal), which is also known as the ***GI tract*** (**gastr/o** means stomach, **intestin** means intestine, and **-al** means pertaining to). These organs work in cooperation with ***accessory organs*** (Figure 8.1).

- The ***upper GI tract*** consists of the mouth, pharynx (throat), esophagus, and stomach. This transports food from the entry into the body until digestion begins in the stomach.
- The ***lower GI tract***, which is sometimes referred to as the ***bowels***, is made up of the small and large intestines plus the rectum and anus. Here digestion is completed, and waste material is prepared for expulsion from the body.
- The accessory organs of the digestive system include the liver, gallbladder, and pancreas.

The Oral Cavity

The major structures of the **oral cavity**, also known as the ***mouth***, are the lips, hard and soft palates, salivary glands, tongue, teeth, and the periodontium (Figure 8.2).

The Lips

The **lips**, which are also known as the ***labia***, surround the opening to the oral cavity (singular, *labium*). The term *labia* is also used to describe parts of the female genitalia (see Chapter 14).

- During eating, the lips, tongue, and cheeks hold the food in the mouth.
- The lips also have important roles in breathing, speaking, and the expression of emotions.

The Palate

The **palate** (**PAL**-at), which forms the roof of the mouth, consists of three major parts (Figure 8.2).

- The **hard palate** is the anterior portion of the palate. This area is covered with specialized mucous membrane. ***Rugae*** are irregular ridges or folds in this mucous membrane (singular, *ruga*).
- The **soft palate** is the flexible posterior portion of the palate. During swallowing, it has the important role of closing off the nasal passage to prevent food and liquid from moving upward into the nasal cavity.
- The **uvula** (**YOU**-view-lah) is the third part, and it hangs from the free edge of the soft palate. During swallowing, it moves upward with the soft palate. It also plays an important role in snoring and in the formation of some speech sounds.

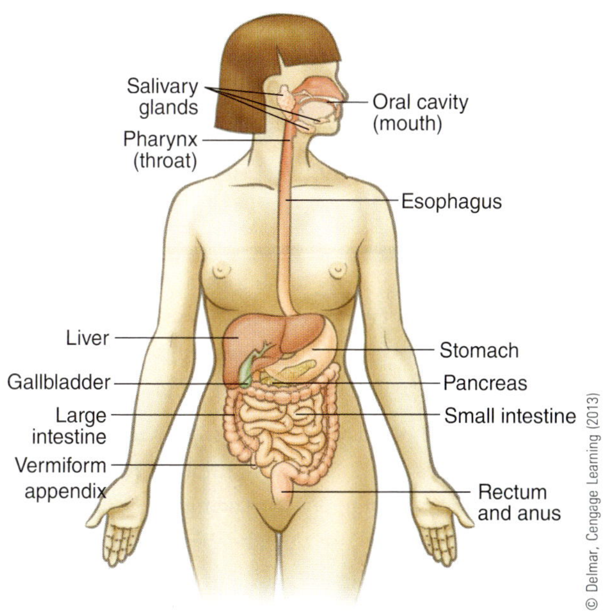

FIGURE 8.1 Major structures and accessory organs of the digestive system.

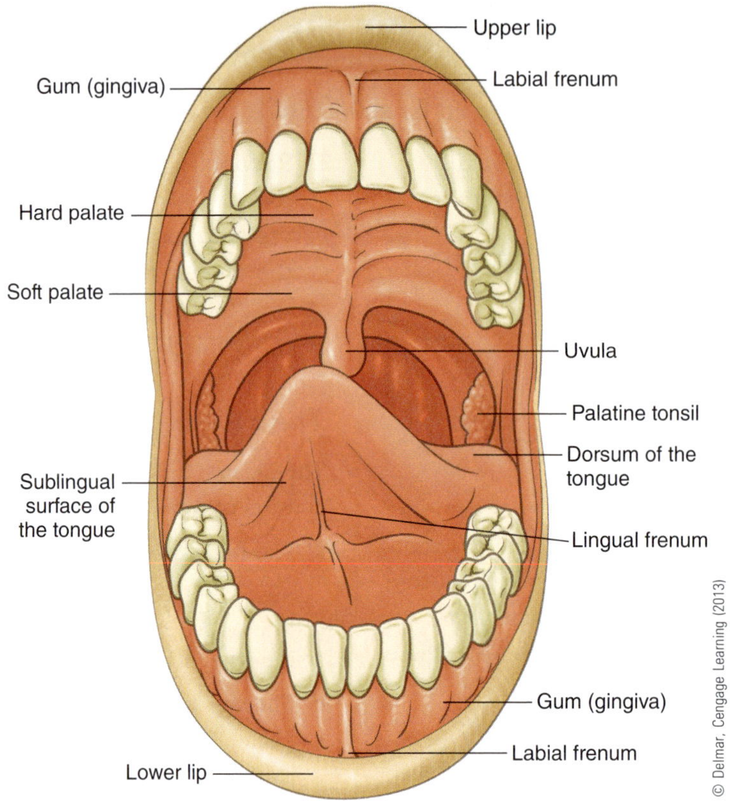

FIGURE 8.2 Structures of the tongue and oral cavity.

The Tongue

The **tongue** is very strong, flexible, and muscular. The posterior portion of the tongue is attached. The anterior end of the tongue moves freely and is flexible. It is the structure of the tongue that makes it so important for chewing, speaking, and swallowing (Figure 8.2).

- The upper surface of the tongue is the ***dorsum***. This surface has a tough protective covering and in some areas, small bumps known as **papillae** (pah-**PILL**-ee) (singular, *papilla*). These papillae contain ***taste buds***, which are the sensory receptors for the sense of taste.
- The ***sublingual surface*** of the tongue and the tissues that lie under the tongue are covered with delicate highly vascular tissues. ***Sublingual*** means under the tongue. ***Highly vascular*** means containing many blood vessels.
- The presence of this rich blood supply under the tongue makes it suitable for administering certain medications sublingually by placing them under the tongue, where they are quickly absorbed into the bloodstream.
- The ***lingual frenum*** is a band of tissue that attaches the tongue to the floor of the mouth. This frenum limits the motion of the tongue.

Soft Tissues of the Oral Cavity

- The term **periodontium** (**pehr**-ee-oh-**DON**-shee-um) describes the structures that surround, support, and are attached to the teeth (**peri-** means surrounding, **odonti** means the teeth, and **-um** is the noun ending). This consists of the bone of the dental arches and the soft tissues that surround and support the teeth.
- The **gingiva** (**JIN**-jih-vah), also known as ***masticatory mucosa*** or the ***gums***, is the specialized mucous membrane that covers the bone of the dental arches and surrounds the neck of the teeth (plural *gingivae*).

The Dental Arches

The **dental arches** are the bony structures of the oral cavity (Figure 8.3 A & B). These arches hold the teeth firmly in position to facilitate chewing and speaking.

- The ***maxillary arch*** is commonly known as the upper jaw and consists of bones of the lower surface of the skull. This arch does not move.
- The ***mandibular arch***, commonly know as the lower jaw, is a separate bone and is the only movable component part of the joint.

- The **temporomandibular joint** (**tem**-poh-roh-man-**DIB**-you-lar), commonly known as the *TMJ*, is formed at the back of the mouth where the maxillary and mandibular arches come together.

The Teeth

The term **dentition** (den-**TISH**-un) refers to the natural teeth arranged in the upper and lower jaws. Human dentition consists of four types of teeth (Figure 8.3). These are the:

- *Incisors* and *canines* (also known as *cuspids*). These teeth are used for biting and tearing.
- *Premolars*, which are also known as *bicuspids*, and *molars*. These teeth are used for chewing and grinding.

Primary and Permanent Dentition

- The primary dentition is also known as the *deciduous dentition*, or *baby teeth*. These 20 teeth erupt during early childhood, are normally lost in late childhood, and are replaced by the permanent teeth. The primary dentition consists of 8 incisors, 4 canines, and 8 molars, but no premolars.
- The permanent dentition consists of 32 teeth designed to last a lifetime. Of these teeth, 20 replace primary teeth and 12 erupt at the back of the mouth. The permanent dentition includes 8 incisors, 4 canines, 8 premolars, and 12 molars.
- The term **occlusion**, as used in dentistry, describes any contact between the chewing surfaces of the upper and lower teeth.

Structures and Tissues of the Teeth

The *crown* is the portion of a tooth that is visible in the mouth. It is covered with *enamel*, which is the hardest substance in the body (Figure 8.4).

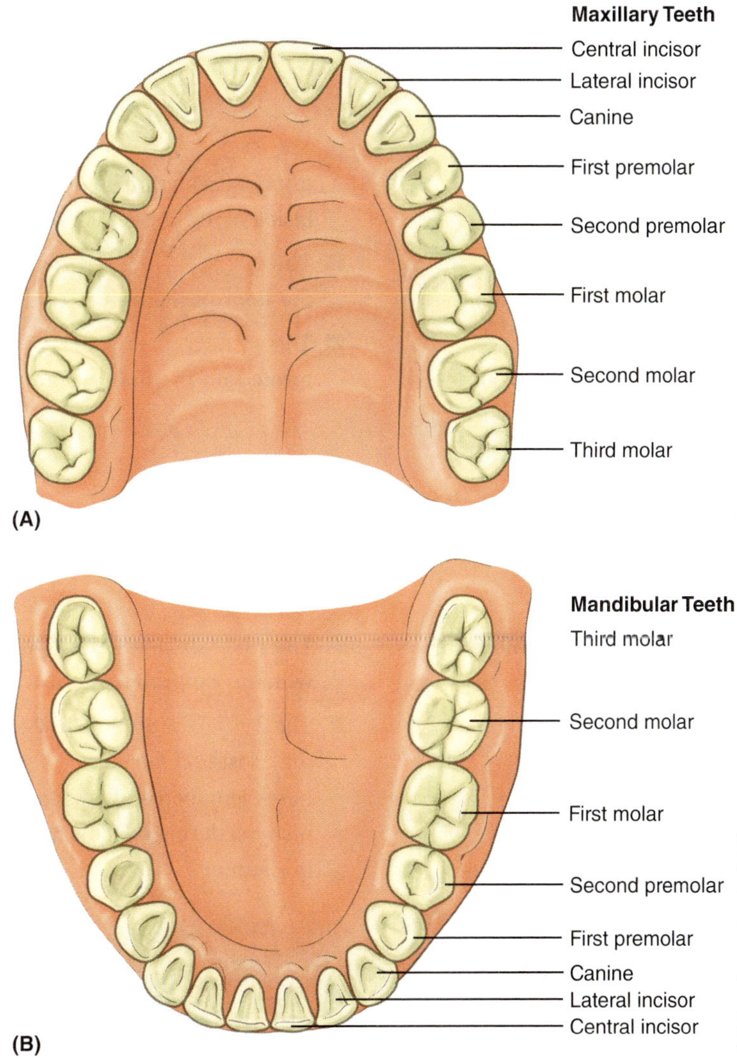

FIGURE 8.3 Four types of teeth make up adult dentition. (A) Maxillary arch. (B) Mandibular arch.

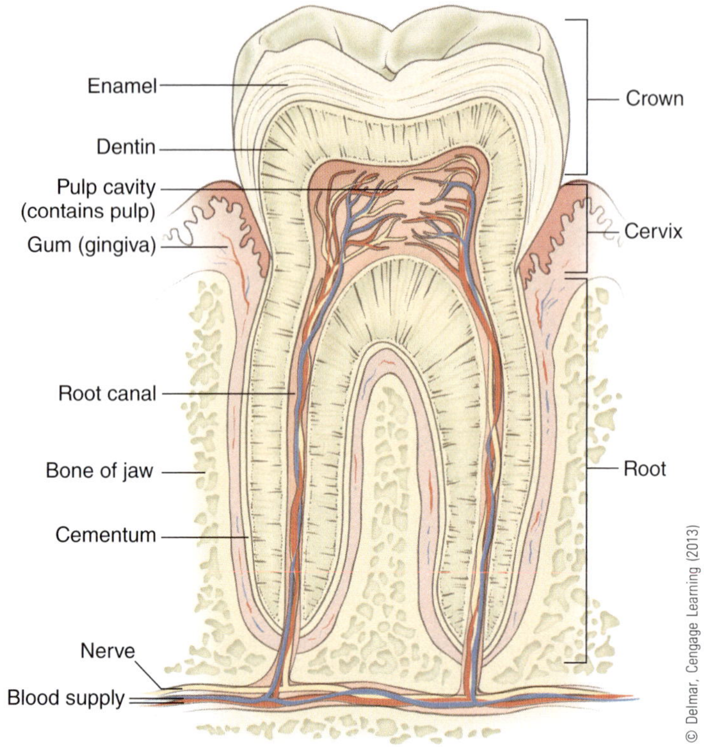

FIGURE 8.4 Structures and tissues of the tooth.

- The *roots* of the tooth hold it securely in place within the dental arch. The roots are protected by *cementum*. This substance is hard, but it is not as strong as enamel.
- The *cervix*, also known as the neck of the tooth, is where the crown and root meet.
- *Dentin* makes up the bulk of the tooth. The portion that is above the gum line is covered with enamel. The root area is covered with cementum.
- The *pulp cavity* is the area within the crown and roots of the tooth that is surrounded by the dentin to protect the delicate pulp of the tooth. In the roots, the pulp continues in the space known as the *root canals*.
- The *pulp* itself consists of a rich supply of blood vessels and nerves that provide nutrients and innervation to the tooth.

Saliva and Salivary Glands

Saliva is a colorless liquid that maintains the moisture in the mouth. It helps maintain the health of the teeth, and it begins the digestive process by lubricating food during chewing and swallowing.

The three pairs of **salivary glands** (**SAL**-ih-ver-ee) secrete saliva that is carried by ducts into the mouth (Figure 8.5).

- The *parotid glands* are located on the face, slightly in front of each ear. The ducts for these glands are on the inside of the cheek near the upper molars.
- The *sublingual glands* and their ducts are located on the floor of the mouth under the tongue.
- The *submandibular glands* and their ducts are located on the floor of the mouth near the mandible.

The Pharynx

The **pharynx** (**FAR**-inks), which is the common passageway for both respiration and digestion, is discussed in Chapter 7.

- The pharynx plays an important role in *deglutition*, which is commonly known as swallowing.
- The *epiglottis* (**ep**-ih-**GLOT**-is) is a lid-like structure that closes off the entrance to the trachea (windpipe) to prevent food and liquids from moving from the pharynx during swallowing. This is discussed further in Chapter 7.

StudyWARE CONNECTION

Watch the **Swallowing Safeguards** animation in the StudyWARE™.

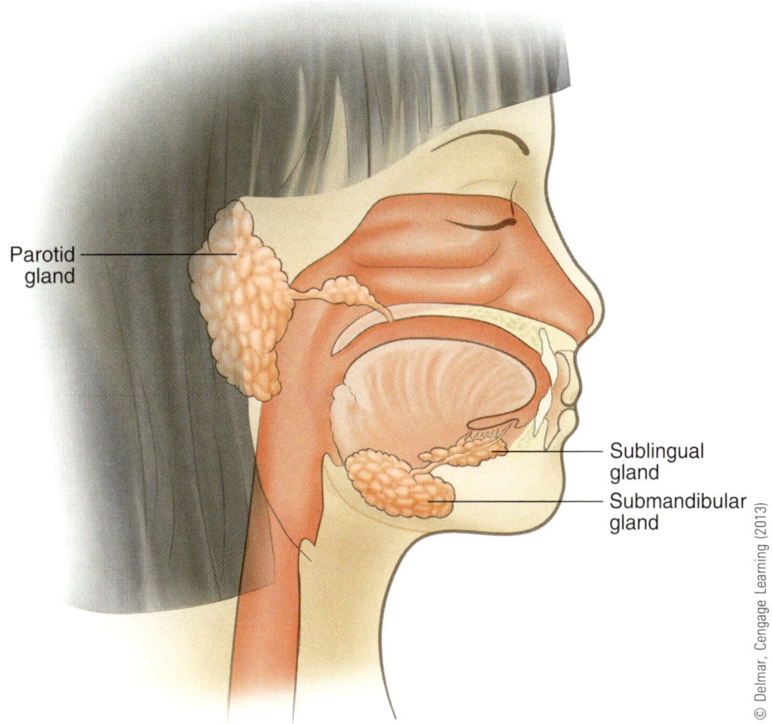

FIGURE 8.5 The salivary glands.

The Esophagus

The **esophagus** (eh-**SOF**-ah-gus) is the muscular tube through which ingested food passes from the pharynx to the stomach (Figure 8.1).

- The **lower esophageal sphincter**, also known as the *cardiac sphincter*, is a muscular ring between the esophagus and stomach. During swallowing, it relaxes to allow food to enter the stomach (Figure 8.6).
- This sphincter normally opens to allow the flow of food into the stomach and closes to prevent the stomach contents from regurgitating into the esophagus. *Regurgitating* means to flow backward.

The Stomach

The **stomach** is a sac-like organ composed of the *fundus* (upper, rounded part), *body* (main portion), and *antrum* (lower part) (Figure 8.6).

- **Rugae** (**ROO**-gay) are the folds in the mucosa lining of the stomach. These folds allow flexibility of the stomach increasing and decreasing in size. Glands located within these folds produce gastric juices.
- **Gastric juices** aid in the beginning of food digestion. Mucus produced by glands in the stomach create a protective coating on the lining of the stomach.
- The **pyloric sphincter** (pye-**LOR**-ick) is the ring-like muscle at the base of the stomach that controls the flow of partially digested food from the stomach to the duodenum of the small intestine.
- The **pylorus** (pye-**LOR**-us) is the narrow passage that connects the stomach with the small intestine.

The Small Intestine

The **small intestine** extends from the pyloric sphincter to the first part of the large intestine. This coiled organ is up to 20 feet in length and consists of three sections where food is digested and the nutrients are absorbed into the bloodstream (see Figure 8.1).

1. The **duodenum** (**dew**-oh-**DEE**-num) is the first portion of the small intestine. The duodenum extends from the pylorus of the stomach to the jejunum.
2. The **jejunum** (jeh-**JOO**-num), which is the middle portion of the small intestine, extends from the duodenum to the ileum.
3. The **ileum** (**ILL**-ee-um), which is the last and longest portion of the small intestine, extends from the jejunum to the cecum of the large intestine.

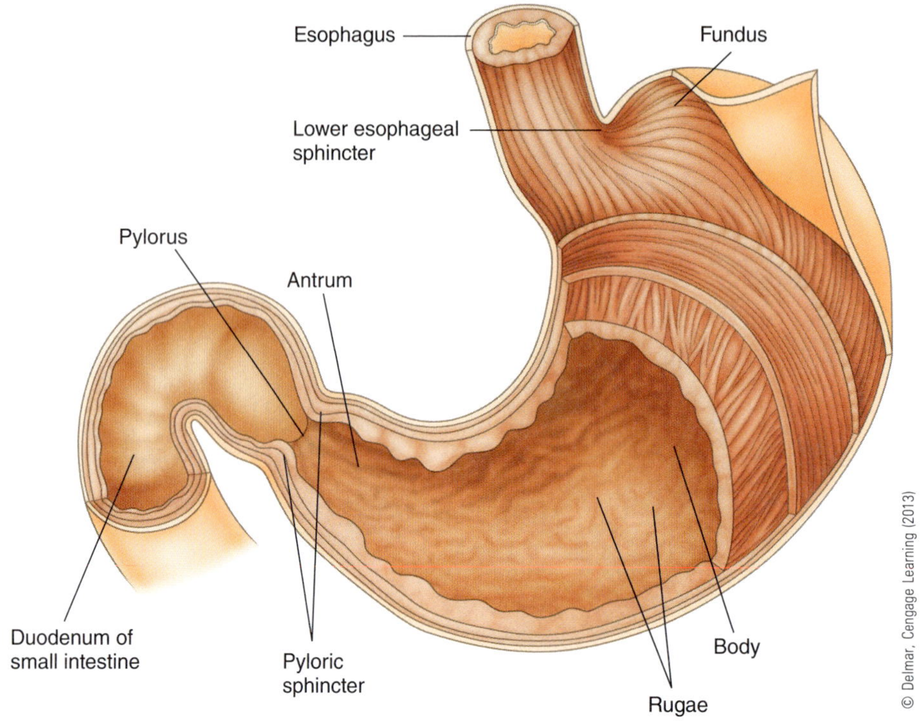

FIGURE 8.6 Structures of the stomach.

The Large Intestine

The **large intestine** extends from the end of the small intestine to the anus. It is about twice as wide as the small intestine; however, it is only one-fourth as long. It is here that the waste products of digestion are processed in preparation for excretion through the anus. The major parts of the large intestine are the cecum, colon, rectum, and anus (Figure 8.7).

The Cecum

The **cecum** (**SEE**-kum) is a pouch that lies on the right side of the abdomen. It extends from the end of the ileum to the beginning of the colon.

- The **ileocecal sphincter** (**ill**-ee-oh-**SEE**-kull) is the ring-like muscle that controls the flow from the ileum of the small intestine into the cecum of the large intestine (Figure 8.7).
- The **vermiform appendix**, commonly called the ***appendix***, hangs from the lower portion of the cecum. The term ***vermiform*** refers to a worm-like shape. The appendix, which consists of lymphoid tissue, is discussed in Chapter 6.

The Colon

The **colon**, which is the longest portion of the large intestine, is subdivided into four parts (Figure 8.7):

- The **ascending colon** travels upward from the cecum to the undersurface of the liver. ***Ascending*** means upward.
- The **transverse colon** passes horizontally across the abdominal cavity from right to left toward the spleen. ***Transverse*** means across.
- The **descending colon** travels down the left side of the abdominal cavity to the sigmoid colon. ***Descending*** means downward.
- The **sigmoid colon** (**SIG**-moid) is an S-shaped structure that continues from the descending colon above and joins the rectum below. ***Sigmoid*** means curved like the letter *S*.

The Rectum and Anus

- The **rectum** is the widest division of the large intestine. It makes up the last 4 inches of the large intestine and ends at the anus.
- The **anus** is the lower opening of the digestive tract. The flow of waste through the anus is controlled by the ***internal anal sphincter*** and the ***external anal sphincter***.
- The term **anorectal** (**ah**-noh-**RECK**-tal) refers to the anus and rectum as a single unit (**an/o** means anus, **rect** means rectum, and **-al** means pertaining to).

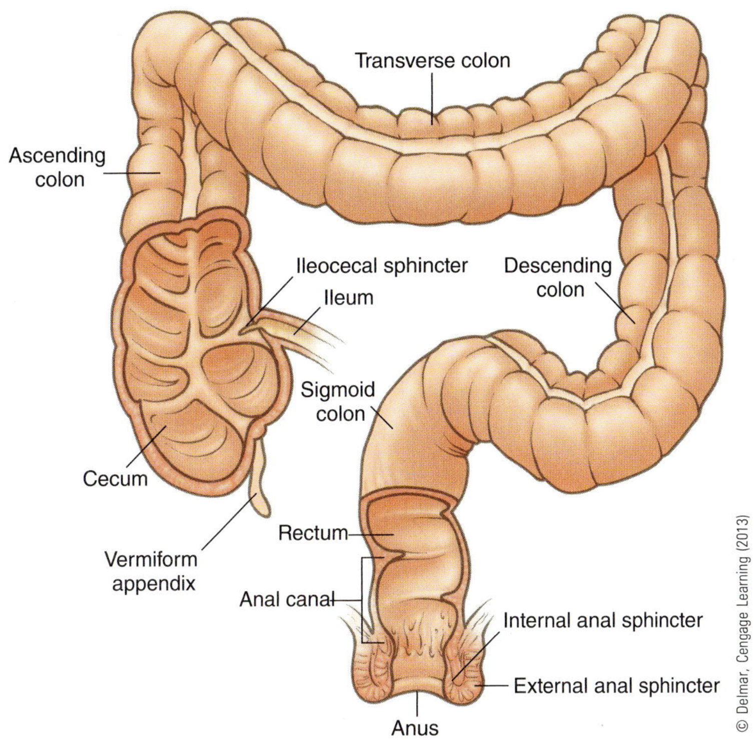

FIGURE 8.7 Structures of the large intestine.

Accessory Digestive Organs

The **accessory organs** of the digestive system are so named because they play a key role in the digestive process, but are not part of the gastrointestinal tract (Figure 8.8). The accessory digestive organs are the liver, gallbladder, and pancreas.

The Liver

The **liver** is the largest organ in the body (Figure 8.8). It has several important functions related to removing toxins from the blood and turning food into the fuel and nutrients the body needs. The term **hepatic** means pertaining to the liver (**hepat** means liver, and **-ic** means pertaining to).

- The liver removes excess ***glucose***, which is commonly known as blood sugar, from the bloodstream and stores it as glycogen. ***Glycogen*** is a form of starch that is stored in the liver. When the blood sugar level is low, the liver converts glycogen back into glucose and releases it for use by the body. Glucose and glycogen are discussed further in Chapter 13.
- **Bilirubin** (bill-ih-**ROO**-bin) is a yellow to green fluid, commonly known as bile, that is manufactured by the liver and is necessary for the digestion of fat. Excessive amounts of bilirubin in the body can lead to jaundice and other diseases.
- **Bile**, which aids in the digestion of fats, is a digestive juice secreted by the liver. Bile travels from the liver to the gallbladder, where it is concentrated and stored.

The Biliary Tree

The **biliary tree** (**BILL**-ee-air-ee) provides the channels through which bile is transported from the liver to the small intestine. ***Biliary*** means pertaining to bile.

- Small ducts in the liver join together like branches to form the biliary tree. The trunk, which is just outside the liver, is known as the ***common hepatic duct***.
- The bile travels from the liver through the common hepatic duct to the gallbladder where it enters and exits through the narrow ***cystic duct***.
- The cystic duct leaving the gallbladder rejoins the common hepatic duct to form the ***common bile duct***. The common bile duct joins the ***pancreatic duct***, and together they enter the duodenum of the small intestine.

The Gallbladder

The **gallbladder** is a pear-shaped organ about the size of an egg located under the liver. It stores and concentrates bile for later use (Figures 8.8 and 8.9).

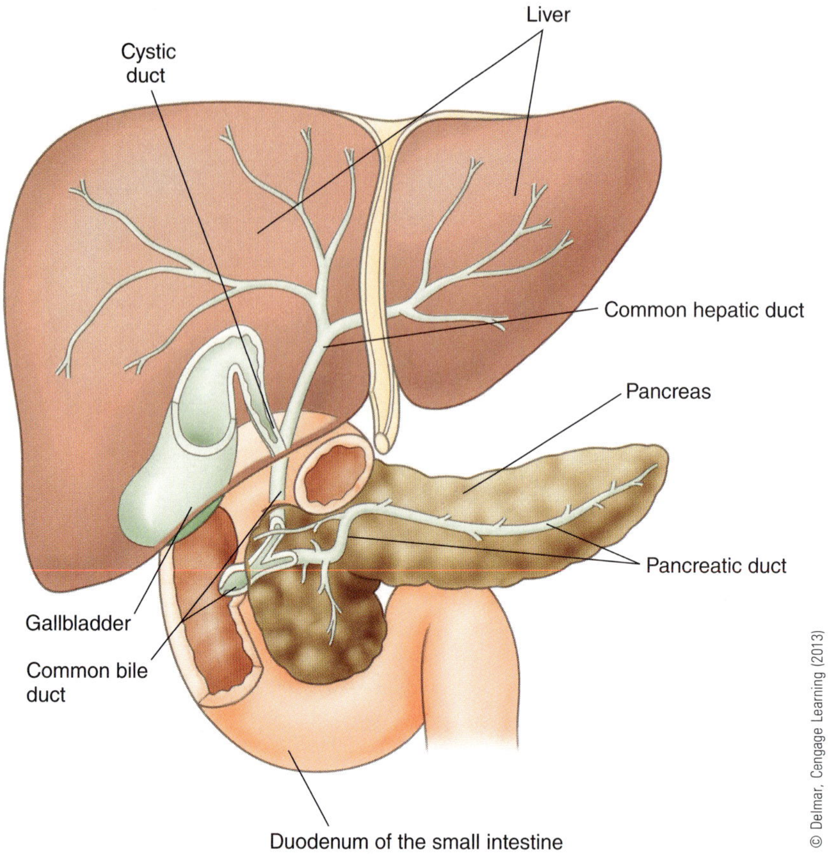

FIGURE 8.8 Accessory digestive organs: the liver, gallbladder, and pancreas.

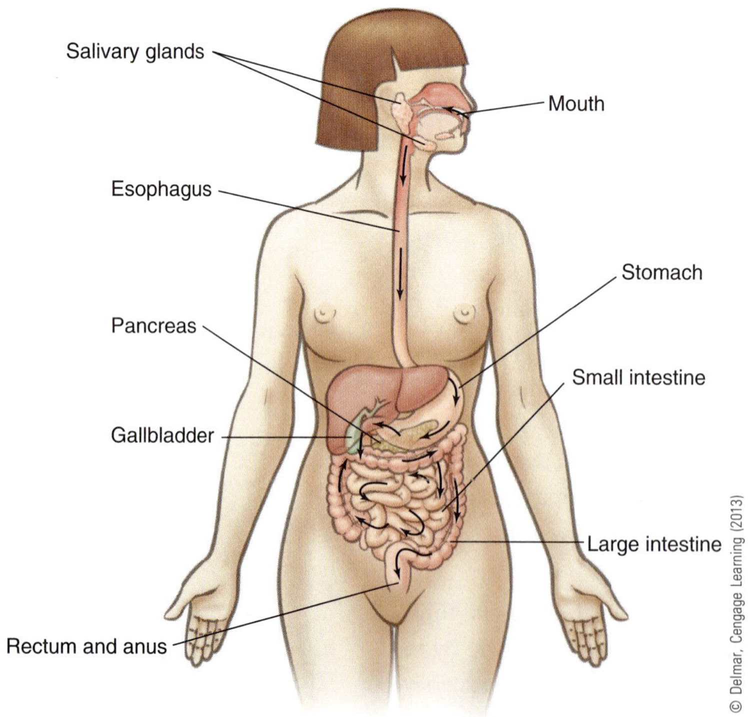

FIGURE 8.9 The pathway of food through the digestive system.

- When bile is needed, the gallbladder contracts, forcing the bile out through the biliary tree.
- The term **cholecystic** (**koh**-luh-**SIS**-tick) means pertaining to the gallbladder (**cholecyst** means gallbladder, and **-ic** means pertaining to).

The Pancreas

The **pancreas** (**PAN**-kree-as) is a soft, 6-inch long oblong gland that is located behind the stomach (Figures 8.8 and 8.9). This gland has important roles in both the digestive and endocrine systems. The digestive functions are discussed here. The endocrine functions, plus the pathology and procedures related to the pancreas, are discussed in Chapter 13.

- The pancreas produces and secretes *pancreatic juices* that aid in digestion and contain digestive enzymes and sodium bicarbonate to help neutralize stomach acids. *Pancreatic* means pertaining to the pancreas.
- The pancreatic juices leave the pancreas through the *pancreatic duct* that joins the *common bile duct* just before the entrance into the duodenum.

DIGESTION

Digestion is the process by which complex foods are broken down into nutrients in a form the body can use. The flow of food through the digestive system is shown in Figure 8.9.

- *Digestive enzymes* are responsible for the chemical changes that break foods down into simpler forms of nutrients for use by the body.
- A *nutrient* is a substance, usually from food, that is necessary for normal functioning of the body. The primary nutrients are *carbohydrates*, *fats*, and *proteins*. *Vitamins* and *minerals* are essential nutrients, which are required only in small amounts.

Metabolism

The term **metabolism** (meh-**TAB**-oh-lizm) includes all of the processes involved in the body's use of nutrients (**metabol** means change, and **-ism** means condition). It consists of two parts: anabolism and catabolism.

- **Anabolism** (an-**NAB**-oh-lizm) is the building up of body cells and substances from nutrients. Anabolism is the opposite of catabolism.
- **Catabolism** (kah-**TAB**-oh-lizm) is the breaking down of body cells or substances, releasing energy and carbon dioxide. Catabolism is the opposite of anabolism.

Absorption

Absorption (ab-**SORP**-shun) is the process by which completely digested nutrients are transported to the cells throughout the body.

- The mucosa that lines the small intestine is covered with finger-like projections called **villi** (**VILL**-eye) (singular, *villus*). Each villus contains blood vessels and lacteals. The blood vessels absorb nutrients directly from the digestive system into the bloodstream for delivery to the cells of the body.
- The *lacteals*, which are specialized structures of the lymphatic system, absorb fats and fat-soluble vitamins that cannot be transported directly by the bloodstream. Instead they absorb these nutrients and transport them via lymphatic vessels. As these nutrients are being transported, they are filtered by the lymph nodes in preparation for their delivery to the bloodstream. (Lacteals are discussed in Chapter 6.)

The Role of the Mouth, Salivary Glands, and Esophagus

- **Mastication** (**mass**-tih-**KAY**-shun), also known as *chewing*, breaks food down into smaller pieces, mixes it with saliva, and prepares it to be swallowed.
- A **bolus** (**BOH**-lus) is a mass of food that has been chewed and is ready to be swallowed. The *term* bolus is also used in relation to the administration of medication and is discussed in Chapter 15.
- During swallowing, food travels from the mouth into the pharynx and on into the esophagus.
- In the esophagus, food moves downward through the action of gravity and peristalsis. **Peristalsis** (**pehr**-ih-**STAL**-sis) is a series of wave-like contractions of the smooth muscles in a single direction that moves the food forward into the digestive system.

The Role of the Stomach

- The gastric juices of the stomach contain hydrochloric acid and digestive enzymes to begin the digestive process. Few nutrients enter the bloodstream through the walls of the stomach.
- The churning action of the stomach works with the gastric juices by converting the food into chyme.

Chyme (**KYM**) is the semifluid mass of partly digested food that passes out of the stomach, through the pyloric sphincter, and into the small intestine.

The Role of the Small Intestine

The conversion of food into usable nutrients is completed as the chyme is moved through the small intestine by peristaltic action.

- In the duodenum, chyme is mixed with pancreatic juice and bile. The bile breaks apart large fat globules so enzymes in the pancreatic juices can digest the fats. This action is called ***emulsification*** and must be completed before the nutrients can be absorbed into the body.
- The jejunum secretes large amounts of digestive enzymes and continues the process of digestion.
- The primary function of the ileum is the absorption of nutrients from the digested food.

The Role of the Large Intestine

The role of the entire large intestine is to receive the waste products of digestion and store them until they are eliminated from the body.

- Food waste enters the large intestine in liquid form. Excess water is reabsorbed into the body through the walls of the large intestine, helping maintain the body's fluid balance, and the remaining waste forms into feces.
- **Feces** (**FEE**-seez), also known as ***solid body wastes***, are expelled through the rectum and anus.
- **Defecation** (**def**-eh-**KAY**-shun), also known as a ***bowel movement (BM)***, is the evacuation or emptying of the large intestine.
- The large intestine contains billions of bacteria, most of them harmless, which help break down organic waste material. This process produces gas.
- **Borborygmus** (**bor**-boh-**RIG**-mus) is the rumbling noise caused by the movement of gas in the intestine.
- **Flatulence** (**FLAT**-you-lens), also known as ***flatus***, is the passage of gas out of the body through the rectum.

StudyWARE CONNECTION

Watch the **Digestion** animation in the StudyWARE™.

MEDICAL SPECIALTIES RELATED TO THE DIGESTIVE SYSTEM

- **Bariatrics** (**bayr**-ee-**AT**-ricks) is the branch of medicine concerned with the prevention and control of obesity and associated diseases.
- A **dentist** holds a doctor of dental surgery (DDS) or doctor of medical dentistry (DMD) degree and specializes in diagnosing and treating diseases and disorders of teeth and tissues of the oral cavity.
- A **gastroenterologist** (**gas**-troh-**en**-ter-**OL**-oh-jist) is a physician who specializes in diagnosing and treating diseases and disorders of the stomach and intestines (**gastr/o** means stomach, **enter** means small intestine, and **-ologist** means specialist).
- An **oral or maxillofacial surgeon** (mack-**sill**-oh-**FAY**-shul) specializes in surgery of the face and jaws to correct deformities, treat diseases, and repair injuries.
- An **orthodontist** (**or**-thoh-**DON**-tist) is a dental specialist who prevents or corrects malocclusion of the teeth and related facial structures (**orth** means straight or normal, **odont** means the teeth, and **-ist** means specialist).
- A **periodontist** (**pehr**-ee-oh-**DON**-tist) is a dental specialist who prevents or treats disorders of the tissues surrounding the teeth (**peri-** means surrounding, **odont** means the teeth, and **-ist** means specialist).
- A **proctologist** (prock-**TOL**-oh-jist) is a physician who specializes in disorders of the colon, rectum, and anus (**proct** means anus and rectum, and **-ologist** means specialist).

PATHOLOGY OF THE DIGESTIVE SYSTEM

Tissues of the Oral Cavity

- **Aphthous ulcers** (**AF**-thus **UL**-serz), also known as ***canker sores*** or ***mouth ulcers***, are gray-white pits with a red border in the soft tissues lining the mouth. Although the exact cause is unknown, the appearance of these very common sores is associated with stress, certain foods, or fever.
- An ***ulcer*** is an open lesion of the skin or mucous membrane resulting in tissue loss around the edges (see Chapter 12).

- **Cheilosis** (kee-**LOH**-sis), also known as ***cheilitis***, is a disorder of the lips characterized by crack-like sores at the corners of the mouth (**cheil** means lips, and **-osis** means abnormal condition or disease).
- **Herpes labialis** (**HER**-peez **lay**-bee-**AL**-iss), also known as ***cold sores*** or ***fever blisters***, are blister-like sores on the lips and adjacent facial tissue that are caused by the *oral herpes simplex virus type 1* (HSV-1). Most adults have been infected by this extremely common virus, and in some, it becomes reactivated periodically, causing cold sores.
- **Leukoplakia** (**loo**-koh-**PLAY**-kee-ah) is an abnormal white precancerous lesion (sore) that develops on the tongue or the inside of the cheek (**leuk/o** means white, and **-plakia** means plaque). These lesions develop in response to chronic irritation in the mouth such as constant rubbing against a broken tooth. Occasionally, leukoplakia patches occur on the genitals, in the digestive system, or in the urinary tract.
- **Stomatitis** (**stoh**-mah-**TYE**-tis) is an inflammation of the mucosa of the mouth (**stomat** means mouth or oral cavity, and **-itis** means inflammation). *Note:* the word *stoma*, which occurs in the later section "Ostomies," refers to an artificial mouth-like opening between an organ and the body's surface.
- **Stomatomycosis** (**stoh**-mah-toh-my-**KOH**-sis) is any disease of the mouth due to a fungus (**stomat/o** means mouth or oral cavity, **myc** means fungus, and **-osis** means abnormal condition or disease).
- **Oral thrush** is a type of stomatomycosis that develops when the fungus *Candida albicans* grows out of control. The symptoms are creamy white lesions on the tongue or inner cheeks. This condition occurs most often in infants, older adults with weakened immune systems, or individuals who have been taking antibiotics.
- The term **trismus** (**TRIZ**-mus) describes any restriction to the opening of the mouth caused by trauma, surgery, or radiation associated with the treatment of oral cancer. This condition causes difficulty in speaking and affects the patient's nutrition due to impaired ability to chew and swallow.
- **Xerostomia** (**zeer**-oh-**STOH**-mee-ah), also known as ***dry mouth***, is the lack of adequate saliva due to diminished secretions by the salivary glands (**xer/o** means dry, **stom** means mouth or oral cavity, and **-ia** means pertaining to). This condition can be due to medications or radiation of the salivary glands, and can cause discomfort, difficulty in swallowing, changes in the taste of food, and dental decay.

Cleft Lip and Cleft Palate

- A **cleft lip**, also known as a ***harelip***, is a birth defect in which there is a deep groove of the lip running upward to the nose as a result of the failure of this portion of the lip to close during prenatal development.
- A **cleft palate** is the failure of the palate to close during the early development of the fetus. This opening can involve the upper lip, hard palate, and/or soft palate. If not corrected, this opening between the nose and mouth makes it difficult for the child to eat and speak. Cleft lip and cleft palate can occur singly or together, and usually can be corrected surgically (Figure 8.10).

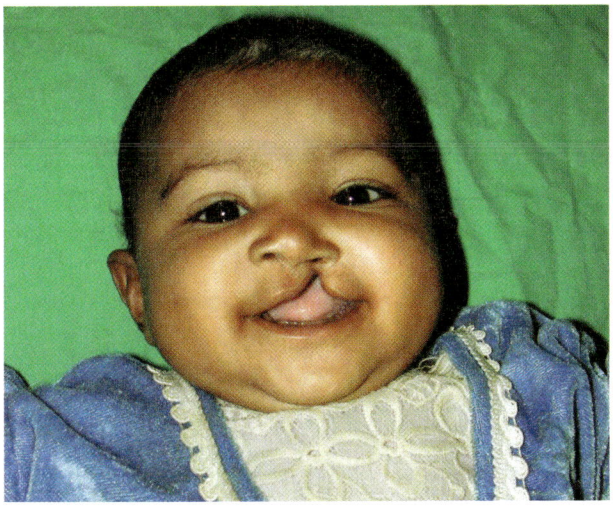

Photo courtesy of The Smile Train: www.smiletrain.org.

(A)

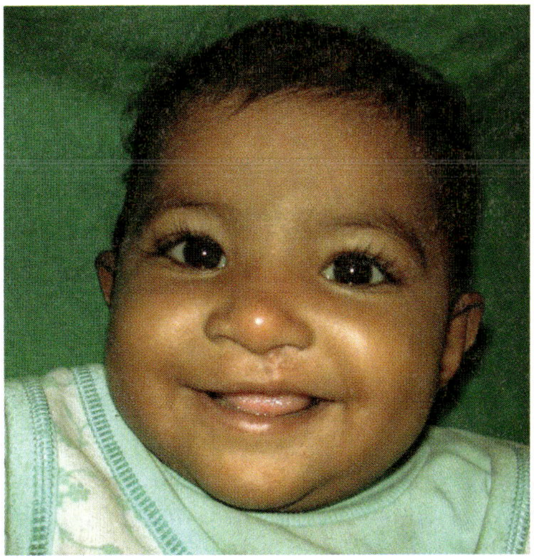

Photo courtesy of The Smile Train: www.smiletrain.org.

(B)

FIGURE 8.10 A child with a cleft palate (A) before and (B) after treatment.

Dental Diseases and Conditions

- **Bruxism** (**BRUCK**-sizm) is the involuntary grinding or clenching of the teeth that usually occurs during sleep and is associated with tension or stress. It can also occur habitually during the day. Bruxism wears away tooth structure, damages periodontal tissues, and injures the temporomandibular joint.
- **Dental caries** (**KAYR**-eez), also known as ***tooth decay*** or a ***cavity***, is an infectious disease caused by bacteria that destroy the enamel and dentin of the tooth. If the decay process is not arrested, the pulp can be exposed and become infected.
- **Dental plaque** (**PLACK**), which is a major cause of dental caries and periodontal disease, forms as soft deposits in sheltered areas near the gums and between the teeth. Dental plaque consists of bacteria and bacterial by-products. In contrast, the ***plaque*** associated with heart conditions consists of deposits of cholesterol that form within blood vessels.
- **Edentulous** (ee-**DEN**-too-lus) means without teeth. This term describes the situation after the natural permanent teeth have been lost.
- **Halitosis** (hal-ih-**TOH**-sis), also known as ***bad breath***, is an unpleasant odor coming from the mouth that can be caused by dental diseases or respiratory or gastric disorders (**halit** means breath, and **-osis** means abnormal condition or disease).
- **Malocclusion** (**mal**-oh-**KLOO**-zhun) is any deviation from the normal positioning of the upper teeth against the lower teeth.

Periodontal Disease

Periodontal disease, also known as ***periodontitis***, is an inflammation of the tissues that surround and support the teeth (**peri-** means surrounding, **odont** means tooth or teeth, and **-al** means pertaining to). This progressive disease is classified according to the degree of tissue involvement. In severe cases, the gums and bone surrounding the teeth are involved.

- **Dental calculus** (**KAL**-kyou-luhs), also known as ***tartar***, is dental plaque that has calcified (hardened) on the teeth. These deposits irritate the surrounding tissues and cause increasingly serious periodontal diseases. The term ***calculus*** is also used to describe hard deposits, such as gallstones or kidney stones, that form in other parts of the body.
- **Gingivitis** (**jin**-jih-**VYE**-tis) is the earliest stage of periodontal disease, and the inflammation affects only the gums (**gingiv** means gums, and **-itis** means inflammation).
- **Acute necrotizing ulcerative gingivitis** (ANUG), also known as ***trench mouth***, is caused by the abnormal growth of bacteria in the mouth. As this condition progresses, the inflammation, bleeding, deep ulceration, and the death of gum tissue become more severe. ***Necrotizing*** means causing ongoing tissue death.

The Esophagus

- **Dysphagia** (dis-**FAY**-jee-ah) is difficulty in swallowing (**dys-** means difficult, and **-phagia** means swallowing).
- **Gastroesophageal reflux disease** (**gas**-troh-eh-**sof**-ah-**JEE**-al **REE**-flucks), also known as ***GERD***, is the upward flow of acid from the stomach into the esophagus (**gastr/o** means stomach, **esophag** means esophagus, and **-eal** means pertaining to). ***Reflux*** means a backward or return flow. When this occurs, the stomach acid irritates and damages the delicate lining of the esophagus.
- **Barrett's esophagus** is a condition that occurs when the cells in the epithelial tissue of the esophagus are damaged by chronic acid exposure. Some patients with chronic GERD develop this complication, which increases the risk of esophageal cancer.
- **Pyrosis** (pye-**ROH**-sis), also known as ***heartburn***, is the burning sensation caused by the return of acidic stomach contents into the esophagus (**pyr** means fever or fire, and **-osis** means abnormal condition or disease).
- **Esophageal varices** (eh-**sof**-ah-**JEE**-al **VAYR**-ih-seez) are enlarged and swollen veins at the lower end of the esophagus (singular, *varix*). Severe bleeding occurs if one of these veins ruptures.
- A **hiatal hernia** (high-**AY**-tal **HER**-nee-ah) is an anatomical abnormality in which a portion of the stomach protrudes upward into the chest, through an opening in the diaphragm (**hiat** means opening, and **-al** means pertaining to). A ***hernia*** is the protrusion of a part or structure through the tissues that normally contain it. This condition can cause GERD and pyrosis (Figure 8.11).

The Stomach

- **Gastritis** (gas-**TRY**-tis) is a common inflammation of the stomach lining that is often caused by the bacterium *Helicobacter pylori* (**gastr** means stomach, and **-itis** means inflammation).

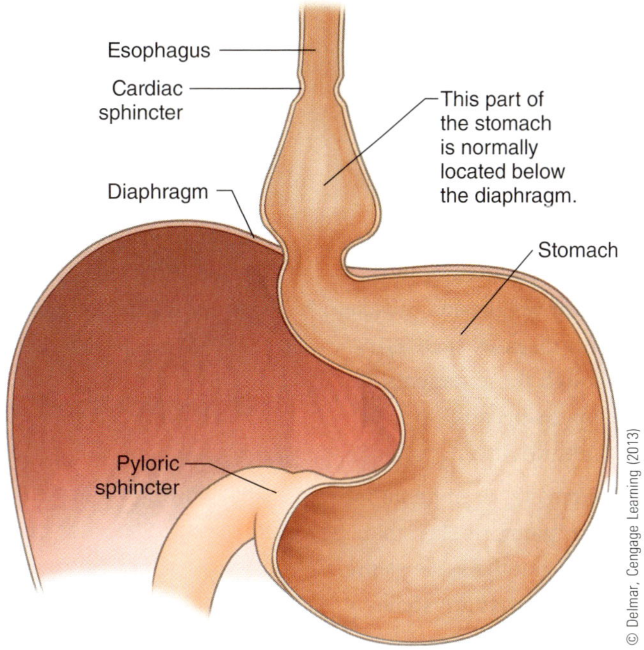

FIGURE 8.11 In a hiatal hernia, part of the stomach protrudes through the esophageal opening in the diaphragm.

- **Gastroenteritis** (**gas**-troh-en-ter-**EYE**-tis) is an inflammation of the mucous membrane lining the stomach and intestines (**gastr/o** means stomach, **enter** means small intestine, and **-itis** means inflammation).
- **Gastrorrhea** (**gas**-troh-**REE**-ah) is the excessive secretion of gastric juice or mucus in the stomach (**gastr/o** is stomach, and **-rrhea** means flow or discharge).

Peptic Ulcers

Peptic ulcers (**UL**-serz) are sores that affect the mucous membranes of the digestive system (**pept** means digestion, and **-ic** means pertaining to). Peptic ulcers are caused by the bacterium *Helicobacter pylori* or by medications, such as aspirin, that irritate the mucous membranes (Figure 8.12). The condition of having peptic ulcers is referred to as *peptic ulcer disease.*

- ***Gastric ulcers*** are peptic ulcers that occur in the stomach.
- ***Duodenal ulcers*** are peptic ulcers that occur in the upper part of the small intestine.
- A ***perforating ulcer*** is a complication of a peptic ulcer in which the ulcer erodes through the entire thickness of the organ wall.

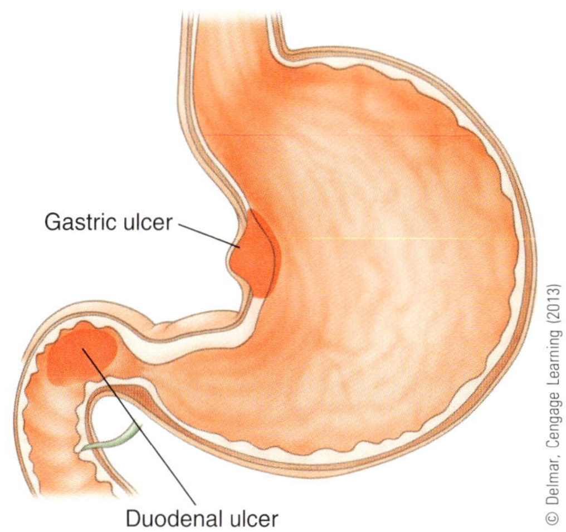

FIGURE 8.12 The locations of peptic ulcers, gastric and duodenal.

Eating Disorders

- **Anorexia** (**an**-oh-**RECK**-see-ah) is the loss of appetite for food, especially when caused by disease.
- **Anorexia nervosa** (**an**-oh-**RECK**-see-ah ner-**VOH**-sah) is an eating disorder characterized by a false perception of body appearance. This leads to an intense fear of gaining weight and refusal to maintain a normal body weight. Voluntary starvation and excessive exercising often cause the patient to become emaciated. ***Emaciated*** means abnormally thin.

- **Bulimia nervosa** (byou-**LIM**-ee-ah ner-**VOH**-sah) is an eating disorder characterized by frequent episodes of binge eating followed by compensatory behaviors such as self-induced vomiting or the misuse of laxatives, diuretics, or other medications. The term ***bulimia*** means continuous, excessive hunger.
- **Cachexia** (kah-**KEKS**-eeh-ah) is a condition of physical wasting away due to the loss of weight and muscle mass that occurs in patients with diseases such as advanced cancer or AIDS. Although these patients are eating enough, the wasting happens because their bodies are unable to absorb the nutrients.
- **Pica** (**PYE**-kah) is an abnormal craving or appetite for nonfood substances, such as dirt, paint, or clay, that lasts for at least one month. Pica is not the same as the short-lasting abnormal food cravings that are sometimes associated with pregnancy.

Nutritional Conditions

- **Dehydration** is a condition in which fluid loss exceeds fluid intake and disrupts the body's normal electrolyte balance (**de-** means removal, **hydra** means water, and **-tion** means the process of).
- **Malnutrition** is a lack of proper food or nutrients in the body due to a shortage of food, poor eating habits, or the inability of the body to digest, absorb, and distribute these nutrients. **Mal-** is a prefix meaning bad or poor.
- **Malabsorption** (**mal**-ab-**SORP**-shun) is a condition in which the small intestine cannot absorb nutrients from food that passes through it.

Obesity

Obesity (oh-**BEE**-sih-tee) is an excessive accumulation of fat in the body. The term ***obese*** is usually used to refer to individuals who are more than 20 to 30% over the established weight standards for their height, age, and gender. The term ***gender*** refers to the differences between men and women.

- **Morbid obesity** (**MOR**-bid oh-**BEE**-sih-tee), also known as ***severe obesity***, is the condition of weighing two times or more than the ideal weight or having a body mass index value greater than 40. As used here, the term ***morbid*** means a diseased state.
- The **body mass index** (BMI) is a number that shows body weight adjusted for height. The results fall into one of these categories: underweight, normal, overweight, or obese. A high BMI is one of many factors related to developing chronic diseases such as heart disease, cancer, or diabetes.
- Obesity is frequently present as a comorbidity with conditions such as hypertension (Chapter 5) or diabetes (Chapter 13). ***Comorbidity*** describes the presence of more than one disease or health condition in an individual at a given time.

Indigestion and Vomiting

- **Aerophagia** (**ay**-er-oh-**FAY**-jee-ah) is the excessive swallowing of air while eating or drinking, and is a common cause of gas in the stomach (**aer/o** means air, and **-phagia** means swallowing).
- **Dyspepsia** (dis-**PEP**-see-ah), also known as ***indigestion***, is pain or discomfort in digestion (**dys-** means painful, and **-pepsia** means digestion).
- **Emesis** (**EM**-eh-sis), also known as ***vomiting***, is the reflex ejection of the stomach contents outward through the mouth. Emesis is used either as a standalone term or as the suffix **-emesis**.
- **Eructation** (eh-ruk-**TAY**-shun) is the act of belching or raising gas orally from the stomach.
- **Hematemesis** (**hee**-mah-**TEM**-eh-sis) is the vomiting of blood (**hemat** means blood, and **-emesis** means vomiting). The substance that is vomited often resembles coffee grounds.
- **Hyperemesis** (**high**-per-**EM**-eh-sis) is extreme, persistent vomiting that can cause dehydration (**hyper-** means excessive, and **-emesis** means vomiting). During the early stages of pregnancy, this is known as ***morning sickness***.
- **Nausea** (**NAW**-see-ah) is the urge to vomit.
- **Regurgitation** (ree-**gur**-jih-**TAY**-shun) is the return of swallowed food into the mouth.

Intestinal Disorders

- **Celiac disease** (**SEE**-lee-ak) is an inherited autoimmune disorder, also known as ***gluten intolerance***, characterized by a severe reaction to foods containing gluten. *Gluten* is a class of proteins found in grains such as wheat, barley, rye, and possibly oats. This disorder damages the villi of the small intestine and can lead to the failure of the body to absorb these substances properly.

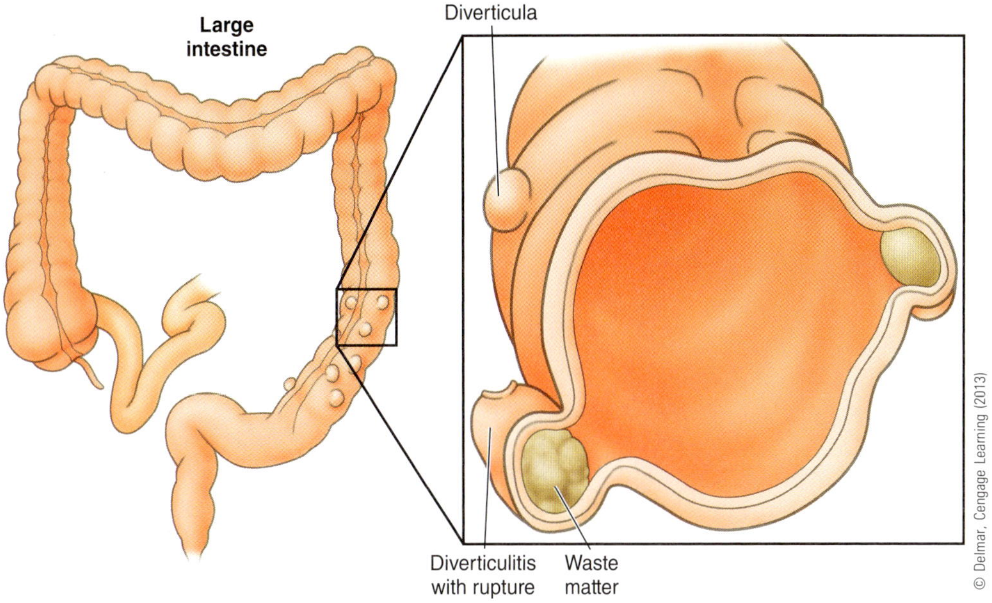

FIGURE 8.13 Diverticulitis is the inflammation of one or more diverticula in the colon.

- **Colorectal carcinoma**, commonly known as ***colon cancer***, often first manifests itself in polyps in the colon (Figure 6.13).
- A **polyp** (**POL**-up) is a mushroom-like growth from the surface of a mucous membrane. Not all polyps are malignant.
- **Diverticulosis** (**dye**-ver-tick-you-**LOH**-sis) is the chronic presence of an abnormal number of diverticula in the colon (**diverticul** means diverticulum, and **-osis** means abnormal condition or disease). Diverticulosis, which often has no symptoms, is believed to be related to a low-fiber diet.
- A **diverticulum** (**dye**-ver-**TICK**-you-lum) is a small pouch, or sac, found in the lining or wall of a tubular organ such as the colon (plural, *diverticula*).
- **Diverticulitis** (**dye**-ver-tick-you-**LYE**-tis), which sometimes develops as a result of diverticulosis, is the inflammation or infection of one or more diverticulum in the colon (**diverticul** means diverticulum, and **-itis** means inflammation). Symptoms of this condition can include sudden abdominal pain, cramping, and nausea (Figure 8.13).
- **Enteritis** (**en**-ter-**EYE**-tis) is an inflammation of the small intestine caused by eating or drinking substances contaminated with viral and bacterial pathogens (**enter** means small intestine, and **-itis** means inflammation).
- **Ischemic colitis** (is-**KEY**-mick koh-**LYE**-tis) occurs when part of the large intestine is partially or completely deprived of blood. If this lack of blood lasts for more than a day, this shortage of blood leads to inflammation or permanent damage of the affected area.

Ileus

Ileus (**ILL**-ee-us) is the partial or complete blockage of the small or large intestine. This condition is also known as ***paralytic ileus***, and it is caused by the stopping of the normal peristalsis of this area of the intestine. Symptoms of ileus can include severe pain, cramping, abdominal distention, vomiting, and the failure to pass gas or stools.

Postoperative ileus is a temporary impairment (stoppage) of bowel action that is considered to be a normal response to abdominal surgery. It is often present for 24 to 72 hours, depending on which part of the digestive system was treated.

Irritable Bowel Syndrome

Irritable bowel syndrome (IBS), which is also known as ***spastic colon***, is a common condition of unknown cause with symptoms that can include intermittent cramping, abdominal pain, bloating, constipation, and diarrhea. This condition, which is usually aggravated by stress and by eating certain foods, is *not* caused by pathogens (bacteria or viruses) or by structural changes.

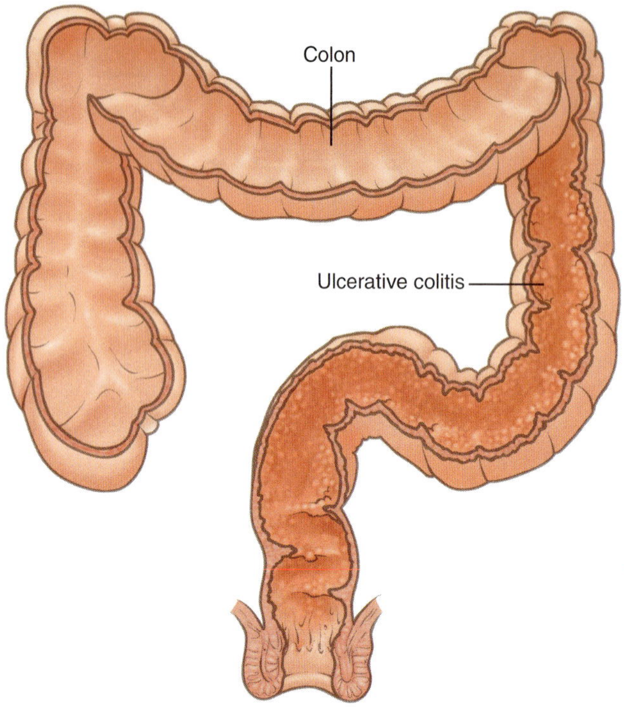

FIGURE 8.14 Ulcerative colitis causes ulcers and irritation in the rectum and large intestine.

Inflammatory Bowel Diseases

Inflammatory bowel disease (IBD) is the general name for diseases that cause inflammation and swelling in the intestines. The two most common inflammatory bowel diseases are ulcerative colitis and Crohn's disease.

- These conditions are grouped together because both are chronic and incurable, and can affect the large and small intestines. They also have similar symptoms, which include abdominal pain, weight loss, fatigue, fever, rectal bleeding, and diarrhea.
- These conditions tend to occur at intervals of active disease known as *flares* alternating with periods of remission. Flares of these disorders are treated with medication and surgery to remove diseased portions of the intestine.

Ulcerative Colitis

Ulcerative colitis (**UL**-ser-**ay**-tiv koh-**LYE**-tis) is a chronic condition of unknown cause in which repeated episodes of inflammation in the rectum and large intestine cause ulcers (lesions in the mucous membrane) and irritation (**col** means colon, and **-itis** means inflammation) (Figure 8.14).

- Ulcerative colitis usually starts in the rectum and progresses upward to the lower part of the colon; however, it can affect the entire large intestine.
- Ulcerative colitis affects only the innermost lining and not the deep tissues of the colon.

Crohn's Disease

Crohn's disease (CD) is a chronic autoimmune disorder that can occur anywhere in the digestive tract; however, it is most often found in the ileum and in the colon.

In contrast to *ulcerative colitis*, Crohn's disease generally penetrates every layer of tissue in the affected area. This can result in scarring and thickening of the walls of the affected structures. The most common complication of Crohn's disease is blockage of the intestine due to swelling and scarring.

Intestinal Obstructions

An **intestinal obstruction** is the partial or complete blockage of the small or large intestine caused by a physical obstruction. This blockage can result from many causes such as scar tissue or a tumor.

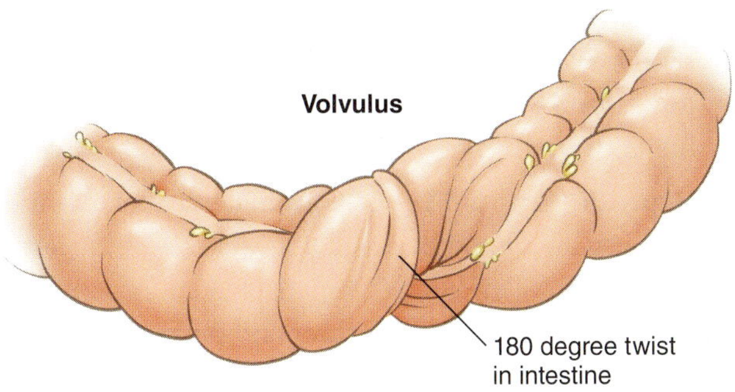

FIGURE 8.15 Volvulus is the twisting of the bowel on itself.

- ***Intestinal adhesions*** abnormally hold together parts of the intestine that normally should be separate. This condition, which is caused by inflammation or trauma, can lead to intestinal obstruction.
- In a ***strangulating obstruction***, the blood flow to a segment of the intestine is blocked. This can lead to gangrene or perforation. ***Gangrene*** is tissue death that is associated with a loss of normal circulation. As used here, ***perforation*** describes a hole through the wall of a structure.
- **Volvulus** (**VOL**-view-lus) is the twisting of the intestine on itself, causing an obstruction. *Volvulus* is a Latin word meaning rolled up or twisted. This condition can cause necrosis of the affected segment of the bowel (Figure 8.15).
- **Intussusception** (**in**-tus-sus-**SEP**-shun) is the telescoping of one part of the small intestine into the opening of an immediately adjacent part (**intussuscept** means to take up or to receive within, and **-ion** means condition). This rare but serious condition is sometimes found in children between three months and six years of age.
- An **inguinal hernia** (**ING**-gwih-nal **HER**-nee-ah) is the protrusion of a small loop of bowel through a weak place in the lower abdominal wall or groin (**inguin** means groin, and **-al** means pertaining to). This condition can be caused by obesity, pregnancy, heavy lifting, or straining to pass a stool.
- A **strangulated hernia** occurs when a portion of the intestine is constricted inside the hernia, causing ischemia (insufficient oxygen) in this tissue by cutting off its blood supply.

Infectious Diseases of the Intestines

Infectious diseases of the intestines can be transmitted through contaminated food and water or through poor sanitation practices. The more common of these infectious diseases include:

- ***Clostridium difficile*** (klos-**TRID**-ee-um dif-us-**SEEL**), also known as ***C. diff***, is a bacterial infection common to older adults in hospitals or long-term care facilities, typically following the use of antibiotics that wipe out competing bacteria. This disease causes diarrhea and can lead to inflammation of the colon. Infection control measures such as hand-scrubbing or wearing gloves can help prevent its spread.
- **Dysentery** (**DIS**-en-**ter**-ee), which is bacterial infection, occurs most frequently in hot countries where it is spread through food or water contaminated by human feces.
- ***E. coli***, which is caused by the bacterium *Escherichia coli*, is transmitted through contaminated foods that have not been cooked properly.
- **Salmonellosis** (**sal**-muh-nel-**LOH**-sis), also referred to as ***salmonella***, is transmitted by feces, either through direct contact with animals, or by eating contaminated raw or undercooked meats and eggs or unpasteurized milk and cheese products.

Anorectal Disorders

- An **anal fissure** is a small crack-like sore in the skin of the anus that can cause severe pain during a bowel movement. As used here, a ***fissure*** is a groove or crack-like sore of the skin.
- **Bowel incontinence** (in-**KON**-tih-nents) is the inability to control the excretion of feces. (*Urinary incontinence* is discussed in Chapter 9.)
- **Constipation** is defined as having a bowel movement fewer than three times per week. With constipation, stools are usually hard, dry, small in size, and difficult to eliminate.
- **Diarrhea** (**dye**-ah-**REE**-ah) is an abnormally frequent flow of loose or watery stools that can lead to dehydration (**dia-** means through, and **-rrhea** means flow or discharge).
- **Hemorrhoids** (**HEM**-oh-roids) occur when a cluster of veins, muscles, and tissues slip near or through the anal opening. These veins can become inflamed, resulting in pain, fecal leakage, itching, and bleeding.
- A **rectocele** (**RECK**-toh-seel) is a bulging of the front wall of the rectum into the vagina, usually as the result of childbirth or pregnancy (**rect/o** means rectum, and **-cele** means hernia).

Abnormal Stools

- **Hematochezia** (hee-**mat**-oh-**KEE**-zee-uh) is the flow of bright red blood in the stool. This bright red color usually indicates that the blood is coming from the lower part of the gastrointestinal tract.
- **Melena** (meh-**LEE**-nah), in contrast to *hematochezia*, is the passage of black, tarry, and foul-smelling stools (**melan** means black or dark, and **-a** is a noun ending). This appearance of the stools is caused by the presence of digested blood and often indicates an injury or disorder in the upper part of the gastrointestinal tract.
- **Steatorrhea** (**stee**-at-oh-**REE**-ah) is the presence of an excess of fat in the stool (**steat/o** means fat and **-rrhea** means flow or discharge). This condition, which results in frothy, foul-smelling feces, is usually caused by pancreatic disease, the removal of the gallbladder, or malabsorption disorders.

The Liver

Liver disorders are a major concern because the functioning of the liver is essential to the digestive process.

- **Ascites** (ah-**SIGH**-teez) is an abnormal accumulation of serous fluid in the peritoneal cavity. This condition is usually the result of severe liver disease. As used here, the term ***serous*** means a substance having a watery consistency.
- **Hepatomegaly** (**hep**-ah-toh-**MEG**-ah-lee) is the abnormal enlargement of the liver (**hepat/o** means liver, and **-megaly** means enlargement).
- **Jaundice** (**JAWN**-dis) is a yellow discoloration of the skin, mucous membranes, and the eyes. This condition is caused by greater-than-normal amounts of bilirubin in the blood.
- **Hepatitis** (**hep**-ah-**TYE**-tis) is an inflammation of the liver usually caused by a viral infection (**hepat** means liver, and **-itis** means inflammation). Viral hepatitis is the leading cause of liver cancer and the most common reason for liver transplants. The three most common varieties of viral hepatitis are shown in Table 8.1.

Cirrhosis

Cirrhosis (sih-**ROH**-sis) is a chronic degenerative disease of the liver characterized by scarring (**cirrh** means yellow or orange, and **-osis** means abnormal condition or disease). ***Degenerative*** means progressive deterioration resulting in the loss of tissue or organ function.

- Cirrhosis is often caused by excessive alcohol abuse or by viral hepatitis B or C.
- The progress of cirrhosis is marked by the formation of areas of scarred liver tissue that are filled with fat. The liver damage causes abnormal conditions throughout the other body systems (Figure 8.16).

Nonalcoholic Fatty Liver Disease

The term **nonalcoholic fatty liver disease** (NAFLD) describes the accumulation of fat in the liver of people who drink little or no alcohol. Those with this condition, which usually has no signs or symptoms, is most common in middle-aged individuals who are obese, have type 2 diabetes, have high cholesterol, or have a combination of these.

TABLE 8.1
The ABCs of Hepatitis

HAV	**Hepatitis A virus** is the most prevalent type of hepatitis. This condition is caused by the highly contagious HAV virus and is transmitted mainly through contamination of food and water with infected fecal matter. A vaccine is available to provide immunity against HAV.
HBV	**Hepatitis B virus** is a bloodborne disease that is transmitted through contact with blood and other body fluids that are contaminated with this virus. A vaccine is available to provide immunity against HBV.
HCV	**Hepatitis C virus** is a bloodborne disease that is spread through contact with blood and other body fluids that are contaminated with this virus. HCV is described as a silent epidemic because it can be present in the body for years, and destroy the liver, before any symptoms appear. There is no vaccine available to prevent this form of hepatitis.

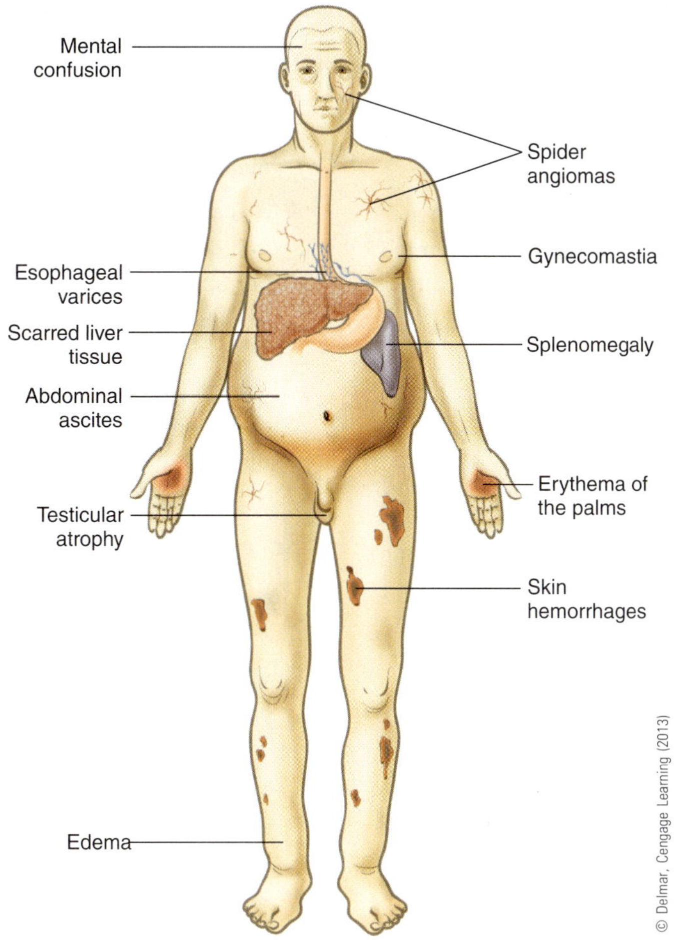

FIGURE 8.16 Clinical conditions associated with cirrhosis of the liver.

Nonalcoholic steatohepatitis (**stee**-ah-toh-hep-ah-**TYE**-tis) (NASH) is a more serious form of this condition since it consists of fatty accumulations plus liver-damaging inflammation (**steat/o** means fat, **hepat** means liver, and **-itis** mean inflammation). In some cases, this will progress to cirrhosis, irreversible liver scarring, or liver cancer.

The Gallbladder

- **Cholangitis** (**koh**-lan-**JIGH**-tis) is an acute inflammation of the bile duct characterized by pain in the upper-right quadrant of the abdomen, fever, and jaundice (**cholang** means bile duct, and **-itis** means inflammation). The most common cause is a bacterial infection.
- **Cholecystitis** (**koh**-luh-sis-**TYE**-tis) is inflammation of the gallbladder, usually associated with gallstones blocking the flow of bile (**cholecyst** means gallbladder, and **-itis** means inflammation).
- A **gallstone**, also known as a ***cholelith***, is a hard deposit formed in the gallbladder and bile ducts due to the concretion of bile components (plural, *calculi*). The formation of stones is discussed further in Chapter 9.
- **Cholelithiasis** (**koh**-leh-lih-**THIGH**-ah-sis) is the presence of gallstones in the gallbladder or bile ducts (**chole** means bile or gall, and **-lithiasis** means presence of stones).
- Pain caused by the passage of a gallstone through the bile duct is called ***biliary colic***.

The Pancreas

Disorders of the pancreas are discussed in Chapter 13.

DIAGNOSTIC PROCEDURES OF THE DIGESTIVE SYSTEM

- **Abdominal computed tomography** (CT) is a radiographic procedure that produces a detailed cross-section of the tissue structure within the abdomen, showing, for example, the presence of a tumor or obstruction. CT scans are discussed in Chapter 15.
- An **abdominal ultrasound** is a noninvasive test used to visualize internal organs by using very-high-frequency sound waves.
- **Cholangiography** (koh-**LAN**-jee-**og**-rah-fee) is a radiographic examination of the bile ducts with the use of a contrast medium (**cholangi/o** means bile duct, and **-graphy** means the process of recording). This test is used to identify obstructions in the liver or bile ducts that slow or block the flow of bile from the liver. The resulting record is a ***cholangiogram***.
- An **enema** (**EH**-neh-ma) is the placement of a solution into the rectum and colon to empty the lower intestine through bowel activity. An enema is sometimes part of the preparation for an endoscopic examination; however, enemas are also used to treat severe constipation and as a means of injecting medication into the body.
- An **esophagogastroduodenoscopy** (eh-**sof**-ah-goh-**gas**-troh-**dew**-oh-deh-**NOS**-koh-pee) is an endoscopic procedure that allows direct visualization of the upper GI tract (**esophag/o** means esophagus, **gastr/o** means stomach, **duoden/o** means duodenum, and **-scopy** means visual examination). This includes the esophagus, stomach, and upper duodenum.
- An **upper GI series** and a **lower GI series** are radiographic studies to examine the digestive system. A contrast medium is required to make these structures visible. A ***barium swallow*** is used for the upper GI series, and a ***barium enema*** is used for the lower GI series.
- **Stool samples** are specimens of feces that are examined for content and characteristics. For example, fatty stools might indicate the presence of pancreatic disease. Cultures of the stool sample can be examined in the laboratory for the presence of bacteria or ***O & P***. This abbreviation stands for ova (parasite eggs) and parasites.

Endoscopic Procedures

An **endoscope** (**EN**-doh-**skope**) is an instrument used for visual examination of internal structures (**endo-** means within, and **-scope** means an instrument for visual examination).

- An **anoscopy** (ah-**NOS**-koh-pee) is the visual examination of the anal canal and lower rectum (**an/o** means anus, and **-scopy** means visual examination).
- A **capsule endoscopy** is the use of a tiny video camera in a capsule that the patient swallows (Figure 8.17). For approximately eight hours, as it passes through the small intestine, this camera transmits images of the walls of the small intestine. The images are detected by sensor devices attached to the patient's abdomen and transmitted to a data recorder worn on the patient's belt.

Screening for Colorectal Carcinoma

The following diagnostic tests are used for the early detection of polyps that may be cancerous.

- **Colonoscopy** (**koh**-lun-**OSS**-koh-pee) is the direct visual examination of the inner surface of the entire colon from the rectum to the cecum (**colon/o** means colon, and **-scopy** means visual examination). A ***virtual colonoscopy*** uses x-rays and computers to produce two- and three-dimensional images of the colon.
- **Sigmoidoscopy** (**sig**-moi-**DOS**-koh-pee) is the endoscopic examination of the interior of the rectum, sigmoid colon, and possibly a portion of the descending colon (**sigmoid/o** means sigmoid colon, and **-scopy** is the visual examination).
- A **Hemoccult test** (**HEE**-moh-kult), also known as the ***fecal occult blood test***, is a laboratory test for hidden blood in the stools (**hem** means blood, and **-occult** means hidden). This test kit is used to obtain the specimens at home, and these are then evaluated in a laboratory. *Note:* the term Hemoccult is capitalized because it is the name of the manufacturer.

TREATMENT PROCEDURES OF THE DIGESTIVE SYSTEM

Medications

- **Antacids**, which neutralize the acids in the stomach, are taken to relieve the discomfort of conditions such as pyrosis or to help peptic ulcers heal.
- **Proton pump inhibitors** decrease the amount of acid produced by the stomach. These medications are used to treat the symptoms of GERD.

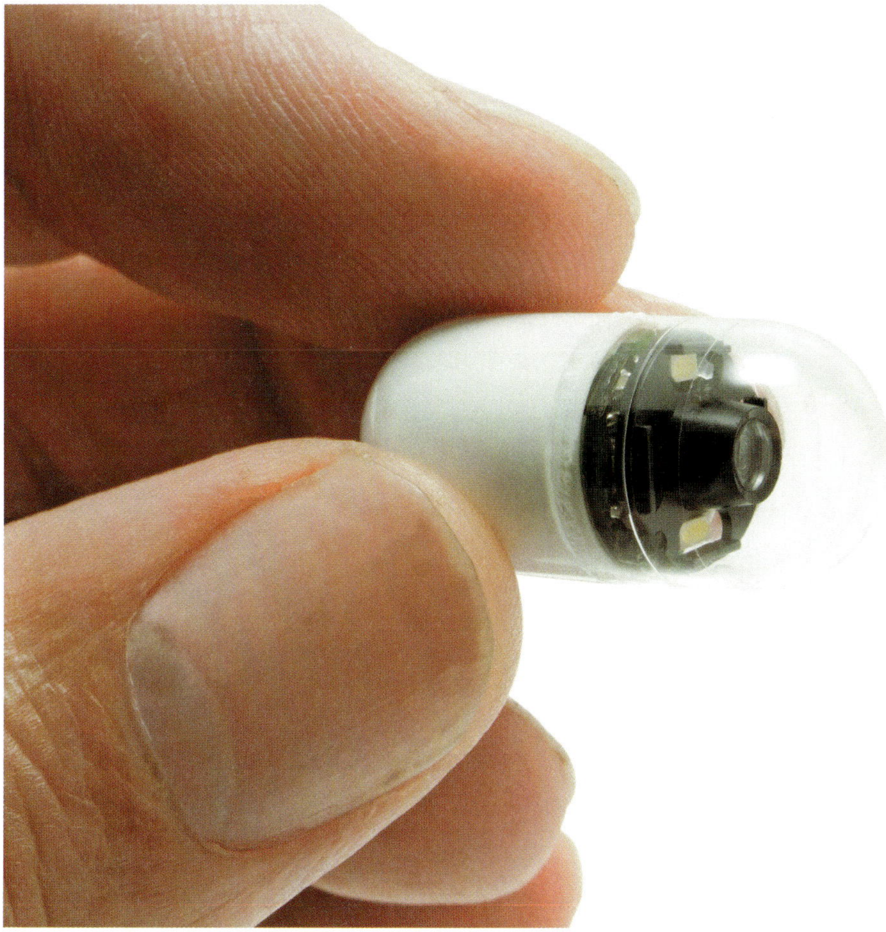

FIGURE 8.17 The capsule endoscopy camera is swallowed by the patient so that it can transmit images from the small intestine to a sensor device.

- An **antiemetic** (**an**-tih-ee-**MET**-ick) is a medication that is administered to prevent or relieve nausea and vomiting (**anti-** means against, **emet** means vomit, and **-ic** means pertaining to).
- **Laxatives** are medications or foods given to stimulate bowel movements. ***Bulk-forming laxatives***, such as bran, treat constipation by helping fecal matter retain water and remain soft as it moves through the intestines.
- **Intravenous fluids** (**in**-trah-**VEE**-nus) (IV) are administered to combat the effects of dehydration (**intra-** means within, **ven/o** means vein, and **-us** is the noun ending).
- **Oral rehydration therapy** (ORT) is a treatment in which a solution of electrolytes is administered in a liquid preparation to counteract the dehydration that can accompany severe diarrhea, especially in young children (**re-** means back or again, **hydra** means water, and **-tion** is the process of).

The Oral Cavity and Esophagus

- A **dental prophylaxis** (**proh**-fih-**LACK**-sis) is the professional cleaning of the teeth to remove plaque and calculus. The term ***prophylaxis*** also refers to a treatment intended to prevent a disease or stop it from spreading. Examples include vaccination to provide immunity against a specific disease.
- A **gingivectomy** (**jin** -jih-**VECK**-toh-mee) is the surgical removal of diseased gingival tissue (**gingiv** means gingival tissue, and **-ectomy** means surgical removal).
- **Maxillofacial surgery** (mack-**sill**-oh-**FAY**-shul) is specialized surgery of the face and jaws to correct deformities, treat diseases, and repair injuries.
- **Palatoplasty** (**PAL**-ah-toh-**plas**-tee) is surgical repair of a cleft palate, also used to refer to the repair of a cleft lip (**palat/o** means palate, and **-plasty** means surgical repair) (Figure 8.10).

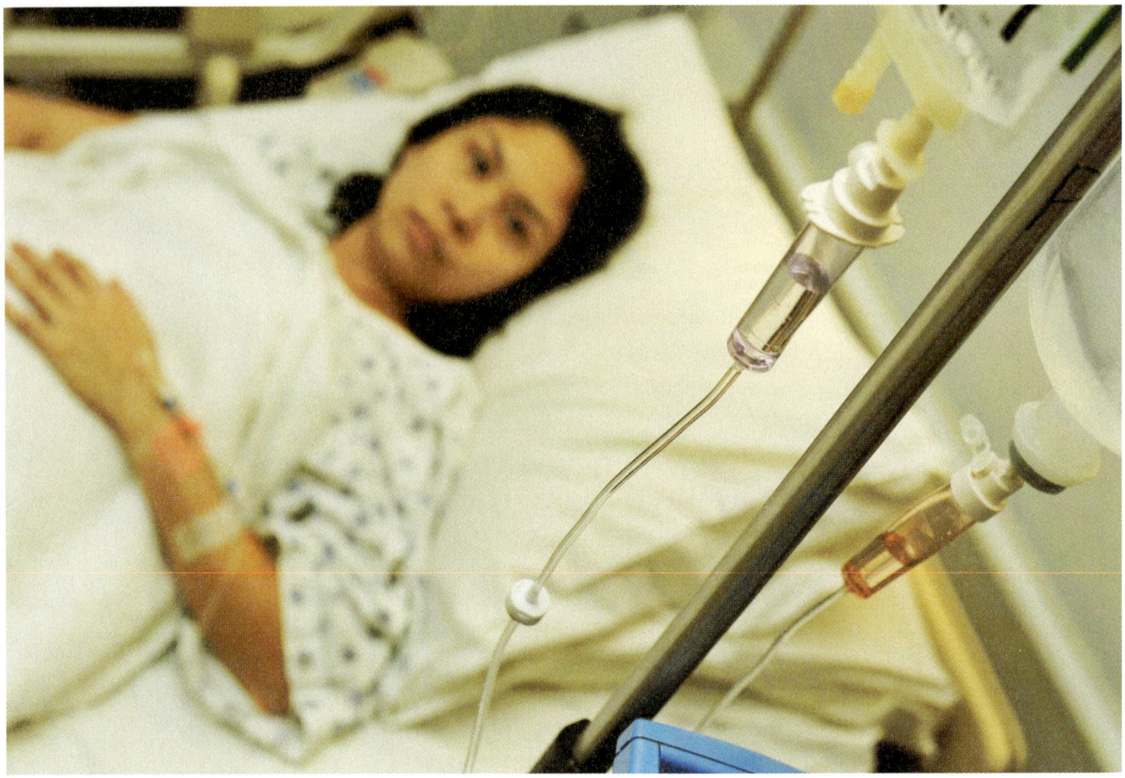

iStockphoto/dblight

FIGURE 8.18 Fluids are administered intravenously to combat the effects of dehydration.

The Stomach

- A **gastrectomy** (gas-**TRECK**-toh-mee) is the surgical removal of all or a part of the stomach (**gastr** means stomach, and **-ectomy** means surgical removal).
- **Nasogastric intubation** (**nay**-zoh-**GAS**-trick **in**-too-**BAY**-shun) is the placement of a feeding tube through the nose and into the stomach (**nas/o** means nose, **gastr** means stomach, and **-ic** means pertaining to). This tube, which is placed temporarily, provides nutrition for patients who cannot take sufficient nutrients by mouth (Figure 8.19).
- A **gastrostomy tube** (gas-**TROS**-toh-mee) is a surgically placed feeding tube from the exterior of the body directly into the stomach (**gastr** means stomach, and **-ostomy** means surgically creating an opening). This is also known as a ***G-tube*** and it is permanently placed, to provide nutrition for patients who cannot swallow or take sufficient nutrients by mouth (Figure 8.19).
- **Total parenteral nutrition** (pah-**REN**-ter-al) (TPN) is administered to patients who cannot or should not get their nutrition through eating. All of the patient's nutritional requirements are met through a specialized solution administered intravenously. ***Parenteral*** means not in or through the digestive system.

Bariatric Surgery

Bariatric surgery is performed to treat morbid obesity by restricting the amount of food that can enter the stomach and be digested. These procedures limit food intake and force dietary changes that enable weight reduction.

- ***Gastric bypass surgery*** makes the stomach smaller, usually by stapling a section to create a small pouch, and causes food to bypass the first part of the small intestine. This procedure, which is the most common bariatric surgery, is not reversible.

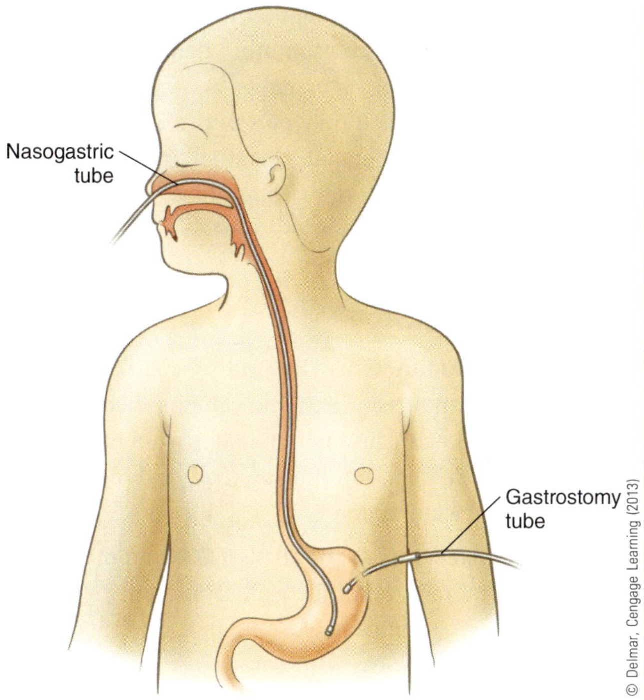

FIGURE 8.19 Nasogastric and gastrostomy tubes can be used to supply nutrition to a child who cannot eat by mouth.

- The ***lap-band adjustable gastric banding*** (LAGB) procedure involves placing a band around the exterior of the stomach to restrict the amount of food that can enter (Figure 8.20). This procedure has the advantage of being reversible through the removal of the band.

The Intestines

- A **colectomy** (koh-**LECK**-toh-mee) is the surgical removal of all or part of the colon (**col** means colon, and **-ectomy** means surgical removal).
- A **colotomy** (koh-**LOT**-oh-mee) is a surgical incision into the colon (**col** means colon, and **-otomy** means a surgical incision).
- A **diverticulectomy** (**dye**-ver-**tick**-you-**LECK**-toh-mee) is the surgical removal of a diverticulum (**diverticul** means diverticulum, and **-ectomy** means surgical removal).
- A **gastroduodenostomy** (**gas**-troh-**dew**-oh-deh-**NOS**-toh-mee) is the establishment of an anastomosis between the upper portion of the stomach, and the duodenum (**gastr/o** means stomach, **duoden** means first part of the small intestine, and **-ostomy** means surgically creating an opening). This procedure is performed to treat stomach cancer or to remove a malfunctioning pyloric valve.

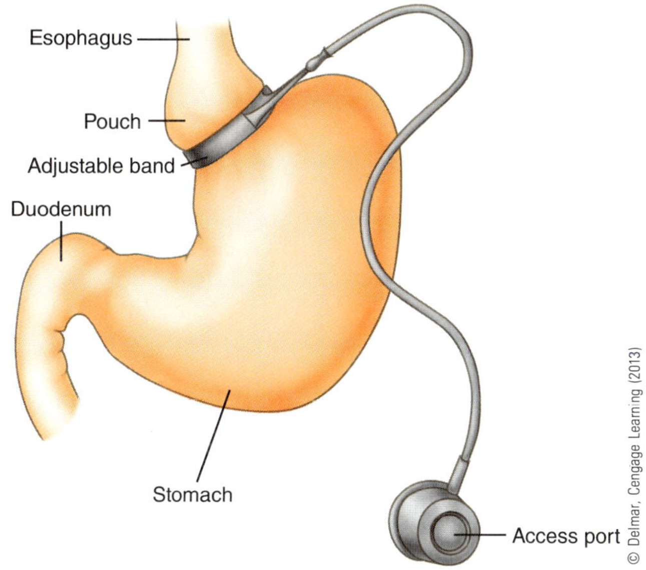

FIGURE 8.20 Lap-band adjustable gastric banding is one type of bariatric surgery.

- An **anastomosis** (ah-**nas**-toh-**MOH**-sis) is a surgical connection between two hollow, or tubular, structures (plural, *anastomoses*).
- An **ileectomy** (**ill**-ee-**ECK**-toh-mee) is the surgical removal of the ileum (**ile** means the ileum, and **-ectomy** means surgical removal. Note: This term is spelled with a double *e*.)

Ostomies

An **ostomy** (**OSS**-toh-mee) is a surgical procedure to create an artificial opening between an organ and the body surface. This artificial opening is also known as a ***stoma***. Ostomy can be used alone as a noun to describe a procedure or as a suffix with the word part that describes the organ involved.

- An **ileostomy** (**ill**-ee-**OS**-toh-mee) is the surgical creation of an artificial excretory opening between the ileum, at the end of the small intestine, and the outside of the abdominal wall (**ile** means small intestine, and **-ostomy** means surgically creating an opening).
- A **colostomy** (koh-**LAHS**-toh-mee) is the surgical creation of an artificial excretory opening between the colon and the body surface (**col** means colon, and **-ostomy** means surgically creating an opening). The segment of the intestine below the ostomy is usually removed, and the fecal matter flows through the stoma into a disposable bag. A colostomy can be temporary to divert feces from an area that needs to heal (Figure 8.21).

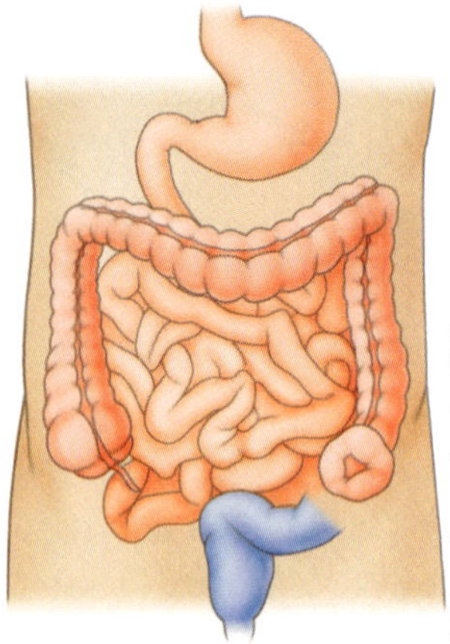

FIGURE 8.21 Colostomy sites are named for portion of the bowel removed. Shown here is a sigmoid colostomy. The stoma is located at the end of the remaining intestine, which is shown in brown. The portion that has been removed is shown in blue.

The Rectum and Anus

- A **hemorrhoidectomy** (**hem**-oh-roid-**ECK**-toh-mee) is the surgical removal of hemorrhoids (**hemorrhoid** means piles, and **-ectomy** means surgical removal). ***Rubber band ligation*** is often used instead of surgery. Rubber bands cut off the circulation at the base of the hemorrhoid, causing it to eventually fall off. ***Ligation*** means the tying off of blood vessels or ducts.
- **Proctopexy** (**PROCK**-toh-**peck**-see) is the surgical fixation of a prolapsed rectum to an adjacent tissue or organ (**proct/o** means rectum, and **-pexy** means surgical fixation). ***Prolapse*** means the falling or dropping down of an organ or internal part.

The Liver

- A **hepatectomy** (**hep**-ah-**TECK**-toh-mee) is the surgical removal of all or part of the liver (**hepat** means liver, and **-ectomy** means surgical removal).
- A **liver transplant** is an option for a patient whose liver has failed for a reason other than liver cancer. Because liver tissue regenerates, a ***partial liver transplant***, in which only part of the organ is donated, can be adequate. A partial liver can be donated by a living donor whose blood and tissue types match.

The Gallbladder

- A **choledocholithotomy** (koh-**led**-oh-koh-lih-**THOT**-oh-mee) is an incision into the common bile duct for the removal of a gallstone (**choledoch/o** means the common bile duct, **lith** means stone, and **-otomy** means surgical incision).
- A **cholecystectomy** (**koh**-luh-sis-**TECK**-toh-mee) is the surgical removal of the gallbladder (**chole-** means gallbladder, **cyst** means bladder, and **-ectomy** means surgical removal). An ***open cholecystectomy*** is performed through an incision in the right side of the upper abdomen. A ***laparoscopic cholecystectomy***, also known as a ***lap choley***, is the surgical removal of the gallbladder using a laparoscope and other instruments inserted through three or four small incisions in the abdominal wall.

ABBREVIATIONS RELATED TO THE DIGESTIVE SYSTEM

Table 8.2 presents an overview of the abbreviations related to the terms introduced in this chapter. Note: To avoid errors or confusion, always be cautious when using abbreviations.

TABLE 8.2
Abbreviations Related to the Digestive System

body mass index = BMI	**BMI** = body mass index
colonoscopy = COL	**COL** = colonoscopy
esophagogastroduodenoscopy = EGD	**EGD** = esophagogastroduodenoscopy
gastroesophageal reflux disease = GERD	**GERD** = gastroesophageal reflux disease
gastrointestinal = GI	**GI** = gastrointestinal
inguinal hernia = IH	**IH** = inguinal hernia
inflammatory bowel disease = IBD	**IBD** = inflammatory bowel disease
irritable bowel syndrome = IBS	**IBS** = irritable bowel syndrome
nasogastric tube = NG tube	**NG tube** = nasograstric tube
peptic ulcer disease = PUD	**PUD** = peptic ulcer disease
total parenteral nutrition = TPN	**TPN** = total parenteral nutrition
ulcerative colitis = UC	**UC** = ulcerative colitis

StudyWARE CONNECTION

For more practice and to test your mastery of this material, go to the StudyWARE™ to play interactive games and complete the quiz for this chapter.

DELMAR MOBILE MEDIA

Downloadable audio is available for selected medical terms in this chapter to enhance your learning of medical terminology.

Workbook Practice

Go to your workbook, and complete the exercises for this chapter.

CHAPTER 8 LEARNING EXERCISES

MATCHING WORD PARTS 1

Write the correct answer in the middle column.

	Definition	Correct Answer	Possible Answers
8.1.	anus	________________	chol/e
8.2.	bile, gall	________________	an/o
8.3.	large intestine	________________	col/o
8.4.	swallowing	________________	enter/o
8.5.	small intestine	________________	-phagia

MATCHING WORD PARTS 2

Write the correct answer in the middle column.

	Definition	Correct Answer	Possible Answers
8.6.	stomach	________________	cholecyst/o
8.7.	liver	________________	esophag/o
8.8.	gallbladder	________________	gastr/o
8.9.	esophagus	________________	hepat/o
8.10.	presence of stones	________________	-lithiasis

MATCHING WORD PARTS 3

Write the correct answer in the middle column.

	Definition	Correct Answer	Possible Answers
8.11.	sigmoid colon	________________	-pepsia
8.12.	anus and rectum	________________	-emesis

8.13. digestion ______________________ **proct/o**

8.14. vomiting ______________________ **rect/o**

8.15. rectum ______________________ **sigmoid/o**

DEFINITIONS

Select the correct answer, and write it on the line provided.

8.16. The visual examination of the anal canal and lower rectum is known as ______________.

anoscopy colonoscopy proctoscopy sigmoidoscopy

8.17. The term ______________ means any disease of the mouth due to a fungus.

salmonellosis stomatomycosis stomatitis steatorrhea

8.18. The ______________ is the last and longest portion of the small intestine.

cecum ileum jejunum pylorus

8.19. The inability to control the excretion of feces is called ______________.

bowel incontinence constipation anal fissure hematochezia

8.20. The liver secretes ______________, which is stored in the gallbladder for later use.

bile glycogen insulin pepsin

8.21. The ______________ travels upward from the cecum to the undersurface of the liver.

ascending colon descending colon sigmoid colon transverse colon

8.22. The process of the building up of body cells and substances from nutrients is known as ______________.

anabolism catabolism defecation mastication

8.23. The receptors of taste are located on the dorsum of the ______________.

hard palate rugae tongue uvula

8.24. The bone and soft tissues that surround and support the teeth are known as the ______________.

dentition gingiva occlusion periodontium

8.25. The condition characterized by the telescoping of one part of the intestine into another is ________________.

borborygmus flatus intussusception volvulus

MATCHING STRUCTURES

Write the correct answer in the middle column.

Definition	Correct Answer	Possible Answers
8.26. connects the small and large intestine	________________	cecum
8.27. S-shaped structure of the large intestine	________________	duodenum
8.28. widest division of the large intestine	________________	jejunum
8.29. middle portion of the small intestine	________________	rectum
8.30. first portion of the small intestine	________________	sigmoid colon

WHICH WORD?

Select the correct answer, and write it on the line provided.

8.31. The medical term meaning vomiting blood is ________________.

hematemesis hyperemesis

8.32. The ________________ virus is transmitted mainly through contamination of food and water with infected fecal matter.

hepatitis A hepatitis B

8.33. ________________ is characterized by a severe reaction to foods containing gluten.

celiac disease Crohn's disease

8.34. The medical term meaning inflammation of the small intestine is ____________________.

colitis enteritis

8.35. The ____________________ hangs from the free edge of the soft palate.

rugae uvula

SPELLING COUNTS

Find the misspelled word in each sentence. Then write that word, spelled correctly, on the line provided.

8.36. An ilectomy is the surgical removal of the last portion of the ileum. ____________________

8.37. The bacterial infection disentary occurs mostly in hot countries and is spread through food or water contaminated by human feces. ____________________

8.38. The chronic degenerative disease of the liver characterized by scarring is known as serosis. ____________________

8.39. A proctoplexy is the surgical fixation of the rectum to some adjacent tissue or organ. ____________________

8.40. The lack of adequate saliva due to the absence of or diminished secretions by the salivary glands is known as zerostomia. ____________________

ABBREVIATION IDENTIFICATION

In the space provided, write the words that each abbreviation stands for.

8.41. **UC** ____

8.42. **COL** ____

8.43. **GERD** ____

8.44. **IBS** ____

8.45. **PUD** ____

TERM SELECTION

Select the correct answer, and write it on the line provided.

8.46. The surgical removal of all or part of the stomach is a ________________.

gastrectomy gastritis gastroenteritis gastrotomy

8.47. The medical term meaning difficulty in swallowing is ________________.

anorexia dyspepsia dysphagia pyrosis

8.48. The involuntary grinding or clenching of the teeth is called ________________.

bruxism edentulous malocclusion dental caries

8.49. The chronic degeneration of the liver often caused by excessive alcohol abuse is called ________________.

cirrhosis hepatitis C hepatitis A hepatomegaly

8.50 The pigment manufactured by the liver and necessary for the digestion of fat is called ________________.

bile bilirubin hydrochloric acid pancreatic juice

SENTENCE COMPLETION

Write the correct term or terms on the lines provided.

8.51. The excessive swallowing of air while eating or drinking is known as ________________.

8.52. The return of swallowed food to the mouth is known as ________________.

8.53. A yellow discoloration of the skin caused by greater-than-normal amounts of bilirubin in the blood is called ________________.

8.54. The ________________ is the ring-like muscle that controls the flow from the stomach to the small intestine.

8.55. The medical term for the solid body wastes that are expelled through the rectum is ________________.

WORD SURGERY

Divide each term into its component word parts. Write these word parts, in sequence, on the lines provided. When necessary use a slash (/) to indicate a combining vowel. (You may not need all of the lines provided.)

8.56. An **esophagogastroduodenoscopy** is an endoscopic procedure that allows direct visualization of the upper GI tract.

__________ __________ __________ __________

8.57. A **periodontist** is a dental specialist who prevents or treats disorders of the tissues surrounding the teeth.

__________ __________ __________ __________

8.58. A **sigmoidoscopy** is the endoscopic examination of the interior of the rectum, sigmoid colon, and possibly a portion of the descending colon.

__________ __________ __________ __________

8.59. An **antiemetic** is a medication that is administered to prevent or relieve nausea and vomiting.

__________ __________ __________ __________

8.60. A **gastroduodenostomy** is the establishment of an anastomosis between the upper portion of the stomach and the duodenum.

__________ __________ __________ __________

TRUE/FALSE

If the statement is true, write **True** on the line. If the statement is false, write **False** on the line.

8.61. ________________ Cholangitis is an acute infection of the bile duct characterized by pain in the upper right quadrant of the abdomen, fever, and jaundice.

8.62. ________________ Cholangiography is an endoscopic diagnostic procedure.

8.63. ________________ Acute necrotizing ulcerative gingivitis is caused by the abnormal growth of bacteria in the mouth.

8.64. ________________ Bruxism means to be without natural teeth.

8.65. ________________ A choledocholithotomy is an incision in the common bile duct for the removal of gallstones.

CLINICAL CONDITIONS

Write the correct answer on the line provided.

8.66. James Ridgeview was diagnosed as having ________________, which is the partial or complete blockage of the small or large intestine.

8.67. Chang Hoon suffers from ________________. This condition is an abnormal accumulation of serous fluid in the peritoneal cavity.

8.68. Rita Martinez is a dentist. She described her patient Mr. Espinoza as being ________________, which means that he was without natural teeth.

8.69. Baby Kilgore was vomiting almost continuously. The medical term for this excessive vomiting is ________________.

8.70. A/An ________________ was performed on Mr. Schmidt to create an artificial excretory opening between his colon and body surface.

8.71. After eating, Mike Delahanty often complained about heartburn. The medical term for this condition is ________________.

8.72. After the repeated passage of black, tarry, and foul-smelling stools, Catherine Baldwin was diagnosed as having ________________. This condition is caused by the presence of digested blood in the stools.

8.73. Alberta Roberts was diagnosed as having an inflammation of one or more diverticula. The medical term for this condition is ________________.

8.74. Carlotta Hansen has blister-like sores on her lips and adjacent facial tissue. She says they are cold sores; however, the medical term for this condition is________________ .

8.75. Lisa Wilson saw her dentist because she was concerned about bad breath. Her dentist refers to this condition as ________________.

WHICH IS THE CORRECT MEDICAL TERM?

Select the correct answer, and write it on the line provided.

8.76. The ________________ test detects hidden blood in the stools.

anoscopy colonoscopy enema Hemoccult

8.77. A/An ______________ is a surgical connection between two hollow or tubular structures.

anastomosis ostomy stoma sphincter

8.78. The eating disorder characterized by voluntary starvation and excessive exercising because of an intense fear of gaining weight is known as______________.

anorexia anorexia nervosa bulimia bulimia nervosa

8.79. The hardened deposit that forms on the teeth and irritate the surrounding tissues is known as dental ______________.

calculus caries decay plaque

8.80. The surgical removal of all or part of the liver is known as ______________.

anoplasty palatoplasty proctopexy hepatectomy

CHALLENGE WORD BUILDING

These terms are *not* found in this chapter; however, they are made up of the following familiar word parts. If you need help in creating the term, refer to your medical dictionary.

col/o	**-algia**
enter/o	**-ectomy**
esophag/o	**-itis**
gastr/o	**-megaly**
hepat/o	**-ic**
proct/o	**-pexy**
sigmoid/o	**-rrhaphy**

8.81. Surgical suturing of a stomach wound is known as ______________.

8.82. Pain in the esophagus is known as ______________.

8.83. The surgical removal of all or part of the sigmoid colon is a/an ______________.

8.84. Pain in and around the anus and rectum is known as ______________.

8.85. The surgical fixation of the stomach to correct displacement is a/an ______________.

8.86. Inflammation of the sigmoid colon is known as ______________.

8.87. The surgical removal of all or part of the esophagus and stomach is a/an ______________.

8.88. The term meaning relating to the liver and intestines is ______________.

8.89. Abnormal enlargement of the liver is known as ______________.

8.90. Inflammation of the stomach, small intestine, and colon is known as ______________.

LABELING EXERCISES

Identify the numbered items on the accompanying figure.

8.91. ______________ glands

8.92. ______________

8.93. ______________

8.94. ______________

8.95. ______________

8.96. ______________

8.97. ______________ intestine

8.98. vermiform ______________

8.99. ______________ intestine

8.100. ______________ and anus

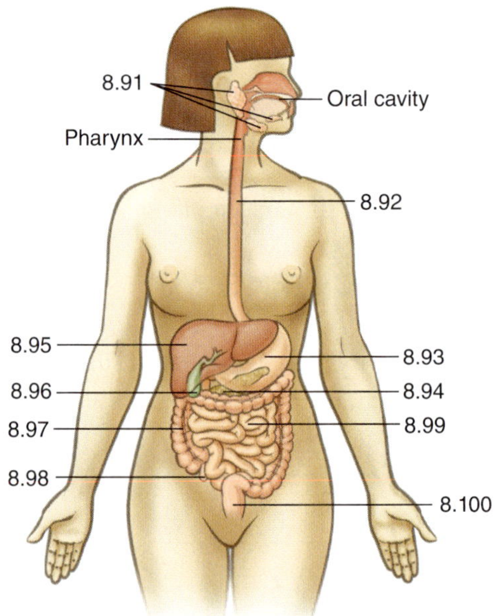

CHAPTER 9

The Urinary System

Overview of STRUCTURES, COMBINING FORMS, AND FUNCTIONS OF THE URINARY SYSTEM

Major Structures	Related Combining Forms	Primary Functions
Kidneys	**nephr/o**, **ren/o**	Filter the blood to remove waste products, maintain electrolyte concentrations, and remove excess water to maintain the fluid volume within the body.
Renal Pelvis	**pyel/o**	Collects urine produced by the kidneys.
Urine	**ur/o**, **urin/o**	Liquid waste products to be excreted.
Ureters	**ureter/o**	Transport urine from the kidneys to the bladder.
Urinary Bladder	**cyst/o**	Stores urine until it is excreted.
Urethra	**urethr/o**	Transports urine from the bladder through the urethral meatus, where it is excreted.
Prostate	**prostat/o**	A gland of the male reproductive system that surrounds the male urethra. Disorders of this gland can disrupt the flow of urine.

Vocabulary Related to **THE URINARY SYSTEM**

This list contains essential word parts and medical terms for this chapter. These terms are pronounced in the student StudyWARE™ and Audio CDs that are available for use with this text. These and the other important **primary terms** are shown in boldface throughout the chapter. *Secondary terms*, which appear in *orange* italics, clarify the meaning of primary terms.

Word Parts

- ☐ **-cele** hernia, tumor, swelling
- ☐ **cyst/o** urinary bladder, cyst, sac of fluid
- ☐ **dia-** through, between, apart, complete
- ☐ **-ectasis** stretching, dilation, enlargement
- ☐ **glomerul/o** glomerulus
- ☐ **lith/o** stone, calculus
- ☐ **-lysis** breakdown, separation, setting free, destruction, loosening
- ☐ **nephr/o** kidney
- ☐ **-pexy** surgical fixation
- ☐ **pyel/o** renal pelvis, bowl of kidney
- ☐ **-tripsy** to crush
- ☐ **ur/o** urine, urinary tract
- ☐ **ureter/o** ureter
- ☐ **urethr/o** urethra
- ☐ **-uria** urination, urine

Medical Terms

- ☐ **ablation** (ab-**LAY**-shun)
- ☐ **anuria** (ah-**NEW**-ree-ah)
- ☐ **benign prostatic hyperplasia** (bee-**NINE** pros-**TAT**-ick **high**-per-**PLAY**-zee-ah)
- ☐ **chronic kidney disease**
- ☐ **cystitis** (sis-**TYE**-tis)
- ☐ **cystocele** (**SIS**-toh-seel)
- ☐ **cystolith** (**SIS**-toh-lith)
- ☐ **cystopexy** (**SIS**-toh-**peck**-see)
- ☐ **cystoscopy** (sis-**TOS**-koh-pee)
- ☐ **dialysis** (dye-**AL**-ih-sis)
- ☐ **diuresis** (**dye**-you-**REE**-sis)
- ☐ **end-stage renal disease**
- ☐ **enuresis** (**en**-you-**REE**-sis)
- ☐ **epispadias** (**ep**-ih-**SPAY**-dee-as)
- ☐ **extracorporeal shockwave lithotripsy** (**ecks**-trah-kor-**POUR**-ee-al **LITH**-oh-**trip**-see)
- ☐ **glomerulonephritis** (gloh-**mer**-you-loh-neh-**FRY**-tis)
- ☐ **hemodialysis** (**hee**-moh-dye-**AL**-ih-sis)
- ☐ **hydronephrosis** (**high**-droh-neh-**FROH**-sis)
- ☐ **hydroureter** (**high**-droh-**YOUR**-eh-ter)
- ☐ **hyperproteinuria** (**high**-per-**proh**-tee-in-**YOU**-ree-ah)
- ☐ **hypoproteinemia** (**high**-poh-**proh**-tee-in-**EE**-mee-ah)
- ☐ **hypospadias** (**high**-poh-**SPAY**-dee-as)
- ☐ **incontinence** (in-**KON**-tih-nents)
- ☐ **interstitial cystitis** (**in**-ter-**STISH**-al sis-**TYE**-tis)
- ☐ **intravenous pyelogram** (**in**-trah-**VEE**-nus **PYE**-eh-loh-**gram**)
- ☐ **nephrolith** (**NEF**-roh-lith)
- ☐ **nephrolithiasis** (**nef**-roh-lih-**THIGH**-ah-sis)
- ☐ **nephrolysis** (neh-**FROL**-ih-sis)
- ☐ **nephrons** (**NEF**-ronz)
- ☐ **nephropathy** (neh-**FROP**-ah-thee)
- ☐ **nephroptosis** (**nef**-rop-**TOH**-sis)
- ☐ **nephropyosis** (**nef**-roh-pye-**OH**-sis)
- ☐ **nephrostomy** (neh-**FROS**-toh-me)
- ☐ **nephrotic syndrome** (neh-**FROT**-ick)
- ☐ **neurogenic bladder** (new-roh-**JEN**-ick)
- ☐ **nocturia** (nock-**TOO**-ree-ah)
- ☐ **nocturnal enuresis** (nock-**TER**-nal **en**-you-**REE**-sis)
- ☐ **oliguria** (**ol**-ih-**GOO**-ree-ah)
- ☐ **percutaneous nephrolithotomy** (**per**-kyou-**TAY**-nee-us **nef**-roh-lih-**THOT**-oh-mee)
- ☐ **peritoneal dialysis** (**pehr**-ih-toh-**NEE**-al dye-**AL**-ih-sis)
- ☐ **polycystic kidney disease** (**pol**-ee-**SIS**-tick)
- ☐ **polyuria** (**pol**-ee-**YOU**-ree-ah)
- ☐ **prostatism** (**PROS**-tah-tizm)
- ☐ **pyeloplasty** (**PYE**-eh-loh-**plas**-tee)
- ☐ **pyelotomy** (**pye**-eh-**LOT**-oh-mee)
- ☐ **suprapubic catheterization** (**soo**-prah-**PYOU**-bick **kath**-eh-ter-eye-**ZAY**-shun)
- ☐ **uremia** (you-**REE**-mee-ah)
- ☐ **ureterectasis** (you-**reh**-ter-**ECK**-tah-sis)
- ☐ **ureterolith** (you-**REE**-ter-oh-**lith**)
- ☐ **ureterorrhagia** (you-**ree**-ter-oh-**RAY**-jee-ah)
- ☐ **ureterorrhaphy** (you-**reet**-eh-**ROAR**-ah-fee)
- ☐ **urethritis** (**you**-reh-**THRIGH**-tis)
- ☐ **urethropexy** (you-**REE**-throh-**peck**-see)
- ☐ **urethrorrhagia** (you-**ree**-throh-**RAY**-jee-ah)
- ☐ **urethrostenosis** (you-**ree**-throh-steh-**NOH**-sis)
- ☐ **urethrotomy** (**you**-reh-**THROT**-oh-mee)
- ☐ **urinary catheterization** (**kath**-eh-ter-eye-**ZAY**-shun)
- ☐ **vesicovaginal fistula** (**ves**-ih-koh-**VAJ**-ih-nahl **FIS**-tyou-lah)
- ☐ **voiding cystourethrography** (**sis**-toh-you-ree-**THROG**-rah-fee)
- ☐ **Wilms tumor**

LEARNING GOALS

On completion of this chapter, you should be able to:

1. Identify and describe the major functions and structures of the urinary system.
2. Identify the medical specialists who treat disorders of the urinary system.
3. Recognize, define, spell, and pronounce the primary terms related to the pathology and the diagnostic and treatment procedures of the urinary system.

FUNCTIONS OF THE URINARY SYSTEM

The urinary system performs many functions that are important in maintaining homeostasis. ***Homeostasis*** is the process through which the body maintains a constant internal environment (**home/o** means constant, and **-stasis** means control). These functions include:

- Maintaining the proper balance of water, salts, and acids in the body by filtering the blood as it flows through the kidneys.
- Constantly filtering the blood to remove urea, creatinine, uric acid, and other waste materials from the bloodstream. **Urea** (you-**REE**-ah) is the major waste product of protein metabolism. ***Creatinine*** is a waste product of muscle metabolism.
- Converting these waste products and excess fluids into **urine** in the kidneys and excrete them from the body via the urinary bladder.

STRUCTURES OF THE URINARY SYSTEM

The urinary system, also referred to as the ***urinary tract***, consists of two kidneys, two ureters, one bladder, and a urethra (Figures 9.1 and 9.4). The adrenal glands, which are part of the endocrine system, are located on the top of the kidneys.

The urinary tract is located in close proximity to the reproductive organs, so these two body systems are sometime referred to together as the ***genitourinary tract***.

The Kidneys

The **kidneys** constantly filter the blood to remove waste products and excess water. These are excreted as urine, which is 95% water and 5% urea and other body wastes.

About 200 quarts of blood are processed every day, producing an average of 2 quarts of urine. The kidneys also help the body maintain the proper level of fluid, produce hormones that control blood pressure and make red blood cells, and activate vitamin D to maintain healthy bones.

- The term **renal** (**REE**-nal) means pertaining to the kidneys (**ren** means kidney or kidneys, and **-al** means pertaining to).
- The two bean-shaped kidneys are located in the retroperitoneal space, with one on each side of the vertebral column below the diaphragm and the lower edge of the rib cage. ***Retroperitoneal*** means behind the peritoneum, which is the membrane that lines the abdominal cavity.
- The **renal cortex** (**REE**-nal **KOR**-tecks) is the outer region of the kidney. This layer of tissue contains more than one million microscopic units called nephrons. The term ***cortex*** means the outer portion of an organ.
- The **medulla** (meh-**DULL**-ah) is the inner region of the kidney, and it contains most of the urine-collecting tubules. A ***tubule*** is a small tube.

Nephrons

The **nephrons** (**NEF**-ronz) are the microscopic functional units of each kidney. It is here that urine is produced through the processes of filtration, reabsorption, and secretion (Figure 9.2). ***Reabsorption*** is the return to the blood of some of the substances that were removed during filtration.

- Each nephron contains a **glomerulus** (gloh-**MER**-you-lus), which is a cluster of capillaries (plural, *glomeruli*), surrounded by a cup-shaped membrane called the Bowman's capsule, and a **renal tubule**.
- Blood enters the kidney through the **renal artery** and flows into the nephrons.

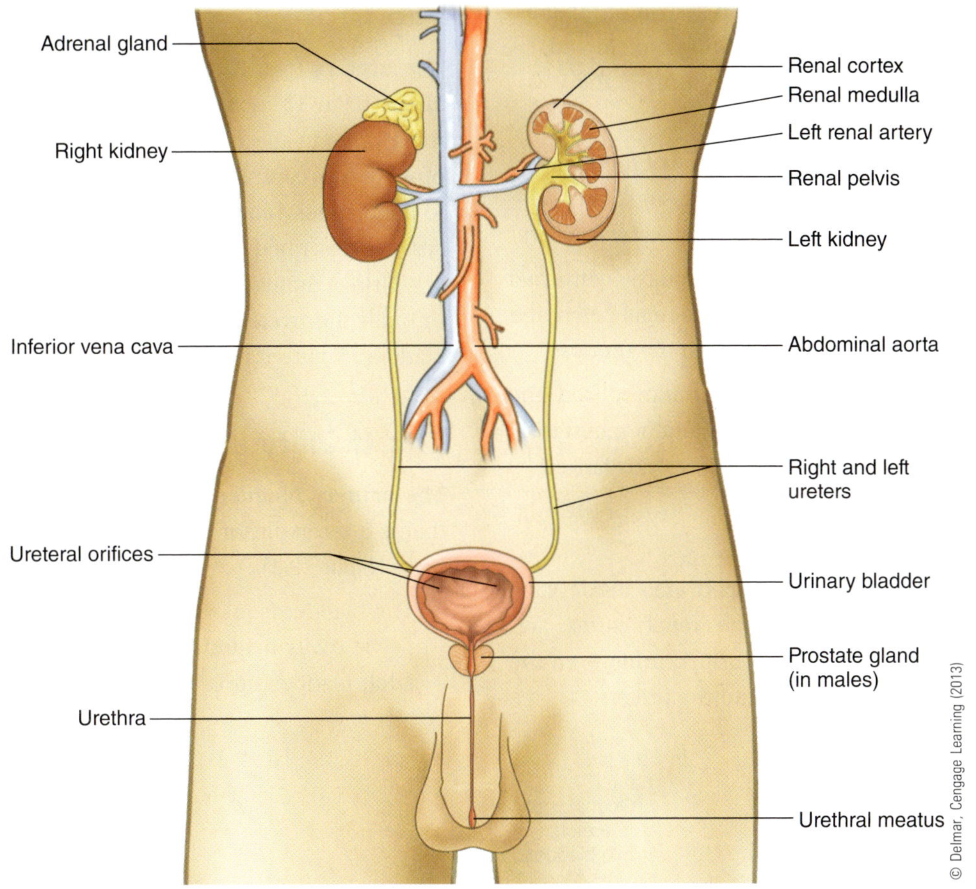

FIGURE 9.1 The primary structures of the urinary system, as shown here in a male, are the kidneys, ureters, urinary bladder, and urethra. The adrenal gland, positioned on top of each kidney, is a structure of the endocrine system. The prostrate gland, which is part of the male reproductive system, surrounds the urethra.

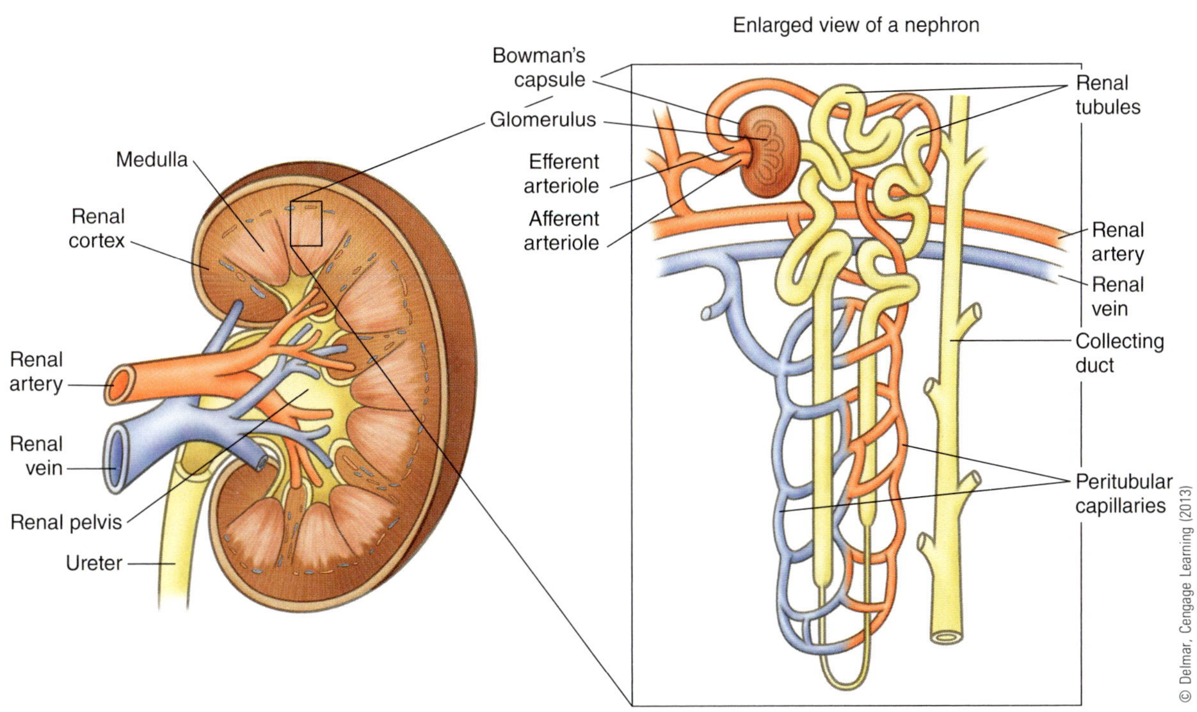

FIGURE 9.2 A nephron and its associated structures.

- After passing through the filtration system of the glomerulus, the filtered blood containing protein and blood cells leaves the kidney and returns to the bloodstream through the **renal vein**.
- The remaining filtrate flows into the renal tubules, where elements, including some water, sugar, and salts, are returned to the bloodstream via a nearby capillary.
- Remaining waste products are continuously converted into urine, which is transported to the renal pelvis and collected in preparation for entry into the ureters.
- If waste products are not efficiently removed from the bloodstream, the body cannot maintain homeostasis, with a stable balance of salts and other substances.

The Renal Pelvis

The **renal pelvis** is the funnel-shaped area inside each kidney that is surrounded by the renal cortex and medulla. This is where the newly formed urine from the nephrons collects before it flows into the ureters.

The Ureters

The **ureters** (you-**REE**-ters) are two narrow tubes, each about 10 to 12 inches long, which transport urine from the kidney to the bladder. ***Peristalsis***, which is a series of wave-like contractions, moves urine down each ureter to the bladder. (Peristalsis is also part of the digestive process, as described in Chapter 8.)

Urine drains from the ureters into the bladder through the **ureteral orifices** in the wall of the urinary bladder (Figure 9.1). ***Orifice*** means opening.

The Urinary Bladder

The **urinary bladder** is an oval, hollow muscular organ that is a reservoir for urine before it is excreted from the body (Figure 9.3).

- The bladder is located in the anterior portion of the pelvic cavity behind the pubic symphysis. The average adult bladder stores more than one pint of urine.

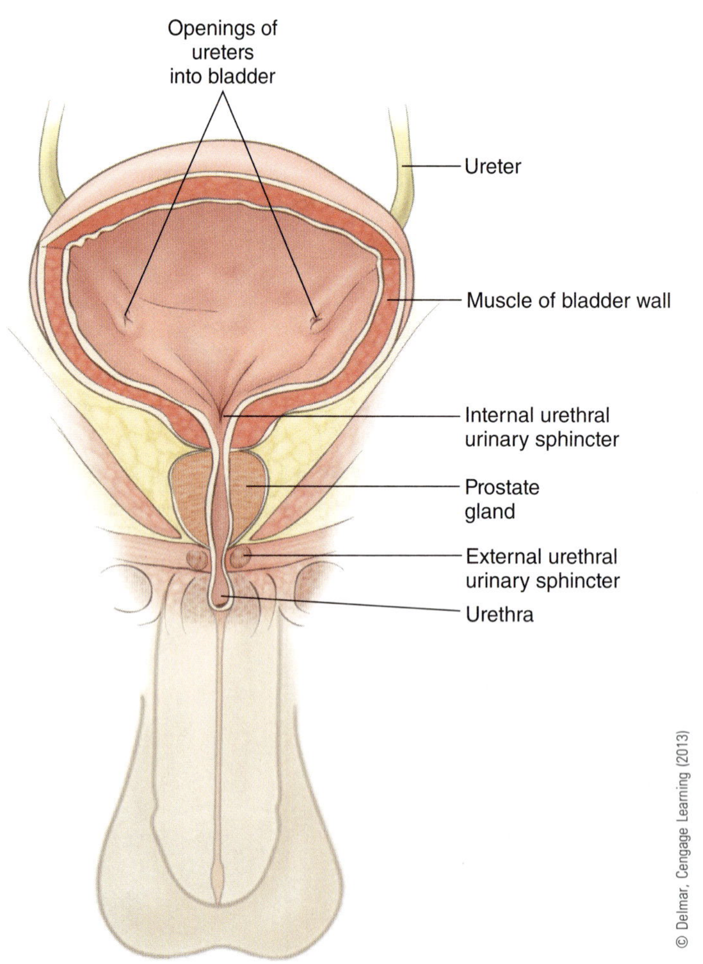

FIGURE 9.3 The structures of the male urinary bladder.

- Like the stomach, the bladder is lined with *rugae*. These folds allow it to expand when full and contract when empty.

The Urethra

The **urethra** (you-**REE**-thrah) is the tube extending from the bladder to the exterior of the body. Caution: the spellings of *ureter* and *urethra* are very similar! You may find it helpful to remember that the ureter comes first, both anatomically and alphabetically.

- There are two *urinary sphincters*, one located at either end of the urethra. These muscular rings control the flow of urine from the bladder into the urethra, and out of the urethra through the urethral meatus. A *sphincter* is a ring-like muscle that closes a passageway (Figure 9.3).
- The **urethral meatus** (you-**REE**-thrahl mee-**AY**-tus), also known as the *urinary meatus*, is the external opening of the urethra. The term *meatus* means the external opening of a canal.
- The **female urethra** is approximately 1.5 inches long, and the urethral meatus is located between the clitoris and the opening of the vagina (see Chapter 14). In the female, the urethra conveys only urine.
- The **male urethra** is approximately 8 inches long, and the urethral meatus is located at the tip of the penis (Figure 9.1). This urethra transports both urine and semen.
- The **prostate gland** (**PROS**-tayt), which is part of the male reproductive system, surrounds the urethra (Figure 9.3). Most disorders of the prostate affect the male's ability to urinate. For more information about the role of the prostate gland in reproduction, see Chapter 14.

THE EXCRETION OF URINE

Urination, also known as *voiding* or *micturition*, is the normal process of excreting urine.

- As the bladder fills up with urine, pressure is placed on the base of the urethra, resulting in the urge to **urinate** or *micturate*.
- Urination requires the coordinated contraction of the bladder muscles and relaxation of the sphincters. This action forces the urine through the urethra and out through the urethral meatus.

StudyWARE™ CONNECTION

Watch the **Urine Formation** animation in the StudyWARE™.

MEDICAL SPECIALTIES RELATED TO THE URINARY SYSTEM

- A **nephrologist** (neh-**FROL**-oh-jist) is a physician who specializes in diagnosing and treating diseases and disorders of the kidneys (**nephr** means kidney, and **-ologist** means specialist).

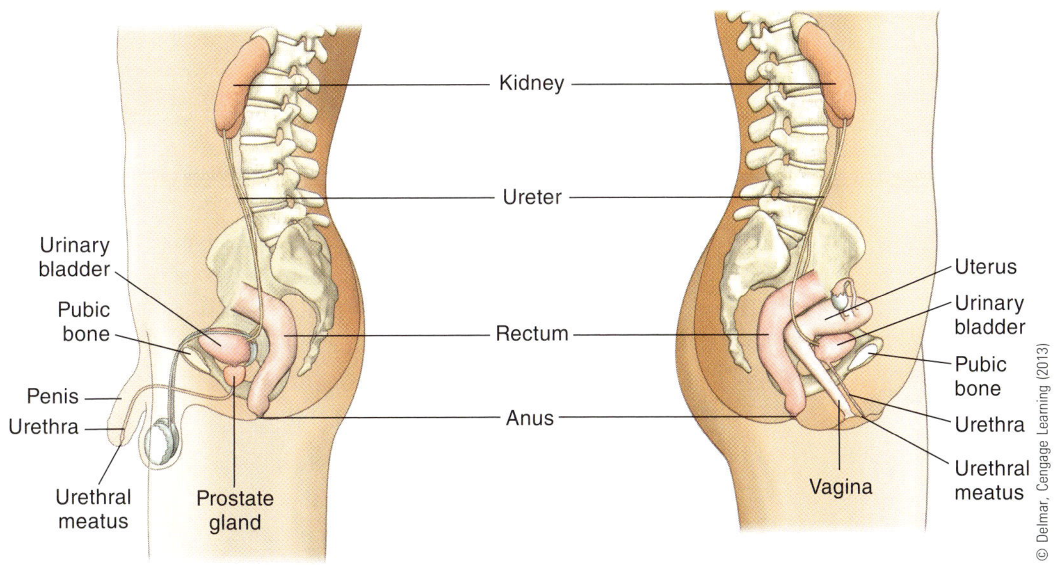

FIGURE 9.4 Cross-sections of the male and female urinary systems.

- A **urologist** (you-**ROL**-oh-jist) is a physician who specializes in diagnosing and treating diseases and disorders of the urinary system of females and the genitourinary system of males (**ur** means urine, and **-ologist** means specialist).

PATHOLOGY OF THE URINARY SYSTEM

Nephropathy

The term **nephropathy** (neh-**FROP**-ah-thee) means any disease of the kidney (**nephr/o** means kidney, and **-pathy** means disease). This definition includes both degenerative and inflammatory conditions. ***Diabetic nephropathy*** is kidney disease resulting from late-stage diabetes mellitus.

Renal Failure

Renal failure, also known as ***kidney failure***, is the inability of one or both of the kidneys to perform their functions. The body cannot replace damaged nephrons, and when too many nephrons have been destroyed, the result is kidney failure.

- **Uremia** (you-**REE**-mee-ah), also known as ***uremic poisoning***, is a toxic condition resulting from renal failure in which kidney function is compromised and urea and other waste products normally secreted in the urine are retained in the blood (**ur** means urine, and **-emia** means blood condition).
- **Acute renal failure** (ARF) has sudden onset and is characterized by uremia. It can be fatal if not reversed promptly. This condition can be caused by the kidneys not receiving enough blood to filter due to dehydration or a sudden drop in blood volume or blood pressure because of injury, burns, or a severe infection.
- **Chronic kidney disease** (CKD), also known as ***chronic renal disease***, or ***kidney failure***, is the progressive loss of renal function over months or years. This common condition, which can be life-threatening, may result from diabetes mellitus, hypertension, or a family history of kidney disease.
- The buildup of waste in the blood from chronic kidney disease can be a contributing factor in heart attacks and strokes.
- **End-stage renal disease** (ESRD) is the final stage of chronic kidney disease, and this condition is fatal unless the functions of the failed kidneys are successfully replaced by dialysis, or with a successful kidney transplant.

Nephrotic Syndrome

Nephrotic syndrome (neh-**FROT**-ick), also known as ***nephrosis***, is a group of conditions in which excessive amounts of protein are lost through the urine. This condition, which is usually caused by damage to the kidney's glomeruli, results in abnormally low levels of protein in the blood (**nephr/o** means kidney, and **-tic** means pertaining to).

- **Edema** (eh-**DEE**-mah) is excessive fluid accumulation in body tissues that can be symptomatic of nephrotic syndrome and other kidney diseases. This swelling can be in the area around the eyes, the abdomen, or the legs and feet.
- **Hyperproteinuria** (**high**-per-**proh**-tee-in-**YOU**-ree-ah) is the presence of abnormally high concentrations of protein in the *urine* (**hyper-** means excessive, **protein** means protein, and **-uria** means urine).
- **Hypoproteinemia** (**high**-poh-**proh**-tee-in-**EE**-mee-ah) is the presence of abnormally low concentrations of protein in the *blood* (**hypo-** means deficient or decreased, **protein** means protein, and **-emia** means blood condition). This condition is often associated with hyperproteinuria.
- Causes of nephrotic syndrome include diabetes mellitus, infection, and kidney disorders. ***Minimal change disease***, so called because the nephrons look normal under a regular microscope, is the most common cause of nephrotic syndrome in children.

Additional Kidney Conditions

- **Hydronephrosis** (**high**-droh-neh-**FROH**-sis) is the dilation (swelling) of one or both kidneys (**hydr/o** means water, **nephr** means kidney, and **-osis** means abnormal condition or disease). This condition can be caused by problems associated with the backing up of urine due to an obstruction such as a nephrolith (kidney stone) or a stricture (narrowing) in the ureter (Figure 9.5).
- **Nephritis** (neh-**FRY**-tis) is an inflammation of the kidney or kidneys (**nephr** means kidney, and **-itis** means inflammation). The most common causes of nephritis are toxins, infection, or an autoimmune disease.

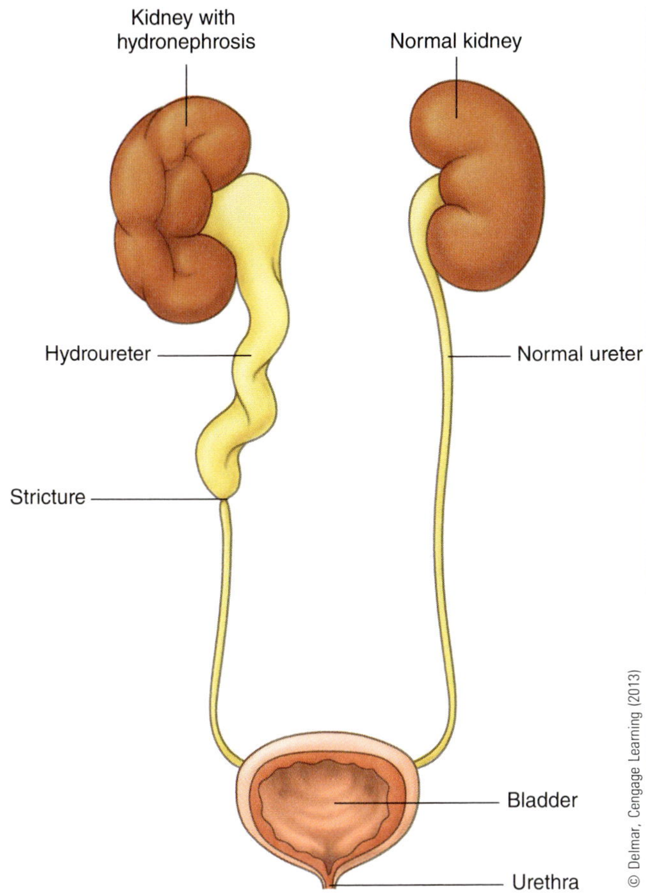

FIGURE 9.5 A stricture of the ureter can cause both hydronephrosis and hydroureter.

- **Glomerulonephritis** (gloh-**mer**-you-loh-neh-**FRY**-tis) is a type of nephritis caused by inflammation of the glomeruli that causes red blood cells and proteins to leak into the urine (**glomerul/o** means glomeruli, **nephr** means kidney, and **-itis** means inflammation).
- **Nephroptosis** (**nef**-rop-**TOH**-sis), also known as a ***floating kidney***, is the prolapse, or dropping down, of a kidney into the pelvic area when the patient stands. (**nephr/o** means kidney, and **-ptosis** means droop or sag). ***Prolapse*** means slipping or falling out of place.
- **Nephropyosis** (**nef**-roh-pye-**OH**-sis), also known as ***pyonephrosis***, is suppuration of the kidney (**nephr/o** means kidney, **py** means pus, and **-osis** means abnormal condition or disease). ***Suppuration*** means the formation or discharge of pus.
- **Polycystic kidney disease** (PKD) (**pol**-ee-**SIS**-tick) is a genetic disorder characterized by the growth of numerous fluid-filled cysts in the kidneys (**poly-** means many, **cyst** means cyst, and **-ic** means pertaining to). These cysts, which slowly replace much of the mass of the kidney, reduce the kidney function, and this eventually leads to kidney failure (Figure 9.6).
- **Renal colic** (**REE**-nal **KOLL**-ick) is an acute pain in the kidney area that is caused by blockage during the passage of a nephrolith (kidney stone). ***Colic*** means spasms of pain in the abdomen. Renal colic pain sometimes comes in waves due to the peristaltic movement of the ureters.

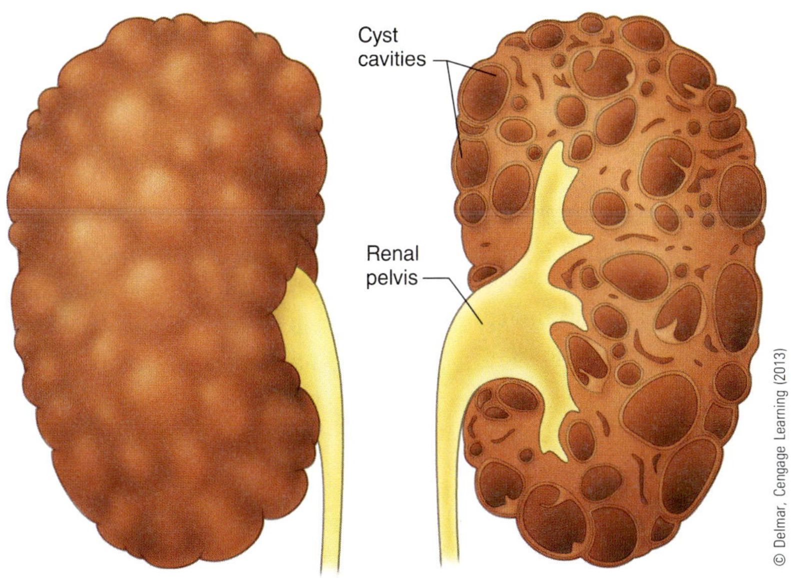

FIGURE 9.6 Polycystic kidney disease: On the left is the exterior of a kidney with polycystic disease. On the right is a cross-section view of a kidney with polycystic disease.

- A **Wilms tumor** is a rare type of malignant tumor of the kidney that occurs in young children. There is a high cure rate for this condition when treated promptly.

Stones

A **stone**, also known as *calculus*, is an abnormal mineral deposit that has formed within the body and is named for the organ or tissue where it is located (plural, *calculi*). These stones vary in size from small sand-like granules that pass through the body unnoticed to stones the size of marbles that can become lodged, causing acute pain.

- In the urinary system, stones form when waste products in the urine separate and crystallize (Figure 9.7). Normally urine contains chemicals to prevent this from happening; however, dehydration and other factors may also disrupt this balance.
- The term **nephrolithiasis** (**nef**-roh-lih-**THIGH**-ah-sis) describes the presence of stones in the kidney (**nephr/o** means kidney, and **-lithiasis** means the presence of stones). As these stones travel with the flow of urine, they are named for the location where they become lodged.
- A **nephrolith** (**NEF**-roh-lith), also known as a *kidney stone* or a *renal calculus*, is found in the kidney (**nephr/o** means kidney, and **-lith** means stone).
- A **ureterolith** (you-**REE**-ter-oh-**lith**) is a stone located anywhere along the ureter (**ureter/o** means ureter, and **-lith** means stone).
- A **cystolith** (**SIS**-toh-lith) is a stone located within the urinary bladder (**cyst/o** means bladder, and **-lith** means stone).

The Ureters

- **Hydroureter** (**high**-droh-**YOUR**-eh-ter) is the condition of the distention (swelling) of the ureter with urine that cannot flow because the ureter is blocked (**hydr/o** means water, and **-ureter** means ureter) (Figure 9.5). Hydroureter always accompanies hydronephrosis, discussed earlier.
- **Ureterectasis** (you-**reh**-ter-**ECK**-tah-sis) is the distention (enlargement) of a ureter (**ureter** means ureter, and **-ectasis** means enlargement).
- **Ureterorrhagia** (you-**ree**-ter-oh-**RAY**-jee-ah) is the discharge of blood from the ureter (**ureter/o** means ureter, and **-rrhagia** means bleeding).

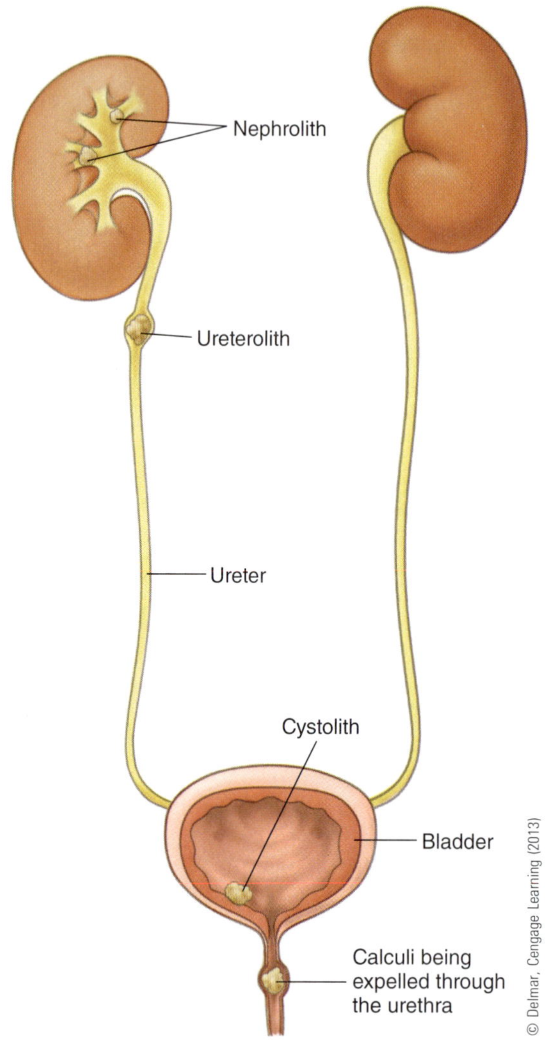

FIGURE 9.7 Potential locations of renal stones (calculi) as they move through the urinary system.

The Urinary Bladder

- **Cystalgia** (sis-**TAL**-jee-ah) and *cystodynia* both mean pain in the bladder (**cyst** means bladder, and **-algia** means pain).
- A **cystocele** (**SIS**-toh-seel), also known as a *prolapsed bladder*, is a hernia of the bladder through the vaginal wall (**cyst/o** means bladder, and **-cele** means hernia). This sometimes occurs as a result of pregnancy or childbirth.
- **Interstitial cystitis** (**in**-ter-**STISH**-al sis-**TYE**-tis) is a chronic inflammation within the walls of the bladder. The symptoms of this condition are similar to those of cystitis; however, they do not respond to traditional treatment. *Interstitial* means relating to spaces within a tissue or organ.

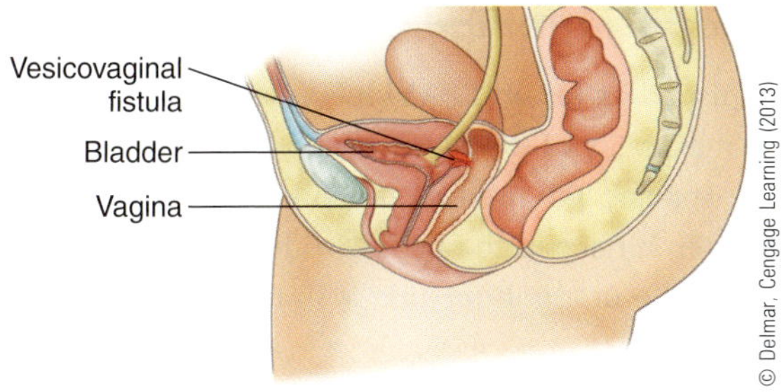

FIGURE 9.8 A vesicovaginal fistula allows urine to flow into the vagina.

- A **vesicovaginal fistula** (**ves**-ih-koh-**VAJ**-ih-nahl **FIS**-tyou-lah) is an abnormal opening between the bladder and vagina that allows constant involuntary flow of urine from the bladder into the vagina (**vesic/o** means bladder, **vagin** means vagina, and **-al** means pertaining to). A ***fistula*** is an abnormal passage between two internal organs (Figure 9.8). A vesicovaginal fistula may be caused by prolonged labor during childbirth or surgery such as a hysterectomy.

Neurogenic Bladder

Neurogenic bladder (new-roh-**JEN**-ick) is a urinary problem caused by interference with the normal nerve pathways associated with urination (**neur/o** means nerve, and **-genic** means created by). Normal urinary function depends on nerves to sense when the bladder is full, and to control the muscles that either retain the urine or allow the bladder to empty.

- Depending on the type of neurological disorder causing the problem, the bladder may empty spontaneously, resulting in incontinence, which is discussed in a later section.
- In contrast, the problem can prevent the bladder from emptying at all or from emptying completely. This can result in urinary retention with overflow leakage.
- Some of the causes of this condition are a tumor of the nervous system, trauma, neuropathy, or an inflammatory condition such as multiple sclerosis. ***Neuropathy*** is any disease or damage to a nerve.

The Prostate Gland

- **Benign prostatic hyperplasia (BPH)**, (bee-**NINE** pros-**TAT**-ick **high**-per-**PLAY**-zee-ah), also known as ***benign prostatic hypertrophy*** or ***enlarged prostate***, is an enlargement of the prostate gland that most often occurs in men older than age 50 (Figure 9.9). This condition can make urination difficult and causes other urinary tract problems for men. ***Hyperplasia*** is an increase in cell numbers typically associated with tumor growth; however, in this case, it is not caused by cancer or infection.
- **Prostatism** (**PROS**-tah-tizm) is a disorder resulting from the compression or obstruction of the urethra due to benign prostatic hyperplasia (**prostat** means prostate gland, and **-ism** means condition of). This can produce difficulties with urination and with urinary retention.

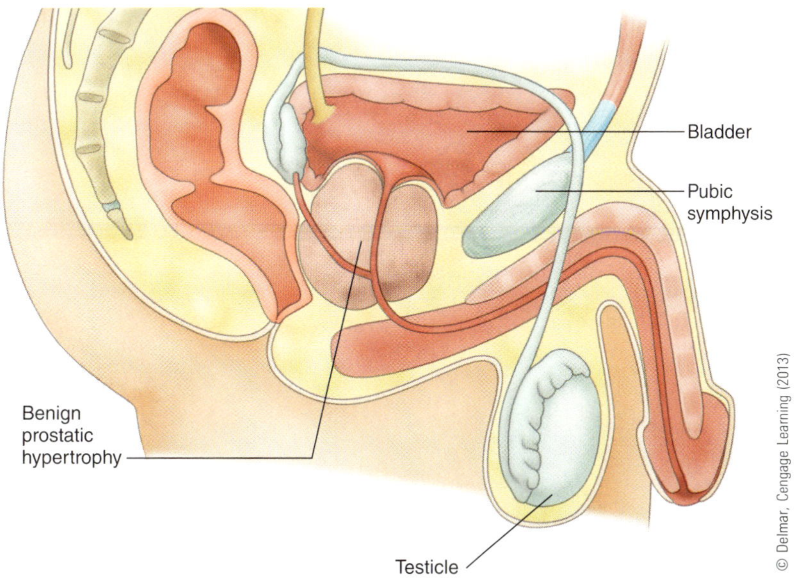

FIGURE 9.9 In benign prostatic hyperplasia, the enlarged prostate presses against the bladder and slows the flow of urine through the urethra.

- **Prostate cancer** is one of the most common cancers among men. The disease can grow slowly with no symptoms, or it can grow aggressively and spread throughout the body.
- **Prostatitis** (**pros**-tah-**TYE**-tis) is a group of disorders characterized by the inflammation of the prostate gland (**prostat** means prostate gland, and **-itis** means inflammation).
  - The most common type is ***chronic nonbacterial prostatitis***, with no single known cause.
  - ***Bacterial prostatitis*** usually results from bacteria transported in the urine.

The Urethra

- **Urethrorrhagia** (you-**ree**-throh-**RAY**-jee-ah) is bleeding from the urethra (**urethr/o** means urethra, and **-rrhagia** means bleeding).
- **Urethrorrhea** (you-**ree**-throh-**REE**-ah) is an abnormal discharge from the urethra (**urethr/o** means urethra, and **-rrhea** means flow or discharge). This condition is associated with some sexually transmitted diseases (see Chapter 14).
- **Urethrostenosis** (you-**ree**-throh-steh-**NOH**-sis), or ***urethral stricture***, is narrowing of the urethra (**urethr/o** means urethra, and **-stenosis** means tightening or narrowing). This condition occurs almost exclusively in men and is caused by scarring from infection or injury.

Abnormal Urethral Openings

- **Epispadias** (**ep**-ih-**SPAY**-dee-as) is a congenital abnormality of the urethral opening. In the male with epispadias, the urethral opening is located on the upper surface of the penis. In the female with epispadias, the urethral opening is in the region of the clitoris.
- **Hypospadias** (**high**-poh-**SPAY**-dee-as) is a congenital abnormality of the urethral opening. In the male with hypospadias, the urethral opening is on the ventral surface (underside) of the penis. In the female with hypospadias, the urethra opens into the vagina.

Urinary Tract Infections

A **urinary tract infection (UTI)** usually begins in the bladder; however, such an infection can affect all parts of the urinary system. These common infections are caused by bacteria, most often *E. coli*, entering the urinary system through the urethra. They occur more frequently in women because the urethra is short and located near the opening to the rectum.

- **Cystitis** (sis-**TYE**-tis) is an inflammation of the bladder (**cyst** mean bladder, and **-itis** means inflammation) (Figure 9.10A). See also *interstitial cystitis* in the earlier section on the urinary bladder.
- **Pyelitis** (**pye**-eh-**LYE**-tis) is an inflammation of the renal pelvis (**pyel** means renal pelvis, and **-itis** means inflammation) (Figure 9.10B).

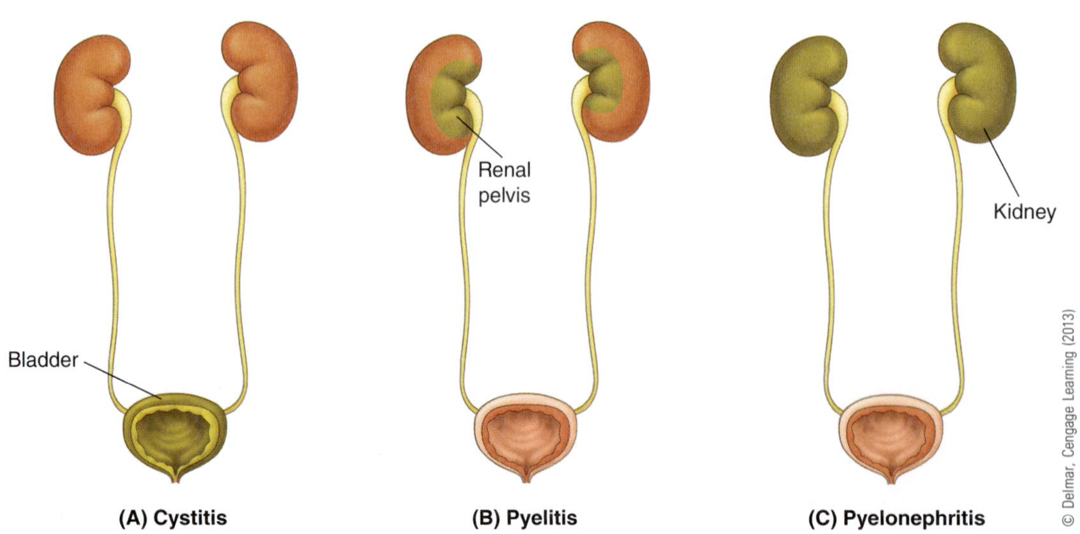

FIGURE 9.10 Infections of the urinary tract, indicated in green: (A) cystitis; (B) pyelitis; and (C) pyelonephritis.

- **Pyelonephritis** (**pye**-eh-loh-neh-**FRY**-tis) is an inflammation of both the renal pelvis and of the kidney (**pyel/o** means renal pelvis, **nephr** means kidney, and **-itis** means inflammation). This is usually caused by a bacterial infection that has spread upward from the bladder (Figure 9.10C).
- **Urethritis** (**you**-reh-**THRIGH**-tis) is an inflammation of the urethra (**urethr** means urethra, and **-itis** means inflammation).

Urination

- **Anuria** (ah-**NEW**-ree-ah) is the absence of urine formation by the kidneys (**an-** means without, and **-uria** means urine). This condition is often caused by a failure in kidney function, or a urinary tract obstruction.
- **Diuresis** (**dye**-you-**REE**-sis) is the increased output of urine (**diur** means increasing the output of urine, and **-esis** means an abnormal condition).
- **Dysuria** (dis-**YOU**-ree-ah) is difficult, or painful urination (**dys-** means painful, and **-uria** means urination). This condition is frequently associated with urinary tract infections.
- **Enuresis** (**en**-you-**REE**-sis) is the involuntary discharge of urine (**en-** means into, and **-uresis** means urination).
- **Nocturnal enuresis** (nock-**TER**-nal **en**-you-**REE**-sis) is urinary incontinence during sleep. It is also known as ***bed-wetting***. ***Nocturnal*** means pertaining to night.
- **Nocturia** (nock-**TOO**-ree-ah) is frequent and excessive urination during the night (**noct** means night, and **-uria** means urination).
- **Oliguria** (**ol**-ih-**GOO**-ree-ah) means scanty urination (**olig** means scanty, and **-uria** means urination). This can be caused by dehydration, renal failure, or a urinary tract obstruction. Oliguria is the opposite of polyuria.
- **Polyuria** (**pol**-ee-**YOU**-ree-ah) means excessive urination and is a common symptom of diabetes (**poly-** means many, and **-uria** means urination). Polyuria is the opposite of oliguria.
- **Urinary hesitancy** is difficulty in starting a urinary stream. This condition is most common in older men with enlarged prostate glands. In younger people, the inability to urinate when another person is present is known as ***bashful bladder syndrome***.
- **Urinary retention**, also known as ***ischuria***, is the inability to completely empty the bladder when attempting to urinate. This condition is also more common in men and is frequently associated with an enlarged prostate gland.

Incontinence

Incontinence (in-**KON**-tih-nents) is the inability to control the excretion of urine, feces, or both.

- **Urinary incontinence** is the inability to control the voiding of urine.
- **Overflow incontinence** is continuous leaking from the bladder either because it is full or because it does not empty completely. It is usually caused by a blocked urethra and is prevalent in older men with enlarged prostates.
- **Stress incontinence** is the inability to control the voiding of urine under physical stress such as running, lifting, sneezing, laughing, or coughing. This condition occurs much more often in women than in men.
- **Overactive bladder** (OAB), also known as ***urge incontinence***, occurs when the muscles of the bladder contract involuntarily even though the bladder is not actually full enough to indicate the need to urinate. The urinary sphincters' relaxation in response to this urgent need to urinate may result in urinary frequency or accidental urination. This is a common condition in adults older than 40 and may be caused by excessive consumption of caffeine or alcohol, urinary tract infections, neurological diseases, or bladder or prostate problems.

DIAGNOSTIC PROCEDURES OF THE URINARY SYSTEM

- **Urinalysis** (**you**-rih-**NAL**-ih-sis) is the examination of urine to determine the presence of abnormal elements (**urin** means urine, and **-analysis** means a study of the parts). These tests, which are used to diagnose diseases as well as to detect the presence of substances such as illegal drugs, are discussed further in Chapter 15.
- A **bladder ultrasound** is the use of a handheld ultrasound transducer to look for stones or for elevation of the bladder by an enlarged prostate, and to measure the residual amount of urine remaining in the bladder after urination. A normal bladder holds between 300 and 400 mL of urine. When more than this amount is still present after urination, the bladder is described as being ***distended***, or enlarged.

- **Urinary catheterization** (**kath**-eh-ter-eye-**ZAY**-shun) is the insertion of a tube into the bladder to procure a sterile specimen for diagnostic purposes. It is also used to drain urine from the bladder when the patient is unable to urinate for other reasons. Another use is to place medication into the bladder. (See the later section "Treatment Procedures for the Urinary Bladder.")
- **Cystoscopy** (sis-**TOS**-koh-pee) is the visual examination of the urinary bladder with the use of a specialized type of endoscope known as a cystoscope (**cyst/o** means bladder, and **-scopy** means visual examination) (Figure 9.11). An ***endoscope*** is an instrument used for visual examination of internal structures. A specialized cystoscope is also used for treatment procedures such as the removal of tumors or the reduction of an enlarged prostate gland.
- **Voiding cystourethrography** (**sis**-toh-you-ree-**THROG**-rah-fee) is a diagnostic procedure in which a fluoroscope is used to examine the flow of urine from the bladder and through the urethra (**cyst/o** means bladder, **urethr/o** means urethra, and **-graphy** means the process of producing a picture or record). This procedure is often performed after cystography.
- **Computed tomography**, also known as a ***CAT scan***, is more commonly used as a primary tool for evaluation of the urinary system because it can be rapidly performed and provides additional imaging of the abdomen, which may reveal other potential sources for the patient's symptoms. ***Nephrotomography*** is the use of a CAT scan to examine the kidneys.

StudyWARE™ CONNECTION

Watch the **Cystoscopy** animation in the StudyWARE™.

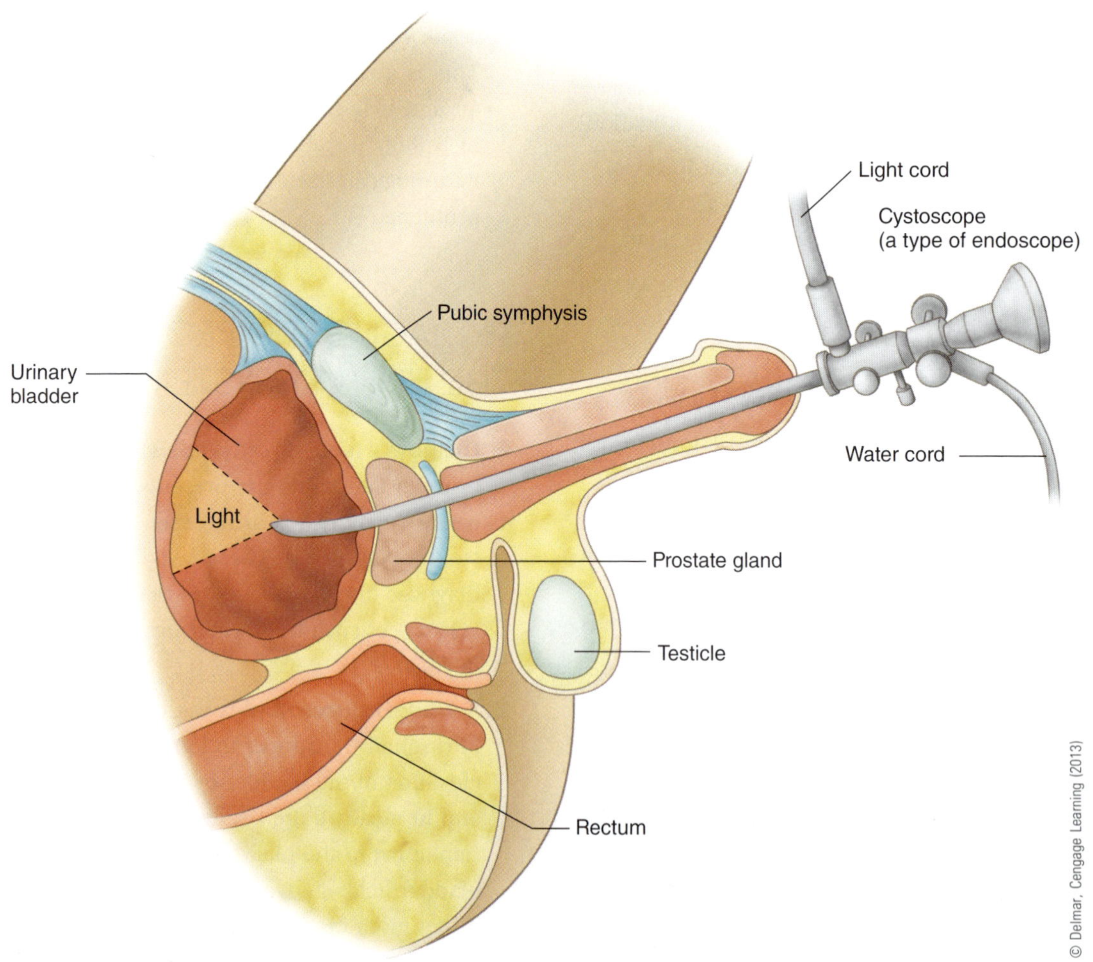

FIGURE 9.11 Use of a cystoscope to examine the interior of the bladder in a male.

Radiographic Examinations of the Urinary System

- **Cystography** (sis-**TOG**-rah-fee) is a radiographic, or x-ray, examination of the bladder after a contrast medium is instilled via a urethral catheter (**cyst/o** means bladder, and **-graphy** means the process of creating a picture or record). The resulting film is a ***cystogram***.
- An **intravenous pyelogram** (**in**-trah-**VEE**-nus **PYE**-eh-loh-**gram**) (IVP), also known as ***excretory urography***, is a radiographic study of the kidneys and ureters (**pyel/o** means renal pelvis, and **-gram** means a picture or record). A contrast medium is administered intravenously to clearly define these structures in the resulting image. This examination is used to diagnose changes in the urinary tract resulting from nephroliths, infections, enlarged prostate, tumors, and internal injuries after an abdominal trauma (Figure 9.12).
- A **KUB** (Kidneys, Ureters, Bladder) is a radiographic study without the use of a contrast medium. This study, also referred to as a ***flat-plate of the abdomen***, is used to detect bowel obstructions and nephroliths. Despite its name, a KUB x-ray does not show the ureters.

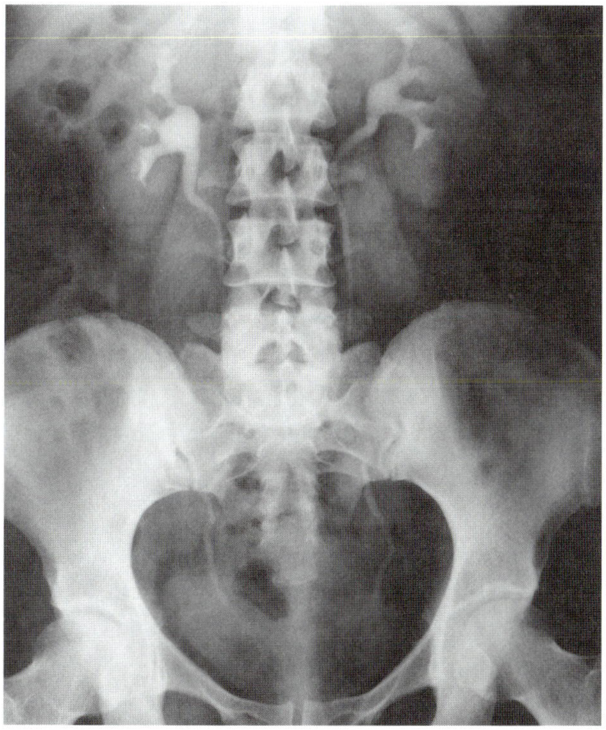

FIGURE 9.12 This normal, intravenous pyelogram shows the urinary tract, including the ureters, a kidney, and the bladder.

- **Retrograde urography** is a radiograph of the urinary system taken after a contrast medium has been placed in the urethra through a sterile catheter and caused to flow upward through the urinary tract (**ur/o** means urine, and **-graphy** means the process of creating a picture or record). ***Retrograde*** means moving backward.

Diagnostic Procedures of the Prostate Gland

- A **digital rectal examination** is performed on men by using a lubricated, gloved finger placed in the rectum to palpate the prostate gland to detect prostate enlargement and to look for indications of prostate cancer or tumors of the rectum. In this context, the term ***digital*** means using a finger. ***Palpate*** means the use of touch to examine a body part.
- The **prostate-specific antigen (PSA)** blood test is used to screen for prostate cancer. This test measures the amount of prostate-specific antigen that is present in a blood specimen. The ***prostate-specific antigen*** is a protein produced by the cells of the prostate gland to help liquefy semen. The higher a man's PSA level, the more likely cancer is present.

TREATMENT PROCEDURES OF THE URINARY SYSTEM

Medications

- **Diuretics** (**dye**-you-**RET**-icks) are medications administered to increase urine secretion, primarily to rid the body of excess water and salt. Some foods and drinks, such as coffee, tea, and alcoholic beverages, also have a diuretic effect.
- Other drugs used to treat urinary tract problems include ***antibiotics*** for urinary tract infections and ***antispasmodics*** to block the signals that cause urinary incontinence.

Dialysis

Dialysis (dye-**AL**-ih-sis) is a procedure to remove waste products, such as urea, creatinine, as well as excess water from the blood of a patient whose kidneys no longer function (**dia-** means complete or through, and **-lysis** means separation). The two types of dialysis in common use are *hemodialysis* and *peritoneal dialysis*. Patients can sometimes choose the type of long-term dialysis they prefer.

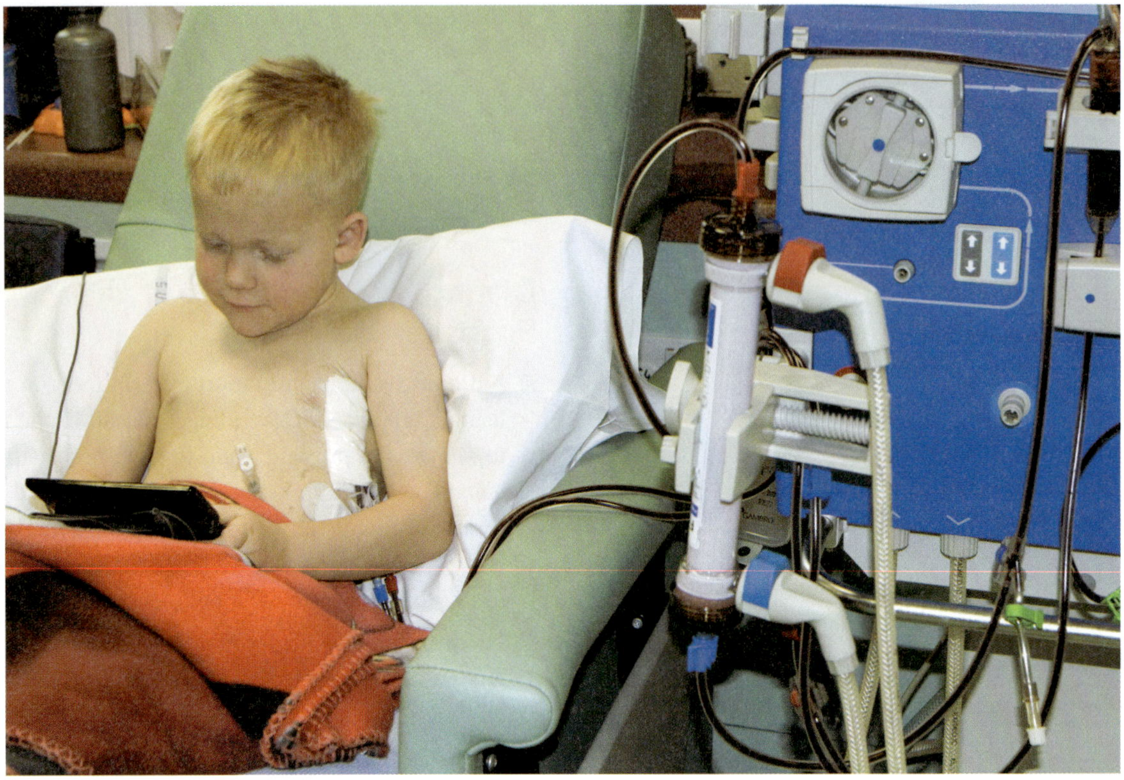

FIGURE 9.13 In a hemodialysis unit, waste is filtered from the patient's blood. The filtered blood is then returned to the patient's body.

Hemodialysis

Hemodialysis (**hee**-moh-dye-**AL**-ih-sis) is the process by which waste products are filtered directly from the patient's blood (**hem/o** means blood, **dia** means complete or through, and **-lysis** means separation). Treatment is performed on an external hemodialysis unit commonly referred to as an ***artificial kidney*** (Figure 9.13). Hemodialysis is the most common type of dialysis.

- A shunt implanted in the patient's arm is connected to the hemodialysis unit, and arterial blood flows through the filters of the unit. A ***shunt*** is an artificial passage that allows the blood to flow between the body and the hemodialysis unit.
- The filters contain ***dialysate***, which is a sterilized solution made up of water and electrolytes. This solution cleanses the blood by removing waste products and excess fluids.
- ***Electrolytes*** are the salts that conduct electricity and are found in the body fluid, tissue, and blood.
- The cleansed blood is returned to the body through a vein.
- These treatments each take several hours and must be repeated about three times a week.

Peritoneal Dialysis

In **peritoneal dialysis** (**pehr**-ih-toh-**NEE**-al dye-**AL**-ih-sis) the lining of the peritoneal cavity acts as the filter to remove waste from the blood. The dialysate, which is a sterile solution containing glucose, flows into the peritoneal cavity around the intestine through a catheter implanted in the abdominal wall. This fluid is left in for a period of time to absorb waste products and then drained out through the tube.

The process is normally repeated several times during the day and can be done using an automated system. This type of dialysis has some advantages: for example, it can be done at home by the patient. However, it is considered less effective than hemodialysis (Figure 9.14).

- ***Continuous ambulatory peritoneal dialysis*** provides ongoing dialysis as the patient goes about his or her daily activities. In this procedure, a dialysate solution is instilled from a plastic container worn under the patient's clothing. About every 4 hours, the used solution is drained back into this bag and the bag is discarded. A new bag is then attached, the solution is instilled, and the process continues.

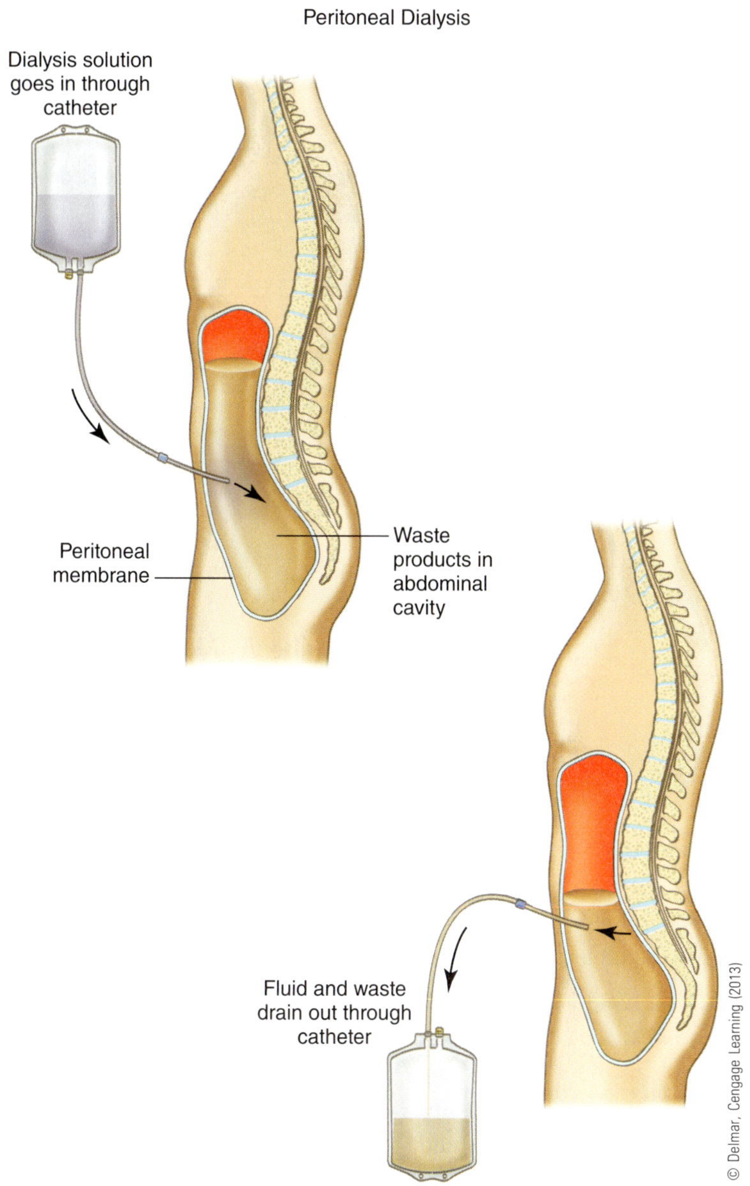

FIGURE 9.14 Peritoneal dialysis removes waste through a fluid exchange in the peritoneal cavity.

- ***Continuous cycling peritoneal dialysis*** uses a machine to cycle the dialysate fluid during the night while the patient sleeps.

The Kidneys

- **Nephrolysis** (neh-**FROL**-ih-sis) is the surgical freeing of a kidney from adhesions (**nephr/o** means kidney, and **-lysis** means setting free). An ***adhesion*** is a band of fibers that holds structures together abnormally.
- Note: The suffix **-lysis** means setting free; however, it also means destruction. Therefore, the term *nephrolysis* can also describe a pathologic condition in which there is destruction of renal cells.
- A **nephropexy** (**NEF**-roh-**peck**-see), also known as ***nephrorrhaphy***, is the surgical fixation of nephroptosis, or a floating kidney (**nephr/o** means kidney, and **-pexy** means surgical fixation).
- A **nephrostomy** (neh-**FROS**-toh-mee) is the placement of a catheter to maintain an opening from the pelvis of one or both kidneys to the exterior of the body (**nephr** means kidney, and **-ostomy** means creating an opening). In a kidney affected by hydronephrosis, this allows urine from the kidney to be drained directly through the lower back. Nephrostomy tubes are also used to gain access to the kidneys for diagnostic procedures.

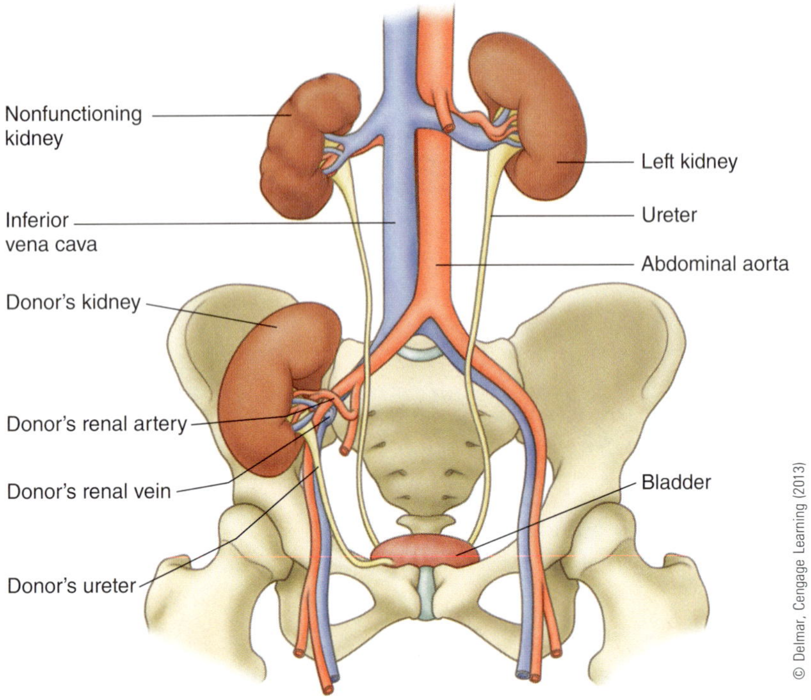

FIGURE 9.15 In a kidney transplant, the nonfunctioning kidney is usually not removed. Instead, the donor kidney and its associated structures are sutured into place at a lower point in the abdomen.

- **Pyeloplasty** (**PYE**-eh-loh-**plas**-tee) is the surgical repair of the ureter and renal pelvis (**pyel/o** means the renal pelvis, and **-plasty** means surgical repair). Hydronephrosis can cause damage to the ureter and renal pelvis.
- A **pyelotomy** (**pye**-eh-**LOT**-oh-mee) is a surgical incision into the renal pelvis (**pyel** means the renal pelvis, and **-otomy** means surgical incision). This procedure is performed to correct obstructions such as a stone lodged in the junction between the renal pelvis and the ureter.
- **Renal transplantation**, commonly known as a ***kidney transplant***, is the grafting of a donor kidney, from either a living or nonliving donor, into the body to replace the recipient's failed kidneys. Kidney donors need to be genetically similar to the recipient, although a tissue match increases the success rate. A single transplanted kidney is capable of adequately performing all kidney functions and frees the patient from the need for dialysis (Figure 9.15).

Treatment of Nephroliths

Most small nephroliths (kidney stones) pass out of the urinary tract naturally over a period of two days to three weeks. This process can be quite painful and is sometimes accompanied by vomiting due to the pain. Larger stones may require surgical intervention.

- **Extracorporeal shockwave lithotripsy** (**ecks**-trah-kor-**POUR**-ee-al **LITH**-oh-**trip**-see) (ESWL) is the most common kidney stone treatment (**lith/o** means stone, and **-tripsy** means to crush). High-energy ultrasonic waves traveling through water or gel are used to break up the stone into fragments, which are then excreted in the urine. ***Extracorporeal*** means situated or occurring outside the body (Figure 9.16).
- Lithotripsy is also used to break up calculi in the ureter, bladder, or urethra.
- A **percutaneous nephrolithotomy** (**per**-kyou-**TAY**-nee-us **nef**-roh-lih-**THOT**-oh-mee) is the surgical removal of a nephrolith through a small incision in the back (**nephr/o** means kidney, **lith** means stone, and **-otomy** means surgical incision). A small tube is temporarily inserted through the incision into the kidney. First urine is removed; then the stone is crushed and the pieces are removed. This procedure is used if ESWL has not been successful, if an infection is present, or if the stone is particularly large. ***Percutaneous*** means performed through the skin.

The Ureters

- A **ureterectomy** (**you**-reh-ter-**ECK**-toh-mee) is the surgical removal of a ureter (**ureter** means ureter, and **-ectomy** means surgical removal).

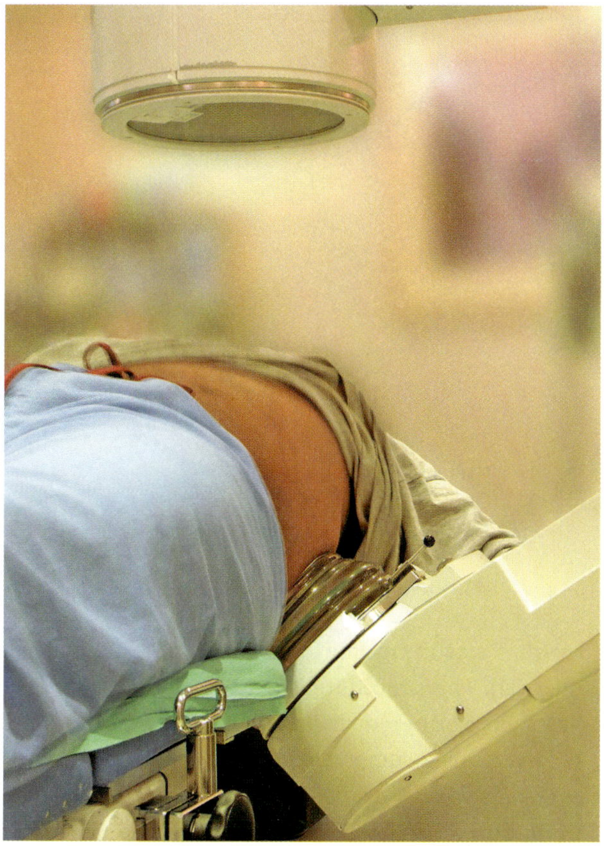

FIGURE 9.16 Extracorporeal shockwave lithotripsy uses shock waves traveling through water or a gel to destroy kidney stones.

- **Ureteroplasty** (you-**REET**-er-oh-**plas**-tee) is the surgical repair of a ureter (**ureter/o** means ureter, and **-plasty** means surgical repair).
- **Ureterorrhaphy** (you-**reet**-eh-R**OAR**-ah-fee) is the surgical suturing of a ureter (**ureter/o** means ureter, and **-rrhaphy** means surgical suturing).
- **Ureteroscopy** (you-**reet**-eh-**ROS**-koh-pee) is a treatment for a nephrolith lodged in the ureter (**ureter/o** means ureter, and **-scopy** means visual examination). A specialized instrument called a ***ureteroscope*** is inserted through the urethra and bladder into the ureter. If possible, the nephrolith is removed intact through the scope. If the stone is too large, a laser is used to break it up and the pieces are then removed.

The Urinary Bladder

- A **cystectomy** (sis-**TECK**-toh-mee) is the surgical removal of all or part of the urinary bladder. This procedure is usually performed to treat bladder cancer (**cyst** means bladder, and **-ectomy** means surgical removal).
- A **neobladder** (**NEE**-oh-**blad**-er) is a replacement for the missing bladder created by using about 20 inches of the small intestine. It allows patients to avoid having an abdominal stoma.
- An **ileal conduit** (**ill**-ee-al **KON**-doo-it), or ***ileostomy***, is the use of a small piece of intestine to convey urine to the ureters and to a stoma in the abdomen (**ile** means ileum or small intestine, and **-al** means pertaining to).
- **Cystopexy** (**sis**-toh-**peck**-see) is the surgical fixation of the bladder to the abdominal wall (**cyst/o** means bladder, and **-pexy** means surgical fixation).
- **Cystorrhaphy** (sis-**TOR**-ah-fee) is the surgical suturing of a wound or defect in the bladder (**cyst/o** means bladder, and **-rrhaphy** means surgical suturing).
- A **lithotomy** (lih-**THOT**-oh-mee) is a surgical incision for the removal of a nephrolith from the bladder (**lith** means stone, and **-otomy** means surgical incision). Although this surgery is no longer common, its name is still used to describe a physical examination position for procedures involving the pelvis and lower abdomen (see Chapter 15).

Urinary Catheterization

Urinary catheterization, also known as ***cathing***, is performed to withdraw urine for diagnostic purposes, to allow urine to drain freely, or to place a fluid such as a chemotherapy solution into the bladder (Figure 9.16). Note that the term *catheterization* may also refer to inserting a tube into the heart (see Chapter 5).

- An **indwelling catheter** remains inside the body for a prolonged time based on need (Figure 9.17A). ***Indwelling*** means residing within. This can be either a urethral or a suprapubic catheter.
- **Urethral catheterization** is performed by inserting a plastic tube called a ***catheter*** though the urethra and into the bladder.
- **Suprapubic catheterization** (**soo**-prah-**PYOU**-bick **kath**-eh-ter-eye-**ZAY**-shun) is the placement of a catheter into the bladder through a small incision made through the abdominal wall just above the pubic bone (Figure 9.17B).
- A **Foley catheter** is the most common type of indwelling catheter. This device is made of a flexible tube with a balloon filled with sterile water at the end to hold it in place in the bladder. It is commonly used on postsurgical patients.

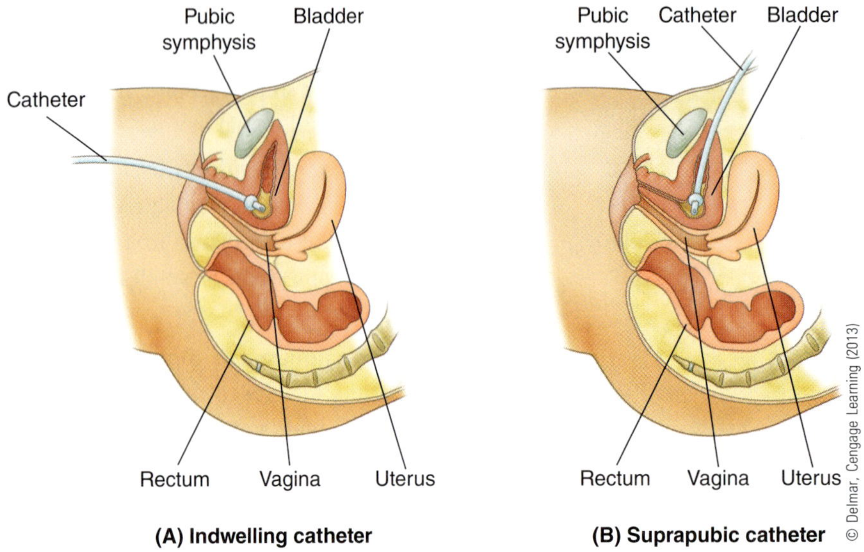

FIGURE 9.17 Types of urinary catheterization.

- An **intermittent catheter**, also known as a ***short-term catheter***, is inserted as needed several times a day to drain urine from the bladder.

The Urethra

- A **meatotomy** (**mee**-ah-**TOT**-oh-mee) is a surgical incision made in the urethral meatus to enlarge the opening (**meat** means meatus, and **-otomy** means surgical incision).
- **Urethropexy** (you-**REE**-throh-**peck**-see) is the surgical fixation of the urethra to nearby tissue (**urethr/o** means urethra, and **-pexy** means surgical fixation). This procedure is usually performed to correct urinary stress incontinence.
- A **urethrotomy** (**you**-reh-**THROT**-oh-mee) is a surgical incision into the urethra for relief of a stricture (**urethr** means urethra, and **-otomy** means surgical incision). A ***stricture*** is an abnormal narrowing of a bodily passage.

Prostate Treatment

- **Ablation** (ab-**LAY**-shun) is the term used to describe some types of treatment of prostate cancer. This treatment involves the removal of a body part or the destruction of its function through the use of surgery, hormones, drugs, heat, chemicals, electrocautery, or other methods. ***Electrocautery*** is the use of high-frequency electrical current to destroy tissue.
- A **prostatectomy** (**pros**-tah-**TECK**-toh-mee) is the surgical removal of part or all of the prostate gland (**prostat** means prostate, and **-ectomy** means surgical removal). This procedure is performed to treat prostate cancer or to reduce an enlarged prostate gland; however, this treatment can lead to erectile difficulties.
  - A ***radical prostatectomy*** is the surgical removal of the entire prostate gland in cases where it is extremely enlarged or when cancer is suspected.
  - A **transurethral prostatectomy**, also known as a ***TURP***, is the removal of excess tissue from an enlarged prostate gland with the use of a resectoscope. A ***resectoscope*** is a specialized endoscopic instrument that resembles a cystoscope (Figure 9.18).
- **Retrograde ejaculation** is when an orgasm results in semen flowing backward into the bladder instead of out through the penis. This is a common side effect of the transurethral prostatectomy. ***Retrograde*** means moving backward.
- ***Radiation therapy*** and ***hormone therapy*** are additional treatments used to control prostate cancer. ***Watchful waiting*** is often the prescribed course of action in older patients because this disease normally progresses slowly.

Urinary Incontinence Treatment

- **Kegel exercises**, which were named for Dr. Arnold Kegel, are a series of pelvic muscle exercises used to strengthen the muscles of the pelvic floor. They are used to control urinary stress incontinence in both sexes, in men to treat prostate pain and swelling, and in women to condition the muscles so that they will recover quickly after childbirth.

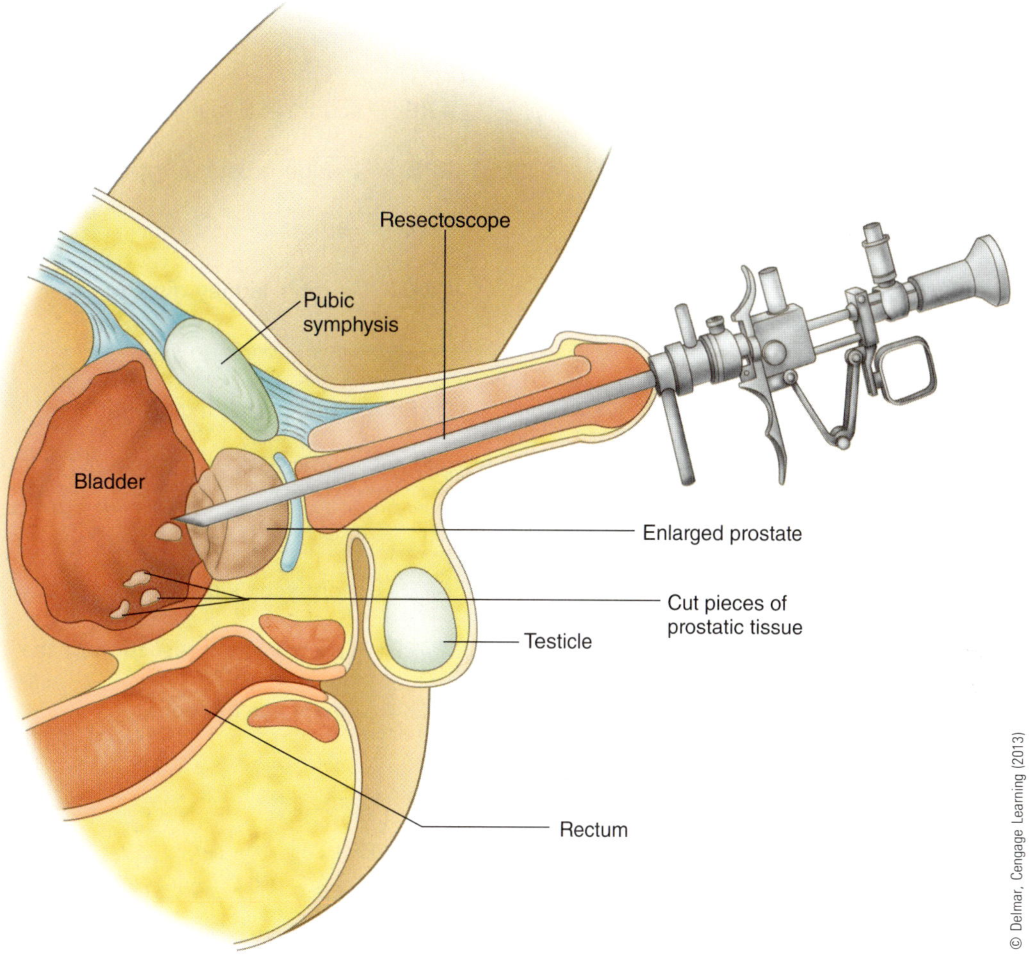

FIGURE 9.18 A transurethral prostatectomy (TURP) being performed with the use of a resectoscope.

- **Bladder retraining** is behavioral therapy in which the patient learns to urinate on a schedule, with increasingly longer time intervals as the bladder increases its capacity. The goal is to reestablish voluntary bladder control and to break the cycle of frequency and urgency that results from urge incontinence.

ABBREVIATIONS RELATED TO THE URINARY SYSTEM

Table 9.1 presents an overview of the abbreviations related to the terms introduced in this chapter. Note: To avoid errors or confusion, always be cautious when using abbreviations.

TABLE 9.1
Abbreviations Related to the Urinary System

acute renal failure = ARF	**ARF** = acute renal failure
benign prostatic hyperplasia = BPH	**BPH** = benign prostatic hyperplasia
catheterization = cath	**cath** = catheterization
chronic kidney disease = CKD	**CKD** = chronic kidney disease
cystoscopy = cysto	**cysto** = cystoscopy
digital rectal examination = DRE	**DRE** = digital rectal examination
end-stage renal disease = ESRD	**ESRD** = end-stage renal disease
intravenous pyelogram = IVP	**IVP** = intravenous pyelogram
polycystic kidney disease = PKD	**PKD** = polycystic kidney disease
transurethral resection of the prostate = TURP	**TURP** = transurethral resection of the prostate
urinary tract infection = UTI	**UTI** = urinary tract infection

StudyWARE CONNECTION

For more practice and to test your mastery of this material, go to the StudyWARE™ to play interactive games and complete the quiz for this chapter.

Workbook Practice

Go to your workbook, and complete the exercises for this chapter.

DELMAR MOBILE MEDIA

Downloadable audio is available for selected medical terms in this chapter to enhance your learning of medical terminology.

CHAPTER 9

LEARNING EXERCISES

MATCHING WORD PARTS 1

Write the correct answer in the middle column.

	Definition	Correct Answer	Possible Answers
9.1.	bladder	________________	-cele
9.2.	glomerulus	________________	cyst/o
9.3.	hernia, tumor, cyst	________________	glomerul/o
9.4.	kidney	________________	lith/o
9.5.	stone, calculus	________________	nephr/o

MATCHING WORD PARTS 2

Write the correct answer in the middle column.

	Definition	Correct Answer	Possible Answers
9.6.	urine, urinary tract	________________	-tripsy
9.7.	renal pelvis	________________	pyel/o
9.8.	setting free, separation	________________	-ur/o
9.9.	surgical fixation	________________	-pexy
9.10.	to crush	________________	-lysis

MATCHING WORD PARTS 3

Write the correct answer in the middle column.

	Definition	Correct Answer	Possible Answers
9.11.	complete, through	________________	-uria
9.12.	enlargement, stretching	________________	urethr/o

9.13. ureter ______________________ **ureter/o**

9.14. urethra ______________________ **-ectasis**

9.15. urination, urine ______________________ **dia-**

DEFINITIONS

Select the correct answer, and write it on the line provided.

9.16. Urine is carried from the kidneys to the urinary bladder by the ______________________.

glomeruli nephrons urethras ureters

9.17. A stone in the urinary bladder is known as a ______________________.

cholelith cystolith nephrolith ureterolith

9.18. The increased output of urine is known as ______________________.

anuria diuresis dysuria oliguria

9.19. Before entering the ureters, urine collects in the ______________________.

glomeruli renal cortex renal pelvis urinary bladder

9.20. Urine leaves the bladder through the ______________________.

prostate kidney ureter urethra

9.21. Urine is produced in microscopic functional units of each kidney called ______________________.

uremia ureters urethra nephrons

9.22. In the male, the ______________________ carries both urine and semen.

prostate gland renal pelvis ureter urethra

9.23. A specialist who treats the genitourinary system of males is a/an ______________________.

gynecologist nephrologist neurologist urologist

9.24. In ______________________, the urethral opening is on the upper surface of the penis.

epispadias hyperspadias hypospadias urethritis

9.25. The term ______________________ describes treatment in which a body part is removed or its function is destroyed. This type of procedure is frequently used to treat prostate cancer.

ablation adhesion lithotomy meatotomy

MATCHING STRUCTURES

Write the correct answer in the middle column.

	Definition	Correct Answer	Possible Answers
9.26.	the opening through which urine leaves the body	________________________	urethral meatus
9.27.	the portion of a nephron that is active in filtering urine	________________________	urethra
9.28.	the outer region of the kidney	________________________	ureters
9.29.	the tube from the bladder to the outside of the body	________________________	renal cortex
9.30.	the tubes that carry urine from the kidney to the bladder	________________________	glomerulus

WHICH WORD?

Select the correct answer, and write it on the line provided.

9.31. A surgical incision into the renal pelvis is ________________________.

pyelotomy pyeloplasty

9.32. The discharge of blood from the ureter is ________________________.

ureterorrhagia urethrorrhagia

9.33. The term meaning excessive urination is ________________________.

incontinence polyuria

9.34. The term meaning inflammation of the bladder is ________________________.

cystitis pyelitis

9.35. The major waste product of protein metabolism is ________________________.

urea urine

SPELLING COUNTS

Find the misspelled word in each sentence. Then write that word, spelled correctly, on the line provided.

9.36. A Willms tumor is a malignant tumor of the kidney that occurs in children. ______________________

9.37. Being unable to control excretory functions is known as incontinance. ______________________

9.38. The process of withdrawing urine from the bladder is known as urinary cathaterization. ______________________

9.39. Keagel exercises are a series of pelvic muscle exercises used to strengthen the muscles of the pelvic floor to control urinary stress incontinence. ______________________

9.40. A vesicovaginel fistula is an abnormal opening between the bladder and vagina. ______________________

ABBREVIATION IDENTIFICATION

In the space provided, write the words that each abbreviation stands for.

9.41. **BPH** ______________________________________

9.42. **ESRD** ______________________________________

9.43. **ESWL** ______________________________________

9.44. **IVP** ______________________________________

9.45. **OAB** ______________________________________

TERM SELECTION

Select the correct answer, and write it on the line provided.

9.46. The absence of urine formation by the kidneys is known as ______________________.

anuria | nocturia | oliguria | polyuria

9.47. The surgical suturing of the bladder is known as ______________________.

cystorrhaphy | cystorrhagia | cystorrhexis | nephrorrhaphy

9.48. The term meaning the freeing of a kidney from adhesions is ______________________.

nephrolithiasis | nephrolysis | anuria | pyelitis

9.49. The term meaning scanty urination is ______________________.

diuresis | dysuria | enuresis | oliguria

9.50. The process of artificially filtering waste products from the patient's blood is known as ____________________.

diuresis   hemodialysis   homeostasis   hydroureter

SENTENCE COMPLETION

Write the correct term or terms on the lines provided.

9.51. An inflammation of the kidney, most commonly caused by toxins, infection, or an autoimmune disease is called ____________________.

9.52. A stone located anywhere along the ureter is known as a ____________________.

9.53. The placement of a catheter into the bladder through a small incision made through the abdominal wall just above the pubic bone is known as ____________________.

9.54. The surgical fixation of the bladder to the abdominal wall is a/an ____________________.

9.55. A/An ____________________ (TURP) is the removal of excess tissue from the prostate with the use of a resectoscope.

WORD SURGERY

Divide each term into its component word parts. Write these word parts, in sequence, on the lines provided. When necessary, use a slash (/) to indicate a combining vowel. (You may not need all of the lines provided.)

9.56. **Hyperproteinuria** is abnormally high concentrations of protein in the urine.

__________ __________ __________ __________

9.57. **Hydronephrosis** is the dilation of one or both kidneys.

__________ __________ __________ __________

9.58. Voiding **cystourethrography** is a diagnostic procedure in which a fluoroscope is used to examine the flow of urine from the bladder and through the urethra.

__________ __________ __________ __________

9.59. A percutaneous **nephrolithotomy** is the surgical removal of a kidney stone through a small incision in the back.

__________ __________ __________ __________

9.60. **Ureterorrhaphy** means the surgical suturing of a ureter.

__________ __________ __________ __________

TRUE/FALSE

If the statement is true, write **True** on the line. If the statement is false, write **False** on the line.

9.61. ________ Stress incontinence is the inability to control the voiding of urine under physical stress such as running, sneezing, laughing, or coughing.

9.62. ________ Prostatism is a malignancy of the prostate gland.

9.63. ________ Urethrorrhea is bleeding from the urethra.

9.64. ________ Renal colic is an acute pain in the kidney area that is caused by blockage during the passage of a kidney stone.

9.65. ________ Acute renal failure has sudden onset and is characterized by uremia.

CLINICAL CONDITIONS

Write the correct answer on the line provided.

9.66. Mr. Baldridge suffers from excessive urination during the night. The medical term for this is ________________________.

9.67. Rosita LaPinta inherited ________________________ kidney disease. These cysts slowly reduce the kidney function, and this eventually leads to kidney failure.

9.68. Doris Volk has a chronic bladder condition involving inflammation within the wall of the bladder. This is known as ________________________.

9.69. John Danielson has an enlarged prostate gland. This caused narrowing of the urethra, which is known as ________________________.

9.70. Norman Smith was born with the opening of the urethra on the upper surface of the penis. This is known as ________________________.

9.71. Henry Wong's kidneys failed. He is being treated with ________________________ ________________________, which involves the removal of waste from his blood through a fluid exchange in the abdominal cavity.

9.72. Roberta Gridley is scheduled for surgical repair of damage to the ureter. This procedure is a/an ________________________.

9.73. When Lenny Nowicki's ________________ blood test showed a very high PSA level, his physician was concerned about the possibility of prostate cancer.

9.74. Dr. Morita's patient was diagnosed as having ________________. This is a type of kidney disease caused by inflammation of the glomeruli that causes red blood cells and proteins to leak into the urine.

9.75. Mrs. Franklin describes her condition as a floating kidney. The medical term for this condition, in which there is a dropping down of the kidney, is ________________.

WHICH IS THE CORRECT MEDICAL TERM?

Select the correct answer, and write it on the line provided.

9.76. Acute renal failure has sudden onset and is characterized by ________________. This condition can be caused by many factors, including a sudden drop in blood volume or blood pressure due to injury or surgery.

anuria dysuria enuresis uremia

9.77. The term ________________ means urinary incontinence during sleep. It is also known as bed-wetting.

nocturnal enuresis overactive bladder stress incontinence urinary incontinence

9.78. The term meaning the distention of the ureter is ________________.

ureteritis ureterectasis ureterolith urethrostenosis

9.79. The presence of abnormally *low* concentrations of protein in the blood is known as ________________.

hyperplasia hyperproteinuria hypocalcemia hypoproteinemia

9.80. A specialist in diagnosing and treating diseases and disorders of the kidneys is a/an ________________.

gynecologist nephrologist proctologist urologist

CHALLENGE WORD BUILDING

These terms are *not* found in this chapter; however, they are made up of the following familiar word parts. If you need help in creating the term, refer to your medical dictionary.

cyst/o	**-cele**
nephr/o	**-itis**
pyel/o	**-lysis**
ureter/o	**-malacia**
urethr/o	**-ostomy**
	-otomy
	-plasty
	-ptosis
	-rrhexis
	-sclerosis

9.81. The creation of an artificial opening between the urinary bladder and the exterior of the body is a/an ____________________.

9.82. A surgical incision into the kidney is a/an ____________________.

9.83. Abnormal hardening of the kidney is known as ____________________.

9.84. Prolapse of the bladder into the urethra is known as ____________________.

9.85. A prolapse of the female urethra is a/an ____________________.

9.86. The procedure to separate adhesions around a ureter is a/an ____________________.

9.87. Abnormal softening of the kidney is known as ____________________.

9.88. Inflammation of the renal pelvis and kidney is known as ____________________.

9.89. The surgical creation of an outside excretory opening from the urethra is a/an ____________________.

9.90. The surgical repair of the bladder is a/an ____________________.

LABELING EXERCISES

Identify the numbered items on the accompanying figure.

9.91. ____________________ gland

9.92. exterior view of the right ____________________

9.93. inferior ____________________

9.94. ____________________

9.95. renal ____________________

9.96. renal ____________________

9.97. abdominal ____________________

9.98. right and left ____________________

9.99. urinary ____________________

9.100. urethral ____________________

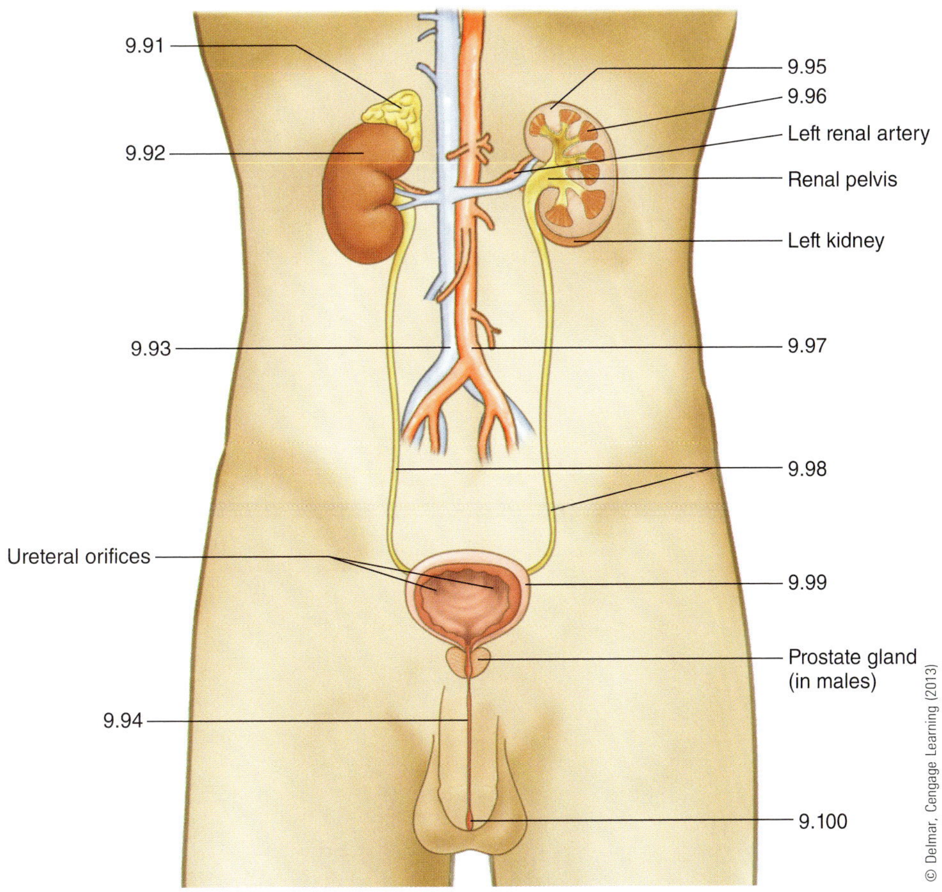

CHAPTER 10

The Nervous System

Overview of STRUCTURES, COMBINING FORMS, AND FUNCTIONS OF THE NERVOUS SYSTEM

Major Structures	Related Combining Forms	Primary Functions
Brain	**cerebr/o**, **encephal/o**	Coordinates all body activities by receiving and transmitting messages throughout the body.
Spinal Cord	**myel/o**	Transmits nerve impulses between the brain, arms and legs, and lower part of the body.
Nerves	**neur/i**, **neur/o**	Receive and transmit messages to and from all parts of the body.
Sensory Organs and Receptors		Receive external stimulation and transmit these stimuli to the sensory neurons.
Eyes (sight)		See Chapter 11.
Ears (hearing)		See Chapter 11.
Nose (smell)		See Chapter 7.
Skin (touch)		See Chapter 12.
Tongue (taste)		See Chapter 8.

Vocabulary Related to **THE NERVOUS SYSTEM**

This list contains essential word parts and medical terms for this chapter. These terms are pronounced in the student StudyWARE™ and Audio CDs that are available for use with this text. These and the other important **primary terms** are shown in boldface throughout the chapter. *Secondary terms*, which appear in *orange* italics, clarify the meaning of primary terms.

Word Parts

- ☐ **caus/o** burning, burn
- ☐ **cerebr/o** cerebrum, brain
- ☐ **concuss/o** shaken together, violently agitated
- ☐ **contus/o** bruise
- ☐ **encephal/o** brain
- ☐ **-esthesia** sensation, feeling
- ☐ **esthet/o** feeling, nervous sensation, sense of perception
- ☐ **-graphy** the process of producing a picture or record
- ☐ **mening/o** membranes, meninges
- ☐ **myel/o** spinal cord, bone marrow
- ☐ **neur/i**, **neur/o** nerve, nerve tissue
- ☐ **phobia** abnormal fear
- ☐ **psych/o** mind
- ☐ **radicul/o** root or nerve root
- ☐ **tropic** having an affinity for

Medical Terms

- ☐ **acrophobia** (**ack**-roh-**FOH**-bee-ah)
- ☐ **Alzheimer's disease** (**ALTZ**-high-merz)
- ☐ **amyotrophic lateral sclerosis** (ah-**my**-oh-**TROH**-fick skleh-**ROH**-sis)
- ☐ **anesthetic** (**an**-es-**THET**-ick)
- ☐ **anesthetist** (ah-**NES**-theh-tist)
- ☐ **anxiety disorders**
- ☐ **autism** (**AW**-tizm)
- ☐ **Bell's palsy** (**PAWL**-zee)
- ☐ **carotid ultrasonography** (kah-**ROT**-id **ul**-trah-son-**OG**-rah-fee)
- ☐ **causalgia** (kaw-**ZAL**-jee-ah)
- ☐ **cerebral contusion** (**SER**-eh-bral kon-**TOO**-zhun)
- ☐ **cerebral palsy** (**seh**-**REE**-bral **PAWL**-zee)
- ☐ **cerebrovascular accident** (**ser**-eh-broh-**VAS**-kyou-lar)
- ☐ **cervical radiculopathy** (rah-**dick**-you-**LOP**-ah-thee)
- ☐ **claustrophobia** (**klaws**-troh-**FOH**-bee-ah)
- ☐ **cognition** (kog-**NISH**-un)
- ☐ **coma** (**KOH**-mah)
- ☐ **concussion** (kon-**KUSH**-un)
- ☐ **cranial hematoma** (**hee**-mah-**TOH**-mah)
- ☐ **delirium** (deh-**LEER**-ee-um)
- ☐ **delirium tremens** (deh-**LEER**-ee-um **TREE**-mens)
- ☐ **delusion** (dih-**LOO**-zhun)
- ☐ **dementia** (dih-**MEN**-shah)
- ☐ **dura mater** (**DOO**-rah **MAH**-ter)
- ☐ **dyslexia** (dis-**LECK**-see-ah)
- ☐ **echoencephalography** (**eck**-oh-en-**sef**-ah-**LOG**-rah-fee)
- ☐ **electroencephalography** (ee-**leck**-troh-en-**sef**-ah-**LOG**-rah-fee)
- ☐ **encephalitis** (**en**-sef-ah-**LYE**-tis)
- ☐ **epidural anesthesia** (**ep**-ih-**DOO**-ral **an**-es-**THEE**-zee-ah)
- ☐ **epilepsy** (**EP**-ih-**lep**-see)
- ☐ **factitious disorder** (fack-**TISH**-us)
- ☐ **Guillain-Barré syndrome** (gee-**YAHN**-bah-**RAY SIN**-drohm)
- ☐ **hallucination** (hah-**loo**-sih-**NAY**-shun)
- ☐ **hemorrhagic stroke** (**hem**-oh-**RAJ**-ick)
- ☐ **hydrocephalus** (high-droh-**SEF**-ah-lus)
- ☐ **hyperesthesia** (**high**-per-es-**THEE**-zee-ah)
- ☐ **hypochondriasis** (**high**-poh-kon-**DRY**-ah-sis)
- ☐ **ischemic stroke** (iss-**KEE**-mick)
- ☐ **lethargy** (**LETH**-ar-jee)
- ☐ **meningitis** (**men**-in-**JIGH**-tis)
- ☐ **meningocele** (meh-**NING**-goh-**seel**)
- ☐ **migraine headache** (**MY**-grayn)
- ☐ **multiple sclerosis** (skleh-**ROH**-sis)
- ☐ **myelitis** (**my**-eh-**LYE**-tis)
- ☐ **myelography** (**my**-eh-**LOG**-rah-fee)
- ☐ **narcolepsy** (**NAR**-koh-**lep**-see)
- ☐ **neurotransmitters** (**new**-roh-trans-**MIT**-erz)
- ☐ **obsessive-compulsive disorder**
- ☐ **panic attack**
- ☐ **paresthesia** (**pair**-es-**THEE**-zee-ah)
- ☐ **Parkinson's disease**
- ☐ **peripheral neuropathy** (new-**ROP**-ah-thee)
- ☐ **post-traumatic stress disorder**
- ☐ **Reye's syndrome** (**RIZE SIN**-drome)
- ☐ **schizophrenia** (**skit**-soh-**FREE**-nee-ah)
- ☐ **sciatica** (sigh-**AT**-ih-kah)
- ☐ **seizure** (**SEE**-zhur)
- ☐ **shaken baby syndrome**
- ☐ **syncope** (**SIN**-koh-pee)
- ☐ **trigeminal neuralgia** (try-**JEM**-ih-nal new- **RAL**-jee-ah)

LEARNING GOALS

On completion of this chapter, you should be able to:

1. Describe the functions and structures of the nervous system.
2. Identify the major divisions of the nervous system, and describe the structures of each by location and function.
3. Identify the medical specialists who treat disorders of the nervous system.
4. Recognize, define, spell, and pronounce the primary terms related to the pathology and the diagnostic and treatment procedures of the nervous system.
5. Recognize, define, spell, and pronounce the primary terms related to the pathology and the diagnostic and treatment procedures of mental health disorders.

FUNCTIONS OF THE NERVOUS SYSTEM

The nervous system, with the brain as its center, coordinates and controls all bodily activities. When the brain ceases functioning, the body dies.

STRUCTURES OF THE NERVOUS SYSTEM

The major structures of the nervous system are the nerves, brain, spinal cord, and sensory organs. The sensory organs, which are the eyes, ears, nose, skin, and tongue, are discussed in other chapters.

Divisions of the Nervous System

For descriptive purposes, the nervous system is divided into two primary parts: the central and peripheral nervous systems (Figure 10.1).

- The **central nervous system** (CNS) includes the brain and spinal cord. The functions of the central nervous system are to receive and process information, and to regulate all bodily activity.
- The **peripheral nervous system** (PNS) includes the 12 pairs of cranial nerves extending from the brain and the 31 pairs of peripheral spinal nerves extending outward from the spinal cord. The function of the peripheral nervous system is to transmit nerve signals to and from the central nervous system.

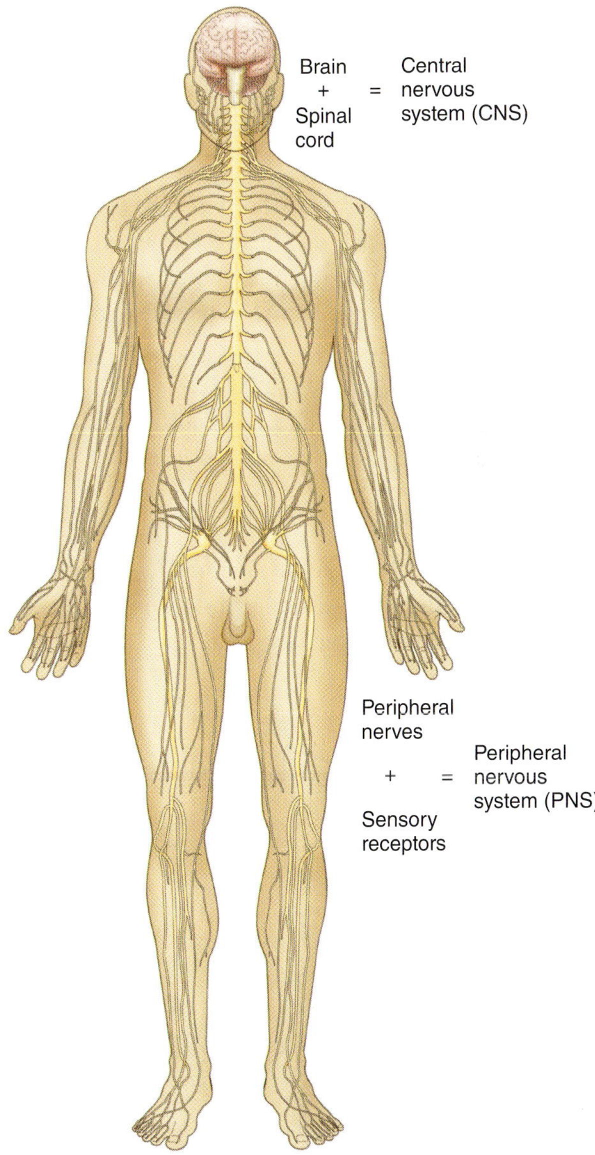

FIGURE 10.1 The structural organization of the central and peripheral nervous systems.

The Nerves

A **nerve** is one or more bundles of *neurons* that connect the brain and the spinal cord with other parts of the body. A **tract** is a bundle or group of nerve fibers located within the brain or spinal cord.

- ***Ascending nerve tracts*** carry nerve impulses *toward* the brain.
- ***Descending nerve tracts*** carry nerve impulses *away from* the brain.
- A **ganglion** (**GANG**-glee-on) is a nerve center made up of a cluster of nerve cell bodies outside the central nervous system (plural, *ganglia* or *ganglions*). Note: The term *ganglion* also describes a benign, tumor-like cyst.
- The term **innervation** (**in**-err-**VAY**-shun) means the supply of nerves to a specific body part.
- A **plexus** (**PLECK**-sus) is a network of intersecting spinal nerves (plural, *plexuses*) (Figure 10.8A). This term also describes a network of intersecting blood or lymphatic vessels.
- **Receptors** are sites in the sensory organs (eyes, ears, skin, nose, and taste buds) that receive external stimulation. The receptors send the stimulus through the sensory neurons to the brain for interpretation.
- A **stimulus** is anything that excites (activates) a nerve and causes an impulse (plural, *stimuli*). An ***impulse*** is a wave of excitation transmitted through nerve fibers and neurons.

The Reflexes

A **reflex** (**REE**-flecks) is an automatic, involuntary response to some change, either inside or outside the body. Examples of reflex actions include:

- Changes in the heart rate, breathing rate, and blood pressure
- Coughing and sneezing
- Responses to painful stimuli

Deep tendon reflexes are discussed in Chapter 4.

The Neurons

Neurons (**NEW**-ronz) are the basic cells of the nervous system that allow different parts of the body to communicate with each other.

- The body has billions of neurons carrying nerve impulses throughout the body via an electrochemical process. In the brain, this process creates patterns of neuron electrical activity known as ***brain waves***. Different types of brain waves are produced during periods of intense activity, rest, and sleep.
- The three types of neurons are described according to their function. The system of naming the neurons is summarized in Table 10.1. The memory aid **A-C-E** will help you remember their names, and **S-A-M** will help you remember their functions.

Neuron Parts

Each neuron consists of a cell body, several dendrites, a single axon, and terminal end fibers (Figure 10.2).

- The **dendrites** (**DEN**-drytes) are the root-like processes that receive impulses and conduct them to the cell body. A ***process*** is a structure that extends out from the cell body.
- The **axon** (**ACK**-son) is a process that conducts impulses away from the nerve cell. An axon can be more than 3 feet long. Many, but not all, axons are protected by a myelin sheath, which is a white fatty tissue covering.

TABLE 10.1
Types of Neurons and Their Functions

Types of Neurons	Neuron functions
"ACE"	"SAM"
Afferent neurons (**AF**-er-ent) ***Afferent*** means toward.	Also known as ***sensory neurons***, these neurons emerge from sensory organs and the skin to carry the impulses from the sensory organs *toward* the brain and spinal cord.
Connecting neurons	Also known as ***associative neurons***, these neurons link afferent and efferent neurons.
Efferent neurons (**EF**-er-ent) ***Efferent*** means away from.	Also known as ***motor neurons***, these neurons carry impulses *away from* the brain and spinal cord and toward the muscles and glands.

- **Terminal end fibers** are the branching fibers at the end of the axon that lead the nervous impulse from the axon to the synapse.
- A **synapse** (**SIN**-apps) is the space between two neurons or between a neuron and a receptor organ. A single neuron can have a few or several hundred synapses.

Neurotransmitters

Neurotransmitters (**new**-roh-trans-**MIT**-erz) are chemical substances that make it possible for messages to cross from the synapse of a neuron to the target receptor. There are between 200 and 300 known neurotransmitters, and each has a specialized function. Examples of neurotransmitters and their roles follow:

- *Acetylcholine* is released at some synapses in the spinal cord and at neuromuscular junctions; it influences muscle action.
- *Dopamine* is released within the brain. It is believed to be involved in mood and thought disorders and in abnormal movement disorders such as Parkinson's disease.
- *Endorphins* are naturally occurring substances that are produced by the brain to help relieve pain.
- *Norepinephrine* affects alertness and arousal, increasing blood pressure and heart rate, and releasing stores of glucose in response to stress. It is also a hormone released by the adrenal gland as part of the body's fight-or-flight response (see Chapter 13).

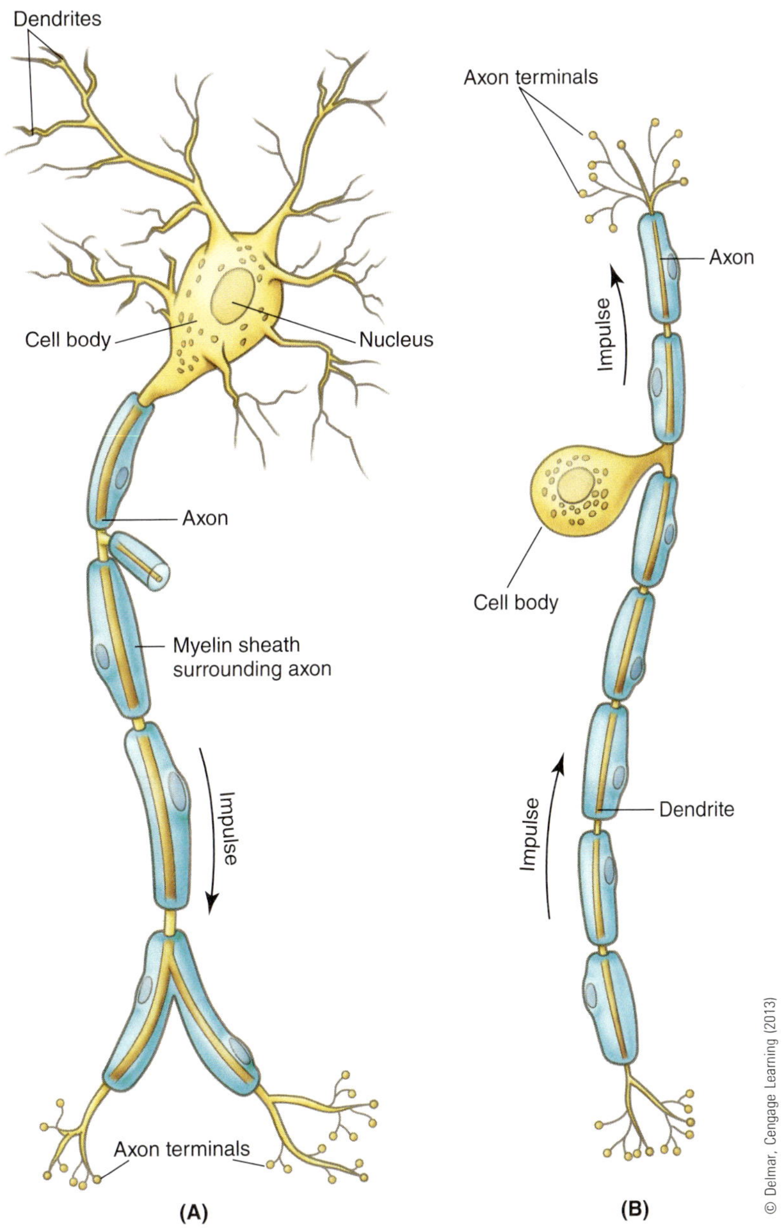

FIGURE 10.2 The structure of two types of neurons. (A) Efferent (motor) neurons. (B) Afferent (sensory) neurons.

- *Serotonin*, which is released in the brain, has roles in sleep, hunger, and pleasure recognition. It is also sometimes linked to mood disorders.

Glial Cells

Glial cells (**GLEE**-ul) provide support and protection for neurons, and their four main functions are (1) to surround neurons and hold them in place, (2) to supply nutrients and oxygen to neurons, (3) to insulate one neuron from another, and (4) to destroy and remove dead neurons.

The Myelin Sheath

A **myelin sheath** (**MY**-eh-lin) is the protective covering made up of glial cells. This white sheath forms the white matter of the brain and covers some parts of the spinal cord and the axon of most peripheral nerves (Figure 10.2).

- The portion of the nerve fibers that are myelinated are known as *white matter*. The term *myelinated* means having a myelin sheath. It is the color of this covering that makes these fibers white.
- The portion of the nerve fibers that are unmyelinated are known as *gray matter*. The term *unmyelinated* means lacking a myelin sheath. It is the lack of the myelin sheath that creates the gray color of the brain and spinal cord.

THE CENTRAL NERVOUS SYSTEM

The **central nervous system** is made up of the brain and spinal cord. These structures are protected externally by the bones of the cranium and the vertebrae of the spinal column, which are discussed in Chapter 3. Within these bony structures, the brain and spinal cord are further protected by the meninges and the cerebrospinal fluid (Figure 10.3).

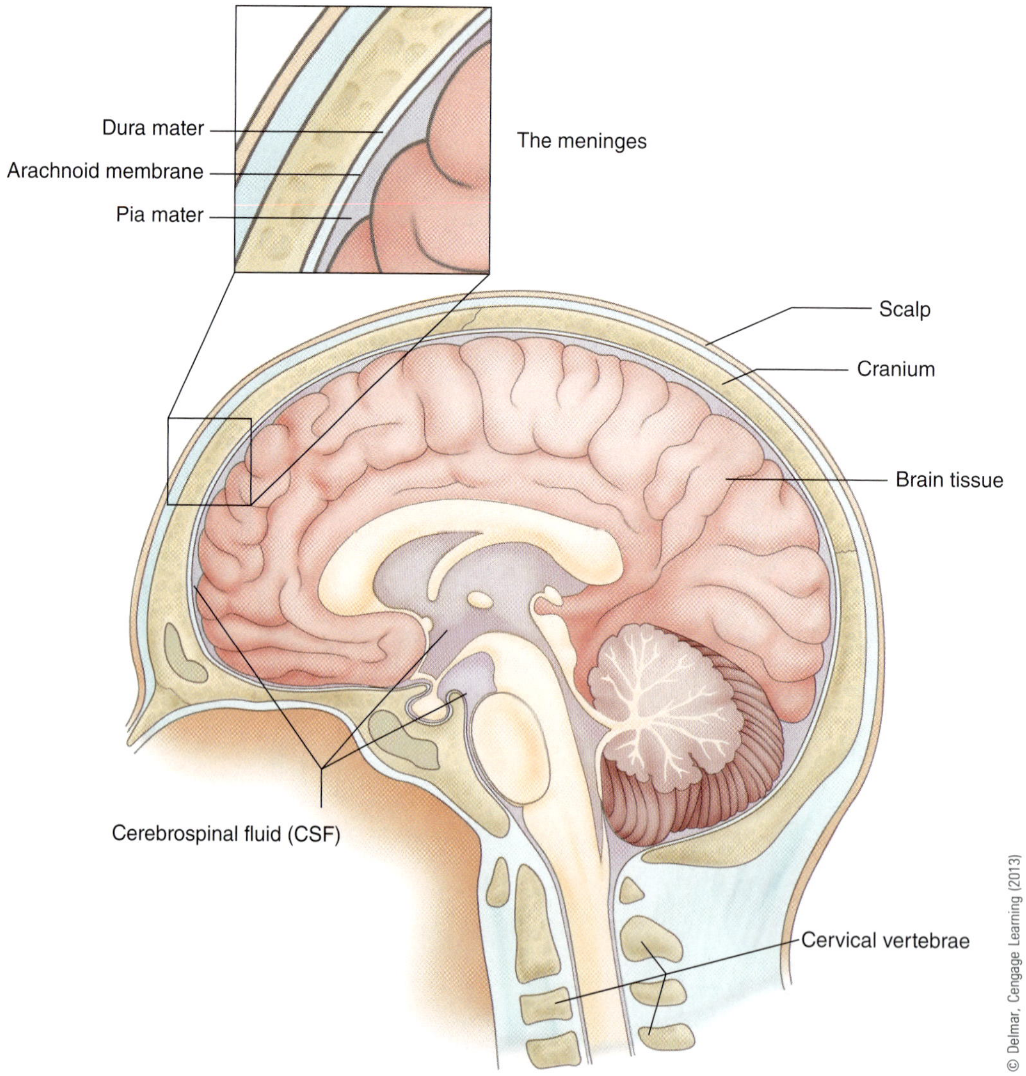

FIGURE 10.3 A cross-section of the brain showing the meninges and the protective coverings. The cerebrospinal fluid is shown in purple.

The Meninges

The **meninges** (meh-**NIN**-jeez) are the system of membranes that enclose the brain and spinal cord (singular *meninx*). The meninges consist of three layers of connective tissue. These are the dura mater, arachnoid membrane, and the pia mater (Figure 10.3).

The Dura Mater

The **dura mater** (**DOO**-rah **MAH**-ter) is the thick, tough, outermost membrane of the meninges. ***Dura*** means hard, and ***mater*** means mother.

- The inner surface of the cranium (skull) is lined with the dura mater.
- The inner surface of the vertebral column is known as the ***epidural space***. This space, which is located between the walls of the vertebral column and the dura mater of the meninges, contains fat and supportive connective tissues to cushion the dura mater.
- In both the skull and vertebral column, the ***subdural space*** is located between the dura mater and the arachnoid membrane.

The Arachnoid Membrane

The **arachnoid membrane** (ah-**RACK**-noid), which resembles a spiderweb, is the second layer of the meninges and is located between the dura mater and the pia mater. ***Arachnoid*** means having to do with spiders.

- The arachnoid membrane is loosely attached to the other meninges to allow space for fluid to flow between the layers.
- The ***subarachnoid space***, which is located below the arachnoid membrane and above the pia mater, contains cerebrospinal fluid.

The Pia Mater

The **pia mater** (**PEE**-ah **MAH**-ter), which is the third layer of the meninges, is located nearest to the brain and spinal cord. It consists of delicate connective tissue that contains a rich supply of blood vessels. ***Pia*** means tender or delicate, and ***mater*** means mother.

StudyWARE CONNECTION

Watch the **Brain Safeguards** animation in the StudyWARE™.

Cerebrospinal Fluid

Cerebrospinal fluid (**ser**-eh-broh-**SPY**-nal), also known as ***spinal fluid***, is produced by special capillaries within the four ventricles located in the middle region of the cerebrum (Figures 10.3 and 10.4). Cerebrospinal fluid is a clear, colorless, and watery fluid that flows throughout the brain and around the spinal cord. The functions of this fluid are to:

- Cool and cushion these organs from shock or injury
- Nourish the brain and spinal cord by transporting nutrients and chemical messengers to these tissues

The Parts of the Brain

The brain parts are shown in Figures 10.4 through 10.6. The body functions that are controlled by these brain parts are summarized in Table 10.2. Notice that the functions most essential to the support of life are located within the most protected portions of the brain.

The Cerebrum

The **cerebrum** (seh-**REE**-brum) is the largest and uppermost portion of the brain. It is responsible for all thought, judgment, memory, and emotion, as well as for controlling and integrating motor and sensory functions. Note that *cerebrum* and *cerebellum* are similar words, but refer to very different parts of the brain. Memory aid: The cere*bel*lum is *bel*ow the cerebrum.

- The term **cerebral** (**see**-**EE**-bral) means pertaining to the cerebrum or to the brain (**cerebr** means brain, and **-al** means pertaining to).
- The **cerebral cortex**, which is made up of gray matter, is the outer layer of the cerebrum and is made up of elevated folds and deep fissures (Figure 10.6).
  - ***Gyri*** (singular ***gyrus***) are the elevated folds of gray matter in the cerebral cortex.
  - ***Sulci*** are the fissures of the cerebral cortex. As used here, a ***fissure*** is a normally occurring deep groove. Skin fissures, which are crack-like sores, are discussed in Chapter 12.

The Cerebral Hemispheres

The cerebrum is divided to create two **cerebral hemispheres** that are connected at the lower midpoint by the ***corpus callosum*** (Figure 10.5).

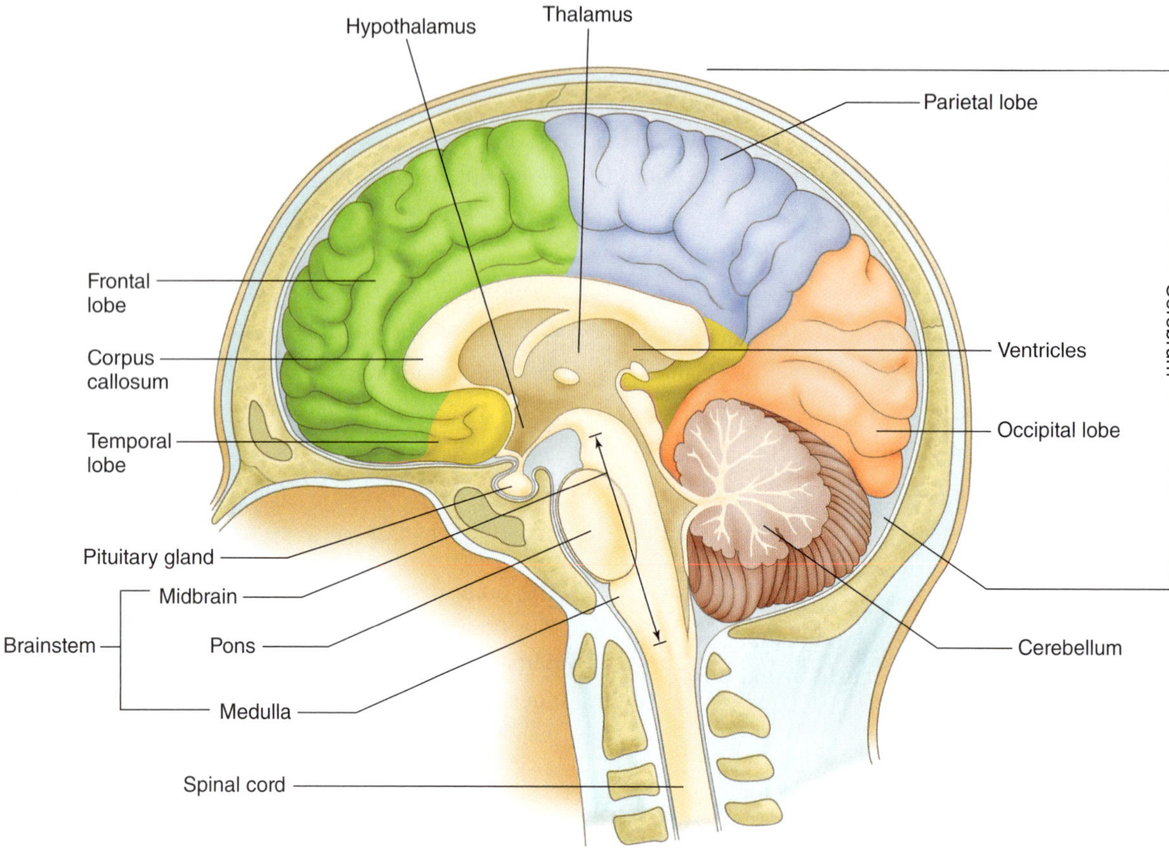

FIGURE 10.4 A cross-section showing the major parts of the brain.

TABLE 10.2
Brain Parts and Their Functions

Brain Part	Functions
The **cerebrum**, which is the largest and uppermost part of the brain, consists of four lobes.	Controls the highest level of thought, including judgment, memory, association, and critical thinking. It also processes sensations and controls all voluntary muscle activity.
The **thalamus** is located below the cerebrum.	Relays sensory stimuli from the spinal cord and midbrain to the cerebral cortex. The thalamus suppresses some stimuli and magnifies others.
The **hypothalamus** is located below the thalamus	Controls vital bodily functions (Table 10.3).
The **cerebellum** is located in the lower back of the cranium below the cerebrum.	Coordinates muscular activity and balance for smooth and steady movements.
The **brainstem** is located in the base of the brain and forms the connection between the brain and spinal cord. It consists of the: • midbrain • pons • medulla oblongata	Controls the functions necessary for survival (breathing, digestion, heart rate, and blood pressure), and for arousal (being awake and alert).

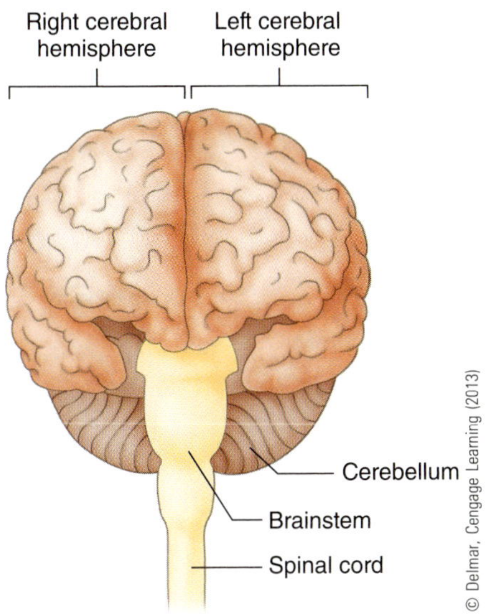

FIGURE 10.5 An anterior view showing how the brain is divided into right and left hemispheres.

- The ***left cerebral hemisphere*** controls the majority of functions on the right side of the body. An injury to the left hemisphere produces sensory and motor deficits on the right side of the body.
- The ***right cerebral hemisphere*** controls most of the functions on the left side of the body. An injury to the right hemisphere produces sensory and motor deficits on the left side of the body.
- The crossing of nerve fibers that makes this arrangement possible occurs in the brainstem (Figure 10.4).

The Cerebral Lobes

Each cerebral hemisphere is subdivided to create pairs of **cerebral lobes**. Each lobe is named for the bone of the cranium that covers it (Figure 10.6).

- The ***frontal lobe*** controls skilled motor functions, memory, and behavior.
- The ***parietal lobe*** receives and interprets nerve impulses from sensory receptors in the tongue, skin, and muscles.
- The ***occipital lobe*** controls eyesight.
- The ***temporal lobe*** controls the senses of hearing and smell, and the ability to create, store, and access new information.

The Thalamus

The **thalamus** (**THAL**-ah-mus), which is located below the cerebrum, produces sensations by relaying impulses to and from the cerebrum and the sense organs of the body.

The Hypothalamus

The **hypothalamus** (**high**-poh-**THAL**-ah-mus) is located below the thalamus (Figure 10.4). The seven major regulatory functions of the hypothalamus are summarized in Table 10.3.

The Cerebellum

The **cerebellum** (**ser**-eh-**BELL**-um) is the second-largest part of the brain. It is located at the back of

TABLE 10.3
Regulatory Functions of the Hypothalamus

1. Regulates and integrates the autonomic nervous system, including controlling heart rate, blood pressure, respiratory rate, and digestive tract activity.
2. Regulates emotional responses, including fear and pleasure.
3. Regulates body temperature.
4. Regulates food intake by controlling hunger sensations.
5. Regulates water balance by controlling thirst sensations.
6. Regulates sleep-wakefulness cycles.
7. Regulates the pituitary gland and endocrine system activity (see Chapter 13).

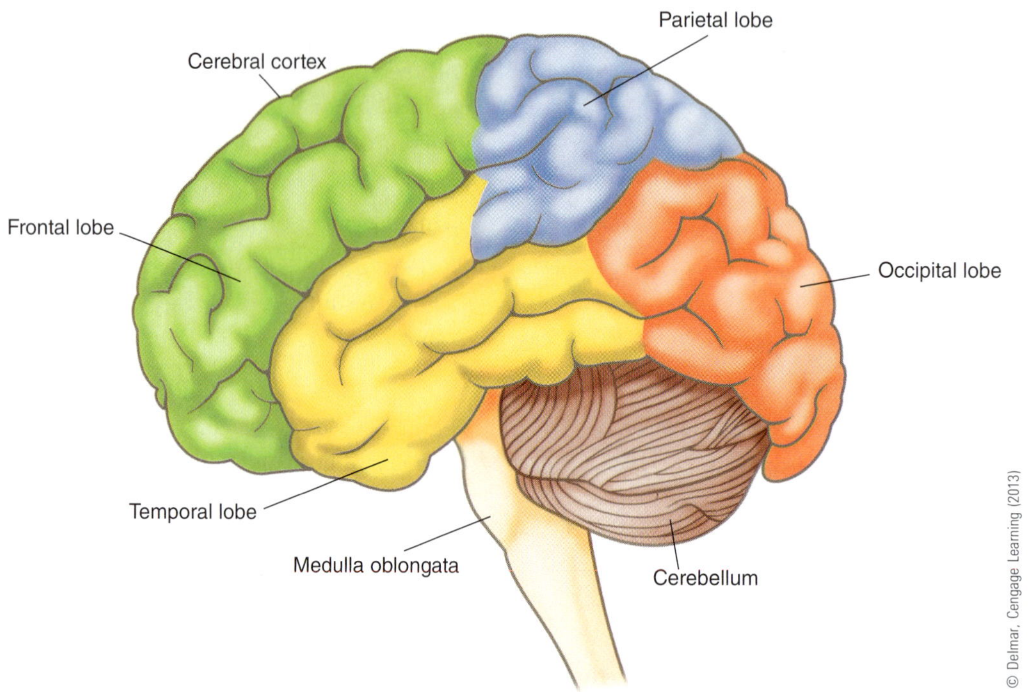

FIGURE 10.6 A left lateral view of the exterior of the brain showing the four lobes of the cerebrum plus the medulla oblongata and the cerebellum. The cerebral cortex is the outer layer of the cerebrum.

the head below the posterior portion of the cerebrum (Figures 10.4 through 10.6).

- The cerebellum receives incoming messages regarding movement within joints, muscle tone, and positions of the body. From here, messages are relayed to the different parts of the brain that control the motions of skeletal muscles.
- The general functions of the cerebellum are to produce smooth and coordinated movements, to maintain equilibrium, and to sustain normal postures.

The Brainstem

The **brainstem** is the stalk-like portion of the brain that connects the cerebral hemispheres with the spinal cord. It is made up of three parts: the midbrain, pons, and medulla oblongata (Figure 10.4).

- The **midbrain** and **pons** (**PONZ**) provide conduction pathways to and from the higher and lower centers in the brain. They also control reflexes for movements of the eyes and head in response to visual and auditory stimuli. (*Pons* is the Latin word for bridge.)
- The **medulla oblongata** (meh-**DULL**-ah **ob**-long-**GAH**-tah), which is located at the lowest part of the brainstem, is connected to the spinal cord. It controls basic survival functions, including the muscles that make possible respiration, heart rate, and blood pressure, as well as reflexes for coughing, sneezing, swallowing, and vomiting.

The Spinal Cord

The **spinal cord** is a long, fragile tube-like structure that begins at the end of the brainstem and continues down almost to the bottom of the spinal column (Figure 10.1).

- The spinal cord contains all the nerves that affect the limbs and lower part of the body, and serves as the pathway for impulses traveling to and from the brain.
- The spinal cord is surrounded and protected by cerebrospinal fluid and the meninges.

THE PERIPHERAL NERVOUS SYSTEM

The **peripheral nervous system** consists of the 12 pairs of cranial nerves that extend from the brain, plus 31 pairs of spinal nerves that extend from the spinal cord. ***Peripheral*** means pertaining to body parts that are away from the center of the body.

Three types of specialized peripheral nerves transmit signals to and from the central nervous system. These are autonomic, sensory, and somatic nerve fibers.

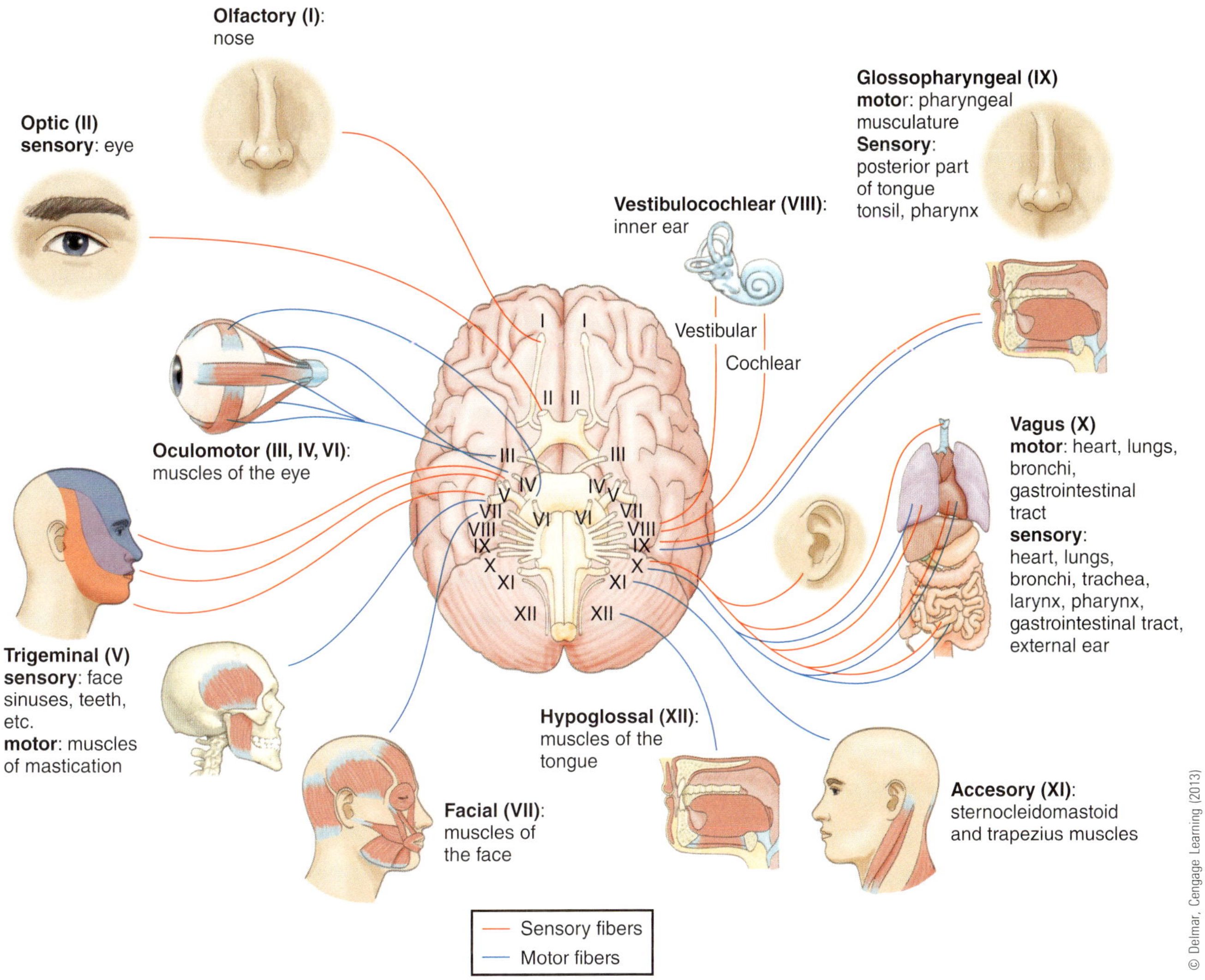

FIGURE 10.7 Cranial nerves are identified with Roman numerals and are named for the area or function they serve.

- ***Autonomic nerve fibers*** carry instructions to the organs and glands from the autonomic nervous system.
- ***Sensory nerve fibers*** receive external stimuli, such as how something feels, and transmit this information to the brain where it is interpreted.
- ***Somatic nerve fibers***, which are also known as ***motor nerve fibers***, convey information that controls the body's voluntary muscular movements.

The Cranial Nerves

The 12 pairs of **cranial nerves** originate from the undersurface of the brain. The two nerves of a pair are identical in function and structure, and each nerve of a pair serves half of the body. These cranial nerves are identified by Roman numerals and are named for the area or function they serve (Figure 10.7).

The Peripheral Spinal Nerves

The 31 pairs of **peripheral spinal nerves** are grouped together and named based on the region of the body they innervate.

- Within each region, the nerves are referred to by number. The cervical nerves are C1–C8, the thoracic nerves are T1–T12, the lumbar nerves are L1–L5, and the sacral nerves are S1–S5 (Figure 10.8B).
- Spinal nerves sometimes join with others to form a plexus to innervate a certain area. The lumbar plexus, as shown in Figure 10.8A, is made up of the first four lumbar nerves (L1–L4) and serves the lower back.

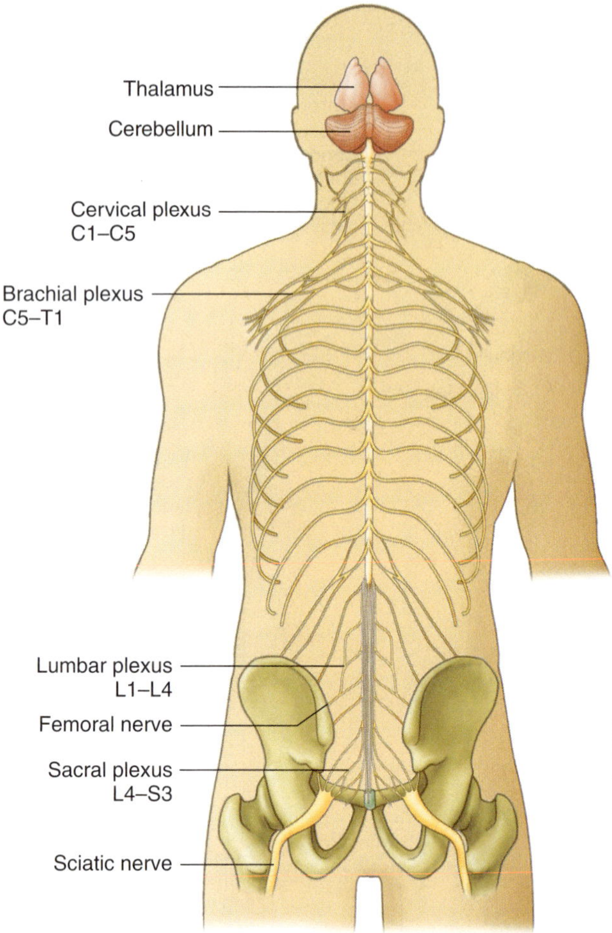

FIGURE 10.8A Most spinal cord plexuses are named for the corresponding vertebrae.

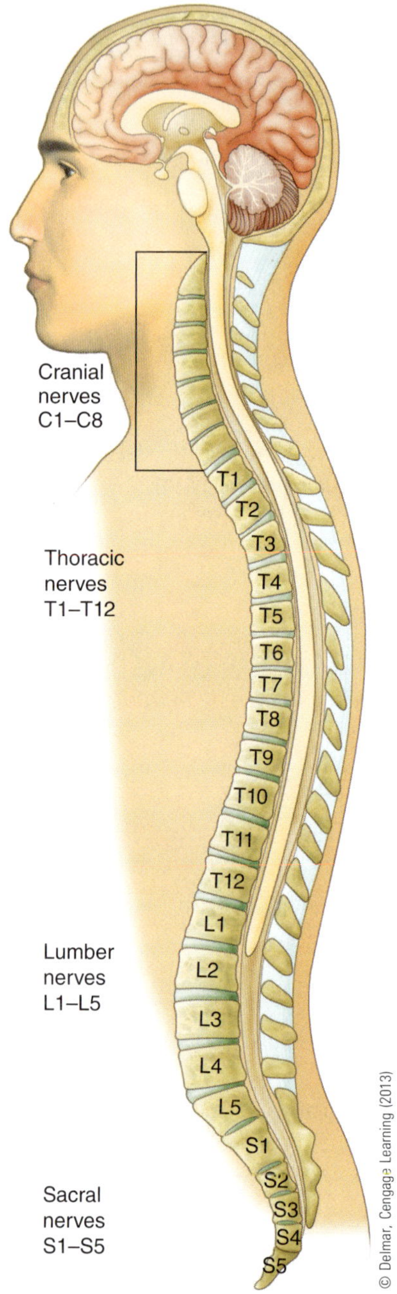

FIGURE 10.8B Within each spinal region, the nerves are referred to by number.

THE AUTONOMIC NERVOUS SYSTEM

The **autonomic nervous system** is organized into two divisions, one comprising *sympathetic nerves* and the other *parasympathetic nerves*. The autonomic nervous system controls the involuntary actions of the body such as the functioning of internal organs. To maintain homeostasis within the body, each division balances the activity of the other division. ***Homeostasis*** is the process of maintaining the constant internal environment of the body (See Chapter 2).

- The **sympathetic nerves** prepare the body for emergencies and stress by increasing the breathing rate, heart rate, and blood flow to muscles. These nerves become aroused as part of the ***fight-or-flight response***, which is the body's natural reaction to real or imaginary danger.
- The **parasympathetic nerves** return the body to normal after a response to stress. They also maintain normal body functions during ordinary circumstances that are not emotionally or physically stressful.

MEDICAL SPECIALTIES RELATED TO THE NERVOUS SYSTEM

- An **anesthesiologist** (**an**-es-**thee**-zee-**OL**-oh-jist) is a physician who specializes in administering anesthetic agents before and during surgery (**an-** means without, **esthesi** means feeling, and **-ologist** means specialist).

- An **anesthetist** (ah-**NES**-theh-tist) is a medical professional who specializes in administering anesthesia, but is not a physician, for example, a nurse anesthetist (**an-** means without, **esthet** means feeling, and **-ist** means specialist).
- A **neurologist** (new-**ROL**-oh-jist) is a physician who specializes in diagnosing and treating diseases and disorders of the nervous system (**neur** means nerve, and **-ologist** means specialist).
- A **neurosurgeon** is a physician who specializes in surgery of the nervous system.
- A **psychiatrist** (sigh-**KYE**-ah-trist) is a physician (MD) who specializes in diagnosing and treating chemical dependencies, emotional problems, and mental illness (**psych** means mind, and **-iatrist** means specialist). A psychiatrist can prescribe medications.
- A **psychologist** (sigh-**KOL**-oh-jist) has a doctoral degree (PhD or PsyD), but is not a medical doctor (MD). This specialist evaluates and treats emotional problems and mental illness (**psych** means mind, and **-ologist** means specialist).

PATHOLOGY OF THE NERVOUS SYSTEM

The Head and Meninges

- **Cephalalgia** (**sef**-ah-**LAL**-jee-ah), also known as a ***headache***, is pain in the head (**cephal** means head, and **-algia** means pain).
- A **migraine headache** (**MY**-grayn), which may be preceded by a warning aura, is characterized by throbbing pain on one side of the head. Migraine headaches primarily affect women and are sometimes accompanied by nausea, vomiting, and sensitivity to light or sound. A ***warning aura*** is a visual disturbance perceived by the patient preceding a migraine headache or epileptic seizure.
- **Cluster headaches** are intensely painful headaches that affect one side of the head and may be associated with tearing of the eyes and nasal congestion. These headaches, which primarily affect men, are named for their repeated occurrence in groups or clusters.
- An **encephalocele** (en-**SEF**-ah-loh-**seel**), also known as a ***craniocele***, is a congenital herniation of brain tissue through a gap in the skull (**encephal/o** means brain, and **-cele** means hernia). ***Congenital*** means present at birth, and ***herniation*** means protrusion of a structure from its normal position. Compare this with a *meningocele.*
- A **meningocele** (meh-**NING**-goh-**seel**) is the congenital herniation of the meninges through a defect in the skull or spinal column (**mening/o** means meninges, and **-cele** means hernia). Compare this with an *encephalocele.*
- **Hydrocephalus** (high-droh-**SEF**-ah-lus) is a condition in which excess cerebrospinal fluid accumulates in the ventricles of the brain (**hydr/o** means water, **cephal** means head, and **-us** is a singular noun ending). This condition can occur at birth or develop later on in life from obstructions related to meningitis, brain tumors, or other causes.
- A **meningioma** (meh-**nin**-jee-**OH**-mah) is a common, slow-growing and usually benign tumor of the meninges (**mening/i** means meninges, and **-oma** means tumor).
- **Meningitis** (**men**-in-**JIGH**-tis), also referred to as ***infectious meningitis***, is an inflammation of the meninges of the brain and spinal cord (**mening** means meninges, and **-itis** means inflammation). This condition, which can be caused by a bacterial or viral infection elsewhere in the body, is characterized by intense headache and flu-like symptoms. Bacterial meningitis, which is less common, is sometimes fatal. Compare with *encephalitis.*

Disorders of the Brain

- The term **cognition** (kog-**NISH**-un) describes the mental activities associated with thinking, learning, and memory. ***Mild cognitive impairment*** is a memory disorder, usually associated with recently acquired information, which may be an early predictor of Alzheimer's disease.
- **Dementia** (dih-**MEN**-shah) is a slowly progressive decline in mental abilities, including memory, thinking, and judgment, that is often accompanied by personality changes. ***Senile dementia*** is dementia of the aged.
- **Vascular dementia** is a form of dementia caused by a stroke or other restriction of the flow of blood to the brain. Although Alzheimer's disease is the primary cause of dementia, vascular dementia accounts for about 10 to 20% of all cases.

- **Encephalitis** (**en**-sef-ah-**LYE**-tis), which is an inflammation of the brain, can be caused by a viral infection such as rabies (**encephal** means brain, and **-itis** means inflammation). Compare with meningitis.
- **Reye's syndrome** (**RIZE**) (RS) is a potentially serious or deadly disorder in children that is characterized by vomiting and confusion. This syndrome sometimes follows a viral illness in which the child was treated with aspirin.
- **Tetanus** (**TET**-ah-nus), also known as ***lockjaw***, is an acute and potentially fatal infection of the central nervous system caused by a toxin produced by the tetanus bacteria. Tetanus can be prevented through immunization. In unimmunized people, this condition is typically acquired through a deep puncture wound.
- **Tourette syndrome** (tuh **RET**) (TS) is a complex neurological disorder characterized by involuntary tics, grunts, and compulsive utterances that sometimes include obscenities.

Neurodegenerative Diseases

The term **neurodegenerative disease** (**new**-roh-deh-**JEN**-er-ah-tiv) is an umbrella term for disorders in which there is a progressive loss of the structure or functions of the neurons.

- **Alzheimer's disease** (**ALTZ**-high-merz) is a group of disorders involving the parts of the brain that control thought, memory, and language (Figure 10.9). It is the leading cause of dementia and is marked by progressive deterioration that affects both the memory and reasoning capabilities of an individual.
- *Huntington's disease* is a genetic disorder that is classified as a neurodegenerative disease (See Chapter 2).
- **Parkinson's disease** (PD) is a chronic, degenerative central nervous disorder characterized by fine muscle tremors, rigidity, and a slow or shuffling gait. ***Gait*** describes the manner of walking. This slow or shuffling gait is caused by gradual progressive loss of control over movements due to inadequate levels of the neurotransmitter dopamine in the brain.

Brain Injuries

- **Amnesia** (am-**NEE**-zee-ah) is a memory disturbance characterized by a total or partial inability to recall past experiences. This condition can be caused by a brain injury, illness, or a psychological disturbance.
- A **concussion** (kon-**KUSH**-un) is a violent shaking up or jarring of the brain (**concuss** means shaken together, and **-ion** means condition or state of). A concussion may result in a temporary loss of awareness and function. Compare with a cerebral contusion.
- A **cerebral contusion** (**SER**-eh-bral kon-**TOO**-zhun) is the bruising of brain tissue as the result of a head injury that causes the brain to bounce against the rigid bone of the skull (**contus** means bruise, and **-ion** means condition). Compare with concussion.

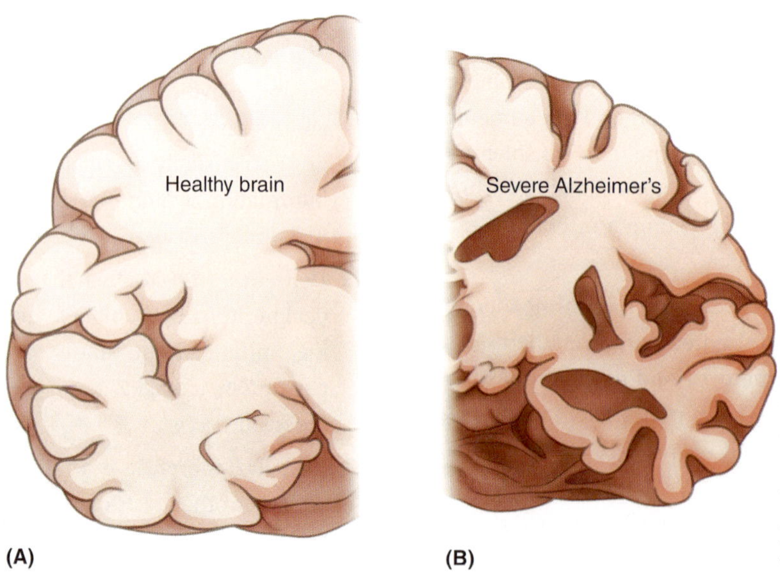

FIGURE 10.9 (A) A healthy brain and (B) the brain of a patient with Alzheimer's disease.

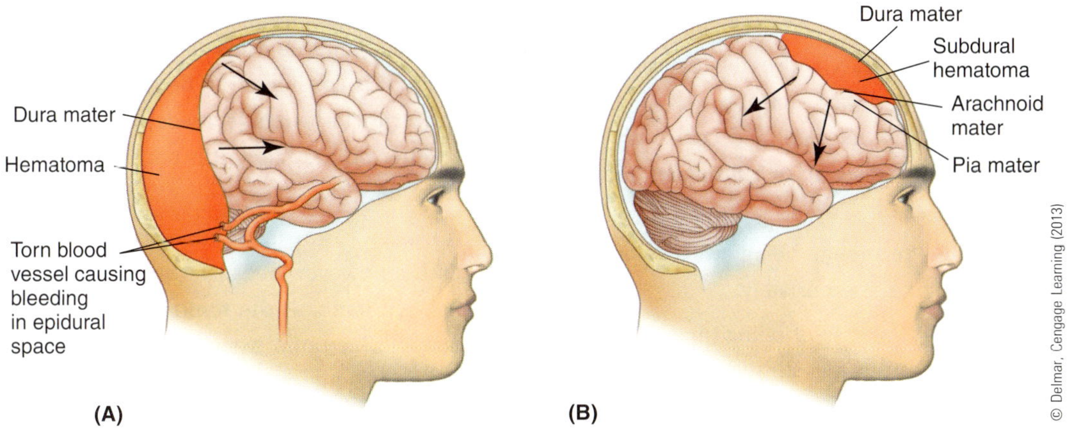

FIGURE 10.10 Cranial hematomas. (A) Epidural hematoma. (B) Subdural hematoma.

- A **cranial hematoma** (**hee**-mah-**TOH**-mah) is a collection of blood trapped in the tissues of the brain (**hemat** means blood, and **-oma** means tumor). Named for their location, the types of cranial hematomas include an ***epidural hematoma*** located above the dura mater or a ***subdural hematoma***, which is located below the dura mater (Figure 10.10). Cranial hematomas may be caused by a major or even minor head injury.

Traumatic Brain Injury

A **traumatic brain injury** is a blow to the head or a penetrating head injury that damages the brain. Not all blows to the head result in damage to the brain. When an injury does occur, it can range from mild, with only a brief change in mental status, to severe, with longer lasting effects.

- The term ***coup*** describes an injury occurring within the skull near the point of impact, such as hitting the windshield in an auto accident. A ***contrecoup***, also described as a ***counterblow***, is an injury that occurs beneath the skull opposite to the area of impact (Figure 10.11).
- **Shaken baby syndrome** describes the results of a child being violently shaken by someone. This action can cause brain injury, blindness, fractures, seizures, paralysis, and death.

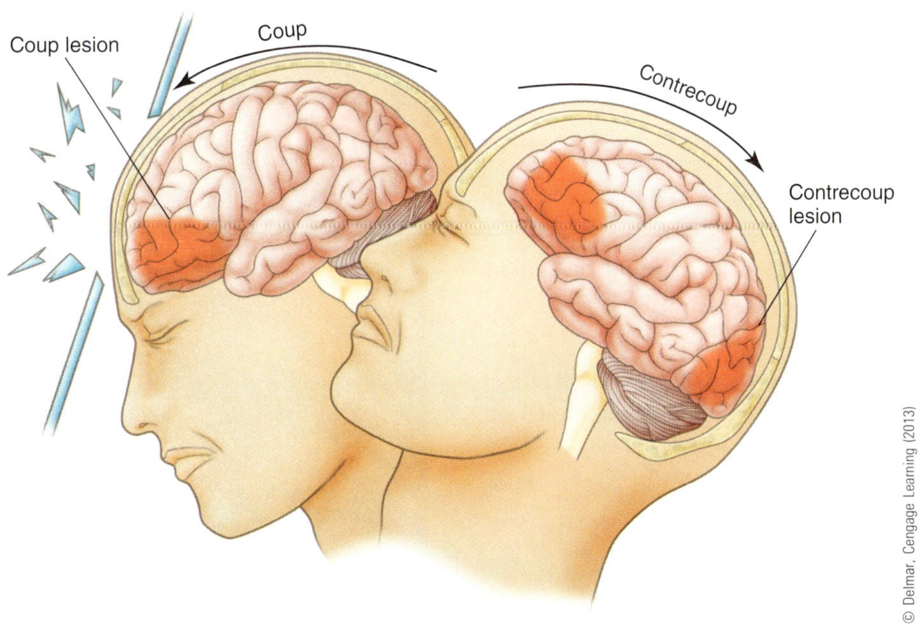

FIGURE 10.11 Coup and contrecoup brain injuries.

Levels of Consciousness

Levels of consciousness (LOC) describe the measurement of response to arousal and stimulus. ***Altered levels of consciousness (ALOC)*** refer to a decrease in consciousness due to injury, disease, or substances such as medication, drugs, or alcohol.

- Being **conscious** is the state of being awake, alert, aware, and responding appropriately.
- Being **unconscious** is a state of being unaware and unable to respond to any stimuli, including pain.
- **Lethargy** (**LETH**-ar-jee) is a lowered level of consciousness marked by listlessness, drowsiness, and apathy. As used here, ***apathy*** means indifference and a reduced level of activity. The term ***lethargic*** refers to a person who is at this level of consciousness.
- A **stupor** (**STOO**-per) is an unresponsive state from which a person can be aroused only briefly despite vigorous, repeated attempts.
- **Syncope** (**SIN**-koh-pee), also known as ***fainting***, is the brief loss of consciousness caused by the decreased flow of blood to the brain.
- A **coma** (**KOH**-mah) is a profound (deep) state of unconsciousness marked by the absence of spontaneous eye movements, no response to painful stimuli, and the lack of speech. The term ***comatose*** refers to a person who is in a coma.
- A **persistent vegetative state** is a type of coma in which the patient exhibits alternating sleep and wake cycles; however, due to severe damage to certain areas of the brain, the person is unconscious even when appearing to be awake.

Delirium

Delirium (deh-**LEER**-ee-um) is an acute condition of confusion, disorientation, disordered thinking and memory, agitation, and hallucinations.

This condition is usually caused by a treatable physical condition, such as a high fever. An individual suffering from this condition is described as being ***delirious***.

Brain Tumors

A **brain tumor** is an abnormal growth located inside the skull (Figure 10.12).

- An invasive ***malignant brain tumor*** destroys brain tissue. When this cancer originates in the brain, it is considered to be the primary site. If this cancer metastasizes (spreads) to the brain from another body system, it is considered to be a secondary site.
- A ***benign brain tumor*** does not invade the brain tissue; however, because this growth is surrounded by rigid bone, as the tumor enlarges, it can damage the brain tissue by placing pressure against the tissues and by increasing the intracranial pressure.
- **Intracranial pressure** is the amount of pressure inside the skull (**intra-** means within, **crani** means cranium, and **-al** means pertaining to). Elevated intracranial pressure can be due to a tumor, an injury, or improper drainage of cerebrospinal fluid.

Strokes

A stroke, or CVA, is properly known as a **cerebrovascular accident** (**ser**-eh-broh-**VAS**-kyou-lar). This condition is damage to the brain that occurs when the blood flow to the brain is disrupted because a blood vessel is either blocked or has ruptured. Strokes are currently the third-leading cause of death and the primary cause of long-term disability.

The location of the disruption determines the symptoms that will be present.

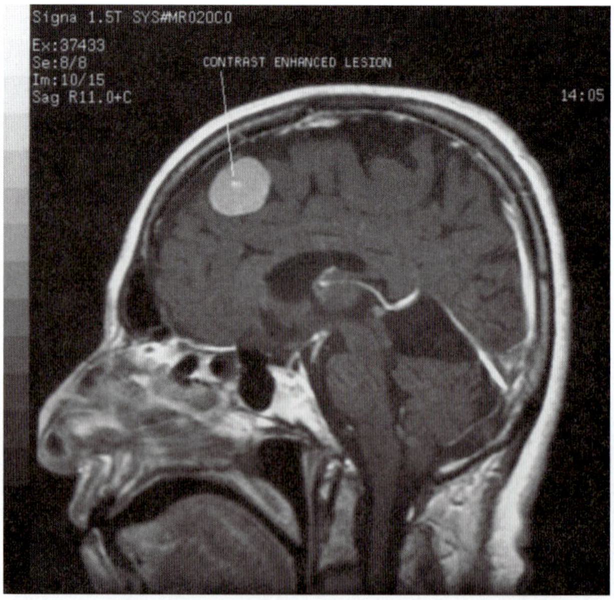

FIGURE 10.12 A brain tumor visualized by magnetic resonance imaging (MRI).

- Damage to the right side of the brain produces symptoms on the left side of the body.
- Damage to the left side of the brain produces symptoms on the right side of the body (Figure 10.13).

Ischemic Stroke

An **ischemic stroke** (iss-**KEE**-mick), which is the most common type of stroke in older people, occurs when the flow of blood to the brain is blocked by the narrowing or blockage of a carotid artery. ***Ischemic*** means pertaining to the disruption of the blood supply (see Chapter 5).

One type of ischemic stroke is a ***thrombotic stroke***, which occurs when a blood clot forms in a carotid artery and blocks it. The other is an ***embolic stroke***, which occurs when a blood clot or other debris forms in a blood vessel somewhere other than the brain and travels through the bloodstream to lodge in the narrower brain arteries.

- A **transient ischemic attack** (TIA), sometimes referred to as a mini-stroke, is the temporary interruption in the blood supply to the brain. ***Transient*** means passing quickly. Symptoms of a TIA include numbness, blurred vision, dizziness, or loss of balance. A TIA passes in less than an hour; however, this incident is often a warning sign that the individual is at risk for a more serious and debilitating stroke.

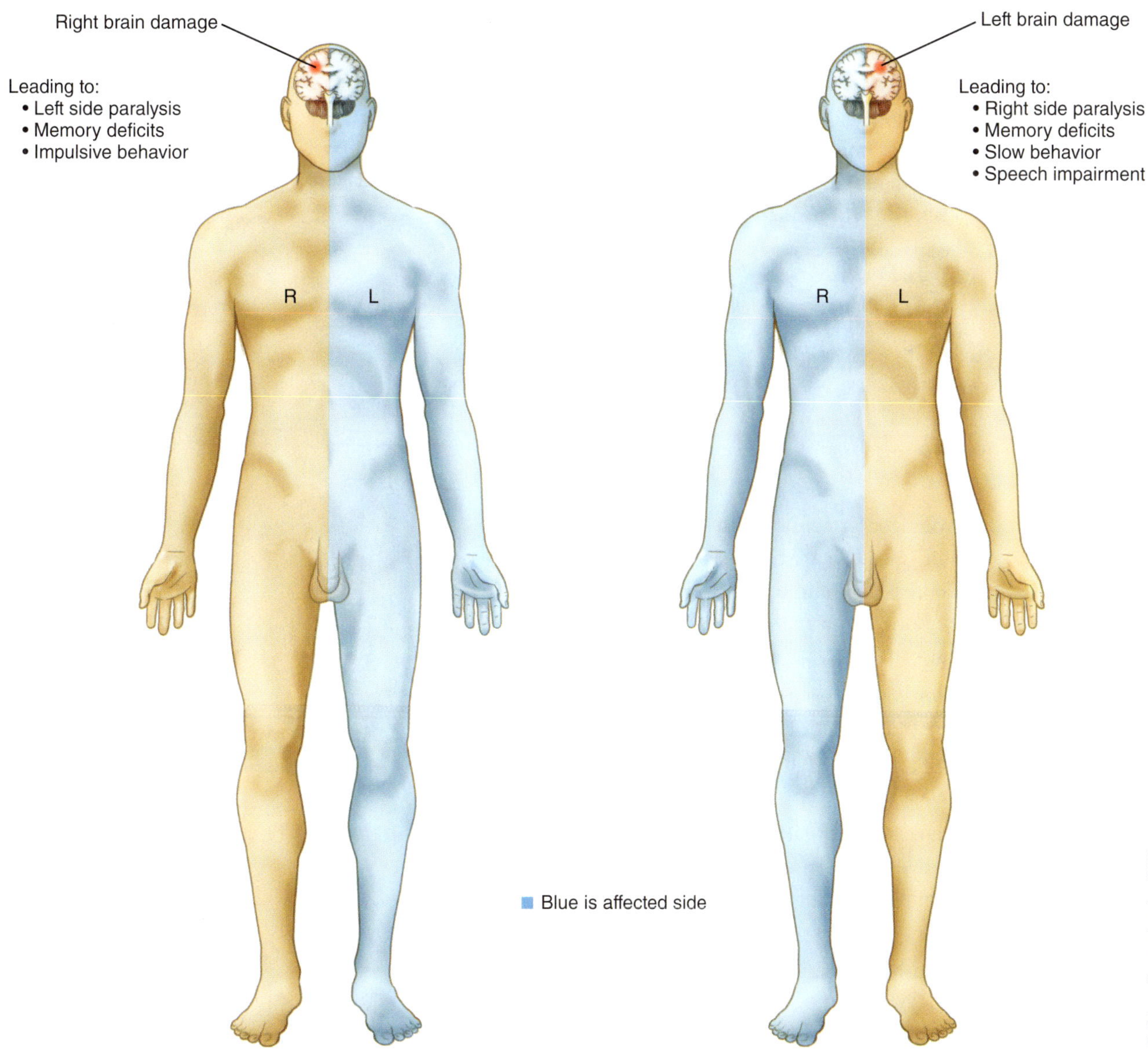

FIGURE 10.13 The location of the damage caused by a cerebrovascular accident depends upon which side of the brain is affected.

■ **Aphasia** (ah-**FAY**-zee-ah), which is often caused by brain damage associated with a stroke, is the loss of the ability to speak, write, and/or comprehend the written or spoken word (**a-** means without, and **-phasia** means speech).

Hemorrhagic Stroke

A **hemorrhagic stroke** (**hem**-oh-**RAJ**-ick), also known as a ***bleed***, occurs when a blood vessel in the brain leaks. A bleed also occurs when an aneurysm within the brain ruptures. An ***aneurysm*** is a localized, weak, balloon-like enlargement of an artery wall. This type of stroke is less common than ischemic strokes and is often fatal. A hemorrhagic stroke affects the area of the brain damaged by the leaking blood (Figures 10.14 and 10.15).

Arteriovenous malformation (ar-**tee**-ree-oh-**VEE**-nus) (AVM) is one of the causes of hemorrhagic strokes. This abnormal connection between the arteries and veins in the brain is usually congenital and can rupture suddenly at any age (**arteri/o** means artery, **ven** means vein, and **-ous** means pertaining to).

StudyWARE CONNECTION

Watch an animation on **Strokes** in the StudyWARE™.

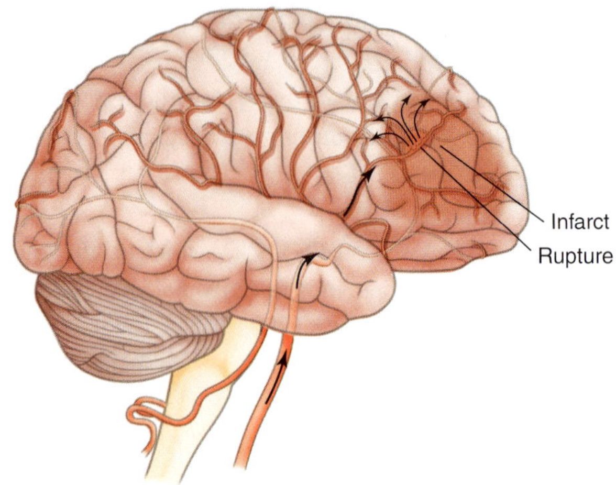

FIGURE 10.14 In a hemorrhagic stroke, the rupture of a blood vessel causes decreased blood flow to an area of the brain tissue. An *infarct* is a localized area of dead tissue caused by a lack of blood.

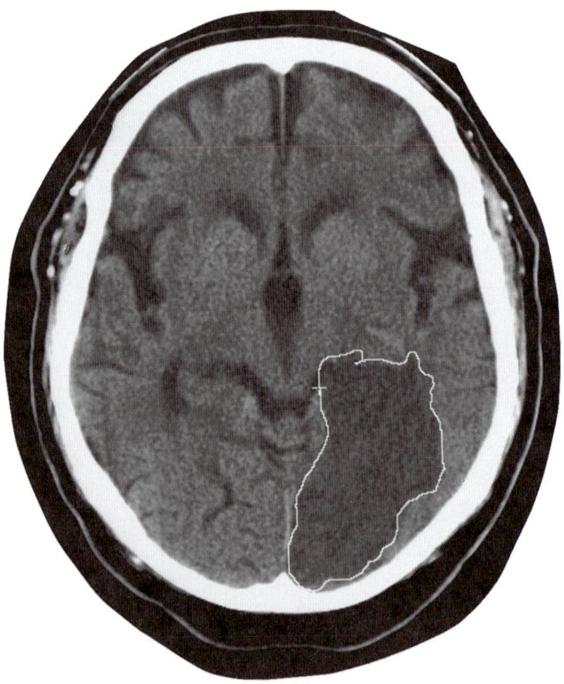

FIGURE 10.15 Magnetic resonance image of a brain with the area of a bleed visible in the lower right.

Sleep Disorders

■ **Insomnia** is the prolonged or abnormal inability to sleep. This condition is usually a symptom of another problem such as depression, pain, or excessive caffeine (**in-** means without, **somn** means sleep, and **-ia** means abnormal condition).

■ **Narcolepsy** (**NAR**-koh-**lep**-see) is a sleep disorder consisting of sudden and uncontrollable brief episodes of falling asleep during the day (**narc/o** means stupor, and **-lepsy** means seizure).

■ **Sleep deprivation** is a sufficient lack of restorative sleep over a cumulative period so as to cause physical or psychiatric symptoms and affect routine performance or tasks.

■ **Somnambulism** (som-**NAM**-byou-lizm), also known as ***sleepwalking*** or ***noctambulism***, is the condition of walking or performing some other activity without awakening (**somn** means sleep, **ambul** means to walk, and **-ism** means condition of).

The Spinal Cord

■ **Myelitis** (**my**-eh-**LYE**-tis) is an inflammation of the spinal cord (**myel** means spinal cord and bone marrow, and **-itis** means inflammation). The term *myelitis* also means inflammation of bone marrow.

- A **myelosis** (**my**-eh-**LOH**-sis) is a tumor of the spinal cord (**myel** means spinal cord and bone marrow, and **-osis** means abnormal condition). *Myelosis* also means an abnormal proliferation of bone marrow tissue.
- **Poliomyelitis** (**poh**-lee-oh-**my**-eh-**LYE**-tis), also known as ***polio***, is a highly contagious viral infection of the brainstem and spinal cord that sometimes leads to paralysis (**poli/o** means gray matter, **myel** means spinal cord and bone marrow, and **-itis** means inflammation). There is no known cure for polio; however, it can be prevented through vaccination.
- ***Post-polio syndrome*** is the recurrence later in life of some polio symptoms in individuals who have had childhood poliomyelitis and have recovered from it.
- **Spinal cord injuries** are discussed in Chapter 4.

Pinched Nerves

Radiculitis (rah-**dick**-you-**LYE**-tis), also known as a ***pinched nerve***, is an inflammation of the root of a spinal nerve that causes pain and numbness radiating down the affected limb (**radicul** means root or nerve root, and **-itis** means inflammation). This term usually applies to that portion of the root that lies between the spinal cord and the intervertebral canal of the spinal column. Figure 3.18 in Chapter 3 shows one cause of this condition.

- **Cervical radiculopathy** (rah-**dick**-you-**LOP**-ah-thee) is nerve pain caused by pressure on the spinal nerve roots in the neck region (**radicul/o** means nerve root, and **-pathy** means disease).
- **Lumbar radiculopathy** is nerve pain in the lower back caused by muscle spasms or by nerve root irritation from the compression of vertebral disks such as a herniated disk.

Multiple Sclerosis

Multiple sclerosis (skleh-**ROH**-sis) is a progressive autoimmune disorder characterized by inflammation that causes demyelination of the myelin sheath. This scars the brain, spinal cord, and optic nerves and disrupts the transmission of nerve impulses. This damage leaves the patient with varying degrees of pain plus physical and cognitive problems.

- ***Demyelination*** is the loss of patches of the protective myelin sheath.
- The disease is characterized by periods of ***exacerbations***, which are episodes of worsening symptoms that are also referred to as ***flares***. Between these episodes, the patient may be in remission. ***Remission*** is a time during which the symptoms ease, but the disease has not been cured.

Nerves

- **Amyotrophic lateral sclerosis** (ah-**my**-oh-**TROH**-fick), also known as ***Lou Gehrig's disease***, is a rapidly progressive neurological disease that attacks the nerve cells responsible for controlling voluntary muscles. Patients affected with this condition become progressively weaker until they are completely paralyzed and die.
- **Bell's palsy** is the temporary paralysis of the seventh cranial nerve that causes paralysis only of the affected side of the face. In addition, paralysis symptoms can include the inability to close the eye, pain, tearing, drooling, hypersensitivity to sound in the affected ear, and impairment of taste.
- **Guillain-Barré syndrome** (gee-**YAHN**-bah-**RAY**), also known as ***infectious polyneuritis***, is an inflammation of the myelin sheath of peripheral nerves, characterized by rapidly worsening muscle weakness that can lead to temporary paralysis. This condition is an autoimmune reaction that can occur after certain viral infections or an immunization.
- **Neuritis** (new-**RYE**-tis) is an inflammation of a nerve accompanied by pain and sometimes loss of function (**neur/o** means nerve, and **-itis** means inflammation).
- **Sciatica** (sigh-**AT**-ih-kah) is inflammation of the sciatic nerve that results in pain, burning, and tingling along the course of the affected sciatic nerve through the thigh, leg, and foot (Figure 10.8A).
- **Trigeminal neuralgia** (try-**JEM**-ih-nal new-**RAL**-jee-ah) is characterized by severe lightning-like pain due to an inflammation of the fifth cranial nerve. These sudden, intense, brief attacks of sharp pain affect the cheek, lips, and gums only on the side of the face innervated by the affected nerve.

Cerebral Palsy

Cerebral palsy (seh-**REE**-bral **PAWL**-zee) is a condition characterized by poor muscle control, spasticity, speech defects, and other neurologic deficiencies due to damage that affects the cerebrum. *Spasticity* is a condition in which certain muscles are continuously contracted. *Palsy* means paralysis of a body part that is often accompanied by loss of feeling and uncontrolled body movements, such as shaking.

- Cerebral palsy occurs most frequently in premature or low-birth-weight infants.
- Cerebral palsy is usually caused by an injury that occurs during pregnancy, birth, or soon after birth.

Epilepsy and Seizures

Epilepsy (**EP**-ih-**lep**-see) is a chronic neurological condition characterized by recurrent episodes of seizures of varying severity. Also known as a *seizure disorder*, epilepsy can usually be controlled with medication.

A **seizure** (**SEE**-zhur) is a sudden surge of electrical activity in the brain that affects how a person feels or acts for a short time. Some seizures can hardly be noticed, whereas others cause a brief loss of consciousness. Seizures are symptoms of different disorders that can affect the brain and also can be caused by extreme high fever, brain injury, or brain lesions.

- A **tonic-clonic seizure**, also called a *grand mal seizure*, involves the entire body. In the tonic phase of the seizure, the body becomes rigid, and in the clonic phase, there is uncontrolled jerking.
- An **absence seizure**, also called a *petit mal seizure*, is a brief disturbance in brain function in which there is a loss of awareness often described as a staring episode.

Abnormal Sensations

- **Causalgia** (kaw-**ZAL**-jee-ah) is persistent, severe burning pain that usually follows an injury to a sensory nerve (**caus** means burning, and **-algia** means pain).
- **Hyperesthesia** (**high**-per-es-**THEE**-zee-ah) is a condition of abnormal and excessive sensitivity to touch, pain, or other sensory stimuli (**hyper-** means excessive, and **-esthesia** means sensation or feeling).
- **Paresthesia** (**pair**-es-**THEE**-zee-ah) refers to a burning or prickling sensation that is usually felt in the hands, arms, legs, or feet, but can also occur in other parts of the body (**par-** means abnormal, and **-esthesia** means sensation or feeling). These sensations may constitute the first symptoms of peripheral neuropathy or may be a drug side effect.
- **Peripheral neuropathy** (new-**ROP**-ah-thee) is a disorder of the peripheral nerves that carry information to and from the brain and spinal cord (**neur/o** means nerve, and **-pathy** means disease). This produces pain, the loss of sensation, and the inability to control muscles, particularly in the arms or legs.
  - *Neuropathy* is any disease or damage to a nerve.
  - *Mononeuropathy* is damage to a singular peripheral nerve, as in carpal tunnel syndrome (see Chapter 4).
  - *Polyneuropathy* is when multiple peripheral nerves are damaged. Diabetes is a common cause of polyneuropathy, along with trauma, vitamin deficiencies, and alcoholism.
- **Restless legs syndrome** (RLS) is a neurological disorder characterized by uncomfortable feelings in the legs, producing a strong urge to move them. The sensation is usually most noticeable at night or when trying to rest.

DIAGNOSTIC PROCEDURES OF THE NERVOUS SYSTEM

- **Magnetic resonance imaging** (MRI) and **computed tomography** (CT) are important neuroimaging tools because they facilitate the examination of the soft tissue structures of the brain and spinal cord (Figures 10.12 and 10.15). These diagnostic techniques are discussed further in Chapter 15.
- A **functional MRI** (fMRI) detects changes in blood flow in the brain when the patient is asked to perform a specific task. This gives a clearer picture of the brain tissue relevant to accomplishing this task.
- **Carotid ultrasonography** (kah-**ROT**-id **ul**-trah-son-**OG**-rah-fee) is an ultrasound study of the carotid artery (**ultra-** means beyond, **son/o** means sound, and **-graphy** means the process of producing a picture or record). This diagnostic test is performed to detect plaque buildup in the artery to predict or diagnose an ischemic stroke.
- **Echoencephalography** (**eck**-oh-en-**sef**-ah-**LOG**-rah-fee) is the use of ultrasound imaging to create a detailed visual image of the brain for diagnostic purposes (**ech/o** means sound, **encephal/o** means brain, and **-graphy** means the process of producing a picture or record).

- **Electroencephalography** (ee-**leck**-troh-en-**sef**-ah-**LOG**-rah-fee) is the process of recording the electrical activity of the brain through the use of electrodes attached to the scalp (**electr/o** means electric, **encephal/o** means brain, and **-graphy** means the process of producing a picture or record). The resulting record is an ***electroencephalogram***. This electrical activity may also be displayed on a monitor as brain waves.
- **Myelography** (**my**-eh-**LOG**-rah-fee) is a radiographic study of the spinal cord after the injection of a contrast medium through a lumbar puncture (**myel/o** means spinal cord, and **-graphy** means the process of producing a picture or record). The resulting record is a ***myelogram***.
- A **lumbar puncture**, also known as a ***spinal tap***, is the process of obtaining a sample of cerebrospinal fluid by inserting a needle into the subarachnoid space of the lumbar region to withdraw fluid. Changes in the composition of the cerebrospinal fluid can be an indication of injury, infection, or disease.

TREATMENT PROCEDURES OF THE NERVOUS SYSTEM

Sedative and Hypnotic Medications

- A **hypnotic** depresses the central nervous system and usually produces sleep.
- An **anticonvulsant** (**an**-tih-kon-**VUL**-sant) is administered to prevent seizures such as those associated with epilepsy.
- **Barbiturates** (bar-**BIT**-you-raytz) are a class of drugs whose major action is a calming or depressed effect on the central nervous system.
  - ***Amobarbital*** is a barbiturate used as a sedative and hypnotic.
  - ***Phenobarbital*** is a barbiturate used as a sedative and as an anticonvulsant.
- A **sedative** depresses the central nervous system to produce calm and diminished responsiveness without producing sleep. ***Sedation*** is the effect produced by a sedative.

Anesthesia

Anesthesia (**an**-es-**THEE**-zee-ah) is the absence of normal sensation, especially sensitivity to pain, that is induced by the administration of an anesthetic agent (**an-** means without, and **-esthesia** means feeling).

- An **anesthetic** (**an**-es-**THET**-ick) is the medication used to induce anesthesia. The anesthetic may be topical, local, regional, or general (**an-** means without, **esthet** means feeling, and **-ic** means pertaining to).
- **Epidural anesthesia** (**ep**-ih-**DOO**-ral **an**-es-**THEE**-zee-ah) is regional anesthesia produced by injecting medication into the epidural space of the lumbar or sacral region of the spine. When administered during childbirth, it numbs the nerves from the uterus and birth passage without stopping labor (Figure 10.16).
- ***General anesthesia*** involves the total loss of body sensation and consciousness induced by anesthetic agents administered primarily by inhalation or intravenous injection.

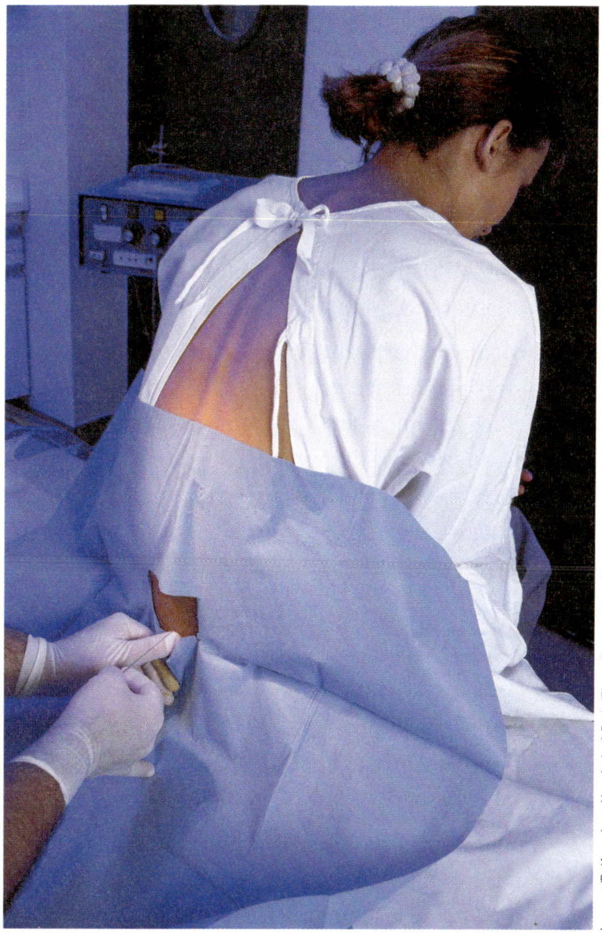

FIGURE 10.16 Epidural anesthesia administered during childbirth numbs the nerves from the uterus and birth passage without stopping labor.

- *Local anesthesia* causes the loss of sensation in a limited area by injecting an anesthetic solution near that area.
- *Regional anesthesia*, the temporary interruption of nerve conduction, is produced by injecting an anesthetic solution near the nerves to be blocked.
- **Spinal anesthesia** is regional anesthesia produced by injecting medication into the subarachnoid space. As with epidural anesthesia, the patient remains conscious. Spinal anesthesia provides numbness from the toes to the waist or lower chest.
- *Topical anesthesia* numbs only the tissue surface and is applied as a liquid, ointment, or spray.

The Brain

- **Deep brain stimulation** (DBS) is a neurosurgical procedure used in the treatment of dystonia, tremors, and Parkinson's disease. A device to stimulate the brain with mild electrical signals is implanted in the brain and is connected to a stimulator implanted near the collar bone. *Dystonia* is the impairment of voluntary muscle movement (see Chapter 4).
- **Gamma knife surgery** is a type of radiation treatment for brain tumors performed without a knife or an incision. The surgeon uses gamma radiation to destroy diseased tissue while preserving the healthy tissue around the tumor. *Gamma radiation*, which is characterized by high energy and a short wavelength, is also used in nuclear medicine (see Chapter 15).
- **Electroconvulsive therapy** (ECT) (ee-**leck**-troh-kon-**VUL**-siv), also known as *electroshock therapy*, is a procedure in which small amounts of electric current are passed through the brain, deliberately triggering a brief seizure in order to reverse symptoms of certain mental illnesses.
- **Light therapy** is exposure to daylight or to specific wavelengths of light in order to counteract seasonal affective disorder (SAD).
- A **lobectomy** (loh-**BECK**-toh-mee) is surgical removal of a portion of the brain to treat brain cancer or seizure disorders that cannot be controlled with medication.
- A **thalamotomy** (**thal**-ah-**MOT**-oh-mee) is a surgical incision into the thalamus (**thalam** means thalamus, and **-otomy** means surgical incision). This procedure, which destroys brain cells, is primarily performed to quiet the tremors of Parkinson's disease.

Nerves

- **Neuroplasty** (**NEW**-roh-**plas**-tee) is the surgical repair of a nerve or nerves (**neur/o** means nerve, and **-plasty** means surgical repair).
- **Neurorrhaphy** (new-**ROR**-ah-fee) is surgically suturing together the ends of a severed nerve (**neur/o** means nerve, and **-rrhaphy** means surgical suturing).
- **Neurotomy** (new-**ROT**-oh-mee) is the surgical division or dissection (cutting) of a nerve (**neur** means nerve, and **-otomy** means a surgical incision).

MENTAL HEALTH

Although described as being disorders of mental health, the causes of the following conditions also include congenital abnormalities, physical changes, substance abuse, medications, or any combination of these factors.

Anxiety Disorders

Anxiety disorders are mental conditions characterized by excessive, irrational dread of everyday situations or fear that is out of proportion to the real danger in a situation. Without treatment, an anxiety disorder can become chronic.

- A **generalized anxiety disorder** (GAD) is characterized by chronic, excessive worrying. Physical symptoms associated with this condition can include muscle tension, sleep disturbance, irritability, trouble concentrating, and restlessness.
- **Obsessive-compulsive disorder** (OCD) is characterized by recurrent *obsessions* (repetitive, intrusive, distressing thoughts or impulses) and/or *compulsions* (repeatedly feeling compelled to do things, like wash or pray). OCD makes someone feel he or she must do compulsive behaviors, such as repeated cleaning or checking, to prevent harm or stop the obsession. Performing compulsions provides only temporary relief, but not performing them temporarily increases anxiety.
- **Panic disorder** is characterized by a fear of panic attacks. Panic disorder can cause people to develop *agoraphobia* or other *phobias* (see following section on phobias).
- A **panic attack** is an unexpected, sudden experience of fear in the absence of danger, accompanied by physical symptoms such as heart palpitations,

shortness of breath, chest tightness, dizziness, sweating, nausea, feelings of unreality, choking sensations, or a combination of these. A panic attack is simply unneeded activation of the body's fight-or-flight response.

- **Post-traumatic stress disorder** (PTSD) may develop after an event involving actual or threatened death or injury to the individual or someone else, during which the person felt intense fear, helplessness, or horror (**post-** means after, **trauma** means injury, and **-tic** means pertaining to). War, natural disasters, or other life-threatening experiences can cause PTSD. Symptoms include emotional numbing, hyperarousal, anxiety, sleep disorders, and persistent reliving of the event (Figure 10.17).

Phobias

A **phobia** (**FOH**-bee-ah) is a persistent irrational fear of a specific thing or situation, strong enough to cause significant distress, to interfere with functioning, and to lead to the avoidance of the thing or situation that causes this reaction. There are countless types of phobias, and they are named by adding **-phobia** to the name of the object.

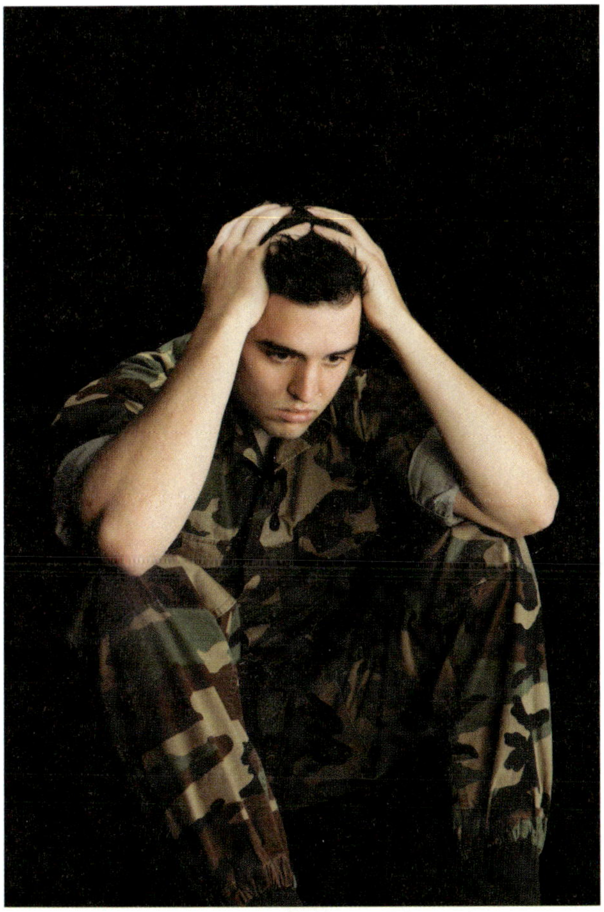

iStockphoto/Steve Jacobs

FIGURE 10.17 Post-traumatic stress disorder may develop after military service as a result of actual or threatened death or injury to the individual or someone else.

- **Acrophobia** (**ack**-roh-**FOH**-bee-ah) is an excessive fear of heights (**acr/o** means top, and **-phobia** means abnormal fear).
- **Agoraphobia** (**ag**-oh-rah-**FOH**-bee-ah) is an excessive fear of environments where the person fears a panic attack might occur. In order to avoid these situations, someone suffering from agoraphobia might not even be able to leave home (**agor/a** means marketplace, and **-phobia** means abnormal fear).
- **Claustrophobia** (**klaws**-troh-**FOH**-bee-ah) is an abnormal fear of being in small or enclosed spaces (**claustr/o** means barrier, and **-phobia** means abnormal fear).
- **Social phobia,** also called ***social anxiety disorder***, is an excessive fear of social situations where the person fears negative evaluation by others and embarrassing himself in front of others.

Developmental Disorders

- An **attention deficit/hyperactivity disorder** (ADHD) is characterized by a short attention span and impulsive behavior that is inappropriate for the child's developmental age. ***Hyperactivity*** is restlessness or a continuing excess of movement. The term ***attention deficit disorder (ADD)*** is sometimes used if hyperactivity is not present. These conditions may persist into adulthood.
- **Dyslexia** (dis-**LECK**-see-ah), also known as a ***developmental reading disorder***, is a learning disability characterized by substandard reading achievement due to the inability of the brain to process symbols.
- **Learning disabilities** are disorders found in children of normal intelligence who have difficulties in learning specific skills such as processing language or grasping mathematical concepts.
- **Mental retardation/intellectual disability** (MR/ID) is a diagnosis of significant below-average intellectual and adaptive functioning present from birth or early infancy. Note: the traditional term *mental retardation* is gradually being replaced by *intellectual disability*; however, during this transition both are used.

Autism Spectrum Disorders

Autistic spectrum disorders (aw-**TIS**-tic) (ASD) describes a group of conditions in which a young child has difficulty developing normal social relationships and communication skills, may compulsively follow repetitive routines, and has narrowly focused, intense interests that are sometimes unusual.

- **Autism** (**AW**-tizm) is a subgroup of autistic spectrum disorders. Children with autism have significant developmental delays, including speech and language. Most children with autism have very minimal verbal skills and lack normal social relationships (Figure 10.18).
- *Asperger's syndrome* is another subgroup of the autism disorders spectrum. Individuals with Asperger's syndrome usually have normal or above-average intelligence but are impaired in social interactions and nonverbal communication.

Dissociative Disorders

Dissociative disorders occur when normal thought is separated from consciousness.

- **Dissociative identity disorder**, formerly known as *multiple personality disorder*, is a mental illness characterized by the presence of two or more distinct personalities, each with its own characteristics, which appear to exist within the same individual.

Factitious Disorders

A **factitious disorder** (fack-**TISH**-us) is a condition in which an individual acts as if he or she has a physical or mental illness when he or she is not really sick. The term *factitious* means artificial, self-induced, or not naturally occurring. Visible symptoms are self-inflicted and seem motivated by a desire for attention and sympathy rather than for external benefits like malingering (see the later section "Somatoform Disorders").

- A **factitious disorder by proxy** is a form of child abuse. Although seeming very concerned about the child's well-being, the mentally ill parent will falsify an illness in a child by making up or inducing symptoms, and then seeking medical treatment, even surgery, for the child.

Impulse Control Disorders

Impulse control disorders are a group of psychiatric disorders characterized by a failure to resist an impulse despite potential negative consequences. In addition to

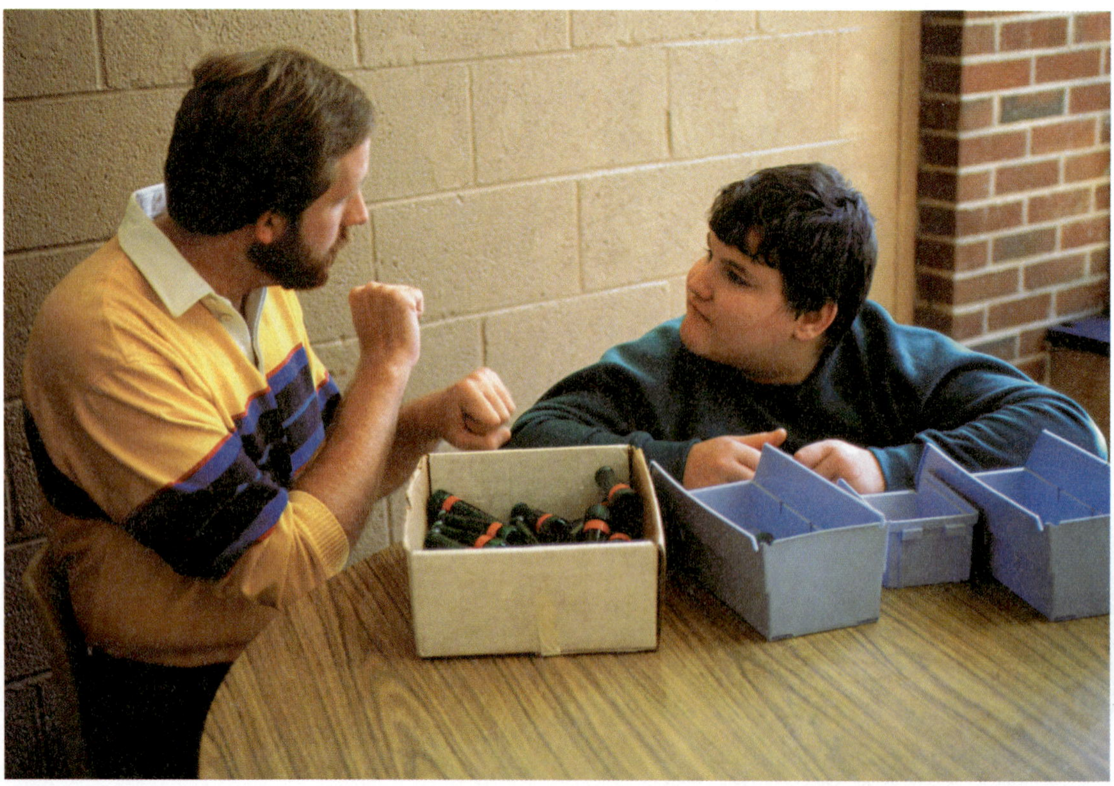

FIGURE 10.18 A therapist works with a boy with autism to develop communication skills.

the examples listed below, this disorder includes compulsive shopping and gambling. The suffix **-mania** means madness.

- ***Kleptomania*** is a disorder characterized by repeatedly stealing objects neither for personal use nor for their monetary value.
- ***Pyromania*** is a disorder characterized by repeated, deliberate fire setting.
- ***Trichotillomania*** is a disorder characterized by the repeated pulling out of one's own hair.

Mood Disorders

- A **bipolar disorder** is a condition characterized by cycles of severe mood changes shifting from highs (manic behavior) and severe lows (depression) that affect a person's attitude, energy, and ability to function.
- **Manic behavior** includes an abnormally elevated mood state, including inappropriate elation, increased irritability, severe insomnia, poor judgment, and inappropriate social behavior.
- **Depression** is a common mood disorder characterized by lethargy and sadness, as well as the loss of interest or pleasure in normal activities. Severe depression may lead to feelings of worthlessness and thoughts of death or suicide. ***Suicide*** is the intentional taking of one's own life.
- **Dysthymia** (dis-**THIGH**-mee-ah), also known as ***dysthymic disorder***, is a low-grade chronic depression with symptoms that are milder than those of severe depression but are present on a majority of days for 2 or more years (**dys-** means bad, **thym** means mind, and **-ia** means condition).
- **Seasonal affective disorder** (SAD) is a seasonal bout of depression associated with the decrease in hours of daylight during winter months.

Personality Disorders

A **personality disorder** is a chronic pattern of inner experience and behavior that causes serious problems with relationships and work. This pattern is pervasive and inflexible, has an onset in adolescence or early adulthood, is stable over time, and leads to distress or impairment.

- An ***antisocial personality disorder*** is a pattern of disregard for and violation of the rights of others. This pattern brings the individual into continuous conflict with society.
- A ***borderline personality disorder*** is characterized by impulsive actions, often with the potential for self-harm, as well as mood instability and chaotic relationships.
- A ***narcissistic personality disorder*** is a pattern of extreme preoccupation with the self and complete lack of empathy for others. ***Empathy*** is the ability to understand another person's mental and emotional state without becoming personally involved.

Psychotic Disorders

A **psychotic disorder** (sigh-**KOT**-ick) is characterized by the loss of contact with reality and deterioration of normal social functioning.

- **Catatonic behavior** (**kat**-ah-**TON**-ick) is marked by a lack of responsiveness, stupor, and a tendency to remain in a fixed posture (Figure 10.19).
- A **delusion** (dee-**LOO**-zhun) is a false personal belief that is maintained despite obvious proof or evidence to the contrary. The belief is not one ordinarily accepted by other members of the individual's culture or religious faith.
- A **hallucination** (hah-**loo**-sih-**NAY**-shun) is a sensory perception (i.e., sight, touch, sound, smell, or taste) experienced in the absence of external stimulation.
- **Schizophrenia** (**skit**-soh-**FREE**-nee-ah) is a psychotic disorder usually characterized by withdrawal from reality, illogical patterns of thinking, delusions, and hallucinations, and accompanied in varying degrees by other emotional, behavioral, or intellectual disturbances (Figure 10.19).

Somatoform Disorders

A **somatoform disorder** (soh-**MAT**-oh-**form**) is characterized by physical complaints or concerns about one's body that are out of proportion to any physical findings or disease.

- A **conversion disorder** is characterized by serious temporary or ongoing changes in function, such as paralysis or blindness, that are triggered by psychological factors rather than by any physical cause.
- **Hypochondriasis** (**high**-poh-kon-**DRY**-ah-sis) is characterized by fearing that one has a serious illness despite appropriate medical evaluation and reassurance. A person exhibiting this syndrome is known as a ***hypochondriac***.

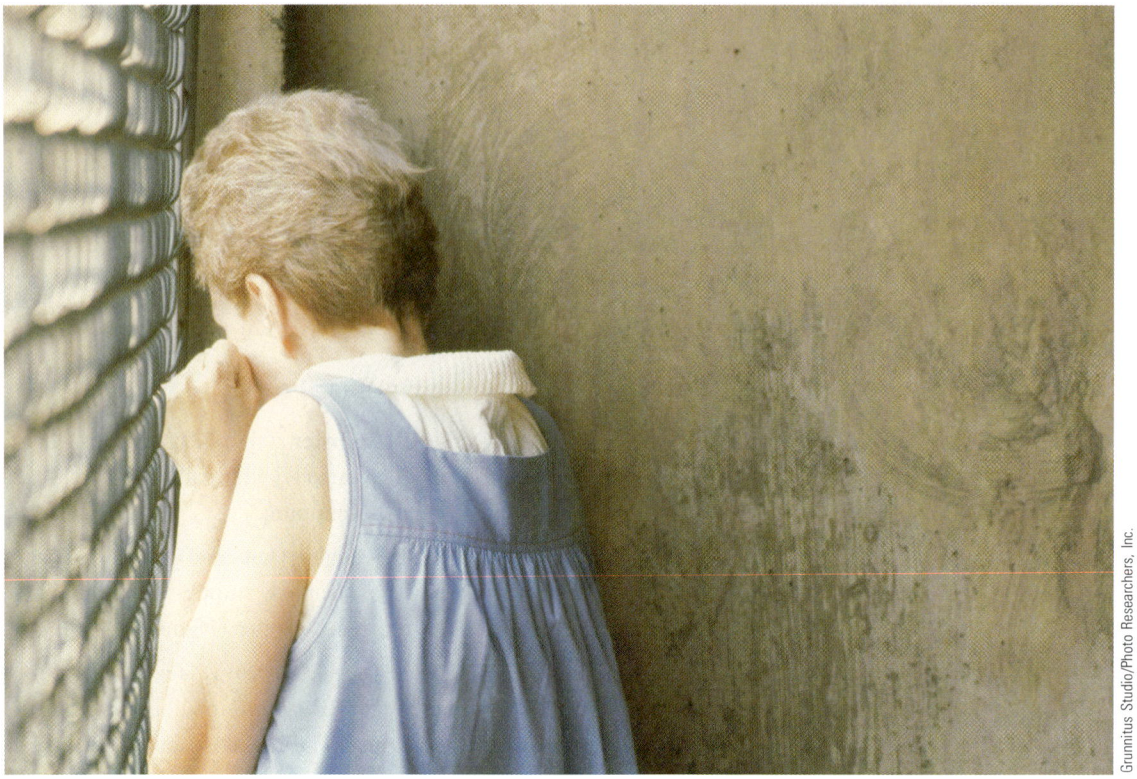

FIGURE 10.19 Schizophrenia is marked by withdrawal from reality and may include catatonic behavior.

- **Malingering** (mah-**LING**-ger-ing) is characterized by the intentional creation of false or grossly exaggerated physical or psychological symptoms. In contrast to a factitious disorder, this condition is motivated by incentives such as avoiding work.

Substance-Related Disorders

Substance abuse is the addictive use of tobacco, alcohol, medications, or illegal drugs. This abuse leads to significant impairment in functioning, danger to one's self or others, and recurrent legal and/or interpersonal problems.

- **Alcoholism** (**AL**-koh-hol-izm) is chronic alcohol dependence with specific signs and symptoms upon withdrawal. ***Withdrawal*** is a psychological or physical syndrome (or both) caused by the abrupt cessation (stopping) of the use of alcohol or a drug in an addicted individual.
- **Delirium tremens** (deh-**LEER**-ee-um **TREE**-mens) (DTs) is a disorder involving sudden and severe mental changes or seizures caused by abruptly stopping the use of alcohol.
- **Drug abuse** is the excessive use of illegal or recreational drugs, or the misuse of prescription drugs. A ***recreational drug*** is one normally used for personal pleasure or satisfaction rather than medical purposes.
- **A drug overdose** is the accidental or intentional use of an illegal drug or prescription medicine in an amount higher than what is safe or normal.

Medications to Treat Mental Disorders

A **psychotropic drug** (**sigh**-koh-**TROP**-pick) acts primarily on the central nervous system, where it produces temporary changes affecting the mind, emotions, and behavior (**psych/o** means mind, and **-tropic** means having an affinity for). These drugs are used as medications to control pain, and to treat narcolepsy and attention disorders.

- An **antidepressant** is administered to prevent or relieve depression. Some of these medications are also used to treat obsessive-compulsive and generalized anxiety disorders and to help relieve chronic pain.
- An **antipsychotic drug** (**an**-tih-sigh-**KOT**-ick) or ***neuroleptic*** is administered to treat symptoms of severe disorders of thinking and mood that are associated with neurological and psychiatric illnesses such as schizophrenia, mania, and delusional disorders (**anti-** means against, **psych/o** means mind, and **-tic** means pertaining to).
- An **anxiolytic drug** (**ang**-zee-oh-**LIT**-ick), also known as an ***antianxiety drug*** or ***tranquilizer***, is administered

to temporarily relieve anxiety and to reduce tension (**anxi/o** means anxiety, and **-lytic** means to destroy).

- **Mood-stabilizing drugs**, such as lithium, are used to treat mood instability and bipolar disorders.
- A **stimulant** works by increasing activity in certain areas of the brain to increase concentration and wakefulness. Drug therapies using stimulants have been effective in treating ADHD and narcolepsy. The overuse of stimulants, including caffeine, can cause sleeplessness and palpitations.

Psychological Therapies to Treat Mental Disorders

Mental disorders are often treated with individual or group therapy by a qualified psychotherapist.

- **Psychoanalysis** (**sigh**-koh-ah-**NAL**-ih-sis) is based on the idea that mental disorders have underlying causes stemming from childhood and can only be overcome by gaining insight into one's feelings and patterns of behavior.
- **Behavioral therapy** focuses on changing behavior by identifying problem behaviors, replacing them with appropriate behaviors and using rewards or other consequences to make the changes.
- **Cognitive therapy** focuses on changing cognitions or thoughts that are affecting a person's emotions and actions. These are identified and then are challenged through logic, gathering evidence, testing in action, or a combination of these. The goal is to change problematic beliefs.
- **Hypnotherapy** is the use of hypnosis to produce an altered state of focused attention in which the patient may be more willing to believe and act on suggestions. It is used for pain relief, anxiety reduction, and behavioral modification.

ABBREVIATIONS RELATED TO THE NERVOUS SYSTEM

Table 10.4 presents an overview of the abbreviations related to the terms introduced in this chapter. Note: To avoid errors or confusion, always be cautious when using abbreviations.

TABLE 10.4
Abbreviations Related to the Nervous System

Alzheimer's disease = AD	**AD** = Alzheimer's disease
amyotrophic lateral sclerosis = ALS	**ALS** = amyotrophic lateral sclerosis
attention-deficit hyperactivity disorder = ADHD	**ADHD** = attention-deficit hyperactivity disorder
cerebral palsy = CP	**CP** = cerebral palsy
cerebrospinal fluid = CSF	**CSF** = cerebrospinal fluid
electroencephalography = EEG	**EEG** = electroencephalography
intracranial pressure = ICP	**ICP** = intracranial pressure
levels of consciousness *or* **loss of consciousness** = LOC	**LOC** = levels of consciousness *or* loss of consciousness
lumbar puncture = LP	**LP** = lumbar puncture
multiple sclerosis = MS	**MS** = multiple sclerosis
obsessive-compulsive disorder = OCD	**OCD** = obsessive-compulsive disorder
post-traumatic stress disorder = PTSD	**PTSD** = post-traumatic stress disorder
seizure = Sz	**Sz** = seizure
transient ischemic attack = TIA	**TIA** = transient ischemic attack

StudyWARE CONNECTION

For more practice and to test your mastery of this material, go to the StudyWARE™ to play interactive games and complete the quiz for this chapter.

Workbook Practice

Go to your workbook, and complete the exercises for this chapter.

DELMAR MOBILE MEDIA

Downloadable audio is available for selected medical terms in this chapter to enhance your learning of medical terminology.

CHAPTER 10

LEARNING EXERCISES

MATCHING WORD PARTS 1

Write the correct answer in the middle column.

	Definition	Correct Answer	Possible Answers
10.1.	feeling	__________	psych/o
10.2.	brain	__________	encephal/o
10.3.	bruise	__________	contus/o
10.4.	mind	__________	concuss/o
10.5.	shaken together	__________	esthet/o

MATCHING WORD PARTS 2

Write the correct answer in the middle column.

	Definition	Correct Answer	Possible Answers
10.6.	brain covering	__________	-esthesia
10.7.	process of producing a picture	__________	-graphy
10.8.	sensation, feeling	__________	radicul/o
10.9.	spinal cord	__________	mening/o
10.10.	nerve root	__________	myel/o

MATCHING WORD PARTS 3

Write the correct answer in the middle column.

	Definition	Correct Answer	Possible Answers
10.11.	abnormal fear	__________	-tropic
10.12.	burning sensation	__________	phobia

10.13. brain ________________ **neur/o**

10.14. nerve, nerves ________________ **cerebr/o**

10.15. having an affinity for ________________ **caus/o**

DEFINITIONS

Select the correct answer, and write it on the line provided.

10.16. The space between two neurons or between a neuron and a receptor organ is known as a ________________.

dendrite ganglion plexus synapse

10.17. The white protective covering over some parts of the spinal cord and the axon of most peripheral nerves is the ________________.

myelin sheath neuroglia neurotransmitter pia mater

10.18. The ________________ are the root-like structures of a nerve that receive impulses and conduct them to the cell body.

axons dendrites ganglions neurotransmitters

10.19. The ________________ is the layer of the meninges that is located nearest to the brain and spinal cord.

arachnoid membrane dura mater meninx pia mater

10.20. Seven vital body functions are regulated by the ________________.

cerebral cortex cerebellum hypothalamus thalamus

10.21. The ________________ nerves are the division of the autonomic nervous system that prepare the body for emergencies and stress.

afferent parasympathetic peripheral sympathetic

10.22. A ________________ is a network of intersecting nerves.

ganglion plexus synapse tract

10.23. Cranial nerves are part of the __________ nervous system.

autonomic central cranial peripheral

10.24. The __________ relays sensory stimuli from the spinal cord and midbrain to the cerebral cortex.

cerebellum hypothalamus medulla oblongata thalamus

10.25. The __________ neurons carry impulses away from the brain and spinal cord.

afferent associative efferent sensory

MATCHING STRUCTURES

Write the correct answer in the middle column.

	Definition	Correct Answer	Possible Answers
10.26.	connects the brain and spinal cord	__________	medulla oblongata
10.27.	controls vital body functions	__________	hypothalamus
10.28.	coordinates muscular activity	__________	cerebrum
10.29.	controls basic survival functions	__________	cerebellum
10.30.	uppermost layer of the brain	__________	brainstem

WHICH WORD?

Select the correct answer, and write it on the line provided.

10.31. A physician who specializes in administering anesthetic agents is an __________.

anesthetist anesthesiologist

10.32. A __________ is a profound state of unconsciousness marked by the absence of spontaneous eye movements, no response to painful stimuli, and the lack of speech.

coma stupor

10.33. An __________ drug is also known as a tranquilizer.

antipsychotic anxiolytic

10.34. A/An ______________ is a sensory perception that has no basis in external stimulation.

delusion hallucination

10.35. An excessive fear of heights is ______________.

acrophobia agoraphobia

SPELLING COUNTS

Find the misspelled word in each sentence. Then write that word, spelled correctly, on the line provided.

10.36. A migrane headache is characterized by throbbing pain on one side of the head. ______________

10.37. Alzhiemer's disease is a group of disorders involving the parts of the brain that control thought, memory, and language. ______________

10.38. An anasthetic is the medication used to induce anesthesia. ______________

10.39. Epalepsy is a chronic neurological condition characterized by recurrent episodes of seizures of varying severity. ______________

10.40. Siatica is a nerve inflammation that results in pain, burning, and tingling through the thigh, leg, and foot. ______________

ABBREVIATION IDENTIFICATION

In the space provided, write the words that each abbreviation stands for.

10.41. **CP** ______________

10.42. **CSF** ______________

10.43. **OCD** ______________

10.44. **PTSD** ______________

10.45. **TIA** ______________

TERM SELECTION

Select the correct answer, and write it on the line provided.

10.46. The acute condition that is characterized by confusion, disorientation, disordered thinking and memory, agitation, and hallucinations is known as ______________________.

delirium dementia lethargy stupor

10.47. The term meaning inflammation of the spinal cord is ______________________. This term also means inflammation of bone marrow.

encephalitis myelitis myelosis radiculitis

10.48. The medical term meaning an abnormal fear of being in small or enclosed spaces is ______________________.

acrophobia claustrophobia kleptomania pyromania

10.49. The condition known as ______________________ is characterized by severe lightning-like pain due to an inflammation of the fifth cranial nerve.

Bell's palsy Guillain-Barré syndrome Lou Gehrig's disease trigeminal neuralgia

10.50. The medical term for the condition also known as a developmental reading disorder is ______________________.

autism dissociative disorder dyslexia mental retardation

SENTENCE COMPLETION

Write the correct term or terms on the lines provided.

10.51. A ______________________ is the bruising of brain tissue as the result of a head injury.

10.52. The mental conditions characterized by excessive, irrational dread of everyday situations or fear that is out of proportion to the real danger in a situation are known as ______________________.

10.53. A low-grade chronic depression with symptoms that are milder than those of severe depression but are present on a majority of days for two or more years is known as ______________________.

10.54. A/An ______________________ disorder is a condition in which an individual acts as if he or she has a physical or mental illness when he or she is not really sick.

10.55. A/An ______________________ drug is administered to treat symptoms of severe disorders of thinking and mood that are associated with neurological and psychiatric illnesses such as schizophrenia, mania, and delusional disorders.

WORD SURGERY

Divide each term into its component word parts. Write these word parts, in sequence, on the lines provided. When necessary, use a slash (/) to indicate a combining vowel. (You may not need all of the lines provided.)

10.56. An **anesthetic** is the medication used to induce anesthesia.

__________ __________ __________ __________

10.57. **Somnambulism** is commonly known as sleepwalking.

__________ __________ __________ __________

10.58. **Electroencephalography** is the process of recording the electrical activity of the brain through the use of electrodes attached to the scalp.

__________ __________ __________ __________

10.59. **Paresthesia** refers to a burning or prickling sensation that is usually felt in the hands, arms, legs, or feet.

__________ __________ __________ __________

10.60. **Poliomyelitis** is a contagious viral infection of the brainstem and spinal cord, which sometimes leads to paralysis.

__________ __________ __________ __________

TRUE/FALSE

If the statement is true, write **True** on the line. If the statement is false, write **False** on the line.

10.61. ______________________ A hemorrhagic stroke occurs when a blood vessel in the brain leaks.

10.62. ______________________ An absence seizure is a brief disturbance in brain function in which there is a loss of awareness.

10.63. ______________________ A sedative is administered to prevent the seizures associated with epilepsy.

10.64. ______________ A patient in a persistent vegetative state sleeps through the night and is awake and conscious during the day.

10.65. ______________ A psychotropic drug acts primarily on the central nervous system where it produces temporary changes affecting the mind, emotions, and behavior.

CLINICAL CONDITIONS

Write the correct answer on the line provided.

10.66. Harvey Ikeman has mood shifts from highs to severe lows that affect his attitude, energy, and ability to function. Harvey's doctor describes this condition as a/an ______________ disorder.

10.67. In the auto accident, Anthony DeNicola hit his head on the windshield. The paramedics were concerned that this jarring of the brain had caused a/an ______________.

10.68. Georgia Houghton suffered a ______________ attack (TIA), and her doctors were concerned that this was a warning of an increased stroke risk.

10.69. To control her patient's tremors caused by Parkinson's disease, Dr. Wang performed a/an ______________. This is a surgical incision into the thalamus.

10.70. Mary Beth Cawthorn was diagnosed as having ______________. This progressive autoimmune disease is characterized by inflammation that causes demyelination of the myelin sheath.

10.71. After several months of being unable to sleep well, Wayne Ladner visited his doctor about this problem. His doctor recorded this condition as being ______________.

10.72. After her stroke, Rosita Valladares was unable to understand written or spoken words. This condition is known as ______________.

10.73. Jill Beck said she fainted. The medical term for this brief loss of consciousness caused by the decreased blood flow to the brain is ______________.

10.74. The Baily baby was born with ______________. This condition is an abnormally increased amount of cerebrospinal fluid in the ventricles of the brain.

10.75. The MRI indicated that Mrs. Hoshi had a collection of blood trapped in the tissues of her brain. This condition, which was caused by a head injury, is called a cranial ______________.

WHICH IS THE CORRECT MEDICAL TERM?

Select the correct answer, and write it on the line provided.

10.76. Persistent, severe burning pain that usually follows an injury to a sensory nerve is known as ____________________.

causalgia hyperesthesia hypoesthesia paresthesia

10.77. The classification of drug that depresses the central nervous system and usually produces sleep is known as a/an ____________________.

anesthetic barbiturate hypnotic sedative

10.78. A/An ____________________ disorder is characterized by serious temporary or ongoing changes in function, such as paralysis or blindness, that are triggered by psychological factors rather than by any physical cause.

anxiety conversion factitious panic

10.79. During childbirth, ____________________ anesthesia is administered to numb the nerves from the uterus and birth passage without stopping labor.

epidural local regional topical

10.80. The condition known as ____________________ is a rapidly progressive neurological disease that attacks the nerve cells responsible for controlling voluntary muscles.

amyotrophic lateral sclerosis cerebral palsy epilepsy multiple sclerosis

CHALLENGE WORD BUILDING

These terms are *not* found in this chapter; however, they are made up of the following familiar word parts. If you need help in creating the term, refer to your medical dictionary.

poly-	**encephal/o**	**-algia**
	mening/o	**-itis**
	myel/o	**-malacia**
	neur/o	**-oma**
		-pathy

10.81. Based on word parts, the term meaning inflammation of the nerves and spinal cord is ________________.

10.82. Abnormal softening of the meninges is known as ________________.

10.83. A benign neoplasm made up of nerve tissue is a/an ________________.

10.84. Based on word parts, the term meaning any degenerative disease of the brain is ________________.

10.85. Pain affecting many nerves is known as ________________.

10.86. Abnormal softening of nerve tissue is known as ________________.

10.87. Inflammation of the meninges and the brain is known as ________________.

10.88. Based on word parts, the term meaning any pathological condition of the spinal cord is ________________.

10.89. Abnormal softening of the brain is known as ________________.

10.90. Inflammation of the meninges, brain, and spinal cord is known as ________________.

LABELING EXERCISES

Identify the numbered items on the accompanying figures.

10.91. ____________________ cortex

10.92. ____________________ lobe

10.93. ____________________ lobe

10.94. ____________________ lobe

10.95. ____________________ lobe

10.96. ____________________

10.97. ____________________

10.98. ____________________

10.99. ____________________ cord

10.100. ____________________

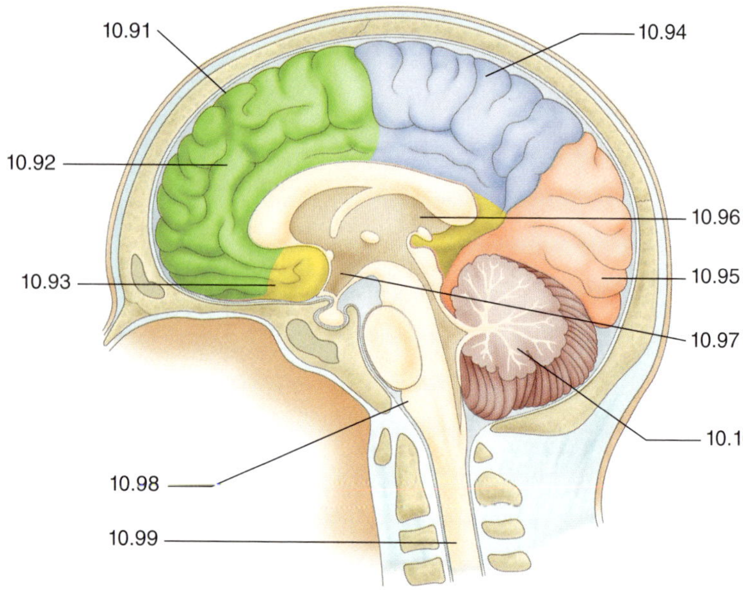

CHAPTER 11

Skin: The Integumentary System

Overview of STRUCTURES, COMBINING FORMS, AND FUNCTIONS OF THE INTEGUMENTARY SYSTEM

Major Structures	Related Combining Forms	Primary Functions
Skin	**cutane/o**, **dermat/o**, **derm/o**	Intact skin is the first line of defense for the immune system. Skin waterproofs the body and is the major receptor for the sense of touch.
Sebaceous Glands	**seb/o**	Secrete sebum (oil) to lubricate the skin and discourage the growth of bacteria on the skin.
Sweat Glands	**hidr/o**	Secrete sweat to regulate body temperature and water content, and these glands excrete some metabolic waste.
Hair	**pil/i**, **pil/o**	Aids in controlling the loss of body heat.
Nails	**onych/o**, **ungu/o**	Protect the dorsal surface of the last bone of each finger and toe.

Vocabulary Related to **THE INTEGUMENTARY SYSTEM**

This list contains essential word parts and medical terms for this chapter. These terms are pronounced in the student StudyWARE™ and Audio CDs that are available for use with this text. These and the other important **primary terms** are shown in boldface throughout the chapter. *Secondary terms*, which appear in *orange* italics, clarify the meaning of primary terms.

Word Parts

- ☐ **cutane/o** skin
- ☐ **derm/o**, **dermat/o** skin
- ☐ **hidr/o** sweat
- ☐ **hirsut/o** hairy, rough
- ☐ **kerat/o** horny, hard
- ☐ **lip/o** fat, lipid
- ☐ **melan/o** black, dark
- ☐ **myc/o** fungus
- ☐ **onych/o** fingernail or toenail
- ☐ **pil/i**, **pil/o** hair
- ☐ **py/o** pus
- ☐ **rhytid/o** wrinkle
- ☐ **seb/o** sebum
- ☐ **urtic/o** rash, hives
- ☐ **xer/o** dry

Medical Terms

- ☐ **actinic keratosis** (ack-**TIN**-ick **kerr**-ah-**TOH**-sis)
- ☐ **albinism** (**AL**-bih-niz-um)
- ☐ **alopecia** (**al**-oh-**PEE**-shee-ah)
- ☐ **blepharoplasty** (**BLEF**-ah-roh-**plas**-tee)
- ☐ **bulla** (**BULL**-ah)
- ☐ **capillary hemangioma** (**KAP**-uh-**ler**-ee hee-**man**-jee-**OH**-mah)
- ☐ **carbuncle** (**KAR**-bung-kul)
- ☐ **cellulitis** (**sell**-you-**LYE**-tis)
- ☐ **chloasma** (kloh-**AZ**-mah)
- ☐ **cicatrix** (sick-**AY**-tricks)
- ☐ **comedo** (**KOM**-eh-doh)
- ☐ **debridement** (dah-**BREED**-ment)
- ☐ **dermatitis** (**der**-mah-**TYE**-tis)
- ☐ **diaphoresis** (**dye**-ah-foh-**REE**-sis)
- ☐ **dysplastic nevi** (dis-**PLAS**-tick **NEE**-vye)
- ☐ **ecchymosis** (**eck**-ih-**MOH**-sis)
- ☐ **eczema** (**ECK**-zeh-mah)
- ☐ **erythema** (**er**-ih-**THEE**-mah)
- ☐ **erythroderma** (eh-**rith**-roh-**DER**-mah)
- ☐ **exanthem** (eck-**ZAN**-thum)
- ☐ **exfoliative dermatitis** (ecks-**FOH**-lee-**ay**-tiv **DER**-mah-**TYE**-tis)
- ☐ **folliculitis** (foh-**lick**-you-**LYE**-tis)
- ☐ **furuncles** (**FYOU**-rung-kulz)
- ☐ **granuloma** (**gran**-you-**LOH**-mah)
- ☐ **hematoma** (**hee**-mah-**TOH**-mah)
- ☐ **hirsutism** (**HER**-soot-izm)
- ☐ **ichthyosis** (**ick**-thee-**OH**-sis)
- ☐ **impetigo** (**im**-peh-**TYE**-goh)
- ☐ **keloid** (**KEE**-loid)
- ☐ **keratosis** (**kerr**-ah-**TOH**-sis)
- ☐ **koilonychia** (**koy**-loh-**NICK**-ee-ah)
- ☐ **lipedema** (lip-eh-**DEE**-mah)
- ☐ **lipoma** (lih-**POH**-mah)
- ☐ **macule** (**MACK**-youl)
- ☐ **malignant melanoma** (mel-ah-**NOH**-mah)
- ☐ **necrotizing fasciitis** (**NECK**-roh-**tiz**-ing **fas**-ee-**EYE**-tis)
- ☐ **onychocryptosis** (**on**-ih-koh-krip-**TOH**-sis)
- ☐ **onychomycosis** (**on**-ih-koh-my-**KOH**-sis)
- ☐ **papilloma** (**pap**-ih-**LOH**-mah)
- ☐ **papule** (**PAP**-youl)
- ☐ **paronychia** (**par**-oh-**NICK**-ee-ah)
- ☐ **pediculosis** (pee-**dick**-you-**LOH**-sis)
- ☐ **petechiae** (pee-**TEE**-kee-ee)
- ☐ **pruritus** (proo-**RYE**-tus)
- ☐ **psoriasis** (soh-**RYE**-uh-sis)
- ☐ **purpura** (**PUR**-pew-rah)
- ☐ **purulent** (**PYOU**-roo-lent)
- ☐ **rhytidectomy** (**rit**-ih-**DECK**-toh-mee)
- ☐ **rosacea** (roh-**ZAY**-shee-ah)
- ☐ **scabies** (**SKAY**-beez)
- ☐ **scleroderma** (**sklehr**-oh-**DER**-mah)
- ☐ **seborrhea** (**seb**-oh-**REE**-ah)
- ☐ **squamous cell carcinoma** (**SKWAY**-mus)
- ☐ **systemic lupus erythematosus** (sis-**TEH**-mik **LOO**-pus er-ih-**thee**-mah-**TOH**-sus)
- ☐ **tinea** (**TIN**-ee-ah)
- ☐ **urticaria** (**ur**-tih-**KARE**-ree-ah)
- ☐ **verrucae** (veh-**ROO**-kee)
- ☐ **vitiligo** (**vit**-ih-**LYE**-goh)
- ☐ **wheal** (**WHEEL**)
- ☐ **xeroderma** (zee-roh-**DER**-mah)

LEARNING GOALS

On completion of this chapter, you should be able to:

1. Identify and describe the functions and structures of the integumentary system.
2. Identify the medical specialists associated with the integumentary system.
3. Recognize, define, spell, and pronounce the primary terms related to the structures and function, pathology, and the diagnostic and treatment procedures of the skin.
4. Recognize, define, spell, and pronounce the primary terms related to the structures and function, pathology, and the diagnostic and treatment procedures of hair, nails, and sebaceous glands.

FUNCTIONS OF THE INTEGUMENTARY SYSTEM

The **integumentary system** (in-**teg**-you-**MEN**-tah-ree), which is made up of the skin and its related structures, performs important functions in maintaining the health of the body. The term ***integument*** comes from the Latin word meaning to cover or enclose.

Functions of the Skin

The **skin** forms the protective outer covering the external surfaces of the entire body.

- The skin waterproofs the body and prevents fluid loss.
- Intact (unbroken) skin plays an important role in the immune system by blocking the entrance of pathogens into the body (see Chapter 6).
- Skin is the major receptor for the sense of touch.
- Skin helps the body synthesize vitamin D, an essential nutrient, from the sun's ultraviolet light, while screening out some harmful ultraviolet radiation.
- The average adult has 2 square yards of skin, making it the largest bodily organ.

Functions of Related Structures

The related structures of the integumentary system are the sebaceous glands, sweat glands, hair, and nails (Figure 12.1).

- The **sebaceous glands** (seh-**BAY**-shus) secrete sebum (oil) that lubricates the skin and discourages the growth of bacteria on the skin.
- The **sweat glands** help regulate body temperature and water content by secreting sweat. A small amount of metabolic waste is also excreted through the sweat glands.
- **Hair** helps control the loss of body heat.
- **Nails** protect the dorsal surface of the last bone of each toe and finger.

THE STRUCTURES OF THE SKIN AND ITS RELATED STRUCTURES

The Skin

The skin is a complex system of specialized tissues made up of three basic layers:

The skin is a complex system of specialized tissues made up of three basic layers: the *epidermis*, *dermis*, and *subcutaneous* layers (Figure 12.1). The term **cutaneous** (kyou-**TAY**-nee-us) means pertaining to the skin (**cutane** means skin, and **-ous** means pertaining to).

The Epidermis

The **epidermis** (**ep**-ih-**DER**-mis), which is the outermost layer of the skin, is made up of several specialized epithelial tissues (**epi-** means above or upon, **derm** means skin, and **-is** is a noun ending).

The epidermis does not contain any blood vessels or connective tissue. It is therefore dependent on lower layers for nourishment.

- **Epithelial tissues** (**ep**-ih-**THEE**-lee-al) form a protective covering for all of the internal *and* external surfaces of the body.

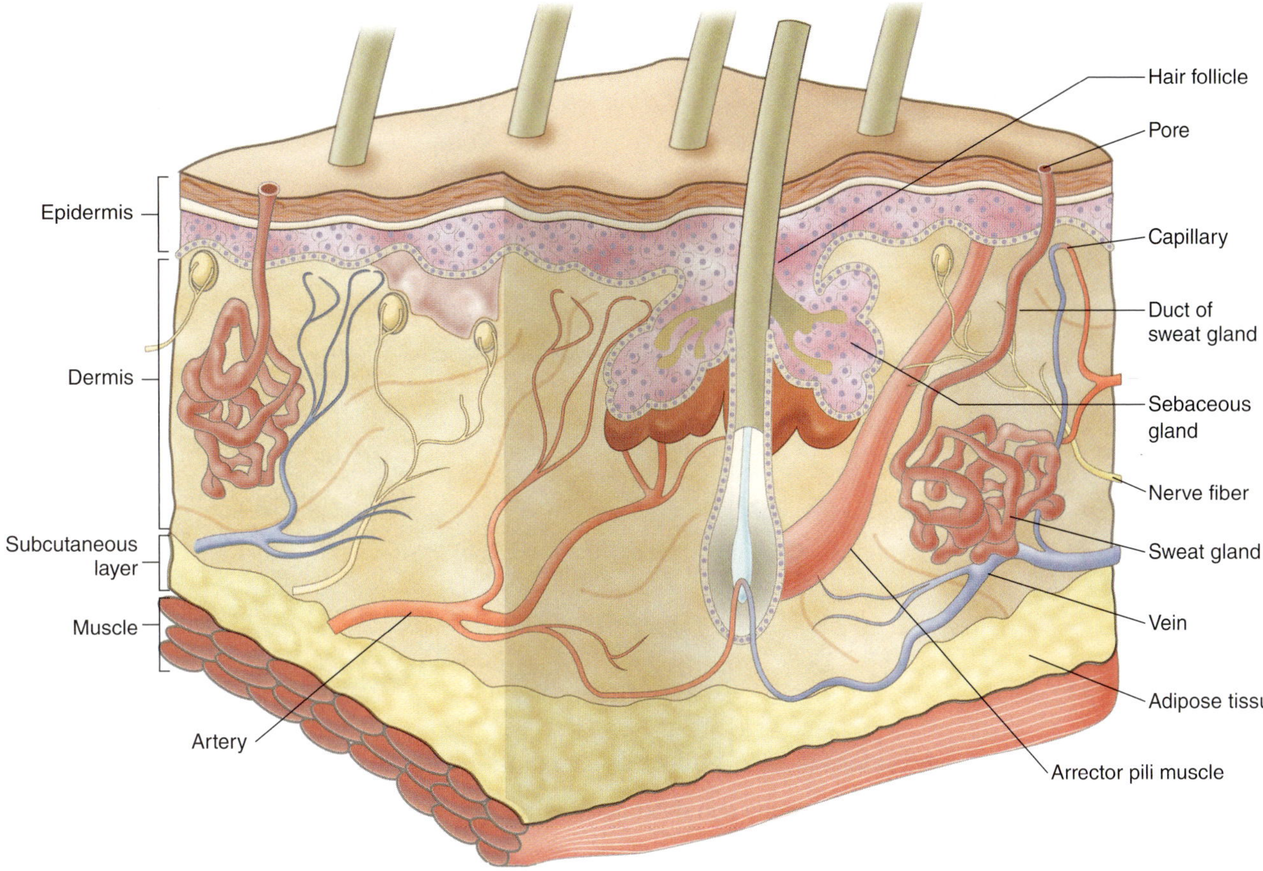

FIGURE 12.1 Structures of the skin. The sweat and sebaceous glands are associated structures of the skin.

- **Squamous epithelial tissue** (**SKWAY**-mus) forms the upper layer of the epidermis. ***Squamous*** means scale-like. This layer consists of flat, scaly cells that are continuously shed.
- The **basal layer** (**BAY**-suhl) is the lowest layer of the epidermis. It is here that new cells are produced and then pushed upward. When these cells reach the surface, they die and become filled with keratin.
- **Keratin** (**KER**-ah-tin) is a fibrous, water-repellent protein. Soft keratin is a primary component of the epidermis. Hard keratin is found in the hair and nails.
- **Melanocytes** (**MEL**-ah-noh-sights) are special cells that are also found in the basal cell layer. These cells produce and contain a dark brown to black pigment known as melanin.
- **Melanin** (**MEL**-ah-nin) is the pigment that determines the color of the skin, which depends upon the type and amount of this pigment that is present (Figure 12.2). Melanin also produces spots of color such as freckles and age spots, which are discussed in later sections.
- Melanin has the important function of protecting the skin against some of the harmful ultraviolet rays of the sun. ***Ultraviolet*** (UV) refers to light that is beyond the visible spectrum at the violet end. Some UV rays help the skin produce vitamin D; however, other rays damage the skin.

The Dermis

The **dermis** (**DER**-mis), also known as the ***corium***, is the thick layer of living tissue directly below the epidermis. It contains connective tissue, blood and lymph vessels, and nerve fibers. Also found in the dermis are the *hair follicles*, *sebaceous glands*, and *sweat glands*, which are the related structures of the integumentary system (as well as the *nails*).

Sensory nerve endings in the dermis are the sensory receptors for stimuli such as touch, temperature, pain, and pressure.

Tissues Within the Dermis

- **Collagen** (**KOL**-ah-jen), which means glue, is a tough, yet flexible, fibrous protein material found in the skin, and also in the bones, cartilage, tendons, and ligaments.

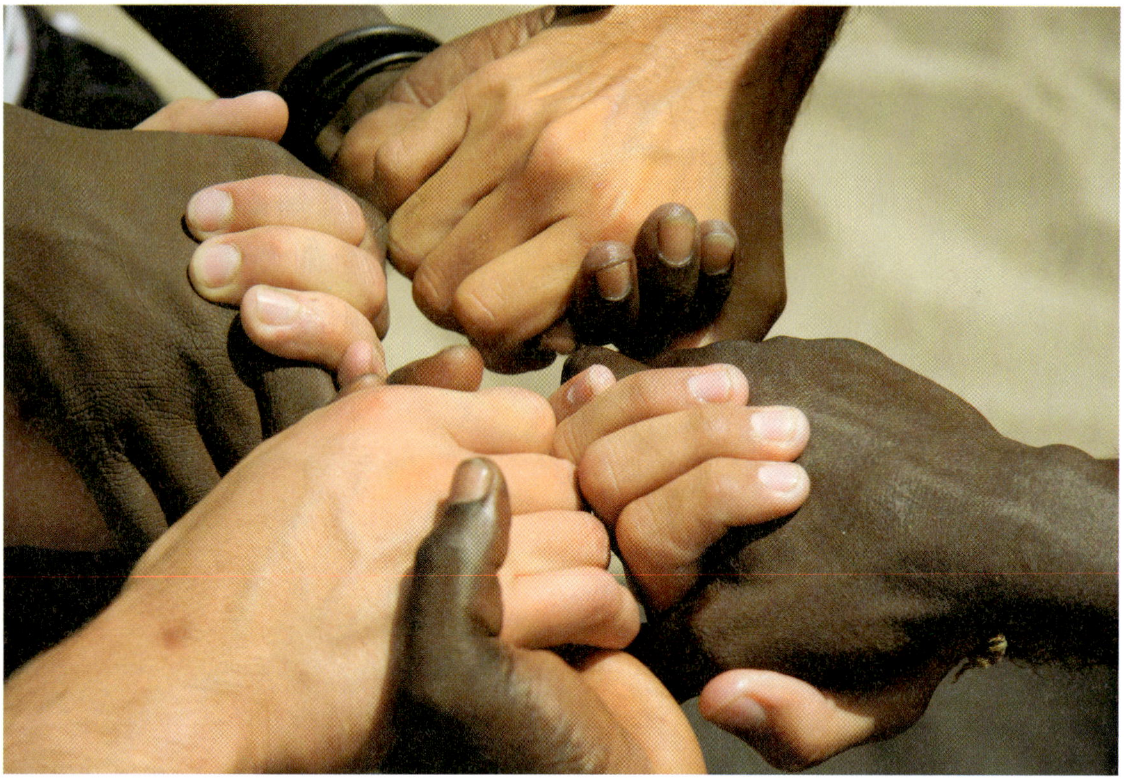

FIGURE 12.2 The amount of melanin present in the skin determines its color.

- **Mast cells**, which are found in the connective tissue of the dermis, respond to injury, infection, or allergy by producing and releasing substances, including heparin and histamine.
- **Heparin** (**HEP**-ah-rin), which is released in response to an injury, is an anticoagulant. An ***anticoagulant*** prevents blood clotting.
- **Histamine** (**HISS**-tah-meen), which is released in response to allergens, causes the signs of an allergic response, including itching and increased mucus secretion.

The Subcutaneous Layer

The **subcutaneous layer** (sub-kyou-**TAY**-nee-us) is located just below the layers of the skin and connects the skin to the surface muscles.

- This layer is made up of loose connective tissue and **adipose tissue** (**AD**-ih-pohs). *Adipose* means fat.
- *Cellulite* is a term used to describe deposits of dimpled fat around the buttocks and thighs. This is not a scientific term, and medical authorities agree that cellulite is simply ordinary fatty tissue. Note: Do not confuse cellulite with *cellulitis*, which is discussed later in this chapter.
- **Lipocytes** (**LIP**-oh-sights), also known as ***fat cells***, are predominant in the subcutaneous layer where they manufacture and store large quantities of fat (**lip/o** means fat, and **-cytes** means cells).

The Sebaceous Glands

Sebaceous glands (seh-**BAY**-shus) are located in the dermis layer of the skin and are closely associated with hair follicles (Figure 12.1).

- These glands secrete **sebum** (**SEE**-bum), which is an oily substance that is released through ducts opening into the hair follicles. From here, the sebum moves onto the surface and lubricates the skin.
- Because sebum is slightly acidic, it discourages the growth of bacteria on the skin.
- The milk-producing **mammary glands**, which are modified sebaceous glands, are sometimes classified with the integumentary system. However, they also are part of the reproductive system and are discussed in Chapter 14.

The Sweat Glands

Sweat glands, also known as ***sudoriferous glands***, are tiny, coiled glands found on almost all body surfaces. They are most numerous in the palms of the hands, the soles of the feet, the forehead, and in the armpits.

- **Pores** are the openings on the surface of the skin that act as the ducts of the sweat glands.
- **Perspiration**, commonly known as ***sweat***, is secreted by sweat glands and is made up of 99% water plus some salt and metabolic waste products.
- Perspiring is one way in which the body excretes excess water.
- As the perspiration evaporates into the air, it also cools the body. Body odor associated with perspiration comes from the interaction of sweat with bacteria on the skin's surface.
- **Hidrosis** (high-**DROH**-sis) is the production and excretion of perspiration.

The Hair

Hair fibers are rod-like structures composed of tightly fused, dead protein cells filled with hard keratin. The darkness and color of the hair is determined by the amount and type of melanin produced by the melanocytes that surround the core of the hair shaft.

- **Hair follicles** (**FOL**-lick-kulz) are the sacs that hold the root of the hair fibers. The shape of the follicle determines whether the hair is straight or curly.
- Although hair is dead tissue, it appears to grow because the cells at the base of the follicle divide rapidly and push the old cells upward. As these cells are pushed upward, they harden and undergo pigmentation.
- The **arrector pili** (ah-**RECK**-tor **PYE**-lye) are tiny muscle fibers attached to the hair follicles that cause the hair to stand erect. In response to cold or fright, these muscles contract, causing raised areas of skin known as goose bumps. This action reduces heat loss through the skin.

The Nails

An **unguis** (**UNG**-gwis), which is commonly known as a fingernail or toenail, is the keratin plate that protects the dorsal surface of the last bone of each finger and toe (plural, *ungues*). Each nail consists of the following parts (Figure 12.3):

- The ***nail body***, which is translucent, is closely molded to the surface of the underlying tissues. It is made up of hard, keratinized plates of epidermal cells.
- The ***nail bed***, which joins the nail body to the underlying connective tissue, nourishes the nail. The blood vessels here give the nail its characteristic pink color.

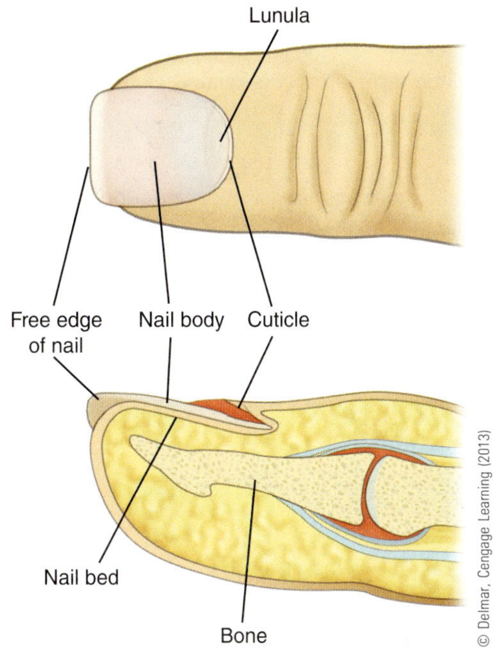

FIGURE 12.3 Structures of the fingernails and toenails.

- The ***free edge***, which is the portion of the nail not attached to the nail bed, extends beyond the tip of the finger or toe.
- The **lunula** (**LOO**-new-lah) is a pale half-moon-shaped region at every nail root, which is generally most easily seen in the thumbnail (plural, *lunulae*). This is the active area of the nail, where new keratin cells form. (**lun** means moon, and **-ula** means little).
- The **cuticle** is a narrow band of epidermis attached to the surface of the nail just in front of the root, protecting the new keratin cells as they form.
- The **nail root** fastens the nail to the finger or toe by fitting into a groove in the skin.

StudyWARE CONNECTION

To see the structures of the skin up close, view the **Skin** animation in the StudyWARE™.

MEDICAL SPECIALTIES RELATED TO THE INTEGUMENTARY SYSTEM

- A **dermatologist** (**der**-mah-**TOL**-oh-jist) is a physician who specializes in diagnosing and treating disorders of the skin (**dermat** means skin, and **-ologist** means specialist).

- A **plastic surgeon** is a physician who specializes in the surgical restoration and reconstruction of body structures. The term ***plastic*** is related to the suffix **-plasty**, meaning surgical repair.
- ***Cosmetic surgeons*** are plastic surgeons who perform operations such as breast augmentation, liposuction, and facelifts that are usually done for aesthetic rather than medical reasons.

PATHOLOGY OF THE INTEGUMENTARY SYSTEM

The Sebaceous Glands

- **Acne vulgaris** (**ACK**-nee vul-**GAY**-ris), commonly known as ***acne***, is a chronic inflammatory disease characterized by pustular eruptions of the skin caused by an overproduction of sebum around the hair shaft. Although often triggered by hormones in puberty and adolescence, it also occurs in adults. ***Vulgaris*** is a Latin term meaning common.
- A **comedo** (**KOM**-eh-doh) is a noninfected lesion formed by the buildup of sebum and keratin in a hair follicle (plural, *comedones*) often associated with acne vulgaris. A comedo with an obstructed opening is called a ***whitehead*** (a closed comedo). A sebum plug that is exposed to air often oxidizes and becomes a ***blackhead*** (an open comedo).
- A **sebaceous cyst** (seh-**BAY**-shus **SIST**) is a closed sac associated with a sebaceous gland that is found just under the skin. These cysts contain yellow, fatty material and are usually found on the face, neck, or trunk.
- **Seborrhea** (**seb**-oh-**REE**-ah) is overactivity of the sebaceous glands that results in the production of an excessive amount of sebum (**seb/o** means sebum, and **-rrhea** means flow or discharge).
- **Seborrheic dermatitis** (**seb**-oh-**REE**-ick **der**-mah-**TYE**-tis) is an inflammation sometimes resulting from seborrhea that causes scaling and itching of the upper layers of the skin or scalp. Extensive ***dandruff*** is a form of seborrheic dermatitis, as is the scalp rash in infants known as ***cradle cap***. In contrast, mild dandruff is usually caused by a yeast-like fungus on the scalp.
- A **seborrheic keratosis** (**seb**-oh-**REE**-ick **kerr**-ah-**TOH**-sis) is a benign skin growth that has a waxy or "pasted-on" look. These growths, which can vary in color from light tan to black, occur most commonly in the elderly.

The Sweat Glands

- **Anhidrosis** (**an**-high-**DROH**-sis) is the abnormal condition of lacking sweat in response to heat (**an-** means without, **hidr** means sweat, and **-osis** means abnormal condition).
- **Diaphoresis** (**dye**-ah-foh-**REE**-sis) is profuse sweating (**dia-** means through or complete, **phor** means movement, and **-esis** means abnormal condition). This is a normal condition when brought on by heat or exertion, but can also be the body's response to emotional or physical distress.
- **Heat rash**, also known as ***prickly heat***, is an intensely itchy rash caused by blockage of the sweat glands by bacteria and dead cells.
- **Hyperhidrosis** (**high**-per-high-**DROH**-sis) is a condition of excessive sweating in one area or over the whole body (**hyper-** means excessive, **hidr** means sweat, and **-osis** means abnormal condition).
- **Sleep hyperhidrosis**, commonly known as ***night sweats***, is the occurrence of hyperhidrosis during sleep. There are many potential causes of this condition, including menopause, certain medications, and some infectious diseases.

The Hair

- **Folliculitis** (foh-**lick**-you-**LYE**-tis) is an inflammation of the hair follicles (**follicul** means the hair follicle, and **-itis** means inflammation). This condition is especially common on arms, legs, and in the beard area of men.
  - One of the causes of folliculitis is a bacterium found in poorly chlorinated hot tubs or whirlpools. This leads to a condition called ***hot tub folliculitis***.
- **Trichomycosis axillaris** (**try**-koh-my-**KOH**-sis **ak**-sih-**LAR**-is) is superficial bacterial infection of the hair shafts in areas with extensive sweat glands, such as the armpits (**trich/o** means hair, **myc** means fungus, and **-osis** means abnormal condition). *Axillaris* is Latin for axillary (**axill** means armpit, and **-ary** means pertaining to.

Excessive Hairiness

Hirsutism (**HER**-soot-izm) is the presence of excessive body and facial hair in women, usually occurring in a male pattern (**hirsut** means hairy, and **-ism** means condition). This condition can be hereditary or caused by a hormonal imbalance.

Abnormal Hair Loss

- **Alopecia** (**al**-oh-**PEE**-shee-ah), also known as ***baldness***, is the partial or complete loss of hair, most commonly on the scalp (**alopec** means baldness, and **-ia** means condition).
- **Alopecia areata** (ah-ree-**AY**-tuh) is an autoimmune disorder that attacks the hair follicles, causing well-defined bald areas on the scalp or elsewhere on the body (Figure 12.4). This condition often begins in childhood. ***Areata*** means occurring in patches.
- **Alopecia totalis** (toh-**TAL**-is), also known as ***alopecia capitis totalis***, is an uncommon condition characterized by the loss of all the hair on the scalp.
- **Alopecia universalis** (**yoo**-nih-vers-**AHL**-is) is the total loss of hair on all parts of the body. ***Universalis*** means total.
- **Female pattern baldness** is a condition in which the hair thins in the front and on the sides of the scalp and sometimes on the crown. This condition rarely leads to total hair loss.
- **Male pattern baldness** is a common hair-loss pattern in men, with the hairline receding from the front to the back until only a horseshoe-shaped area of hair remains in the back and at the temples.

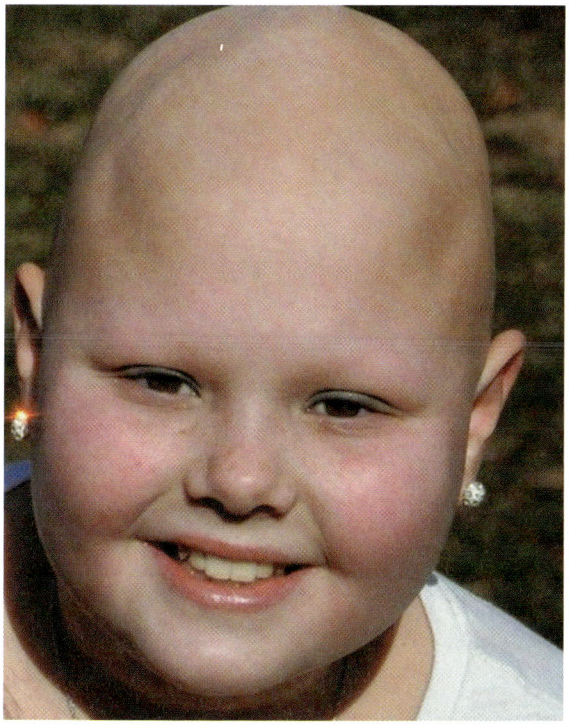

Used with permission from the Children's Alopecia Project.

FIGURE 12.4 Alopecia areata is an autoimmune disorder that often begins in childhood.

The Nails

- **Clubbing** is the abnormal curving of the nails that is often accompanied by enlargement of the fingertips. This condition can be hereditary, but usually is caused by changes associated with oxygen deficiencies related to coronary or pulmonary disease.
- **Koilonychia** (**koy**-loh-**NICK**-ee-ah), also known as ***spoon nail***, is a malformation of the nails in which the outer surface is concave or scooped out like the bowl of a spoon (**koil** means hollow or concave, **onych** means fingernail or toenail, and **-ia** means condition). This condition is often an indication of iron-deficiency anemia (see Chapter 5).
- **Onychia** (oh-**NICK**-ee-ah), also known as ***onychitis***, is an inflammation of the matrix of the nail that often results in the loss of the nail (**onych** means fingernail or toenail, and **-ia** means condition).
- **Onychocryptosis** (**on**-ih-koh-krip-**TOH**-sis) is commonly known as an ***ingrown toenail*** (**onych/o** means fingernail or toenail, **crypt** means hidden, and **-osis** means abnormal condition). The edges of a toenail, usually on the big toe, curve inward and cut into the skin. The affected area is prone to inflammation or infection.
- **Onychomycosis** (**on**-ih-koh-my-**KOH**-sis) is a fungal infection of the nail (**onych/o** means fingernail or toenail, **myc** means fungus, and **-osis** means abnormal condition). Depending on the type of fungus involved, this condition can cause the nails to turn white, yellow, green, or black and to become thick or brittle.
- **Onychophagia** (**on**-ih-koh-**FAY**-jee-ah) means nail biting or nail eating (**onych/o** means fingernail or toenail, and **-phagia** means eating or swallowing).
- **Paronychia** (**par**-oh-**NICK**-ee-ah) is an acute or chronic infection of the skin fold around a nail (**par-** means near, **onych** means fingernail or toenail, and **-ia** means condition).

Skin Pigmentation

- **Age spots,** also known as ***solar lentigines*** or ***liver spots***, are discolorations caused by sun exposure. Although harmless, these spots sometimes resemble skin cancer growths.
- **Albinism** (**AL**-bih-niz-um) is a genetic condition characterized by a deficiency or the absence of pigment in the skin, hair, and irises of the eyes (**albin** means white, and **-ism** means condition).

This condition is the result of a missing enzyme that is necessary for the production of melanin. A person with this condition is known as an *albino*.

- **Chloasma** (kloh-**AZ**-mah), also known as *melasma* or the *mask of pregnancy*, is a pigmentation disorder characterized by brownish spots on the face. This can occur during pregnancy, especially among women with dark hair and fair skin, and usually disappears after delivery.
- **Vitiligo** (**vit**-ih-**LYE**-goh) is a skin condition resulting from the destruction of the melanocytes due to unknown causes. Vitiligo causes irregular patches of white skin, a process known as *depigmentation*. Hair growing in an affected area may also turn white.

Bleeding into the Skin

- A **contusion** (kon-**TOO**-zhun) is an injury to underlying tissues without breaking the skin and is characterized by discoloration and pain (**contus** means bruise, and **-ion** means condition). This discoloration is caused by an accumulation of blood within the skin.
- An **ecchymosis** (**eck**-ih-**MOH**-sis), commonly known as a *bruise*, is a large, irregular area of purplish discoloration due to bleeding under the skin (**ecchym** means pouring out of juice, and **-osis** means abnormal condition) (Figure 12.5). The plural form is *ecchymoses*.
- **Purpura** (**PUR**-pew-rah) is the appearance of multiple purple discolorations on the skin caused by bleeding underneath the skin (**purpur** means purple, and **-a** is a noun ending). These areas of discoloration are smaller than an ecchymosis and larger than petechiae.
- **Petechiae** (pee-**TEE**-kee-ee) are very small, pinpoint hemorrhages that are less than 2 mm in diameter (singular, *petechia*). These hemorrhages sometimes result from high fevers.
- A **hematoma** (**hee**-mah-**TOH**-mah), which is usually caused by an injury, is a swelling of clotted blood trapped in the tissues (**hemat** means blood, and **-oma** means tumor). The body eventually reabsorbs this blood. A hematoma is often named for the area where it occurs. For example, a *subungual hematoma* is blood trapped under a finger or toenail.

Surface Lesions

A **lesion** (**LEE**-zhun) is a pathologic change of the tissues due to disease or injury. Skin lesions are described by their appearance, location, color, and size as measured in centimeters (cm).

- A **crust**, also known as *scab*, is a collection of dried serum and cellular debris (Figure 12.6A).
- **Erosion** (eh-**ROH**-zhun) is the wearing away of a surface, such as the epidermis of the skin or the outer layer of a mucus membrane. This term can also describe the progressive loss of dental enamel.
- A **macule** (**MACK**-youl), also known as a *macula*, is a discolored flat spot that is less than 1 cm in diameter. Freckles, or flat moles, are examples of macules (Figure 12.6B).
- A **nodule** (**NOD**-youl) is a solid, raised skin lesion that is *larger than* 0.5 cm in diameter and deeper than a papule. In acne vulgaris, nodules can cause scarring.

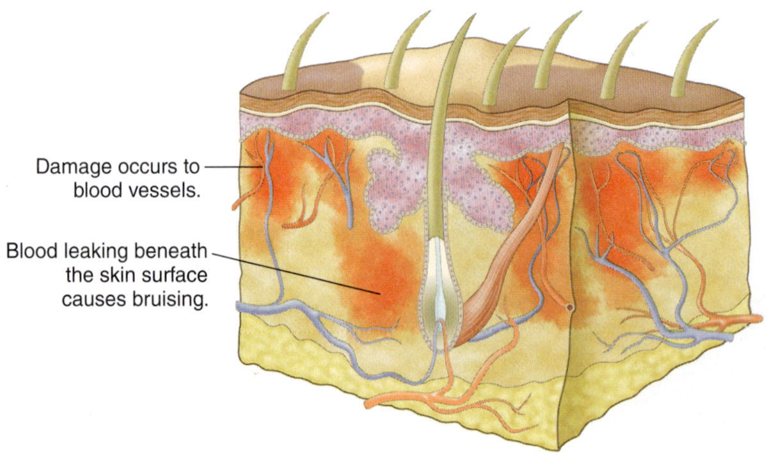

FIGURE 12.5 A cross-section of the skin showing the bleeding under the skin causing ecchymosis.

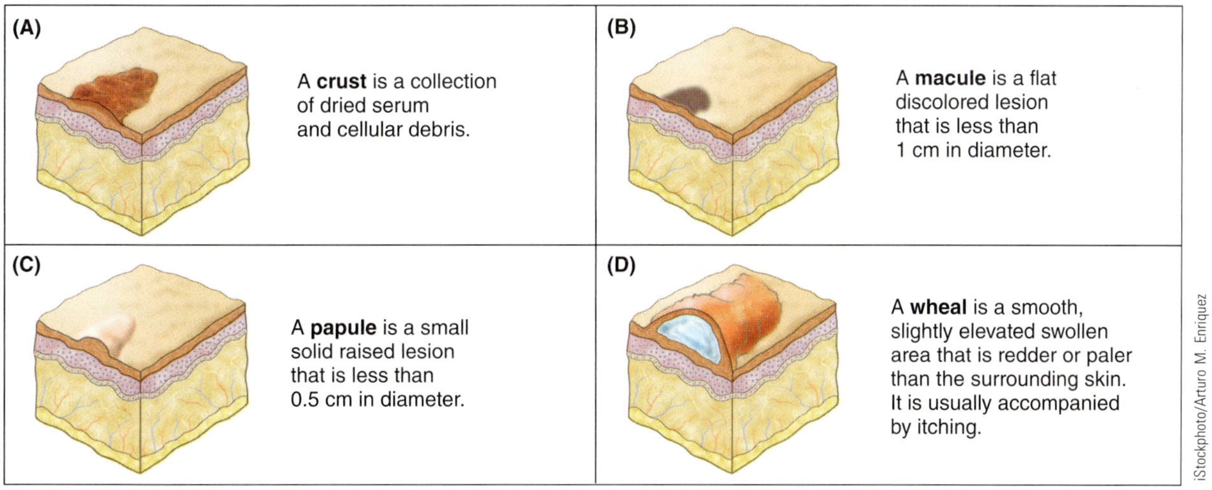

FIGURE 12.6 Surface lesions of the skin. (A) Crust. (B) Macule. (C) Papule. (D) Wheal.

- A **papule** (**PAP**-youl) is a small, raised red lesion that is *less than* 0.5 cm in diameter and does not contain pus. Small pimples and insect bites are types of papules (Figure 12.6C).
- A **plaque** (**PLACK**) is a scaly, solid raised area of closely spaced papules. For example, the lesions of psoriasis are plaques (Figure 12.11). Note: The term *plaque* also means a fatty buildup in the arteries (see Chapter 5) and a soft substance that forms on the teeth (see Chapter 8).
- **Scales** are flakes or dry patches made up of excess dead epidermal cells. Some shedding of these scales is normal; however, excessive shedding is associated with skin disorders such as psoriasis.
- **Verrucae** (veh-**ROO**-kee), also known as ***warts***, are small, hard skin lesions caused by the human papillomavirus (singular, *verruca*). ***Plantar warts*** are verrucae that develop on the sole of the foot. See Chapter 14 for more information on the human papillomavirus.
- A **wheal** (**WHEEL**), also known as a ***welt***, is a small bump that itches. Wheals can appear as *urticaria*, or hives (which are discussed in a later section) as a symptom of an allergic reaction (Figure 12.6D).

Fluid-Filled Lesions

- An **abscess** (**AB**-sess) is a closed pocket containing pus that is caused by a bacterial infection. An abscess can appear on the skin or within other structures of the body.
- **Purulent** (**PYOU**-roo-lent) means producing or containing pus.
- An **exudate** (**ECKS**-you-dayt) is a fluid, such as pus, that leaks out of an infected wound.
- A **cyst** (**SIST**) is an abnormal sac containing gas, fluid, or a semisolid material (Figure 12.7A). The term ***cyst*** can also refer to a sac or vesicle elsewhere in the body. The most common type of skin cyst is a sebaceous cyst.
- A **pustule** (**PUS**-tyoul), also known as a ***pimple***, is a small, circumscribed lesion containing pus (Figure 12.7B). ***Circumscribed*** means contained within a limited area. Pustules can be cause by acne vulgaris, impetigo, or other skin infections.
- A **vesicle** (**VES**-ih-kul) is a small blister, *less than* 0.5 cm in diameter, containing watery fluid (Figure 12.7C). For example, the rash of poison ivy consists of vesicles (Figure 12.10).
- A **bulla** (**BULL**-ah) is a large blister that is usually *more than* 0.5 cm in diameter (plural, *bullae*) (Figure 12.7D).

Lesions Through the Skin

- An **abrasion** (ah-**BRAY**-zhun) is an injury in which superficial layers of skin are scraped or rubbed away.
- A **fissure** (**FISH**-ur) is a groove or crack-like break in the skin. Fissures are, for example, the breaks in the skin between the toes caused by tinea pedis, or athlete's foot (Figure 12.8A). The term ***fissure*** also describes folds in the contours of the brain.
- A **laceration** (**lass**-er-**AY**-shun) is a torn or jagged wound, or an accidental cut wound.
- A **pressure sore**, previously known as a ***decubitus ulcer*** or ***bedsore***, is an open ulcerated wound that is caused by prolonged pressure on an area of skin. Without proper care, these sores quickly become seriously infected and can result in tissue death.

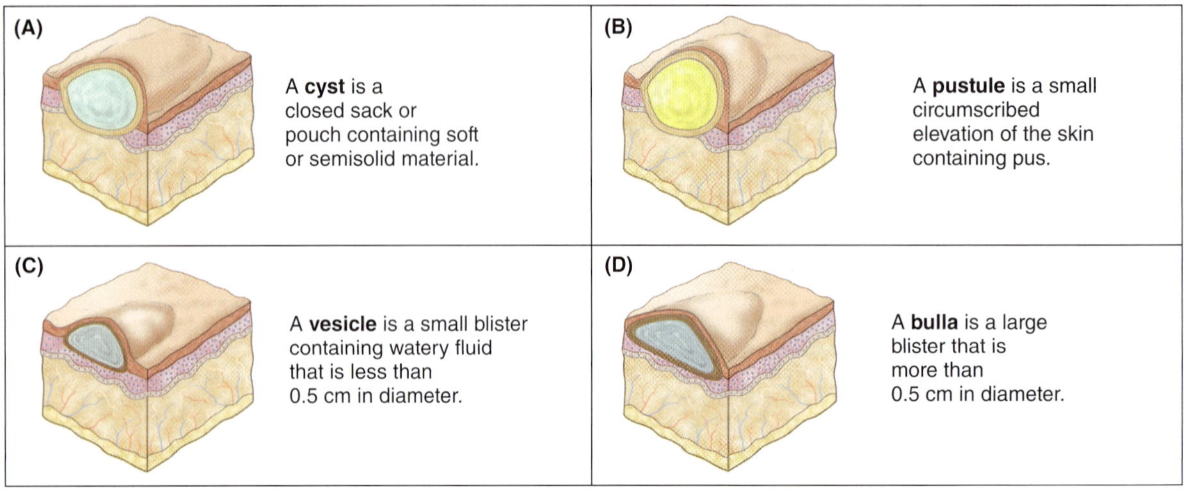

FIGURE 12.7 Fluid-filled lesions in the skin. (A) Cyst. (B) Pustule. (C) Vesicle. (D) Bulla.

- A **puncture wound** is a deep hole made by a sharp object such as a rusty nail or ice pick. This type of percutaneous wound carries a high risk of infection, particularly tetanus (see Chapter 6). ***Percutaneous*** means through the skin.
- A ***needlestick injury*** is an accidental puncture wound caused by a used hypodermic needle, potentially transmitting an infection.
- An **ulcer** (**UL**-ser) is an open lesion of the skin or mucous membrane resulting in tissue loss around the edges (Figure 12.8B). Note: Ulcers also occur inside the body. Those associated with the digestive system are discussed in Chapter 8.

Birthmarks

A birthmark is a mole or blemish on the skin present at birth or shortly thereafter. Some birthmarks marks fade as a child gets older.

- **Pigmented birthmarks** include **nevi**, also known as moles, as well as café-au-lait spots, stork bites, and other irregularities in skin color.
- **Vascular birthmarks** are caused by blood vessels close to the skin's surface.
- A **capillary hemangioma** (**KAP**-uh-**ler**-ee hee-**man**-jee-**OH**-mah), also known as a ***strawberry birthmark***, is a soft, raised, pink or red vascular birthmark (**hem** means blood, **angi** means blood or lymph vessels, and **-oma** means tumor). A ***hemangioma*** is a benign tissue mass made up of newly formed small blood vessels that in birthmarks are visible through the skin (Figure 12.9). (Also see hemangioma in Chapter 5.)
- A **port-wine stain** is a flat vascular birthmark made up of dilated blood capillaries, creating a large, reddish-purple discoloration on the face or neck. This type of birthmark will not resolve without treatment. See the later section "Laser and Light Source Treatments of Skin Conditions."

Dermatitis

The term **dermatitis** (**der**-mah-**TYE**-tis) describes an inflammation of the skin (**dermat** means skin, and **-itis** means inflammation). This condition, which takes many forms, is usually characterized by redness, swelling, and itching.

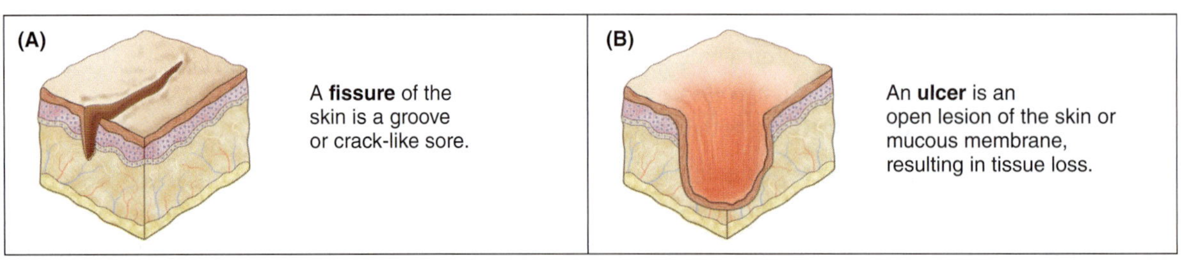

FIGURE 12.8 Lesions extending through the skin. (A) Fissure. (B) Ulcer.

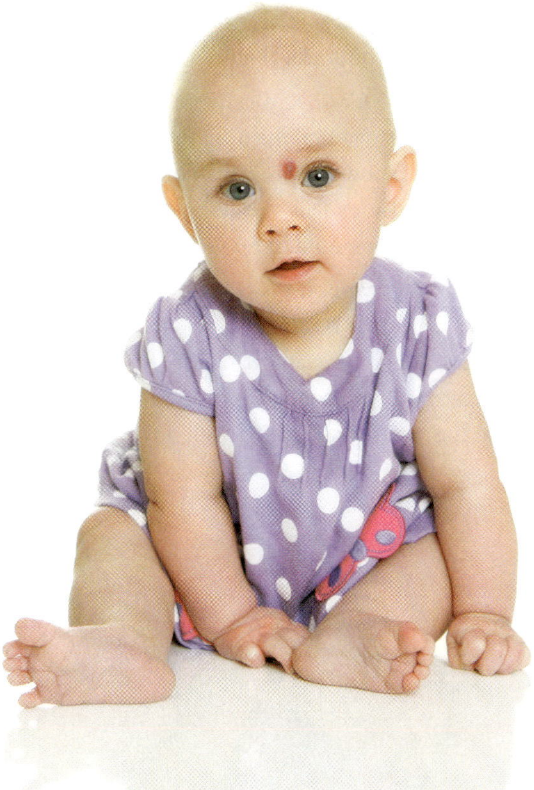

Julie DeGuia/www.Shutterstock.com

FIGURE 12.9 A capillary hemangioma is a raised vascular birthmark made up of newly formed small blood vessels.

- **Contact dermatitis** (CD) is a localized allergic response caused by contact with an irritant, such as diaper rash. It can also be caused by exposure to an allergen, such as poison ivy, or an allergic reaction to latex gloves (Figure 12.10).
- **Eczema** (**ECK**-zeh-mah), also known as ***atopic dermatitis***, is a form of persistent or recurring dermatitis usually characterized by redness, itching, and dryness, with possible blistering, cracking, oozing, or bleeding. This chronic condition, most often seen in infants and children, appears to be the result of a malfunction of the body's immune system.
- **Exfoliative dermatitis** (ecks-**FOH**-lee-**ay**-tiv **der**-mah-**TYE**-tis) is a condition in which there is widespread scaling of the skin. It is often accompanied by pruritus, erythroderma (redness), and hair loss. It may occur in severe cases of many common skin conditions, including eczema, psoriasis, and allergic reactions.

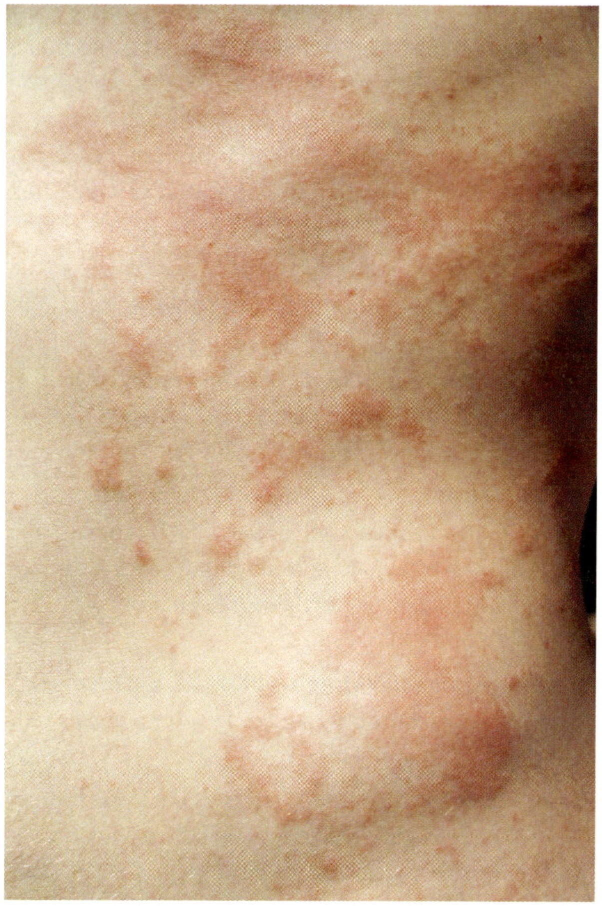

Joy Brown/www.Shutterstock.com

FIGURE 12.10 Contact dermatitis on a young man's torso caused by poison ivy.

- **Pruritus** (proo-**RYE**-tus), also known as ***itching***, is associated with most forms of dermatitis (**prurit** means itching, and **-us** is a singular noun ending). Note that this term ends in *-us*, not *-is*.

Erythema

Erythema (**er**-ih-**THEE**-mah) is redness of the skin due to capillary dilation (**erythem** means flushed, and **-a** is a noun ending). *Dilation* describes the expansion of the capillary.

- ***Erythema infectiosum***, also known as ***fifth disease***, is a mildly contagious viral infection that is common in childhood. This infection produces a red, lace-like rash on the child's face that looks as if the child has been slapped. It is called "fifth disease" because its place on the list of six common childhood diseases that can cause an exanthem (which is discussed in a later bullet). Others include measles and rubella.

- ***Erythema multiforme*** is a skin disorder resulting from a generalized allergic reaction to an illness, infection, or medication. This reaction, which affects the skin, the mucous membranes, or both, is characterized by a rash that may appear as nodules or papules (raised red bumps), macules (flat discolored areas), or vesicles or bullae (blisters).
- ***Erythema pernio***, also known as ***chilblains***, is a purple-red inflammation that occurs when the small blood vessels below the skin are damaged, usually due to exposure to cold and damp weather. When warmth restores full circulation, the affected areas begin to itch; however, they usually heal without treatment.
- ***Sunburn*** is a form of erythema in which skin cells are damaged by exposure to the ultraviolet rays in sunlight. This damage increases the chances of later developing skin cancer.
- **Erythroderma** (eh-**rith**-roh-**DER**-mah) is abnormal redness of the entire skin surface (**erythr/o** means red, and **-derma** means skin).
- **Exanthem** (eck-**ZAN**-thum) refers to a widespread rash, usually in children. A ***rash*** is a breaking out, or eruption, that changes the color or texture of the skin.

General Skin Conditions

- **Dermatosis** (**der**-mah-**TOH**-sis) is a general term used to denote skin lesions or eruptions of any type that are *not* associated with inflammation (**dermat** means skin, and **-osis** means abnormal condition).
- **Ichthyosis** (**ick**-thee-**OH**-sis) is a group of hereditary disorders characterized by dry, thickened, and scaly skin (**ichthy** means dry or scaly, and **-osis** means abnormal condition). These conditions are caused either by the slowing of the skin's natural shedding process or by a rapid increase in the production of the skin's cells.
- **Lipedema** (lip-eh-**DEE**-mah), also known as ***painful fat syndrome***, is a chronic abnormal condition that is characterized by the accumulation of fat and fluid in the tissues just under the skin of the hips and legs (**lip** means fat, and **-edema** means swelling). This condition usually affects women and even with weight loss, this localized excess fat does not go away.
- **Systemic lupus erythematosus** (sis-**TEH**-mik **LOO**-pus er-ih-**thee**-mah-**TOH**-sus) (SLE), also known as ***lupus***, is an autoimmune disorder characterized by a red, scaly rash on the face and upper trunk. In addition to the skin, this condition also attacks the connective tissue in other body systems, especially in the joints.
- **Psoriasis** (soh-**RYE**-uh-sis) is a common skin disorder characterized by flare-ups in which red papules covered with silvery scales occur on the elbows, knees, scalp, back, or buttocks (Figure 12.11).
- **Rosacea** (roh-**ZAY**-shee-ah), which is also known as ***adult acne***, is characterized by tiny red pimples and broken blood vessels. This chronic condition of unknown cause usually develops in individuals with fair skin, between 30 and 60 years of ages.
- **Rhinophyma** (**rye**-noh-**FIGH**-muh), also known as ***bulbous nose***, usually occurs in older men (**rhin/o** means nose, and **-phyma** means growth). This condition is characterized by hyperplasia (overgrowth) of the tissues of the nose and is associated with advanced rosacea.

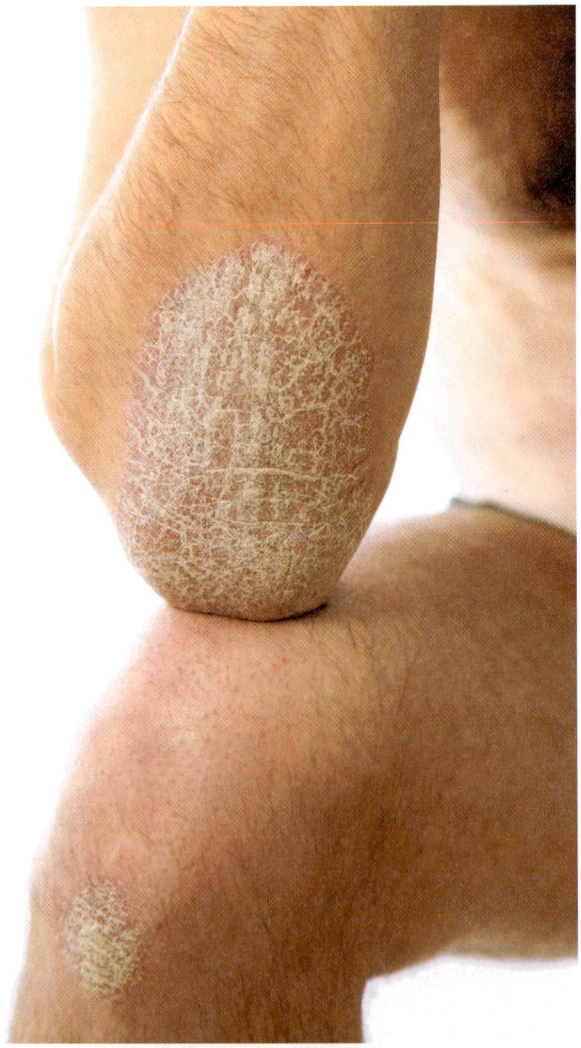

Christine Langer-Pueschel/www.Shutterstock.com

FIGURE 12.11 Psoriasis is characterized by red papules covered with silvery scales.

- **Scleroderma** (**sklehr**-oh-**DER**-mah) is an autoimmune disorder in which the connective tissues become thickened and hardened, causing the skin to become hard and swollen (**scler/o** means hard, and **-derma** means skin). This condition can also affect the joints and internal organs.
- **Urticaria** (**ur**-tih-**KARE**-ree-ah), also known as ***hives***, are itchy wheals caused by an allergic reaction (**urtic** means rash, and **-aria** means connected with).
- **Xeroderma** (zee-roh-**DER**-mah), also known as ***xerosis***, is excessively dry skin (**xer/o** means dry, and **-derma** means skin).

Bacterial Skin Infections

- A **carbuncle** (**KAR**-bung-kul) is a cluster of connected furuncles (boils).
- **Cellulitis** (**sell**-you-**LYE**-tis) is an acute, rapidly spreading bacterial infection within the connective tissues that is characterized by malaise, swelling, warmth, and red streaks. ***Malaise*** is a feeling of general discomfort or uneasiness that is often the first indication of an infection or other disease.
- **Furuncles** (**FYOU**-rung-kulz), also known as ***boils***, are large, tender, swollen areas caused by a staphylococcal infection around hair follicles or sebaceous glands.
- **Gangrene** (**GANG**-green), which is tissue necrosis (death), is most commonly caused by a loss of circulation to the affected tissues. The tissue death is followed by bacterial invasion that causes putrefaction, and if this infection enters the bloodstream, it can be fatal. ***Putrefaction*** is decay that produces foul-smelling odors.
- **Impetigo** (**im**-peh-**TYE**-goh) is a highly contagious bacterial skin infection that commonly occurs in children. This condition is characterized by isolated pustules that become crusted and rupture.
- **Necrotizing fasciitis** (**NECK**-roh-**tiz**-ing **fas**-ee-**EYE**-tis) is a severe infection caused by Group A strep bacteria, which is also known as ***flesh-eating bacteria***. ***Necrotizing*** means causing tissue death, and ***fasciitis*** is inflammation of fascia. These bacteria normally live harmlessly on the skin; however, if they enter the body through a skin wound, this serious infection can result. If untreated, the infected body tissue is destroyed, and the illness can be fatal.
- **Pyoderma** (**pye**-oh-**DER**-mah) is any acute, inflammatory, pus-forming bacterial skin infection such as impetigo (**py/o** means pus, and **-derma** means skin).

Fungal Skin Infections

- **Mycosis** (my-**KOH**-sis) describes any abnormal condition or disease caused by a fungus (**myc** means fungus, and **-osis** means abnormal condition or disease).
- **Tinea** (**TIN**-ee-ah) is a fungal infection that can grow on the skin, hair, or nails. This condition is also known as ***ringworm***, not because a worm is involved, but because as the fungus grows, it spreads out in a worm-like circle, leaving normal-looking skin in the middle (Figure 12.12).
  - ***Tinea capitis*** is found on the scalps of children. ***Capitis*** means head.
  - ***Tinea corporis*** is a fungal infection of the skin on the body. ***Corporis*** means body.
  - ***Tinea cruris***, also known as ***jock itch***, is found in the genital area.
  - ***Tinea pedis***, also known as ***athlete's foot***, is most commonly found between the toes. ***Pedis*** means feet.

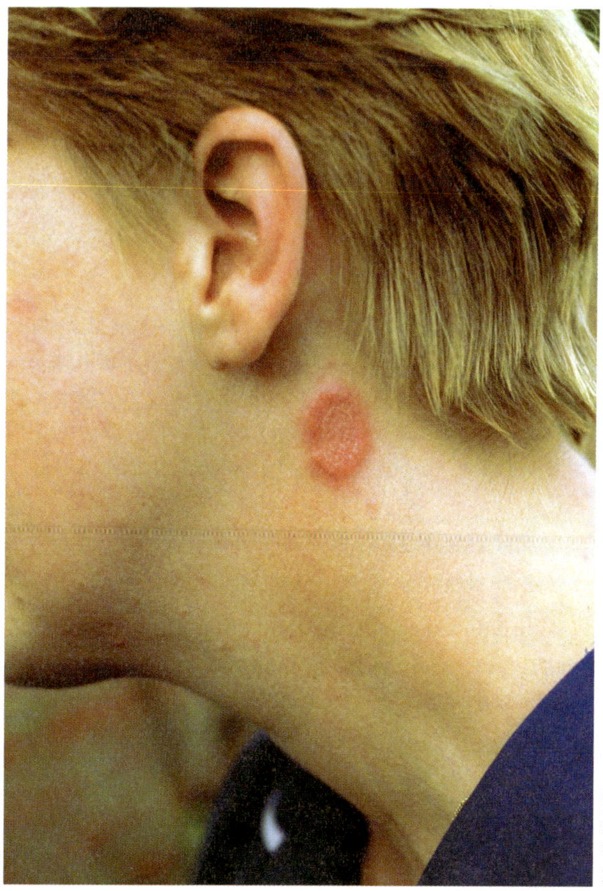

John Hadfield/Photo Researchers, Inc.

FIGURE 12.12 Tinea is a fungal infection also known as ringworm.

- *Tinea versicolor*, also known as *pityriasis versicolor*, is a fungal infection that causes painless, discolored areas on the skin. *Versicolor* means a variety of color.

Parasitic Skin Infestations

An **infestation** is the dwelling of microscopic parasites on external surface tissue. Some parasites live temporarily on the skin. Others lay eggs and reproduce there.

- **Pediculosis** (pee-**dick**-you-**LOH**-sis) is an infestation with *lice* (**pedicul** means lice, and **-osis** means abnormal condition). In order to get rid of the infestation, the lice eggs, which are known as *nits*, must be destroyed. There are three types of lice, each attracted to a specific part of the body:
  - *Pediculosis capitis* is an infestation with head lice.
  - *Pediculosis corporis* is an infestation with body lice.
  - *Pediculosis pubis* is an infestation with lice in the pubic hair and pubic region.
- **Scabies** (**SKAY**-beez) is a skin infection caused by an infestation of *itch mites*. These tiny mites cause small, itchy bumps and blisters by burrowing into the top layer of human skin to lay their eggs. Medications applied to the skin kill the mites; however, itching may persist for several weeks.

Skin Growths

- A **callus** (**KAL**-us) is a thickening of part of the skin on the hands or feet caused by repeated rubbing. Compare with *callus* in Chapter 3. A *clavus*, or *corn*, is a callus in the keratin layer of the skin covering the joints of the toes, usually caused by ill-fitting shoes.
- A **cicatrix** (sick-**AY**-tricks) is a normal scar resulting from the healing of a wound (plural, *cicatrices*).
- **Granulation tissue** is the tissue that normally forms during the healing of a wound. This tissue eventually forms the scar.
- **Granuloma** (**gran**-you-**LOH**-mah) is a general term used to describe a small, knot-like swelling of granulation tissue in the epidermis (**granul** meaning granular, and **-oma** means tumor). Granulomas can result from inflammation, injury, or infection.
- A **keloid** (**KEE**-loid) is an abnormally raised or thickened scar that expands beyond the boundaries of the original incision (**kel** means growth or tumor, and **-oid** means resembling). A tendency to form keloids is often inherited and is more common among people with dark-pigmented skin.
- A **keratosis** (**kerr**-ah-**TOH**-sis) is any skin growth, such as a wart or a callus, in which there is overgrowth and thickening of the skin (**kerat** means hard or horny, and **-osis** means abnormal condition) (plural, *keratoses*). Patches of keratosis in the mouth are known as *leukoplakia*. Note: **kerat/o** also refers to the cornea of the eye. (See Chapter 11.)
- A **lipoma** (lih-**POH**-mah) is a benign, slow-growing fatty tumor located between the skin and the muscle layer (**lip** means fatty, and **-oma** means tumor). This fatty tumor is usually harmless, and treatment is rarely necessary unless the tumor is in a bothersome location, is painful, or is growing rapidly.
- **Nevus** (**NEE**-vus), also known as a *mole*, is a small, dark, skin growth that develops from melanocytes in the skin (plural, *nevi*). Normally, these growths are benign.
- In contrast, **dysplastic nevi** (dis-**PLAS**-tick **NEE**-vye) are atypical moles that can develop into skin cancer.
- A **papilloma** (**pap**-ih-**LOH**-mah) is a benign, superficial wart-like growth on the epithelial tissue or elsewhere in the body, such as in the bladder (**papill** means resembling a nipple, and **-oma** means tumor).
- **Polyp** (**POL**-up) is a general term used most commonly to describe a mushroom-like growth from the surface of a mucous membrane, such as a polyp in the nose. These growths have many causes and are not necessarily malignant.
- **Skin tags** are small, flesh-colored or light-brown polyps that hang from the body by fine stalks. Skin tags are benign and tend to enlarge with age.

Skin Cancer

Skin cancer is a harmful, malignant growth on the skin, which can have many causes, including repeated severe sunburns or long-term exposure to the sun. Skin cancer is becoming very common, affecting about one in five

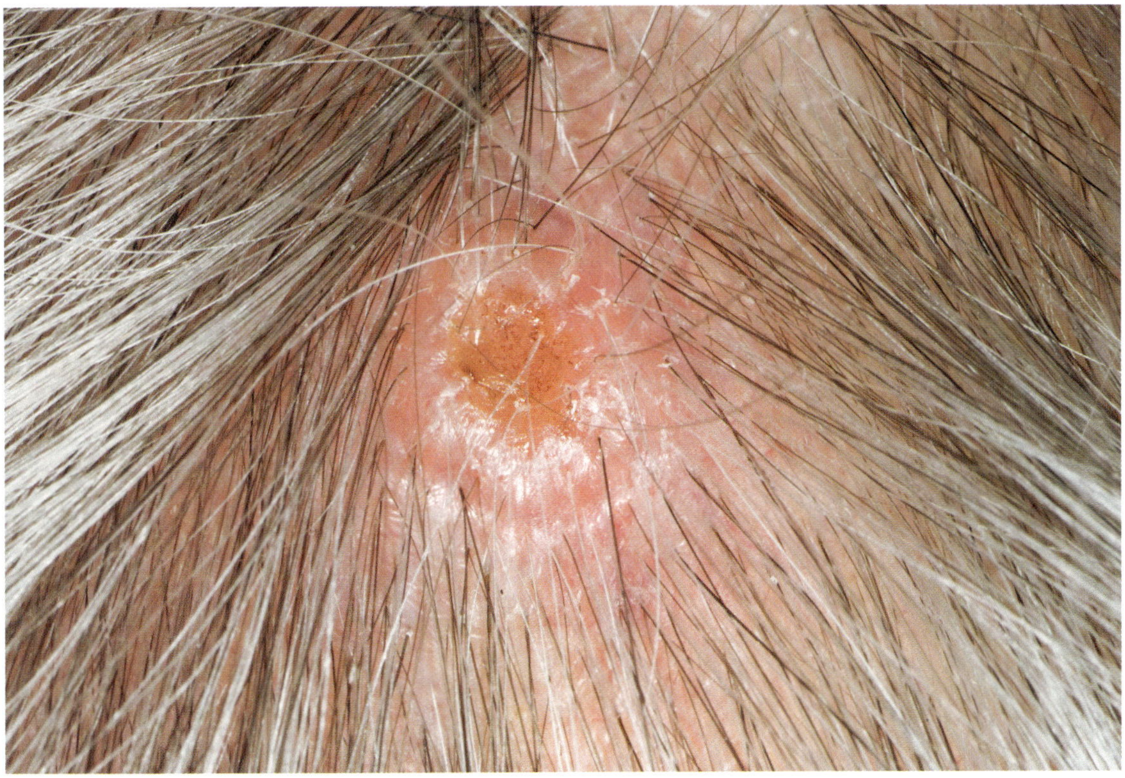

Dr. P. Marazzi/Photo Researchers, Inc.

FIGURE 12.13 Squamous cell carcinoma of the scalp.

Americans in his or her lifetime. There are three main types of skin cancer: basal cell carcinoma, squamous cell carcinoma, and melanoma.

- An **actinic keratosis** (ack-**TIN**-ick **kerr**-ah-**TOH**-sis) is a precancerous skin growth that occurs on sun-damaged skin. It often looks like a red, tan, or pink scaly patch and feels like sandpaper. ***Precancerous*** describes a growth that is not yet malignant; however, if not treated, it is likely to become malignant.
- A **basal cell carcinoma** is a malignant tumor of the basal cell layer of the epidermis. This is the most common and least harmful type of skin cancer because it is slow growing and rarely spreads to other parts of the body. The lesions, which occur mainly on the face or neck and tend to bleed easily, are usually pink, smooth, and are raised with a depression in the center (see carcinoma of the lip in Chapter 6, Figure 6.12).
- **Squamous cell carcinoma** (**SKWAY**-mus) originates as a malignant tumor of the scaly squamous cells of the epithelium; however, it can quickly spread to other body systems. These cancers begin as skin lesions that appear to be sores that will not heal or that have a crusted look (Figure 12.13).
- **Malignant melanoma** (mel-ah-**NOH**-mah), also known as ***melanoma***, is a type of skin cancer that occurs in the melanocytes (**melan** means black, and **-oma** means tumor). This is the most serious type of skin cancer and often the first signs are changes in the size, shape, or color of a mole (Figure 12.14).

Burns

A **burn** is an injury to body tissues caused by heat, flame, electricity, sun, chemicals, or radiation. The severity of a burn is described according to the percentage of the total body skin surface affected (more than 15% is considered serious). It is also described according to the depth or layers of skin involved (Table 12.1 and Figure 12.15).

StudyWARE CONNECTION

Watch an animation on Burns in the StudyWARE™.

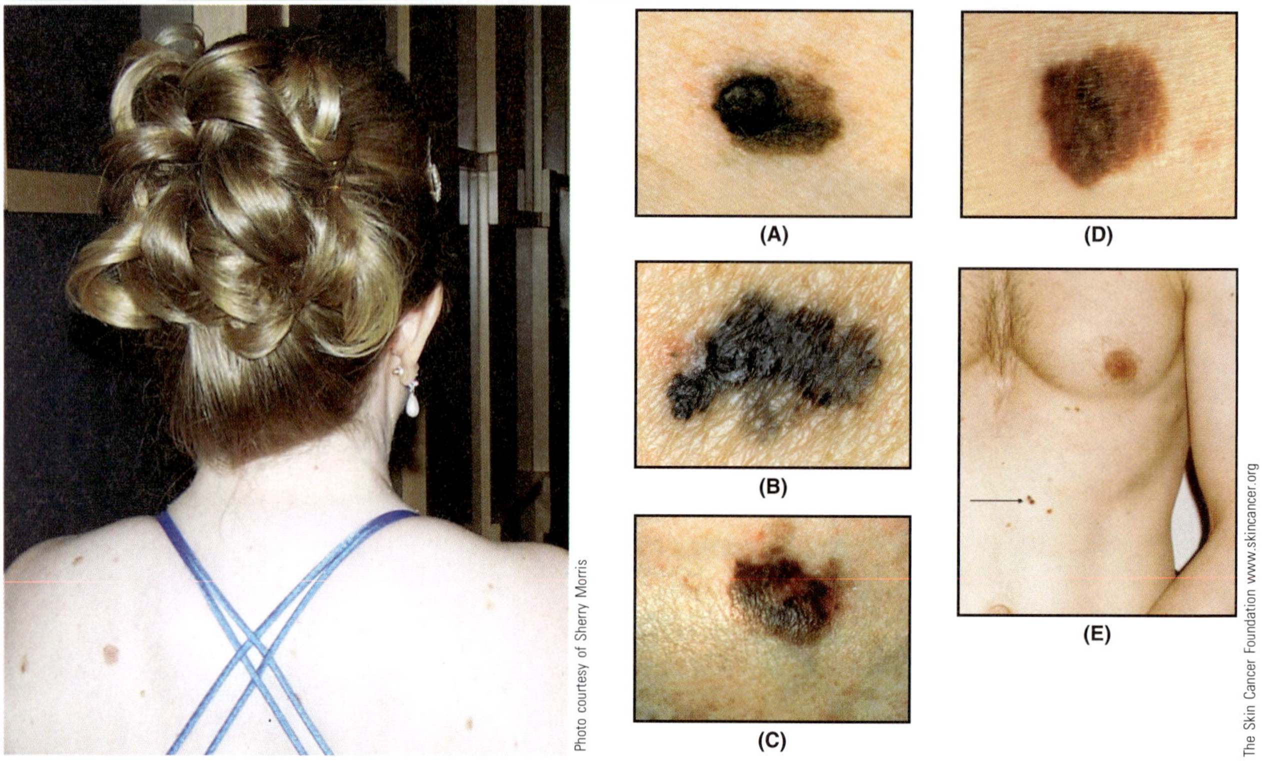

FIGURE 12.14 Left: Melanoma visible on the left shoulder blade. Right: The A-B-C-D-E signs of melanoma are (A) asymmetry, (B) border irregularity, (C) color variation, and (D) diameter larger than a pencil eraser, (E) evolving, or changing in size, shape, or shade of color.

TABLE 12.1
Classification of Burn Severity

Type of Burn	Also Known As	Layers of Skin Involved
First-degree burn	*Superficial burn*	No blisters, superficial damage to the epidermis.
Second-degree burn	*Partial thickness burn*	Blisters, damage to the epidermis, and dermis.
Third-degree burn	*Full thickness burn*	Damage to the epidermis, dermis, and subcutaneous layers, and possibly also the muscle and bone below.

DIAGNOSTIC PROCEDURES OF THE INTEGUMENTARY SYSTEM

A **biopsy** (**BYE**-op-see) is the removal of a small piece of living tissue for examination to confirm or establish a diagnosis (**bi** means pertaining to life, and **-opsy** means view of).

- In an *incisional biopsy*, a piece, but not all, of the tumor or lesion is removed.
- In an *excisional biopsy*, the entire tumor or lesion and a margin of surrounding tissue are removed. *Excision* means the complete removal of a lesion or organ.
- In a *needle biopsy*, a hollow needle is used to remove a core of tissue for examination.
- **Exfoliative cytology** (ecks-**FOH**-lee-**ay**-tiv sigh-TOL-oh-jee) is a technique in which cells are scraped from the tissue and examined under a microscope. *Exfoliation* is the removal of dead epidermal cells,

often through sanding or chemabrasion (which is discussed in the next section), and is sometimes done for cosmetic purposes.

TREATMENT PROCEDURES OF THE INTEGUMENTARY SYSTEM

Preventive Measures

Sunscreen that blocks out the harmful ultraviolet B (UVB) rays is sometimes measured in terms of the strength of the *sun protection factor*. Some sunscreens also give protection against ultraviolet A (UVA rays).

Tissue Removal

- **Cauterization** (**kaw**-ter-eye-**ZAY**-zhun) is the destruction of tissue by burning.
- **Chemabrasion** (**kem**-ah-**BRAY**-zhun), also known as a *chemical peel*, is the use of chemicals to remove the outer layers of skin to treat acne scarring, fine wrinkling, and keratoses.
- **Cryosurgery** (**krye**-oh-**SIR**-jur-ee) is the destruction or elimination of abnormal tissue cells, such as warts or tumors, through the application of extreme cold by using liquid nitrogen (**cry/o** means cold, and **-surgery** means operative procedure).

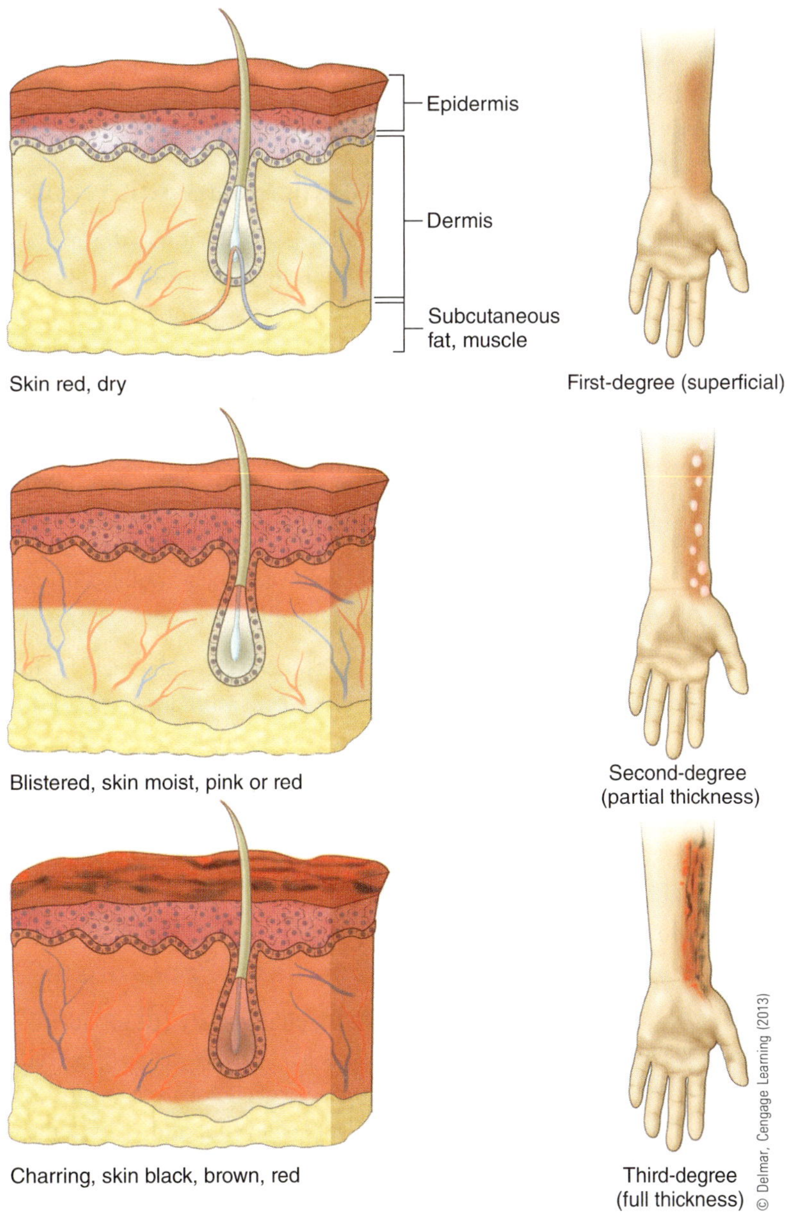

FIGURE 12.15 The degree of a burn is determined by the layers of skin involved.

- **Curettage** (**kyou**-reh-**TAHZH**) is the removal of material from the surface by scraping. One use of this technique is to remove basal cell tumors.
- **Debridement** (dah-**BREED**-ment) is the removal of dirt, foreign objects, damaged tissue, and cellular debris from a wound to prevent infection and to promote healing.
- In an **irrigation and debridement** procedure, pressurized fluid is used to clean out wound debris.
- **Dermabrasion** (**der**-mah-**BRAY**-zhun) is a form of abrasion involving the use of a revolving wire brush or sandpaper. It is used to remove acne and chickenpox scars as well as for facial skin rejuvenation. ***Microdermabrasion*** removes only a fine layer of skin, so the results are temporary.
- **Electrodesiccation** (ee-**leck**-troh-des-ih-**KAY**-shun) is a surgical technique in which tissue is destroyed using an electric spark. It is primarily used to eliminate small superficial growths and to seal off blood vessels.
- An **incision** is a cut made with a surgical instrument. ***Incision and drainage*** (I & D) in an incision (cutting open) of a lesion, such as an abscess, and the draining of the contents.
- **Mohs' surgery** is a technique used to treat various types of skin cancer. Individual layers of cancerous tissue are removed and examined under a microscope one at a time until a margin that is clear of all cancerous tissue has been achieved.

Laser and Light Source Treatments of Skin Conditions

The term **laser** is an acronym in which the letters stand for **L***ight* **A***mplification by* **S***timulated* **E***mission of* **R***adiation*. Lasers are used to treat skin conditions and other disorders of the body.

A laser tube can be filled with a solid, liquid, or gas substance that is stimulated to emit light at a specific wavelength. Some wavelengths are capable of destroying all skin tissue; others target tissue of a particular color.

- *Port-wine stain* is treated using short pulses of laser light to remove the birthmark. Treatment can require many sessions, because only a small section is treated at a time.
- *Rhinophyma* is treated by using a laser to reshape the nose by vaporizing the excess tissue.
- Tattoos are removed by using lasers that target particular colors.
- Some skin cancers, precancer of the lip, and warts that recur around nails and on the soles of feet are treated using lasers.

Photodynamic therapy (PDT) (**foh**-toh-dye-**NAH**-mik) is a technique used to treat damaged and precancerous skin, as well as various types of cancer.

- A *photosensitizing drug* is administered topically or by injection. An incubation period is followed by exposure to a specific wavelength of light, administered either externally or endoscopically.
- When the photosensitizers are thus activated, they produce a form of oxygen that kills nearby cells. PDT is used to treat tumors on or near the surface of the skin, or in the lining of internal organs such as the lungs and esophagus.

Medications for Treatment of the Skin

Retinoids (**RET**-ih-noydz) are a class of chemical compounds derived from vitamin A that are used in skin care and treatment because of their effect on epithelial cell growth. The use of retinoids can, however, make the skin burn more easily.

- ***Isotretinoin***, known by its trade name of Accutane, is a powerful retinoid taken in pill form for the treatment of severe acne.
- ***Tretinoin*** is the active ingredient in Retin-A and Renova, which are used to treat sun-damaged skin, acne, and wrinkles.

Topical steroids such as hydrocortisone and other more potent variations are used in the treatment of various skin disorders and diseases. These drugs, which are derivatives of the natural corticosteroid hormones produced by the adrenal glands, must be used cautiously to avoid potential side effects, which can include irreversible thinning of the skin.

Cosmetic Procedures

- **Blepharoplasty** (**BLEF**-ah-roh-**plas**-tee), also known as a ***lid lift***, is the surgical reduction of the upper and lower eyelids by removing sagging skin (**blephar/o** means eyelid, and **-plasty** means surgical repair) (Figure 12.16). A small amount of fat from the patient's thighs or buttocks is sometimes injected in the hollow below the eye.

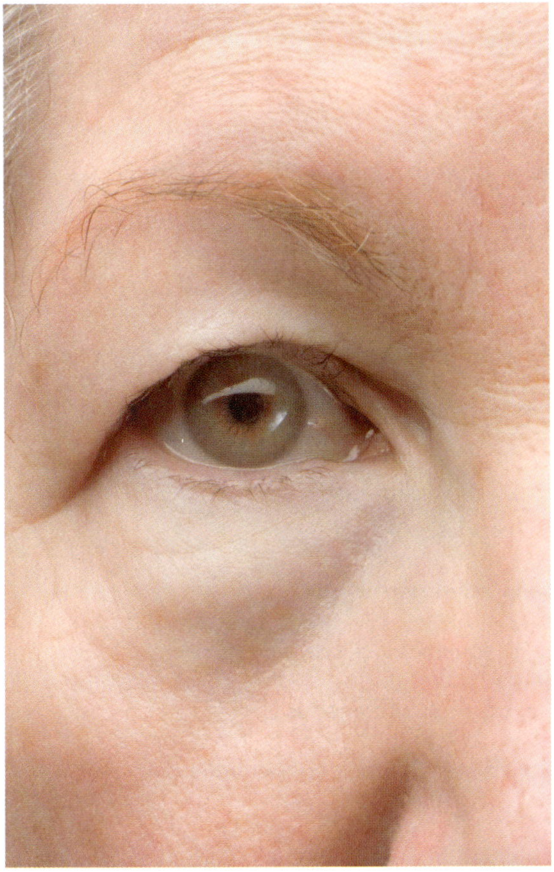

FIGURE 12.16 Blepharoplasty is the surgical reduction of the eyelids by removing sagging skin that can interfere with the field of vision.

- **Botox** is a formulation of *botulinum toxin.* This is the same neurotoxin responsible for the form of food poisoning known as botulism. When small sterile doses are injected into muscles on the forehead, it can temporarily block the nerve signals to the injected muscle for up to 3 to 4 months, reducing moderate to severe *frown lines* between the eyebrows. Botox is now also being used therapeutically to treat migraines and muscle spasms.
- **Collagen replacement therapy** is a form of soft-tissue augmentation used to soften facial lines or scars, or to make lips appear fuller. Tiny quantities of collagen are injected under a line or scar to boost the skin's natural supply of collagen. The effect usually lasts for 3 to 12 months.
- **Dermatoplasty** (**DER**-mah-toh-**plas**-tee), also known as a *skin graft*, is the replacement of damaged skin with healthy tissue taken from a donor site on the patient's body (**dermat/o** means skin, and **-plasty** means surgical repair).
- **Electrolysis** (ee-leck-**TROL**-ih-sis) is the use of electric current to destroy hair follicles in order to produce the relatively permanent removal of undesired hair (**electr/o** means electric, and **-lysis** means destruction).
- **Lipectomy** (lih-**PECK**-toh-mee) is the surgical removal of fat from beneath the skin to improve physical appearance (**lip** means fat, and **-ectomy** means surgical removal).
- **Liposuction** (**LIP**-oh-**suck**-shun), also known as *suction-assisted lipectomy*, is the surgical removal of fat beneath the skin with the aid of suction.
- **Rhytidectomy** (**rit**-ih-**DECK**-toh-mee), also known as a *facelift*, is the surgical removal of excess skin and fat from the face to eliminate wrinkles (**rhytid** means wrinkle, and **-ectomy** means surgical removal).
- **Sclerotherapy** (**sklehr**-oh-**THER**-ah-pee) is the treatment of spider veins by injecting a saline *sclerosing solution* into the vein. This solution irritates the tissue, causing the veins to collapse and disappear. *Spider veins* are small, nonessential veins that can be seen through the skin.

ABBREVIATIONS RELATED TO THE INTEGUMENTARY SYSTEM

Table 12.2 presents an overview of the abbreviations related to the terms introduced in this chapter. Note: To avoid errors or confusion, always be cautious when using abbreviations.

TABLE 12.2

Abbreviations Related to the Integumentary System

basal cell carcinoma = BCC	**BCC** = basal cell carcinoma
cauterization = caut	**caut** = cauterization
eczema = Ecz, Ez	**Ecz, Ez** = eczema
irrigation and debridement = I & D	**I & D** = irrigation and debridement
malignant melanoma = MM	**MM** = malignant melanoma
necrotizing fasciitis = NF	**NF** = necrotizing fasciitis
photodynamic therapy = PDT	**PDT** = photodynamic therapy
psoriasis = Ps	**Ps** = psoriasis
scleroderma = SCD	**SCD** = scleroderma
squamous cell carcinoma = SCC	**SCC** = squamous cell carcinoma
subcutaneous = SC, subq	**SC, subq** = subcutaneous
systemic lupus erythematosus = SLE	**SLE** = systemic lupus erythematosus

StudyWARE CONNECTION

For more practice and to test your mastery of this material, go to the StudyWARE™ to play interactive games and complete the quiz for this chapter.

Workbook Practice

Go to your workbook, and complete the exercises for this chapter.

DELMAR MOBILE MEDIA

Downloadable audio is available for selected medical terms in this chapter to enhance your learning of medical terminology.

CHAPTER 11

LEARNING EXERCISES

MATCHING WORD PARTS 1

Write the correct answer in the middle column.

	Definition	Correct Answer	Possible Answers
12.1.	skin	____________________	**urtic/o**
12.2.	rash	____________________	**rhytid/o**
12.3.	red	____________________	**hidr/o**
12.4.	sweat	____________________	**erythr/o**
12.5.	wrinkle	____________________	**cutane/o**

MATCHING WORD PARTS 2

Write the correct answer in the middle column.

	Definition	Correct Answer	Possible Answers
12.6.	black, dark	____________________	**pedicul/o**
12.7.	fat, lipid	____________________	**melan/o**
12.8.	horny, hard	____________________	**lip/o**
12.9.	lice	____________________	**kerat/o**
12.10.	skin	____________________	**dermat/o**

MATCHING WORD PARTS 3

Write the correct answer in the middle column.

	Definition	Correct Answer	Possible Answers
12.11.	dry	____________________	**xer/o**
12.12.	fungus	____________________	**seb/o**

12.13. hairy, rough ______________________ **onych/o**

12.14. nail ______________________ **myc/o**

12.15. sebum ______________________ **hirsut/o**

DEFINITIONS

Select the correct answer, and write it on the line provided.

12.16. An acute, rapidly spreading bacterial infection within the connective tissues is known as ______________________.

abscess cellulitis fissure ulcer

12.17. Atypical moles that can develop into skin cancer are known as ______________________.

dysplastic nevi lipomas malignant keratoses papillomas

12.18. The autoimmune disorder in which there are well-defined bald areas is known as ______________________.

alopecia areata alopecia capitis alopecia universalis psoriasis

12.19. A/An ______________________ is a swelling of clotted blood trapped in the tissues.

abscess contusion hematoma petechiae

12.20. The term ______________________ means profuse sweating.

anhidrosis diaphoresis hidrosis ecchymosis

12.21. A normal scar resulting from the healing of a wound is called a ______________________.

cicatrix keloid keratosis papilloma

12.22. A large blister that is usually more than 0.5 cm in diameter is known as a/an ______________________.

abscess bulla pustule vesicle

12.23. The removal of dirt, foreign objects, damaged tissue, and cellular debris from a wound is called ______________________.

cauterization curettage debridement dermabrasion

12.24. A ______________________ burn has blisters plus damage only to the epidermis and dermis.

first-degree fourth-degree second-degree third-degree

12.25. Commonly known as warts, ______________ are small, hard skin lesions caused by the human papillomavirus.

nevi   petechiae   scabies   verrucae

MATCHING STRUCTURES

Write the correct answer in the middle column.

	Definition	Correct Answer	Possible Answers
12.26.	fibrous protein found in hair, nails, and skin	______________	unguis
12.27.	fingernail or toenail	______________	sebaceous glands
12.28.	glands secreting sebum	______________	mammary glands
12.29.	milk-producing sebaceous glands	______________	keratin
12.30.	the layer of tissue below the epidermis	______________	dermis

WHICH WORD?

Select the correct answer, and write it on the line provided.

12.31. The medical term for the condition commonly known as an ingrown toenail is ______________.

onychomycosis   onychocryptosis

12.32. The bacterial skin infection characterized by isolated pustules that become crusted and rupture is known as ______________. This highly contagious condition commonly occurs in children.

impetigo   xeroderma

12.33. A torn or jagged wound or an accidental cut wound is known as a ______________.

laceration   lesion

12.34. The lesions of ______________ carcinoma tend to bleed easily.

basal cell   squamous cell

12.35. Group A strep, also known as flesh-eating bacteria, causes ________________________.

systematic lupus erythematosus   necrotizing fasciitis

SPELLING COUNTS

Find the misspelled word in each sentence. Then write that word, spelled correctly, on the line provided.

12.36. Soriasis is a disease of the skin characterized by itching and by red papules covered with silvery scales. ________________________

12.37. Exema is an inflammatory skin disease with possible blistering, cracking, oozing, or bleeding. ________________________

12.38. An absess is a localized collection of pus. ________________________

12.39. Onichia is an inflammation of the nail bed that usually results in the loss of the nail. ________________________

12.40. Schleroderma is an autoimmune disorder in which the connective tissues become thickened and hardened, causing the skin to become hard and swollen. ________________________

ABBREVIATION IDENTIFICATION

In the space provided, write the words that each abbreviation stands for.

12.41. **BCC** ____

12.42. **I & D** ____

12.43. **SLE** ____

12.44. **MM** ____

12.45. **SCC** ____

TERM SELECTION

Select the correct answer, and write it on the line provided.

12.46. A ________________________ is a small, knot-like swelling of granulation tissue in the epidermis.

cicatrix   granuloma   keratosis   petechiae

12.47. An infestation of lice is known as ________________________

pediculosis   itch mites   cicatrix   scabies

12.48. The term ______________ is used to describe any redness of the skin due to dilated capillaries.

dermatitis ecchymosis erythema urticaria

12.49. Flakes or dry patches made up of excess dead epidermal cells are known as ______________.

bullae macules plaques scales

12.50. A cluster of connected boils is known as a/an ______________.

acne vulgaris carbuncle comedo furuncle

SENTENCE COMPLETION

Write the correct term or terms on the lines provided.

12.51. The term meaning producing or containing pus is ______________.

12.52. The term meaning a fungal infection of the nail is ______________.

12.53. Tissue death followed by bacterial invasion and putrefaction is known as ______________.

12.54. A genetic condition characterized by a deficiency or absence of pigment in the skin, hair, and irises is known as ______________.

12.55. Commonly known as hives, ______________ are itchy wheals caused by an allergic reaction.

WORD SURGERY

Divide each term into its component word parts. Write these word parts, in sequence, on the lines provided. When necessary use a slash (/) to indicate a combining vowel. (You may not need all of the lines provided.)

12.56. A **rhytidectomy** is the surgical removal of excess skin for the elimination of wrinkles.

__________ __________ __________ __________

12.57. **Onychomycosis** is a fungal infection of the nail.

__________ __________ __________ __________

12.58. **Folliculitis** is an inflammation of the hair follicles that is especially common on the limbs and in the beard area of men.

__________ __________ __________ __________

12.59. **Pruritus**, which is commonly known as itching, is associated with most forms of dermatitis.

__________ __________ __________ __________

12.60. **Ichthyosis** is a group of hereditary disorders that are characterized by dry, thickened, and scaly skin.

__________ __________ __________ __________

TRUE/FALSE

If the statement is true, write **True** on the line. If the statement is false, write **False** on the line.

12.61. ________________ An actinic keratosis is a precancerous skin growth that occurs on sun-damaged skin.

12.62. ________________ A skin tag is a malignant skin enlargement commonly found on older clients.

12.63. ________________ The arrector pili cause the raised areas of skin known as goose bumps.

12.64. ________________ A keratosis is an abnormally raised scar.

12.65. ________________ Lipedema, which is also known as painful fat syndrome, affects mostly women.

CLINICAL CONDITIONS

Write the correct answer on the line provided.

12.66. Carmella Espinoza underwent ________________ for the treatment of spider veins.

12.67. Jordan Caswell is an albino. This disorder, which is known as ________________, is due to a missing enzyme necessary for the production of melanin.

12.68. Soon after Ying Li hit his thumb with a hammer, a collection of blood formed beneath the nail. This condition is a subungual ________________.

12.69. Trisha Bell fell off her bicycle and scraped off the superficial layers of skin on her knees. This type of injury is known as a/an ________________.

12.70. Molly Malone had a severe fever, and then she developed very small, pinpoint hemorrhages under her skin. The doctor described these as being ________________.

12.71. Many of the children in the Happy Hours Day Care Center required treatment for ________________, a skin infection caused by an infestation of itch mites.

12.72. Dr. Liu treated Jeanette Isenberg's skin cancer with ________________ surgery. With this technique, individual layers of cancerous tissue are removed and examined under a microscope until all cancerous tissue has been removed.

12.73. Mrs. Garrison had cosmetic surgery that is commonly known as a lid lift. The medical term for this surgical treatment is a/an ________________.

12.74. Manuel Fernandez developed a/an ________________. This condition is a closed pocket containing pus that is caused by a bacterial infection.

12.75. Agnes Farrington calls them night sweats; however, the medical term for this condition is ________________.

WHICH IS THE CORRECT MEDICAL TERM?

Select the correct answer, and write it on the line provided.

12.76. The term that refers to an acute infection of the fold of skin around a nail is ________________.

onychia   onychocryptosis   paronychia   vitiligo

12.77. When the sebum plug of a ________________ is exposed to air, it oxidizes and becomes a blackhead.

chloasma   comedo   macule   pustule

12.78. The condition known as ________________ is a skin disorder characterized by flare-ups of red papules covered with silvery scales.

chloasma   psoriasis   rosacea

12.79. The medical term referring to a malformation of the nail is ________________. This condition is also called spoon nail.

clubbing   koilonychia   onychomycosis   paronychia

12.80. Commonly known as a mole, a/an ________________ is a small, dark, skin growth that develops from melanocytes in the skin.

keloid   nevus   papilloma   verrucae

CHALLENGE WORD BUILDING

These terms are *not* found in this chapter; however, they are made up of the following familiar word parts. If you need help in creating the term, refer to your medical dictionary.

an-	**dermat/o**	**-ia**
hypo-	**hidr/o**	**-ectomy**
	melan/o	**-itis**
	myc/o	**-malacia**
	onych/o	**-oma**
	py/o	**-derma**
		-osis
		-pathy
		-plasty

12.81. Abnormal softening of the nails is known as ______________________.

12.82. An abnormal condition resulting in the diminished flow of perspiration is known as ______________________.

12.83. The plastic surgery procedure to change the shape or size of the nose is a/an ______________________.

12.84. A tumor arising from the nail bed is known as ______________________.

12.85. The term meaning any disease marked by abnormal pigmentation of the skin is ______________________.

12.86. The surgical removal of a finger or toenail is a/an ______________________.

12.87. The term meaning pertaining to the absence of fingernails or toenails is ______________________.

12.88. The term meaning any disease of the skin is ______________________.

12.89. Any disease caused by a fungus is ______________________.

12.90. An excess of melanin present in an area of inflammation of the skin is known as ______________________.

LABELING EXERCISES

Identify the numbered items on the accompanying figures.

12.91. ____________________

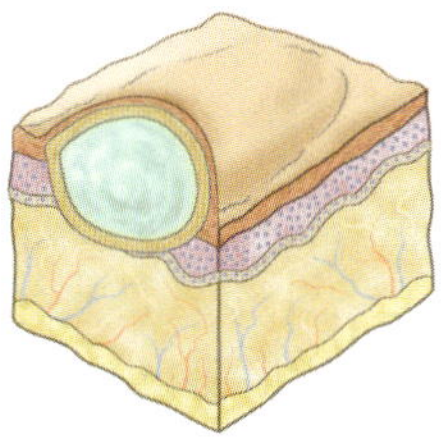

A **12.91** is a closed sack or pouch containing soft or semisolid material.

12.94. ____________________

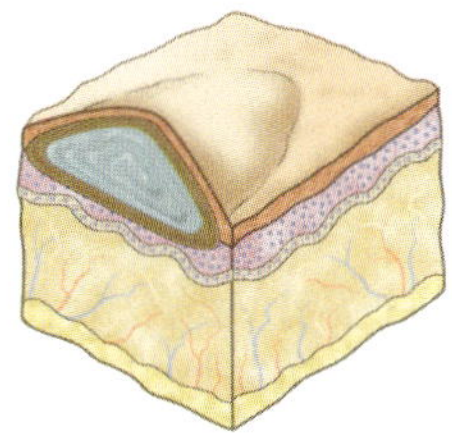

A **12.94** is a large blister that is more than 0.5 cm in diameter.

12.92. ____________________

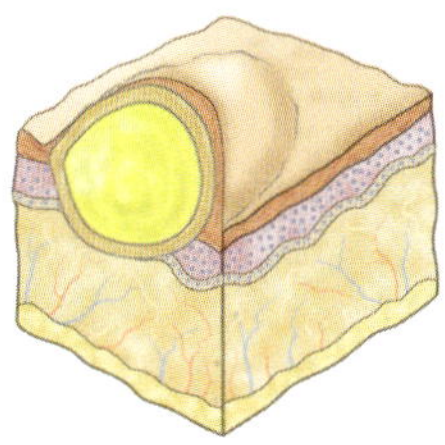

A **12.92** is a small circumscribed elevation of the skin containing pus.

12.95. ____________________

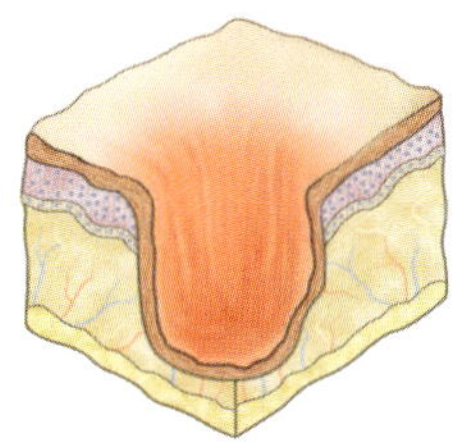

An **12.95** is an open lesion of the skin or mucous membrane, resulting in tissue loss.

12.93. ____________________

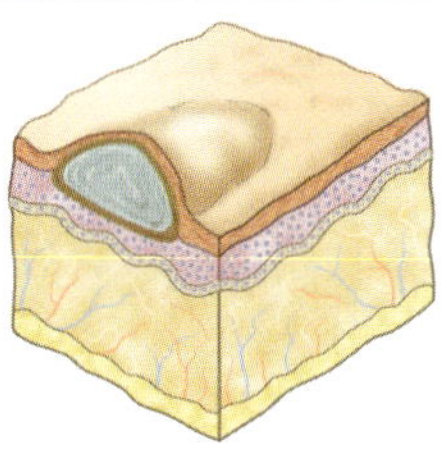

A **12.93** is a small blister containing watery fluid that is less than 0.5 cm in diameter.

12.96. ____________________ layer

12.97. ____________________ layer

12.98. ____________________ tissue

12.99. ____________________ gland

12.100. ____________________ gland

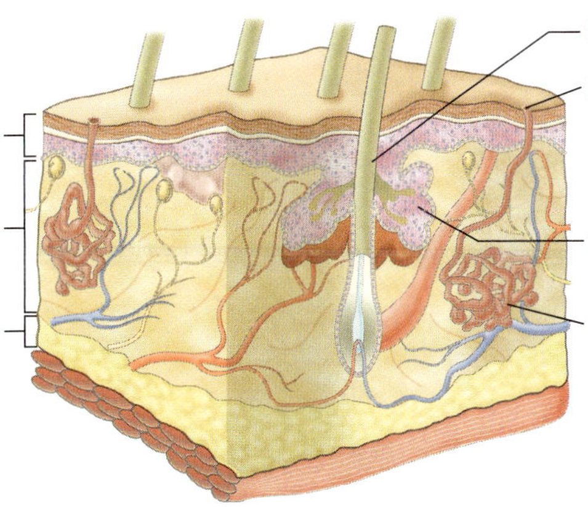

CHAPTER 12

The Endocrine System

Overview of STRUCTURES, COMBINING FORMS, AND FUNCTIONS OF THE ENDOCRINE SYSTEM

Major Structures	Related Combining Forms	Primary Functions
Adrenal Glands	**adren/o**	Regulate electrolyte levels, influence metabolism, and respond to stress.
Gonads	**gonad/o**	Gamete (sex cell) producing glands
Male: Testicles	**testic/o**	Sperm-producing gland
Female: Ovaries	**ovari/o**	Ova (egg) producing gland
Pancreatic Islets	**pancreat/o**	Control blood sugar levels and glucose metabolism.
Parathyroid Glands	**parathyroid/o**	Regulate calcium levels throughout the body.
Pineal Gland	**pineal/o**	Influences the sleep-wakefulness cycle.
Pituitary Gland	**pituit/o**, **pituitar/o**	Secretes hormones that control the activity of the other endocrine glands.
Thymus	**thym/o**	Plays a major role in the immune reaction.
Thyroid Gland	**thyr/o**, **thyroid/o**	Stimulates metabolism, growth, and the activity of the nervous system.

Vocabulary Related to **THE ENDOCRINE SYSTEM**

This list contains essential word parts and medical terms for this chapter. These terms are pronounced in the student StudyWARE™ and Audio CDs that are available for use with this text. These and the other important **primary terms** are shown in boldface throughout the chapter. *Secondary terms*, which appear in *orange* italics, clarify the meaning of primary terms.

Word Parts

- ☐ **acr/o** extremities (hands and feet), top, extreme point
- ☐ **adren/o** adrenal glands
- ☐ **crin/o** secrete
- ☐ **-dipsia** thirst
- ☐ **glyc/o** glucose, sugar
- ☐ **gonad/o** gonad, sex glands
- ☐ **-ism** condition, state of
- ☐ **pancreat/o** pancreas
- ☐ **parathyroid/o** parathyroid glands
- ☐ **pineal/o** pineal gland
- ☐ **pituitar/o** pituitary gland
- ☐ **poly-** many
- ☐ **somat/o** body
- ☐ **thym/o** thymus gland
- ☐ **thyr/o**, **thyroid/o** thyroid gland

Medical Terms

- ☐ **acromegaly** (**ack**-roh-**MEG**-ah-lee)
- ☐ **Addison's disease** (**AD**-ih-sonz)
- ☐ **adrenalitis** (ah-**dree**-nal-**EYE**-tis)
- ☐ **aldosteronism** (al-**DOSS**-teh-roh-**niz**-em)
- ☐ **antidiuretic hormone** (**an**-tih-dye-you-**RET**-ick)
- ☐ **calcitonin** (**kal**-sih-**TOH**-nin)
- ☐ **Conn's syndrome** (**KONS**)
- ☐ **cortisol** (**KOR**-tih-sol)
- ☐ **cretinism** (**CREE**-tin-izm)
- ☐ **Cushing's syndrome** (**KUSH**-ingz)
- ☐ **diabetes insipidus** (**dye**-ah-**BEE**-teez in-**SIP**-ih-dus)
- ☐ **diabetes mellitus** (**dye**-ah-**BEE**-teez **MEL**-ih-tus)
- ☐ **diabetic retinopathy** (**ret**-ih-**NOP**-ah-thee)
- ☐ **electrolytes** (ee-**LECK**-troh-lytes)
- ☐ **epinephrine** (**ep**-ih-**NEF**-rin)
- ☐ **estrogen** (**ES**-troh-jen)
- ☐ **exophthalmos** (**eck**-sof-**THAL**-mos)
- ☐ **follicle-stimulating hormone** (**FOL**-lick-kul)
- ☐ **fructosamine test** (fruck-**TOHS**-ah-meen)
- ☐ **gestational diabetes mellitus** (jes-**TAY**-shun-al **dye**-ah-**BEE**-teez)
- ☐ **gigantism** (jigh-**GAN**-tiz-em)
- ☐ **glucagon** (**GLOO**-kah-gon)
- ☐ **glucose** (**GLOO**-kohs)
- ☐ **Graves' disease** (**GRAYVZ**)
- ☐ **growth hormone**
- ☐ **gynecomastia** (**guy**-neh-koh-**MAS**-tee-ah)
- ☐ **Hashimoto's disease** (hah-shee-**MOH**-tohz)
- ☐ **hypercalcemia** (**high**-per-kal-**SEE**-mee-ah)
- ☐ **hyperglycemia** (**high**-per-glye-**SEE**-mee-ah)
- ☐ **hyperinsulinism** (**high**-per-**IN**-suh-lin-izm)
- ☐ **hyperpituitarism** (**high**-per-pih-**TOO**-ih-tah-rizm)
- ☐ **hyperthyroidism** (**high**-per-**THIGH**-roid-izm)
- ☐ **hypoglycemia** (**high**-poh-gly-**SEE**-mee-ah)
- ☐ **hypothyroidism** (**high**-poh-**THIGH**-roid-izm)
- ☐ **insulin** (**IN**-suh-lin)
- ☐ **insulinoma** (**in**-suh-lin-**OH**-mah)
- ☐ **interstitial cell-stimulating hormone** (**in**-ter-**STISH**-al)
- ☐ **laparoscopic adrenalectomy** (ah-**dree**-nal-**ECK**-toh-mee)
- ☐ **leptin** (**LEP**-tin)
- ☐ **luteinizing hormone** (**LOO**-tee-in-eye-zing)
- ☐ **myxedema** (**mick**-seh-**DEE**-mah)
- ☐ **norepinephrine** (**nor**-ep-ih-**NEF**-rin)
- ☐ **oxytocin** (**ock**-see-**TOH**-sin)
- ☐ **pancreatitis** (**pan**-kree-ah-**TYE**-tis)
- ☐ **parathyroidectomy** (**par**-ah-**thigh**-roi-**DECK**-toh-mee)
- ☐ **pituitary adenoma** (pih-**TOO**-ih-**tair**-ee **ad**-eh-**NOH**-mah)
- ☐ **polydipsia** (**pol**-ee-**DIP**-see-ah)
- ☐ **polyphagia** (**pol**-ee-**FAY**-jee-ah)
- ☐ **polyuria** (**pol**-ee-**YOU**-ree-ah)
- ☐ **prediabetes**
- ☐ **progesterone** (proh-**JES**-ter-ohn)
- ☐ **prolactinoma** (proh-**lack**-tih-**NOH**-mah)
- ☐ **puberty** (**PYU**-ber-tee)
- ☐ **radioactive iodine treatment**
- ☐ **steroids** (**STEHR**-oidz)
- ☐ **testosterone** (tes-**TOS**-teh-rohn)
- ☐ **thymectomy** (thigh-**MECK**-toh-mee)
- ☐ **thymitis** (thigh-**MY**-tis)
- ☐ **thymosin** (**THIGH**-moh-sin)
- ☐ **thyroxine** (thigh-**ROCK**- sin)

LEARNING GOALS

On completion of this chapter, you should be able to:

1. Describe the role of the endocrine glands in maintaining homeostasis.
2. Name and describe the functions of the primary hormones secreted by each of the endocrine glands.
3. Recognize, define, spell, and pronounce the primary terms relating to the pathology and the diagnostic and treatment procedures of the endocrine glands.

FUNCTIONS OF THE ENDOCRINE SYSTEM

The primary function of the endocrine system is to produce hormones that work together to maintain homeostasis. **Homeostasis** (**hoh**-mee-oh-**STAY**-sis) is the processes through which the body maintains a constant internal environment (**home/o** means constant, and **-stasis** means control).

- **Hormones** are chemical messengers that are secreted by endocrine glands directly into the bloodstream (see Chapter 2). This enables them to reach cells and organs throughout the body.
- Each hormone has specialized functions in regulating the activities of specific cells, organs, or both.
- Blood or urine tests are used to measure hormone levels. These tests are discussed in Chapter 15.

STRUCTURES OF THE ENDOCRINE SYSTEM

Endocrine glands (**EN**-doh-krin), which produce hormones, do not have ducts (**endo-** means within, and **-crine** means to secrete).

There are 13 major glands that make up the endocrine system (Figure 13.1):

- One **pituitary gland** (divided into two lobes)
- One **pineal gland**
- One **thyroid gland**
- Four **parathyroid glands**
- One **thymus**
- One **pancreas** (**pancreatic islets**)
- Two **adrenal glands**
- Two **gonads** (either a pair of ovaries in females or a pair of testicles in males)

THE PITUITARY GLAND

The **pituitary gland** (pih-**TOO**-ih-**tair**-ee), or ***hypophysis***, is a pea-sized gland that is divided into two parts, the anterior and the posterior lobes. These lobes hang from a stalk-like structure located below the hypothalamus in the brain (Figure 13.2). The hypothalamus is part of the nervous system that produces hormones that controls many body functions (see Chapter 10).

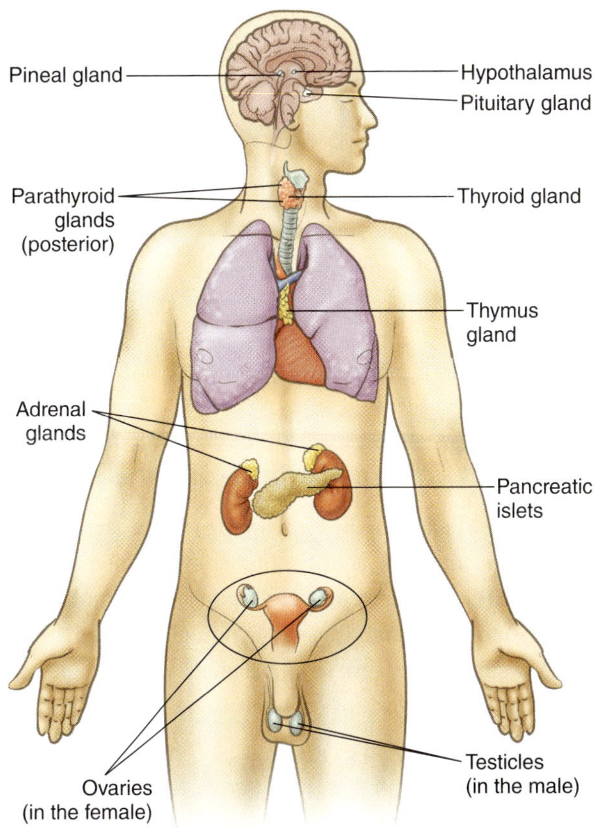

FIGURE 13.1 Structures of the endocrine system.

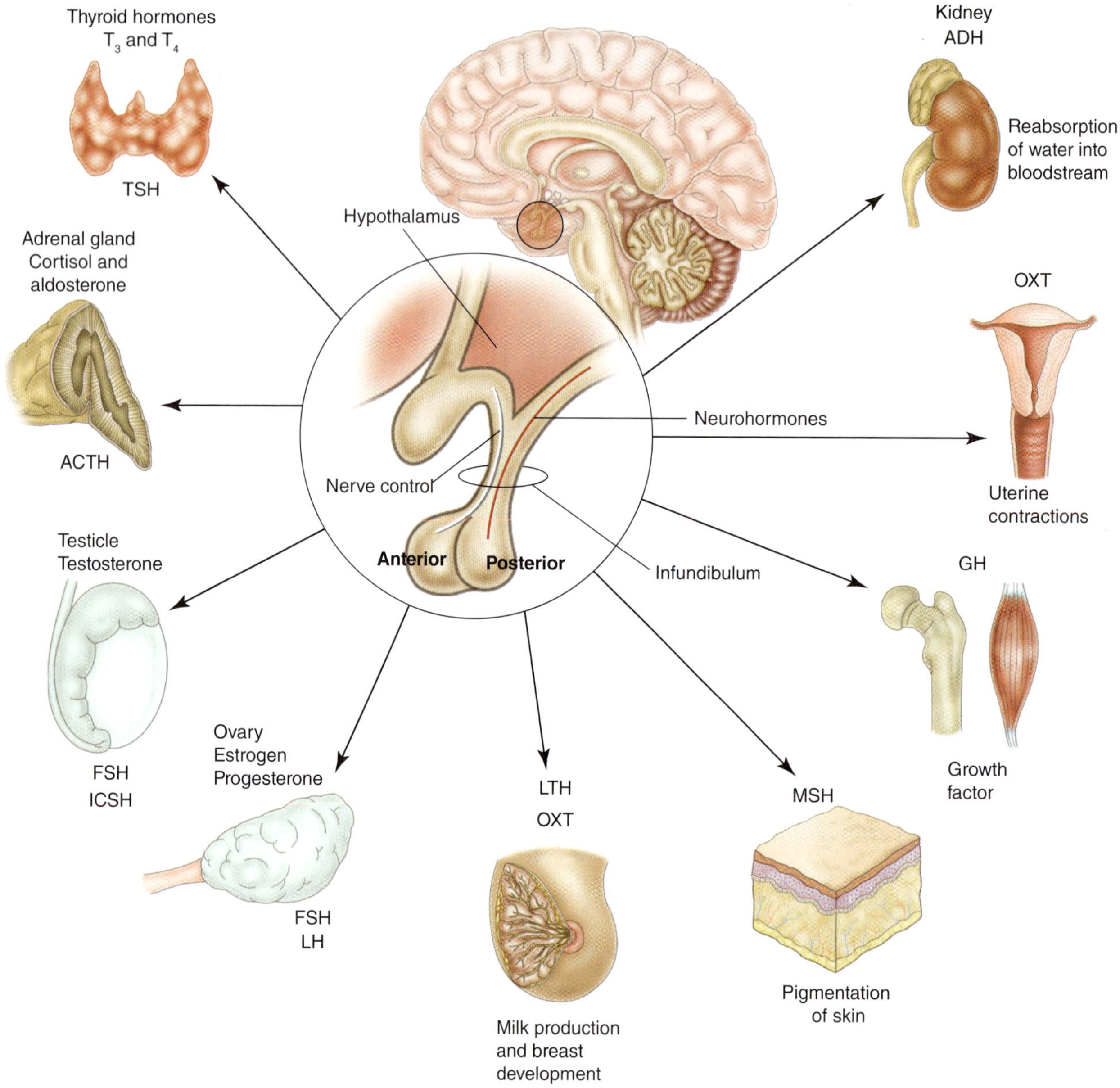

FIGURE 13.2 The pituitary gland secretes hormones that control the activity of other endocrine glands. Hormones are often referred to by their abbreviations, all of which are explained below.

Functions of the Pituitary Gland

The primary function of the pituitary gland is to secrete hormones that control the activity of other endocrine glands.

The pituitary gland acts in response to stimuli from neurohormones secreted by the hypothalamus. This creates a system of checks and balances to maintain an appropriate blood level of each hormone.

Secretions of the Pituitary Gland: Anterior Lobe

- The **adrenocorticotropic hormone** (ACTH) (ah-**DREE**-noh-**kor**-tih-coe-**TROP**-ik) stimulates the growth and secretions of the adrenal cortex (**adren/o** means adrenal, **cortic/o** means cortex, **trop** means change, and **-ic** means pertaining to).
- The **follicle-stimulating hormone** (FSH) stimulates the secretion of estrogen and the growth of ova (eggs) in the ovaries of the female. In the male, it stimulates the production of sperm in the testicles (testes).
- The **growth hormone** (GH), also known as the *somatotropic hormone*, regulates the growth of bone, muscle, and other body tissues (**somat/o** means body, and **-tropic** means having an affinity for).

- The **interstitial cell-stimulating hormone** (ICSH) (**in**-ter-**STISH**-al) stimulates ovulation in the female. In the male, it stimulates the secretion of testosterone.
- The **lactogenic hormone** (LTH), also known as *prolactin*, stimulates and maintains the secretion of breast milk in the mother after childbirth (**lact/o** means milk, **gen** means producing, and **-ic** means pertaining to).
- The **luteinizing hormone** (LH) (**LOO**-tee-in-**eye**-zing) stimulates ovulation in the female. In the male, the luteinizing hormone stimulates the secretion of testosterone.
- The **melanocyte-stimulating hormone** (MSH) (mel-**LAN**-oh-sight) increases the production of melanin in melanocytes, thereby causing darkening of skin pigmentation (see Chapter 12). MSH production usually increases during pregnancy (see Chapter 14).
- The **thyroid-stimulating hormone** (TSH) stimulates the secretion of hormones by the thyroid gland.

Secretions of the Pituitary Gland: Posterior Lobe

- The **antidiuretic hormone** (ADH) (**an**-tih-dye-you-**RET**-ick), which is secreted by the hypothalamus and stored and released in the pituitary gland, helps control blood pressure by reducing the amount of water that is excreted through the kidneys (see Chapter 9). In contrast, a *diuretic* is administered to increase the amount of urine secretion.
- **Oxytocin** (OXT) (**ock**-see-**TOH**-sin) stimulates uterine contractions during childbirth (**oxy-** means swift, and **-tocin** means labor). After childbirth, oxytocin controls postnatal hemorrhage and stimulates the flow of milk from the mammary glands. *Pitocin* is a synthetic form of oxytocin that is administered to induce or speed up labor.

THE PINEAL GLAND

The **pineal gland** (**PIN**-ee-al) is a very small endocrine gland, also known as the *pineal body*. It is located in the central portion of the brain.

Functions and Secretions of the Pineal Gland

The secretions of the pineal gland influence the sleep-wakefulness cycle (Figure 13.3). These secretions include:

- The hormone **melatonin** (**mel**-ah-**TOH**-nin) influences the sleep-wakefulness portions of the circadian cycle. The term *circadian cycle* refers to the biological functions that occur within a 24-hour period.

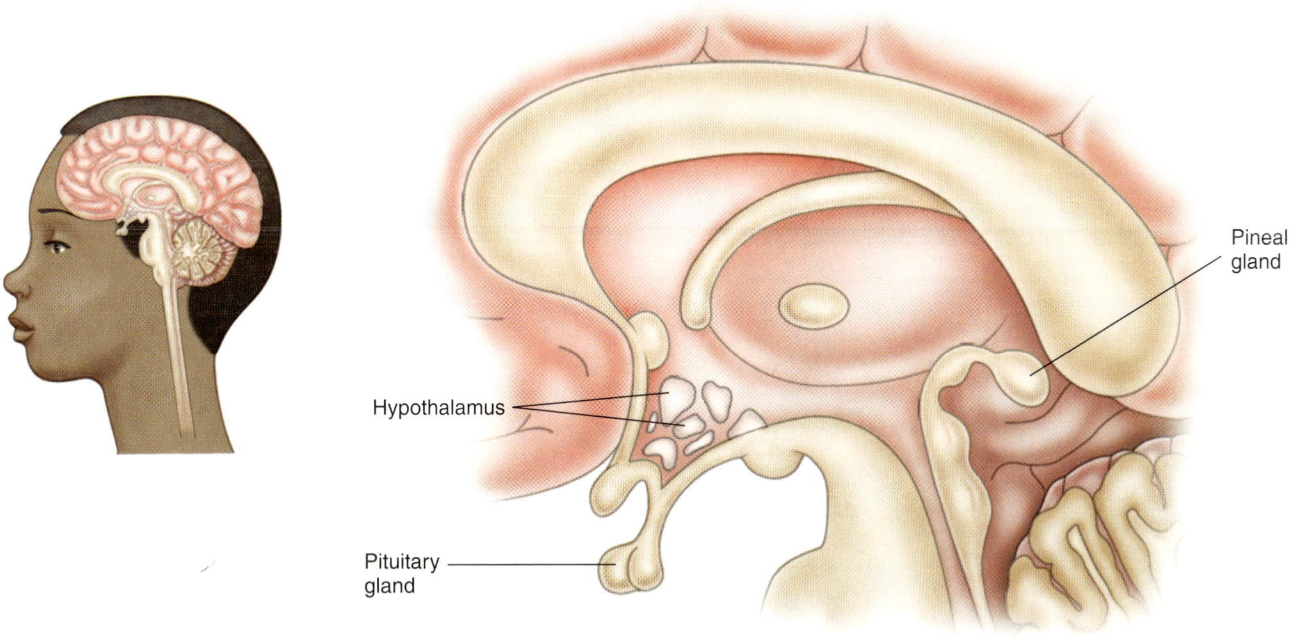

FIGURE 13.3 The pineal gland is located within the brain.

THE THYROID GLAND

The butterfly-shaped **thyroid gland** lies on either side of the larynx, just below the thyroid cartilage (Figure 13.4).

Functions and Secretions of the Thyroid Gland

One of the primary functions of the thyroid gland is to regulate the body's metabolism. The term *metabolism* describes all of the processes involved in the body's use of nutrients, including the rate at which they are used. Thyroid secretions also influence growth and the functioning of the nervous system.

- The two primary thyroid hormones regulate the rate of metabolism and affect the growth and rate of function of many other body systems. They are:
  - **thyroxine** (T_4) (thigh-**ROCK**-seen)
  - **triiodothyronine** (T_3) (try-**eye**-oh-doh-**THIGH**-roh-neen)
- The rate of secretion of these two hormones is controlled by the *thyroid-stimulating hormone* produced by the anterior lobe of the pituitary gland.
- **Calcitonin** (**kal**-sih-**TOH**-nin), which is produced by the thyroid gland, is a hormone that works with the parathyroid hormone to decrease calcium levels in the blood and tissues by moving calcium into storage in the bones and teeth.

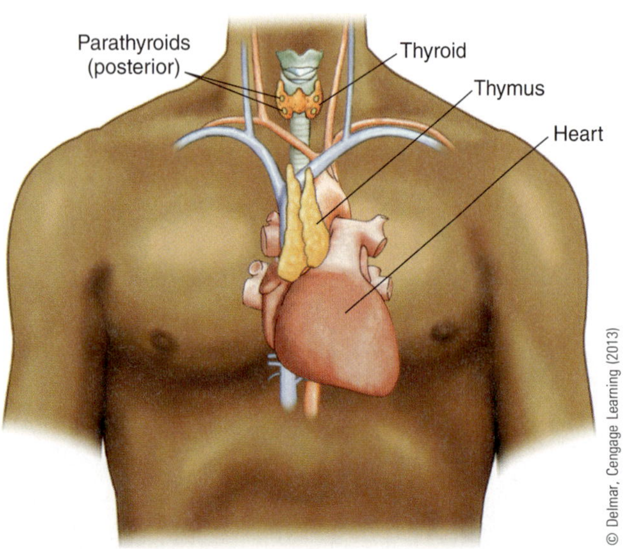

FIGURE 13.4 The thyroid, parathyroid, and thymus glands.

THE PARATHYROID GLANDS

The four **parathyroid glands**, each of which is about the size of a grain of rice, are embedded in the posterior surface of the thyroid gland (Figure 13.4).

Functions and Secretions of the Parathyroid Glands

The primary function of the parathyroid glands is to regulate calcium levels throughout the body. These calcium levels are important to the smooth functioning of the muscular and nervous systems. The secretions of the parathyroid glands include:

- The **parathyroid hormone** (PTH), which works with the hormone *calcitonin* that is secreted by the thyroid gland. Together, they regulate the calcium levels in the blood and tissues.
- Higher-than-normal levels of parathyroid hormone can increase calcium levels in the blood by mobilizing the release of calcium stored in bones and teeth.

THE THYMUS

The **thymus** (**THIGH**-mus) is located near the midline in the anterior portion of the thoracic cavity. It is posterior to (behind) the sternum and slightly superior to (above) the heart (Figure 13.4).

Functions and Secretions of the Thymus

The thymus functions as part of the endocrine system by secreting a hormone that functions as part of the immune system. The secretions of the thymus include:

- **Thymosin** (**THIGH**-moh-sin), which plays an important part in the immune system by stimulating the maturation of lymphocytes into T cells (see Chapter 6).

THE PANCREAS (PANCREATIC ISLETS)

The **pancreas** (**PAN**-kree-as) is a feather-shaped organ located posterior to the stomach that functions as part of both the digestive and the endocrine systems (Figure 13.1).

The **pancreatic islets** (**pan**-kree-**AT**-ick **EYE**-lets) are those parts of the pancreas that have endocrine functions. An *islet* is a small isolated mass, or island, of one type of tissue within a larger mass of a different type.

Functions and Secretions of the Pancreatic Islets

The endocrine functions of these islets are the control of blood sugar levels and glucose metabolism throughout the body. The secretions of the pancreatic islets include:

- **Glucose** (**GLOO**-kohs), also known as *blood sugar*, which is the basic form of energy used by the body.
- **Glucagon** (GCG) (**GLOO**-kah-gon) is the hormone secreted by the *alpha cells* of the pancreatic islets in response to low levels of glucose in the bloodstream. Glucagon increases the glucose level by stimulating the liver to convert glycogen into glucose for release into the bloodstream.
- **Insulin** (**IN**-suh-lin) is the hormone secreted by the *beta cells* of the pancreatic islets in response to high levels of glucose in the bloodstream. Insulin functions in two ways:
  1. When energy is needed, insulin allows glucose to enter the cells to be used as this energy.
  2. When additional glucose is *not* needed, insulin stimulates the liver to convert glucose into glycogen for storage.

StudyWARE CONNECTION

Watch an animation about the **Pancreas** in the StudyWARE™.

THE ADRENAL GLANDS

The **adrenal glands,** which are also known as the *suprarenals*, are so named because they are located with one on top of each kidney. Each of these glands consists of an outer portion, known as the *adrenal cortex*, and the middle portion, which is the *adrenal medulla*. Each of these parts has a specialized role (Figure 13.5).

Functions of the Adrenal Glands

One of the primary functions of the adrenal glands is to control electrolyte levels within the body.

- **Electrolytes** (ee-**LECK**-troh-lytes) are mineral substances, such as sodium and potassium, that are normally found in the blood.
- Other important functions of the adrenal glands include helping regulate metabolism and interacting with the sympathetic nervous system in response to stress (see Chapter 10).

Secretions of the Adrenal Cortex

- **Androgens** are sex hormones secreted by the gonads, the adrenal cortex, and fat cells (see later section on the gonads).
- **Corticosteroids** (**kor**-tih-koh-**STEHR**-oidz) are the steroid hormones produced by the adrenal cortex. The same term describes synthetically produced equivalents that are administered as medications.
  - **Aldosterone** (ALD) (al-**DOSS**-ter-ohn) is a corticosteroid that regulates the salt and water levels in the body by increasing sodium reabsorption and potassium excretion by the kidneys. *Reabsorption* means returning a substance to the bloodstream.

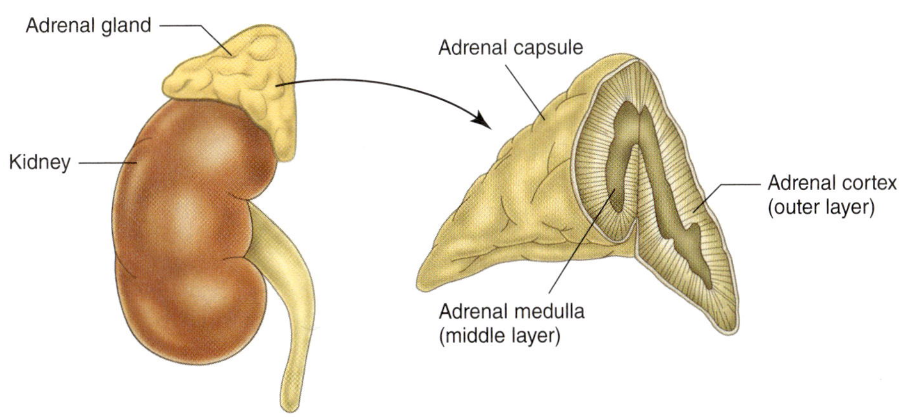

FIGURE 13.5 One adrenal gland is located on top of each kidney. Each adrenal gland consists of the adrenal cortex and adrenal medulla.

- **Cortisol** (**KOR**-tih-sol), also known as *hydrocortisone*, is a corticosteroid that has an anti-inflammatory action. It also regulates the metabolism of carbohydrates, fats, and proteins in the body.

Secretions of the Adrenal Medulla

- **Epinephrine** (Epi, EPI) (**ep**-ih-**NEF**-rin), also known as *adrenaline*, stimulates the sympathetic nervous system in response to physical injury or to mental stress such as fear. It makes the heart beat faster and can raise blood pressure. It also helps the liver release glucose (sugar) and limits the release of insulin.
- **Norepinephrine** (**nor**-ep-ih-**NEF**-rin) is both a hormone and a neurohormone. It is released as a hormone by the adrenal medulla and as a neurohormone by the sympathetic nervous system. It plays an important role in the "fight-or-flight response" by raising blood pressure, strengthening the heartbeat, and stimulating muscle contractions.

THE GONADS

The **gonads** (**GOH**-nadz) are gamete-producing glands. These are ovaries in females and testicles in males.

Functions of the Gonads

The gonads secrete the hormones that are responsible for the development and maintenance of the secondary sex characteristics that develop during puberty. *Secondary sex characteristics* refers to features that distinguish the two sexes, but are not directly related to reproduction. The additional functions of the gonads are discussed in Chapter 14.

- **Puberty** (**PYU**-ber-tee) is the process of physical changes by which a child's body becomes an adult body that is capable of reproducing (Figure 13.6). It is marked by maturing of the genital organs, development of secondary sex characteristics, and by the first occurrence of menstruation in the female. In the United States the average age is 12 for girls and 11 for boys.
- *Precocious puberty* is the early onset of the changes of puberty, usually before age 8 in girls and age 9 in boys. *Precocious* means exceptionally early in development or in occurrence.

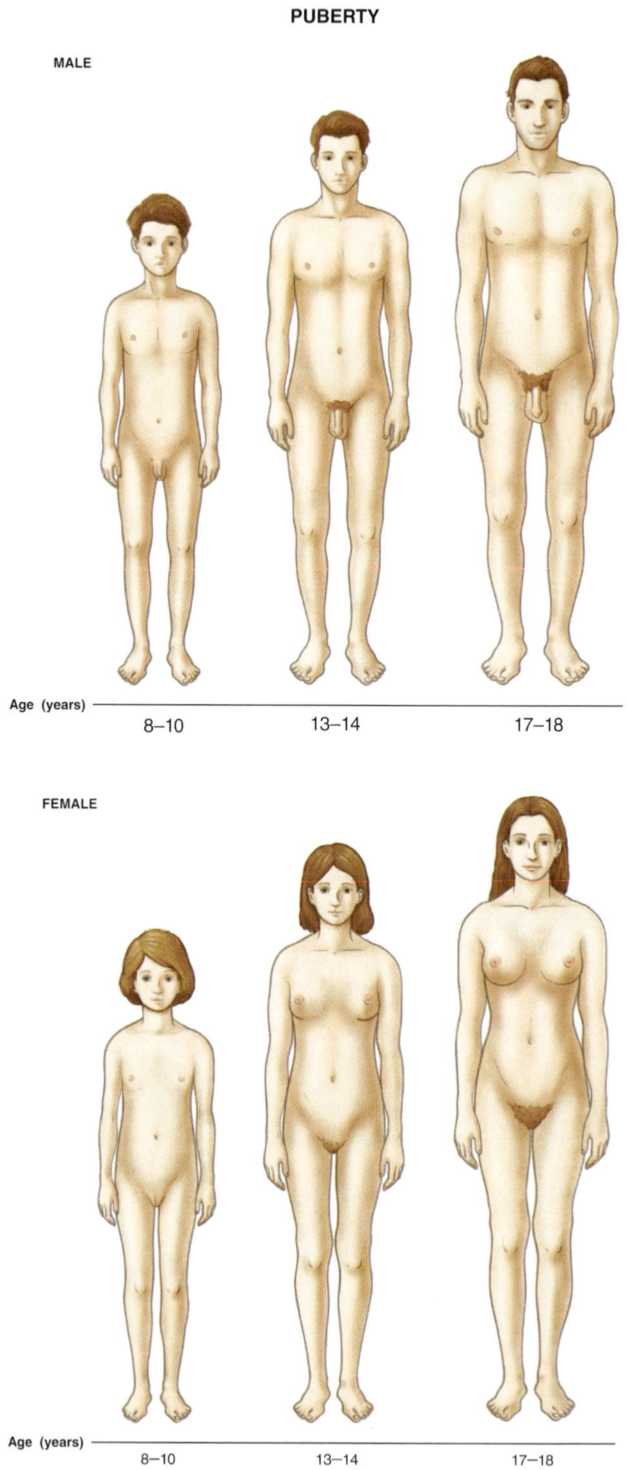

FIGURE 13.6 Puberty is the process through which secondary sex characteristics are gradually developed.

Secretions of the Gonads

- **Estrogen** (E) (**ES**-troh-jen) is a hormone secreted by the ovaries that is important in the development and maintenance of the female secondary sex characteristics and in regulation of the menstrual cycle.

- **Progesterone** (proh-**JES**-ter-ohn) is the hormone released during the second half of the menstrual cycle by the corpus luteum in the ovary. Its function is to complete the preparation of the uterus for possible pregnancy (see Chapter 14).
- A **gamete** (**GAM**-eet) is a reproductive cell. These are *sperm* in the male and *ova* (*eggs*) in the female.
- **Gonadotropin** (**gon**-ah-doh-**TROH**-pin) is any hormone that stimulates the gonads (**gonad/o** means gonad, and **-tropin** means to simulate).
- **Androgens** (**AN**-droh-jenz) are sex hormones, primarily testosterone, secreted by the gonads, the adrenal cortex, and fat cells. Androgens promote the development and maintenance of the male sex characteristics, however, they are present in both men and women.
- **Testosterone** (tes-**TOS**-teh-rohn) is a steroid hormone secreted by the testicles and the adrenal cortex to stimulate the development of male secondary sex characteristics.

StudyWARE™ CONNECTION

Watch the **Endocrine System** animation in the StudyWARE™.

Specialized Types of Hormones

Several specialized types of hormones do not fit the previous hormone definition, either because of their chemical structure or because they are not secreted by endocrine glands directly into the bloodstream.

Steroids

Steroids (**STEHR**-oidz) are a large family of hormone-like substances that share the same fat-soluble chemical structure. Examples of steroids include cholesterol, testosterone, and some anti-inflammatory drugs.

- Steroids are secreted by endocrine glands or artificially produced as medications to relieve swelling and inflammation in conditions such as asthma.
- **Anabolic steroids** (**an**-ah-**BOL**-ick **STEHR**-oidz) are man-made substances that are chemically related to male sex hormones. They are used in the treatment of hormone problems in men and to help the body replace muscle mass lost due to disease. Athletes sometime use these steroids illegally to build muscle mass, a dangerous practice that can lead to lasting damage to the body.

Hormones Secreted by Fat Cells

Adipose tissue is not commonly thought of as an endocrine gland; however, research has shown that fat cells do secrete at least one and possibly more hormones that play important roles in the balance and health of the body.

- **Leptin** (**LEP**-tin) is a protein hormone secreted by fat cells that is involved in the regulation of appetite.
- Leptin leaves the fat cells and travels in the bloodstream to the brain, where it acts on the hypothalamus to suppress appetite and burn fat stored in adipose tissue.

Neurohormones

Neurohormones (**new**-roh-**HOR**-mohnz) are produced and released by neurons in the brain, rather than by the endocrine glands, and delivered to organs and tissues through the bloodstream. One example is neurohormones secreted by the hypothalamus that control the secretions of the pituitary gland (Figure 13.2).

MEDICAL SPECIALTIES RELATED TO THE ENDOCRINE SYSTEM

- An **endocrinologist** (**en**-doh-krih-**NOL**-oh-jist) is a physician who specializes in diagnosing and treating diseases and malfunctions of the endocrine glands (**endocrin** means to secrete within, and **-ologist** means specialist).
- A **certified diabetes educator** (CDE) is a health care professional qualified to teach people with diabetes how to manage their disease.

PATHOLOGY OF THE ENDOCRINE SYSTEM

The Pituitary Gland

- **Acromegaly** (**ack**-roh-**MEG**-ah-lee) is a rare chronic disease characterized by abnormal enlargement of the extremities (hands and feet) caused by the excessive secretion of growth hormone after puberty (**acr/o** means extremities, and **-megaly** means enlargement). Contrast with *gigantism.*
- **Gigantism** (jigh-**GAN**-tiz-em) is abnormal growth of the entire body that is caused by excessive secretion of growth hormone *before* puberty. Contrast with *acromegaly.*

- **Hyperpituitarism** (**high**-per-pih-**TOO**-ih-tah-rizm) is the excess secretion of growth hormone that causes acromegaly and gigantism (**hyper-** means excessive, **pituitar** means pituitary, and **-ism** means condition).
- **Short stature**, formerly known as *dwarfism*, is sometimes caused by deficient secretion of growth hormone (see Chapter 3).
- A **pituitary adenoma** (pih-**TOO**-ih-**tair**-ee **ad**-eh-**NOH**-mah) is also known as a *pituitary tumor*. There are two types of these slow-growing benign tumors of the pituitary gland.
    - *Functioning pituitary tumors* often produce hormones in large and unregulated amounts.
    - *Nonfunctioning pituitary tumors* do not produce any significant amounts of these hormones.
- **Galactorrhea** is a condition in which an excess of prolactin causes the breasts to produce milk spontaneously (see Chapter 14).
- A **prolactinoma** (proh-**lack**-tih-**NOH**-mah) is a benign tumor of the pituitary gland (**pro-** means on behalf of, **lactin** means milk, and **-oma** means tumor). This type of tumor, which causes the pituitary gland to produce too much of the lactogenic hormone known as prolactin, can cause infertility in women and erectile dysfunction in men, and can impair vision.

Antidiuretic Hormone Conditions

- **Diabetes insipidus** (DI) (**dye**-ah-**BEE**-teez in-**SIP**-ih-dus), which is not related to *diabetes mellitus*, is caused by an insufficient production of the antidiuretic hormone ADH or by the inability of the kidneys to respond appropriately to this hormone.
    - When there is an insufficient quantity of ADH, which is secreted by the hypothalamus and stored and released in the pituitary gland, too much fluid is excreted by the kidneys. This causes *polydipsia* (excessive thirst) and *polyuria* (excessive urination). If this problem is not controlled, it can cause severe dehydration.
    - *Insipidus* comes from a Latin word meaning without taste, referring to the relatively low sodium (salt) content of the urine in patients with diabetes insipidus.
- **Syndrome of inappropriate antidiuretic hormone** (SIADH) is caused by the overproduction of the antidiuretic hormone ADH. This is often as a result of cancer or its treatment. High amounts of ADH keep the kidneys from excreting water, resulting in bloating and water retention that can dilute the blood, causing electrolyte imbalances, particularly hyponatremia.

Pathology of the Pineal Gland

- A **pinealoma** (pin-ee-ah-**LOH**-mah) is a tumor of the pineal gland that can disrupt the production of melatonin (**pineal** means pineal gland, and **-oma** means tumor). This tumor can also cause insomnia by disrupting the circadian cycle.

The Thyroid Gland

Thyroid carcinoma, or cancer, is the most common cancer of the endocrine system. This cancer affects more women than men and usually occurs between the ages of 25 and 65 years.

Insufficient Thyroid Secretion

- **Hashimoto's disease** (hah-shee-**MOH**-tohz), also known as *chronic lymphocytic thyroiditis*, is an autoimmune disease in which the body's own antibodies attack and destroy the cells of the thyroid gland. This inflammation often leads to hypothyroidism.
- **Hypothyroidism** (**high**-poh-**THIGH**-roid-izm), also known as an *underactive thyroid*, is caused by a deficiency of thyroid secretion (**hypo-** means deficient, **thyroid** means thyroid, and **-ism** means condition). Symptoms include fatigue, depression, sensitivity to cold, and a decreased metabolic rate.
- **Cretinism** (**CREE**-tin-izm) is a congenital form of hypothyroidism. If treatment is not started soon after birth, cretinism causes arrested physical and mental development.
- **Myxedema** (**mick**-seh-**DEE**-mah), which is also known as *adult hypothyroidism*, is caused by an extreme deficiency of thyroid secretion. Symptoms include swelling, particularly around the eyes and cheeks, fatigue, and a subnormal temperature.

Excessive Thyroid Secretion

- *Thyroid nodules* are lumps in the thyroid that can grow large enough to cause a goiter (see Graves' disease, below). Most nodules are benign; however some are malignant or produce too much thyroxine.
- A **thyroid storm**, also known as a *thyrotoxic crisis*, is a relatively rare, life-threatening condition caused by exaggerated hyperthyroidism. Patients experiencing a thyroid storm may complain of fever, chest pain, palpitations, shortness of breath, tremors, increased sweating, disorientation, and fatigue.

- **Hyperthyroidism** (**high**-per-**THIGH**-roid-izm), also known as *thyrotoxicosis*, is the overproduction of thyroid hormones (**hyper-** means excessive, **thyroid** means thyroid, and **-ism** means condition), which causes an imbalance of the metabolism. This causes symptoms including an increased metabolic rate, sweating, nervousness, and weight loss. The most common cause of hyperthyroidism is Graves' disease.

Graves' Disease

Graves' disease (**GRAYVZ**) is a disorder of unknown cause in which the immune system attacks the thyroid gland and stimulates it to make excessive amounts of thyroid hormone (Figure 13.7). This results in hyperthyroidism and can also cause goiter, exophthalmos, or both. Note: A simple way to remember the difference between Hashimoto's disease (***hypo***thyroidism) and Graves' disease (***hyper***thyroidism) is that the Hashimoto's has an *o* in it and Graves' has an *e* in it.

- **Goiter** (**GOI**-ter), also known as *thyromegaly*, is an abnormal nonmalignant enlargement of the thyroid gland (**thyr/o** means thyroid, and **-megaly** means abnormal enlargement). This enlargement produces a swelling in the front of the neck. A goiter usually occurs when the thyroid gland is not able to produce enough thyroid hormone to meet the body's needs, either due to Graves' disease, other medical conditions, or an iodine deficiency.
- **Exophthalmos** (**eck**-sof-**THAL**-mos) is an abnormal protrusion of the eyeball out of the orbit (**ex-** means out, **ophthalm/o** means eye and **-s** is a noun ending).

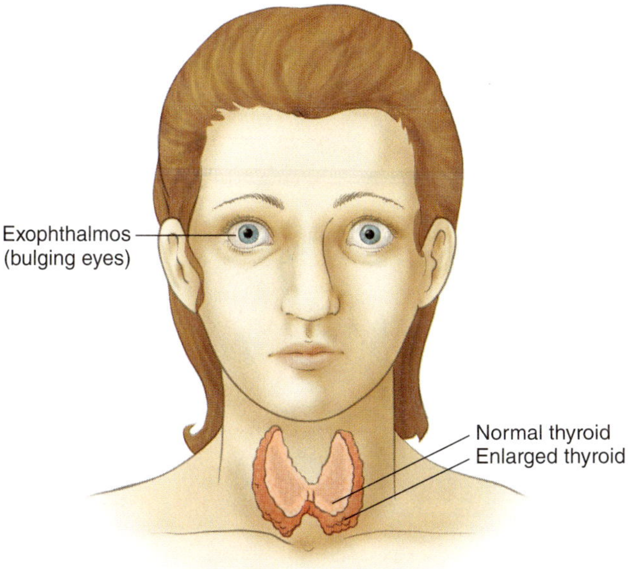

FIGURE 13.7 Graves' disease can cause exophthalmos.

The Parathyroid Glands

- **Hyperparathyroidism** (**high**-per-**par**-ah-**THIGH**-roid-izm), which is the overproduction of the parathyroid hormone, causes the condition known as hypercalcemia (**hyper-** means excessive, **parathyroid** means parathyroid, and **-ism** means condition). Hyperparathyroidism can result from a disorder of the parathyroid gland or from a disorder elsewhere in the body, such as kidney failure. Hyperparathyroidism is the opposite of *hypoparathyroidism.*
- **Hypercalcemia** (**high**-per-kal-**SEE**-mee-ah) is characterized by abnormally *high* concentrations of calcium circulating in the blood instead of being stored in the bones and teeth (**hyper-** means excessive, **calc** means calcium, and **-emia** means blood condition). This can lead to weakened bones and the formation of kidney stones. Hypercalcemia is the opposite of *hypocalcemia.*
- **Hypoparathyroidism** (**high**-poh-**par**-ah-**THIGH**-roid-izm) is caused by an insufficient or absent secretion of the parathyroid hormone (**hypo-** means deficient, **parathyroid** means parathyroid, and **-ism** means condition). This condition causes hypocalcemia, and in severe cases, it leads to tetany. *Tetany* is the condition of periodic, painful muscle spasms and tremors. Hypoparathyroidism is the opposite of *hyperparathyroidism.*
- **Hypocalcemia** (**high**-poh-kal-**SEE**-mee-ah) is characterized by abnormally *low* levels of calcium in the blood (**hypo-** means deficient, **calc** means calcium, and **-emia** means blood condition). Hypocalcemia is the opposite of *hypercalcemia.*

The Thymus

- **Thymitis** (thigh-**MY**-tis) is an inflammation of the thymus gland (**thym** means thymus, and **-itis** means inflammation).

The Pancreas

- An **insulinoma** (**in**-suh-lin-**OH**-mah) is a benign tumor of the pancreas that causes hypoglycemia by secreting additional insulin (**insulin** means insulin, and **-oma** means tumor).
- **Pancreatitis** (**pan**-kree-ah-**TYE**-tis) is an inflammation of the pancreas (**pancreat** means pancreas, and **-itis** means inflammation). A leading cause of pancreatitis is long-term alcohol abuse.

Abnormal Blood Sugar Levels

- **Hyperglycemia** (**high**-per-glye-**SEE**-mee-ah) is an abnormally high concentration of glucose in the blood (**hyper-** means excessive, **glyc** means sugar, and **-emia** means blood condition). Hyperglycemia is seen primarily in patients with diabetes mellitus. The symptoms include polydipsia, polyphagia, and polyuria. Hyperglycemia is the opposite of hypoglycemia.
- **Polydipsia** (**pol**-ee-**DIP**-see-ah) is excessive thirst (**poly-** means many, and **-dipsia** means thirst).
- **Polyphagia** (**pol**-ee-**FAY**-jee-ah) is excessive hunger (**poly-** means many, and **-phagia** means eating).
- **Polyuria** (**pol**-ee-**YOU**-ree-ah) is excessive urination (**poly-** means many, and **-uria** means urination).
- **Hyperinsulinism** (**high**-per-**IN**-suh-lin-izm) is the condition of excessive secretion of insulin in the bloodstream (**hyper-** means excessive, **insulin** means insulin, and **-ism** means condition). Hyperinsulinism can cause *hypoglycemia*.
- **Hypoglycemia** (**high**-poh-glye-**SEE**-mee-ah) is an abnormally low concentration of glucose (sugar) in the blood (**hypo-** means deficient, **glyc** means sugar, and **-emia** means blood condition). Symptoms include nervousness and shakiness, confusion, perspiration, or feeling anxious or weak. Hypoglycemia is the opposite of *hyperglycemia*.

Diabetes Mellitus

Diabetes mellitus (DM) (**dye**-ah-**BEE**-teez **MEL**-ih-tus) is a group of metabolic disorders characterized by hyperglycemia resulting from defects in insulin secretion, insulin action, or both. Diabetes mellitus is not related to diabetes insipidus.

- This condition is described as type 1, type 2, and latent autoimmune diabetes in adults (type 1.5).
- In the past, when a child developed diabetes, this condition was referred to as *juvenile diabetes*; however, the condition in children is now described as being either type 1 or type 2.
- Many patients present with symptoms of both types of diabetes, and their treatment must be modified accordingly. The treatment goals for all types of diabetes are to most effectively control the blood sugar levels and to prevent complications.

- *Metabolic syndrome* is a combination of medical conditions, including increased blood pressure, elevated insulin levels, excess body fat around the waist, or abnormal cholesterol levels. This syndrome increases the patient's risk of heart disease, stroke, and diabetes.

Type 1 Diabetes

Type 1 diabetes is an autoimmune insulin deficiency disorder caused by the destruction of pancreatic islet beta cells. *Insulin deficiency* means that the pancreatic beta cells do not secrete enough insulin. (See Chapter 6 for more information about autoimmune disorders.)

- Symptoms of type 1 diabetes include polydipsia, polyphagia, polyuria, weight loss, blurred vision, extreme fatigue, and slow healing.
- Type 1 diabetes is treated with diet and exercise as well as carefully regulated insulin replacement therapy administered by injection or pump (Figure 13.8).
- The onset of type 1 diabetes is often triggered by a viral infection.

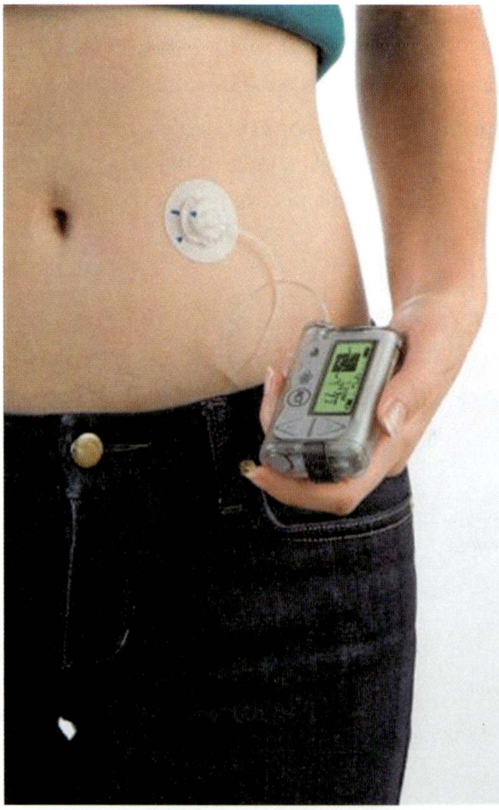

Photos courtesy of Metronic, Inc.

FIGURE 13.8 An insulin pump can be worn on the patient's belt, administering controlled insulin replacement therapy.

Type 2 Diabetes

Type 2 diabetes is an insulin resistance disorder. *Insulin resistance* means that insulin is being produced, but the body does not use it effectively. In an attempt to compensate for this lack of response, the body secretes more insulin. With the rise of childhood obesity, type 2 diabetes is increasingly common in children and young adults. Obese adults are also at high risk for this condition.

- **Prediabetes** is a condition in which the blood sugar level is higher than normal, but not high enough to be classified as type 2 diabetes. However, this condition indicates an increased risk of developing type 2 diabetes, heart disease, and stroke.
- Type 2 diabetics can have no symptoms for years. When symptoms do occur, they include those of type 1 diabetes plus recurring infections, irritability, and a tingling sensation in the hands or feet.
- Type 2 diabetes is usually treated with diet, exercise, and oral medications, which include:
  - *Oral hypoglycemics*, which lower blood sugar by causing the pancreas to release more insulin or increasing the body's sensitivity to insulin.
  - *Glucophage* (*metformin hydrochloride*) and similar medications work within the cells to combat insulin resistance and to help insulin let blood sugar into the cells.

Latent Autoimmune Diabetes in Adults

Latent autoimmune diabetes in adults (LADA), also known as *Type 1.5 diabetes*, is a condition in which type 1 diabetes develops in adults. It shares many of the characteristics of type 2 diabetes; however, autoimmune antibodies are present. *Latent* means present, but not visible.

- LADA usually occurs in adults with a normal weight and family history of type 1 diabetes.
- It is estimated that at least 10% of adults with diabetes have LADA. It is treated with diet, exercise, oral medications, and insulin.

Gestational Diabetes Mellitus

Gestational diabetes mellitus (jes-**TAY**-shun-al **dye**-ah-**BEE**-teez) is a form of diabetes mellitus that occurs during some pregnancies. This condition usually disappears after delivery; however, many of these women have an increased risk to develop type 2 diabetes in later life.

Diabetic Emergencies

Diabetic emergencies are due to either too much or too little blood sugar. Treatment depends on accurately diagnosing the cause of the emergency (Figure 13.9 A & B).

- A **diabetic coma** is caused by very high blood sugar (hyperglycemia). Also known as *diabetic ketoacidosis*, this condition is treated by the prompt administration of insulin.
- **Insulin shock** is caused by very low blood sugar (hypoglycemia). *Oral glucose*, which is a sugary substance that can quickly be absorbed into the bloodstream, is consumed to rapidly raise the blood sugar level.

Diabetic Complications

Most diabetic complications result from the damage to capillaries and other blood vessels due to long-term exposure to excessive blood sugar.

- **Diabetic retinopathy** (**ret**-ih-**NOP**-ah-thee) occurs when diabetes damages the tiny blood vessels in the retina. This causes blood to leak into the posterior segment of the eyeball and produce the damage of the loss of vision (see Chapter 11).
- *Heart disease* occurs because excess blood sugar makes the walls of the blood vessels sticky and rigid. This encourages hypertension and atherosclerosis (see Chapter 5).
- *Kidney disease* can lead to renal failure because damage to the blood vessels reduces blood flow through the kidneys (see Chapter 9).
- *Peripheral neuropathy* is damage to the nerves affecting the hands and feet (see Chapter 10).
- Poorly controlled blood sugar can also slow wound healing and increase the likelihood of wound infections. This can make minor injuries worse and lead to ulcers and gangrene, requiring amputation, particularly in the feet and legs.

The Adrenal Glands

- **Addison's disease** (**AD**-ih-sonz) occurs when the adrenal glands do not produce enough of the hormones cortisol or aldosterone. This condition is characterized by chronic, worsening fatigue and muscle weakness, loss of appetite, low blood pressure, and weight loss.
- **Adrenalitis** (ah-**dree**-nal-**EYE**-tis) is inflammation of the adrenal glands (**adrenal** means adrenal glands, and **-itis** means inflammation).

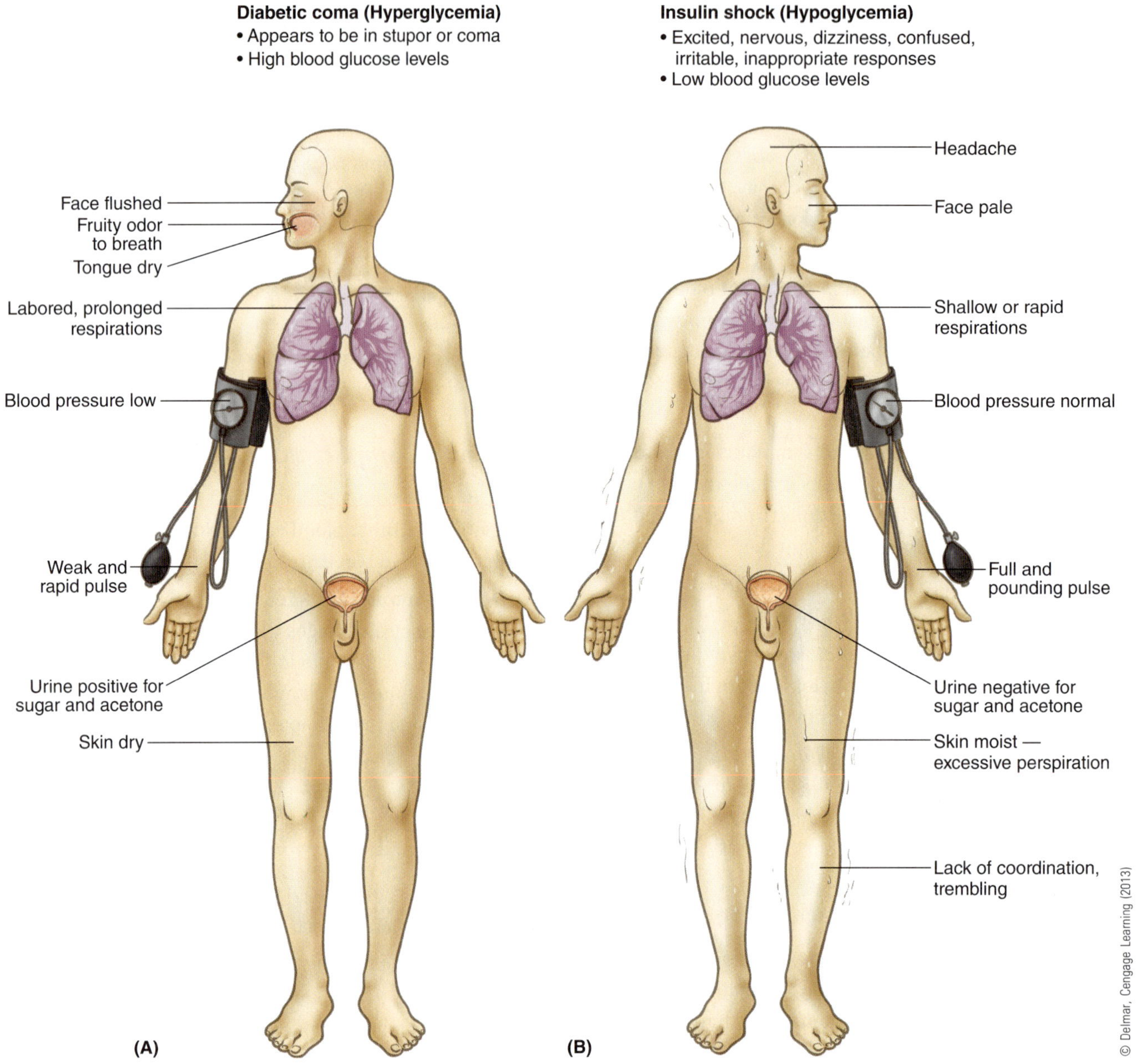

FIGURE 13.9 (A) Diabetic coma (hyperglycemia); (B) Insulin shock (hypoglycemia).

- **Aldosteronism** (al-**DOSS**-teh-roh-**niz**-em) is an abnormality of the electrolyte balance that is caused by the excessive secretion of aldosterone.
- **Conn's syndrome** (**KON**) is a disorder of the adrenal glands that is caused by the excessive production of aldosterone. This disease, which is a form of primary aldosteronism, can cause weakness, cramps, and convulsions.
- A **pheochromocytoma** (fee-oh-**kroh**-moh-sigh-**TOH**-mah) is a rare, benign tumor of the adrenal gland that causes too much release of epinephrine and norepinephrine, which are the hormones that regulate heart rate and blood pressure (**phe/o** means dusky, **chrom/o** means color, **cyt** means cell, and **-oma** means tumor).

Cushing's Syndrome

Cushing's syndrome (**KUSH**-ingz **SIN**-drohm), also known as *hypercortisolism*, is caused by prolonged exposure to high levels of cortisol. Cortisol has an anti-inflammatory action, and it regulates the metabolism of carbohydrates, fats, and proteins in the body. The symptoms include a rounded red "moon" face (Figure 13.10).

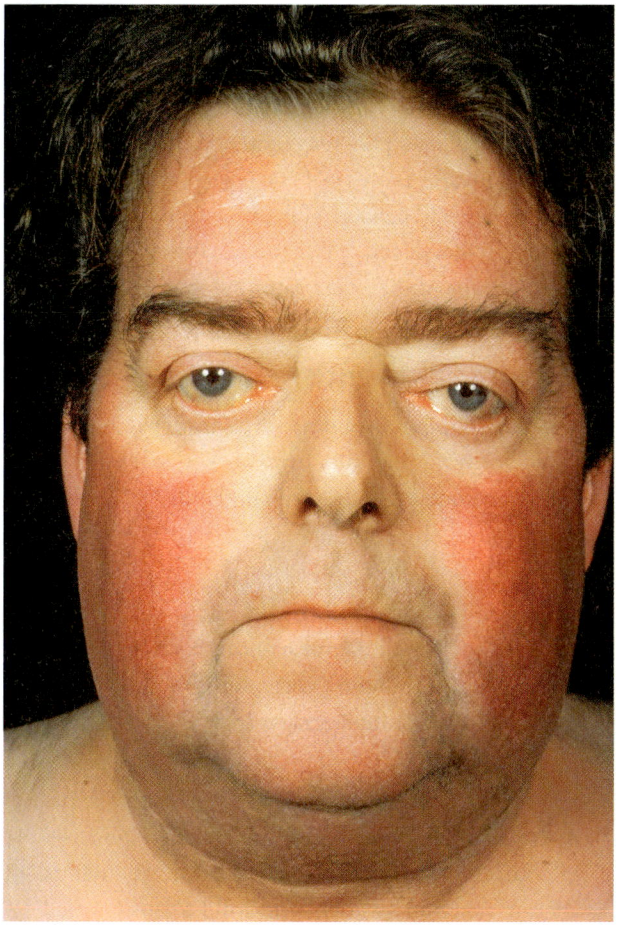

Biophoto Assocociate/Photo Researchers, Inc.

FIGURE 13.10 Cushing's syndrome causes a characteristic rounded, red "moon" face.

This condition can be caused by overproduction of cortisol by the body or by prolonged use of corticosteroids. These steroid hormone medications are used to treat inflammatory diseases such as asthma, lupus, and rheumatoid arthritis and to keep the body from rejecting transplanted organs or tissue.

The Gonads

- **Hypergonadism** (**high**-per-**GOH**-nad-izm) is the condition of excessive secretion of hormones by the sex glands (**hyper-** means excessive, **gonad** means sex gland, and **-ism** means condition). Compare with *hypogonadism*.
- **Hypogonadism** (**high**-poh-**GOH**-nad-izm) is the condition of deficient secretion of hormones by the sex glands (**hypo-** means deficient, **gonad** means sex gland, and **-ism** means condition). Compare with *hypergonadism*.
- **Gynecomastia** (**guy**-neh-koh-**MAS**-tee-ah) is the condition of excessive mammary development in the male (**gynec/o** means female, **mast** means breast, and **-ia** means abnormal condition). This is caused by a decrease in testosterone.

DIAGNOSTIC PROCEDURES RELATED TO THE ENDOCRINE SYSTEM

The Thyroid Gland

- A **radioactive iodine uptake test** (RAIU) uses radioactive iodine administered orally to measure thyroid function. The amount of radioactivity in the thyroid is measured 6 to 24 hours later using a handheld instrument called a gamma probe.
- A **thyroid-stimulating hormone assay** is a diagnostic test to measure the circulating blood level of thyroid-stimulating hormone. This test is used to detect abnormal thyroid activity resulting from excessive pituitary stimulation.
- A **thyroid scan**, which measures thyroid function, is a form of nuclear medicine that is discussed in Chapter 15.

Diabetes Mellitus

- A **fasting blood sugar test**, also known as a *fasting plasma glucose (FPG) test*, measures the glucose (blood sugar) levels after the patient has not eaten for 8 to 12 hours. This test is used to screen for diabetes. It is also used to monitor treatment of this condition.
- An **oral glucose tolerance test** is performed to confirm a diagnosis of diabetes mellitus and to aid in diagnosing hypoglycemia.
- **Home blood glucose monitoring** measures the current blood sugar level. This test, which requires a drop of blood, is performed by the patient.
- **Hemoglobin A1c testing**, also known as *HbA1c*, and pronounced as "*H-B A-one-C*," is a blood test that measures the average blood glucose level over the previous 3 to 4 months.
- The **fructosamine test** (**fruck-TOHS**-ah-meen) measures average glucose levels over the previous 3 weeks. The fructosamine test is able to detect changes more rapidly than the HbA1c test.

TREATMENT PROCEDURES RELATED TO THE ENDOCRINE SYSTEM

The Pituitary Gland

- The **human growth hormone** (HGH) is a synthetic version of the growth hormone that is administered to stimulate growth when the natural supply of growth hormone is insufficient for normal development.

- A **hypophysectomy** (high-**pof**-ih-**SECK**-toh-mee) is the removal of abnormal glandular tissue (**hypophys** refers to the pituitary gland, and **-ectomy** means removal). This surgery is performed through the nasal passages.

The Pineal Gland

- A **pinealectomy** (**pin**-ee-al-**ECK**-toh-mee) is the surgical removal of the pineal gland (**pineal** means pineal gland, and **-ectomy** means surgical removal).

The Thyroid Gland

- An **antithyroid drug** is a medication administered to slow the ability of the thyroid gland to produce thyroid hormones.
- **Radioactive iodine treatment** (RAI) is the oral administration of radioactive iodine to destroy thyroid cells. This procedure, which disables at least part of the thyroid gland, is used to treat thyroid cancer and chronic hyperthyroid disorders such as Graves' disease.
- A **lobectomy** (loh-**BECK**-toh-mee) is the surgical removal of one lobe of the thyroid gland. This term is also used to describe the removal of a lobe of the liver, brain, or lung.
- **Synthetic thyroid hormones** are administered to replace lost thyroid function.

The Parathyroid Glands

- A **parathyroidectomy** (**par**-ah-**thigh**-roi-**DECK**-toh-mee), which is the surgical removal of one or more of the parathyroid glands, is performed to control hyperparathyroidism (**parathyroid** means parathyroid glands and **-ectomy** means surgical removal).

The Thymus

- A **thymectomy** (thigh-**MECK**-toh-mee) is the surgical removal of the thymus gland (**thym** means thymus, and **-ectomy** means surgical removal).

The Pancreas

- A **pancreatectomy** (**pan**-kree-ah-**TECK**-toh-mee) is the surgical removal of all or part of the pancreas (**pancreat** means pancreas, and **-ectomy** means surgical removal). A *total pancreatectomy* is performed to treat pancreatic cancer. This procedure also involves removing the spleen, gallbladder, common bile duct, and portions of the small intestine and stomach.

The Adrenal Glands

- A **laparoscopic adrenalectomy** (ah-**dree**-nal-**ECK**-toh-mee) is a minimally invasive surgical procedure to remove one or both adrenal glands (**adrenal** means adrenal gland, and **-ectomy** means surgical removal).
- **Cortisone** (**KOR**-tih-sohn), also known as *hydrocortisone*, is the synthetic equivalent of corticosteroids produced by the body. Cortisone is administered to suppress inflammation and as an immunosuppressant (see Chapter 6).
- A synthetic version of the hormone epinephrine is used as a vasoconstrictor to cause the blood vessels to contract. It is used to treat conditions such as allergic reactions, shock, and mild asthma. An *epinephrine autoinjector*, also known as an Epi pen, is a device used to inject a measured dose of epinephrine.

ABBREVIATIONS RELATED TO THE ENDOCRINE SYSTEM

Table 13.1 presents an overview of the abbreviations related to the terms introduced in this chapter. Note: To avoid errors or confusion, always be cautious when using abbreviations.

TABLE 13.1
Abbreviations Related to the Endocrine System

aldosterone = ALD	**ALD** = aldosterone
antidiuretic hormone = ADH	**ADH** = antidiuretic hormone
diabetes insipidus = DI	**DI** = diabetes insipidus
diabetes mellitus = DM	**DM** = diabetes mellitus
epinephrine = EPI, Epi	**Epi, EPI** = epinephrine
fasting blood sugar = FBS	**FBS** = fasting blood sugar
fructosamine test = FA	**FA** = fructosamine test
Graves' disease = GD	**GD** = Graves' disease
hypoglycemia = HG	**HG** = hypoglycemia
latent autoimmune diabetes = LADA	**LADA** = latent autoimmune diabetes
leptin = LEP, LPT	**LEP, LPT** = leptin
thyroid stimulating hormone = TSH	**TSH** = thyroid stimulating hormone

StudyWARE CONNECTION

For more practice and to test your mastery of this material, go to the StudyWARE™ to play interactive games and complete the quiz for this chapter.

DELMAR MOBILE MEDIA

Downloadable audio is available for selected medical terms in this chapter to enhance your learning of medical terminology.

Workbook Practice

Go to your workbook, and complete the exercises for this chapter.

CHAPTER 12

LEARNING EXERCISES

MATCHING WORD PARTS 1

Write the correct answer in the middle column.

Definition	Correct Answer	Possible Answers
13.1. adrenal glands	________	acr/o
13.2. extremities	________	adren/o
13.3. ovaries or testicles	________	crin/o
13.4. thirst	________	-dipsia
13.5. to secrete	________	gonad/o

MATCHING WORD PARTS 2

Write the correct answer in the middle column.

Definition	Correct Answer	Possible Answers
13.6. condition	________	pituitar/o
13.7. pancreas	________	pineal/o
13.8. parathyroid glands	________	parathyroid/o
13.9. pineal gland	________	pancreat/o
13.10. pituitary gland	________	-ism

MATCHING WORD PARTS 3

Write the correct answer in the middle column.

Definition	Correct Answer	Possible Answers
13.11. body	________	thym/o
13.12. many	________	thyroid/o

13.13.	sugar	____________	**somat/o**
13.14.	thyroid	____________	**poly-**
13.15.	thymus	____________	**glyc/o**

DEFINITIONS

Select the correct answer, and write it on the line provided.

13.16. The ____________ hormone stimulates ovulation in the female.

estrogen follicle-stimulating lactogenic luteinizing

13.17. The ____________ gland secretes hormones that control the activity of the other endocrine glands.

adrenal hypothalamus pituitary thymus

13.18. The ____________ hormone stimulates the growth and secretions of the adrenal cortex.

adrenocorticotropic growth melanocyte-stimulating thyroid-stimulating

13.19. ____________ gland has functions as part of the endocrine system by secreting a hormone that functions as part of the endocrine and immune systems.

adrenal parathyroid pineal thymus

13.20. The hormone ____________ works with the parathyroid hormone to decrease calcium levels in the blood and tissues.

aldosterone calcitonin glucagon leptin

13.21. Cortisol is secreted by the ____________.

adrenal cortex adrenal medulla pituitary gland thyroid gland

13.22. The amount of glucose in the bloodstream is increased by the hormone ____________.

adrenaline glucagon hydrocortisone insulin

13.23. Norepinephrine is secreted by the ____________.

adrenal cortex adrenal medulla pancreatic islets pituitary gland

13.24. The hormone ____________ stimulates uterine contractions during childbirth.

estrogen oxytocin progesterone testosterone

13.25. The development of the male secondary sex characteristics is stimulated by the hormone ______________________.

parathyroid pitocin progesterone testosterone

MATCHING STRUCTURES

Write the correct answer in the middle column.

	Definition	Correct Answer	Possible Answers
13.26.	controls blood sugar levels	______________________	thyroid gland
13.27.	controls the activity of other endocrine glands	______________________	pituitary gland
13.28.	influences the sleep-wakefulness cycle	______________________	pineal gland
13.29.	regulates electrolyte levels	______________________	pancreatic islets
13.30.	stimulates metabolism	______________________	adrenal glands

WHICH WORD?

Select the correct answer, and write it on the line provided.

13.31. The hormonal disorder that results from too much growth hormone in adults is known as ______________________.

acromegaly gigantism

13.32. The growth hormone is secreted by the ______________________ lobe of the pituitary gland.

anterior lobe posterior lobe

13.33. Diabetes type 2 is an ______________________ disorder.

insulin deficiency insulin resistance

13.34. Insufficient production of ADH causes ______________________.

diabetes insipidus Graves' disease

13.35. ______________________ is caused by prolonged exposure to high levels of cortisol.

Addison's disease Cushing's syndrome

SPELLING COUNTS

Find the misspelled word in each sentence. Then write that word, spelled correctly, on the line provided.

13.36. The lutinizing hormone stimulates ovulation in the female ______________.

13.37. Diabetes mellitas is a group of diseases characterized by defects in insulin production, use secretion, insulin action, or both ______________.

13.38. Myxedemia is also known as adult hypothyroidism ______________.

13.39. The hormone progestarone is released during the second half of the menstrual cycle ______________.

13.40. Thymoxin is secreted by the thymus gland ______________.

ABBREVIATION IDENTIFICATION

In the space provided, write the words that each abbreviation stands for.

13.41. **ACTH** ______________

13.42. **ADH** ______________

13.43. **DM** ______________

13.44. **FBS** ______________

13.45. **FSH** ______________

TERM SELECTION

Select the correct answer, and write it on the line provided.

13.46. A rare life-threatening condition caused by exaggerated hyperthyroidism is called ______________.

thyroid nodules goiter thyroid storm Graves' disease

13.47. The condition known as ______________ is characterized by abnormally high concentrations of calcium circulating in the blood instead of being stored in the bones.

hypercalcemia hyperthyroidism hypocalcemia polyphagia

13.48. The four ________________ glands, each of which is about the size of a grain of rice, are embedded in the posterior surface of the thyroid gland.

adrenal pancreatic parathyroid pineal

13.49. A/An ________________ is a benign tumor of the pituitary gland that causes it to produce too much prolactin.

insuloma pheochromocytoma pituitary adenoma prolactinoma

13.50. The average blood glucose levels over the past 3 weeks is measured by the ________________ test.

blood sugar monitoring fructosamine glucose tolerance hemoglobin A1c

SENTENCE COMPLETION

Write the correct term on the line provided.

13.51. The mineral substances known as ________________ are found in the blood and include sodium and potassium.

13.52. The two primary hormones secreted by the thyroid gland are triiodothyronine (T_3) and ________________ (T_4).

13.53. Damage to the retina of the eye caused by diabetes mellitus is known as diabetic ________________.

13.54. The medical term meaning excessive hunger is ________________.

13.55. Abnormal protrusion of the eye out of the orbit is known as ________________.

WORD SURGERY

Divide each term into its component word parts. Write these word parts, in sequence, on the lines provided. When necessary, use a slash (/) to indicate a combining vowel. (You may not need all of the lines provided.)

13.56. **Hyperpituitarism** is the excess secretion of growth hormone by the pituitary gland, causing acromegaly and gigantism.

________ ________ ________ ________

13.57 **Hypoglycemia** is an abnormally low concentration of glucose in the blood.

________ ________ ________ ________

13.58. **Hyperinsulinism** is the condition of excessive secretion of insulin in the bloodstream.

________ ________ ________ ________

13.59. **Gynecomastia** is the condition of excessive mammary development in the male.

________ ________ ________ ________

13.60. **Hypocalcemia** is characterized by abnormally low levels of calcium in the blood.

________ ________ ________ ________

TRUE/FALSE

If the statement is true, write **True** on the line. If the statement is false, write **False** on the line.

13.61. ____________ The beta cells of the pancreatic islets secrete glucagon in response to low blood sugar levels.

13.62. ____________ A pheochromocytoma is a rare, benign tumor of the adrenal gland that causes too much release of epinephrine and norepinephrine.

13.63. ____________ The hormone melatonin is secreted by the adrenal cortex.

13.64. ____________ An insulinoma is a malignant tumor of the pancreas that causes hypoglycemia by secreting insulin.

13.65. ____________ Polyuria is excessive urination.

CLINICAL CONDITIONS

Write the correct answer on the line provided.

13.66. During his nursing studies, Rodney Milne learned that the ____________ hormone helps control blood pressure by reducing the amount of water that is excreted through the kidneys.

13.67. Eduardo Chavez complained of being thirsty all the time. His doctor noted this excessive thirst on his chart as ____________.

13.68. Mrs. Wei's symptoms included chronic, worsening fatigue, muscle weakness, loss of appetite, and weight loss because her adrenal glands do not produce enough cortisol. Her doctor diagnosed this condition as ____________.

13.69. Linda Thomas was diagnosed as having a/an ________________________. This is a benign tumor of the pancreas that causes hypoglycemia by secreting insulin.

13.70. Patrick Edward has the autoimmune disorder known as ________________________ in which the body's own antibodies attack and destroy the cells of the thyroid gland.

13.71. Because Joe Dean's ultimate goal was to swim in the Olympics, he was tempted to make illegal use of ________________________ steroids to increase his strength and muscle mass.

13.72. Holly Yates was surprised to learn that ________________________, which is a hormone secreted by fat cells, travels to the brain and controls the balance of food intake and energy expenditure.

13.73. As a result of a congenital lack of thyroid secretion, the Vaugh-Eames child suffers from ________________________, which is a condition of arrested physical and mental development.

13.74. Ray Grovenor is excessively tall and large. This condition, which was caused by excessive secretion of growth hormone before puberty, is known as ________________________.

13.75. Rosita DeAngelis required the surgical removal of her pancreas. The medical term for this procedure is a/an ________________________.

WHICH IS THE CORRECT MEDICAL TERM?

Select the correct answer, and write it on the line provided.

13.76. Hormones called ________________________ are produced and released by neurons in the brain, rather than by the endocrine glands, and delivered to organs and tissues through the bloodstream.

hormones neurohormones neurotransmitters steroids

13.77. A/An ________________________ is a slow-growing, benign tumor of the pituitary gland that is a functioning tumor (secreting hormones) or a nonfunctioning tumor (not secreting hormones).

hyperpituitarism hypophysectomy pituitary adenoma prolactinoma

13.78. ________________________ disease, which is an autoimmune disorder caused by hyperthyroidism, is often characterized by goiter, exophthalmos, or both.

Addison's Cushing's Graves' Hashimoto's

13.79. The diabetic emergency caused by very high blood sugar is a/an ________________________.

diabetic coma hypoglycemia insulin shock insuloma

13.80. The hormone ________________, which is secreted by the pineal gland, influences the sleep-wakefulness cycles.

glucagon melatonin parathyroid thymosin

CHALLENGE WORD BUILDING

These terms are *not* found in this chapter; however, they are made up of the following familiar word parts. If you need help in creating the term, refer to your medical dictionary.

endo-	**adren/o**	**-emia**
	crin/o	**-itis**
	insulin/o	**-megaly**
	pancreat/o	**-ology**
	pineal/o	**-oma**
	thym/o	**-otomy**
		-pathy

13.81. The term meaning any disease of the adrenal glands is ________________.

13.82. The study of endocrine glands and their secretions is known as ________________.

13.83. Abnormal enlargement of the adrenal glands is known as ________________.

13.84. The term meaning any disease of the thymus gland is ________________.

13.85. Inflammation of the thyroid gland is known as ________________.

13.86. A surgical incision into the pancreas is a/an ________________.

13.87. A surgical incision into the thyroid gland is a/an ________________.

13.88. The term meaning any disease of the pineal gland is ________________.

13.89. Abnormally high levels of insulin in the blood are known as ________________.

13.90. Inflammation of the adrenal glands is known as ________________.

LABELING EXERCISES

Identify the numbered items on the accompanying figure.

13.91. ______________________ gland

13.92. ______________________ glands

13.93. ______________________ gland

13.94. ______________________ of the female

13.95. ______________________

13.96. ______________________ gland

13.97. ______________________ gland

13.98. ______________________ glands

13.99. ______________________ islets

13.100. ______________________ of the male

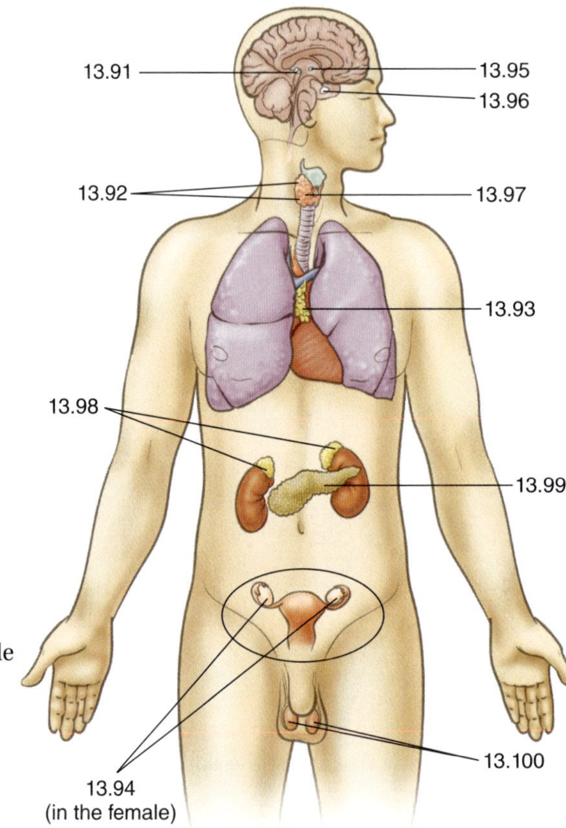

CHAPTER 13

The Reproductive Systems

Overview of STRUCTURES, COMBINING FORMS, AND FUNCTIONS OF THE REPRODUCTIVE SYSTEMS

Major Structures	Related Combining Forms	Primary Functions
Male		
Penis	**pen/i**, **phall/i**	Used for sexual intercourse and urination.
Testicles	**orch/o**, **orchid/o**, **test/i**, **test/o**	Produce sperm and the hormone testosterone.
Female		
Ovaries	**oophor/o**, **ovari/o**	Produce ova (eggs) and female hormones.
Fallopian Tubes	**salping/o**	Catch the mature ovum (egg) and transport it to the uterus. Also the site of fertilization.
Uterus	**hyster/o**, **metr/o**, **metri/o**, **uter/o**	Protects and supports the developing child.
Vagina	**vagin/o**, **colp/o**	Used for sexual intercourse, acts as channel for menstrual flow, and functions as the birth canal.
Placenta	**placent/o**	Exchanges nutrients and waste between the mother and fetus during pregnancy.

Vocabulary Related to **THE REPRODUCTIVE SYSTEMS**

This list contains essential word parts and medical terms for this chapter. These terms are pronounced in the student StudyWARE™ and Audio CDs that are available for use with this text. These and the other important **primary terms** are shown in boldface throughout the chapter. *Secondary terms*, which appear in *orange* italics, clarify the meaning of primary terms.

Word Parts

- ☐ **cervic/o** cervix (neck of uterus)
- ☐ **colp/o** vagina
- ☐ **-gravida** pregnant
- ☐ **gynec/o** woman, female
- ☐ **hyster/o** uterus
- ☐ **mast/o** breast
- ☐ **men/o** menstruation, menses
- ☐ **orchid/o** testicles
- ☐ **ov/o** egg, ovum
- ☐ **ovari/o** ovary
- ☐ **-para** to give birth
- ☐ **-pexy** surgical fixation
- ☐ **salping/o** uterine (fallopian) tube
- ☐ **test/i** testicle, testis
- ☐ **vagin/o** vagina

Medical Terms

- ☐ **amenorrhea** (ah-**men**-oh-**REE**-ah)
- ☐ **amniocentesis** (**am**-nee-oh-sen-**TEE**-sis)
- ☐ **andropause** (**AN**-droh-pawz)
- ☐ **Apgar score**
- ☐ **azoospermia** (ay-**zoh**-oh-**SPER**-mee-ah)
- ☐ **cervical dysplasia** (**SER**-vih-kal dis-**PLAY**-see-ah)
- ☐ **cervicitis** (**ser**-vih-**SIGH**-tis)
- ☐ **chlamydia** (klah-**MID**-ee-ah)
- ☐ **chorionic villus sampling** (**kor**-ee-**ON**-ick **VIL**-us)
- ☐ **colostrum** (kuh-**LOS**-trum)
- ☐ **colpopexy** (**KOL**-poh-**peck**-see)
- ☐ **colporrhaphy** (kol-**POR**-ah-fee)
- ☐ **colposcopy** (kol-**POS**-koh-pee)
- ☐ **dysmenorrhea** (**dis**-men-oh-**REE**-ah)
- ☐ **eclampsia** (eh-**KLAMP**-see-ah)
- ☐ **ectopic pregnancy** (eck-**TOP**-ick)
- ☐ **endocervicitis** (**en**-doh-**ser**-vih-**SIGH**-tis)
- ☐ **endometriosis** (**en**-doh-**mee**-tree-**OH**-sis)
- ☐ **epididymitis** (**ep**-ih-did-ih-**MY**-tis)
- ☐ **episiotomy** (eh-**piz**-ee-**OT**-oh-mee)
- ☐ **fibroadenoma** (**figh**-broh-**ad**-eh-**NOH**-mah)
- ☐ **fibrocystic breast disease** (**figh**-broh-**SIS**-tick)
- ☐ **galactorrhea** (gah-**lack**-toh-**REE**-ah)
- ☐ **gonorrhea** (**gon**-oh-**REE**-ah)
- ☐ **hematospermia** (**hee**-mah-toh-**SPER**-mee-ah)
- ☐ **hydrocele** (**HIGH**-droh-seel)
- ☐ **hypomenorrhea** (**high**-poh-men-oh-**REE**-ah)
- ☐ **hysterectomy** (**hiss**-teh-**RECK**-toh-mee)
- ☐ **hysterosalpingography** (**hiss**-ter-oh-**sal**-pin-**GOG**-rah-fee)
- ☐ **hysteroscopy** (**hiss**-ter-**OSS**-koh-pee)
- ☐ **leukorrhea** (**loo**-koh-**REE**-ah)
- ☐ **mastalgia** (mass-**TAL**-jee-ah)
- ☐ **mastopexy** (**MAS**-toh-**peck**-see)
- ☐ **menarche** (meh-**NAR**-kee)
- ☐ **menometrorrhagia** (**men**-oh-**met**-roh-**RAY**-jee-ah)
- ☐ **metrorrhea** (**mee**-troh-**REE**-ah)
- ☐ **neonate** (**NEE**-oh-nayt)
- ☐ **nulligravida** (**null**-ih-**GRAV**-ih-dah)
- ☐ **nullipara** (nuh-**LIP**-ah-rah)
- ☐ **obstetrician** (**ob**-steh-**TRISH**-un)
- ☐ **oligomenorrhea** (**ol**-ih-goh-**men**-oh-**REE**-ah)
- ☐ **oophorectomy** (**oh**-ahf-oh-**RECK**-toh-mee)
- ☐ **orchidectomy** (**or**-kih-**DECK**-toh-mee)
- ☐ **orchiopexy** (**or**-keeoh-**PECK**-see)
- ☐ **ovariorrhexis** (oh-**vay**-ree-oh-**RECK**-sis)
- ☐ **perimenopause** (pehr-ih-**MEN**-oh-pawz)
- ☐ **Peyronie's disease** (pay-roh-**NEEZ**)
- ☐ **placenta previa** (plah-**SEN**-tah **PREE**-vee-ah)
- ☐ **polycystic ovary syndrome** (**pol**-ee-**SIS**-tick)
- ☐ **preeclampsia** (**pree**-ee-**KLAMP**-see-ah)
- ☐ **priapism** (**PRYE**-ah-**piz**-em)
- ☐ **primigravida** (**prye**-mih-**GRAV**-ih-dah)
- ☐ **primipara** (prye-**MIP**-ah-rah)
- ☐ **pruritus vulvae** (proo-**RYE**-tus **VUL**-vee)
- ☐ **salpingo-oophorectomy** (sal-**ping**-goh oh-**ahf**-oh-**RECK**-toh-mee)
- ☐ **syphilis** (**SIF**-ih-lis)
- ☐ **trichomoniasis** (**trick**-oh-moh-**NYE**-ah-sis)
- ☐ **uterine prolapse** (proh-**LAPS**)
- ☐ **varicocele** (**VAR**-ih-koh-**seel**)
- ☐ **vasovasostomy** (**vay**-soh-vah-**ZOS**-toh-mee)

LEARNING GOALS

On completion of this chapter, you should be able to:

1. Identify and describe the major functions and structures of the male reproductive system.
2. Recognize, define, spell, and pronounce the terms related to the pathology and the diagnostic and treatment procedures of the male reproductive system.
3. Name at least six sexually transmitted diseases.
4. Identify and describe the major functions and structures of the female reproductive system.
5. Recognize, define, spell, and pronounce the primary terms related to the pathology and the diagnostic and treatment procedures of the female reproductive system, and a woman during pregnancy, childbirth, and the postpartum period.

TERMS RELATED TO THE REPRODUCTIVE SYSTEMS OF BOTH SEXES

The **genitalia** (**jen**-ih-**TAY**-lee-ah) are the organs of reproduction and their associated structures.

- *External genitalia* are reproductive organs located outside of the body cavity.
- *Internal genitalia* are reproductive organs protected within the body.

The **perineum** (pehr-ih-**NEE**-um) is the external surface region in both males and females between the pubic symphysis and the coccyx.

- The tissue of the *male perineum* extends from the scrotum to the area around the anus.
- The tissue of the *female perineum* extends from the pubic symphysis to the area around the anus. (Figure 14.6).

FUNCTIONS OF THE MALE REPRODUCTIVE SYSTEM

The primary function of the male reproductive system is to produce sperm and deliver them into the female body so that one sperm can unite with a single ovum (egg) to create a new life. Some structures of the male reproductive system also function as part of the urinary system. These are discussed in Chapter 9.

STRUCTURES OF THE MALE REPRODUCTIVE SYSTEM

- The *external male genitalia* are the penis and the scrotum, which contains two testicles.
- The *internal male genitalia* include the remaining structures of the male reproductive system (Figures 14.1 and 14.2).

The Scrotum and Testicles

The **scrotum** (**SKROH**-tum) is the sac-like structure that surrounds, protects, and supports the testicles. The scrotum is suspended from the pubic arch behind the penis and lies between the thighs.

The **testicles**, also known as *testes*, are the two small, egg-shaped glands that produce the sperm (singular, *testis*). These glands develop within the abdomen of the male fetus and normally descend into the scrotum before or soon after birth.

- Sperm are formed within the **seminiferous tubules** (**see**-mih-**NIF**-er-us **TOO-byouls**) of each testicle (Figure 14.2).
- The **epididymis** (**ep**-ih-**DID**-ih-mis) is a coiled tube at the upper part of each testicle. This tube runs down the length of the testicle, then turns upward toward the body. Here, it narrows to form the tube known as the *vas deferens*.

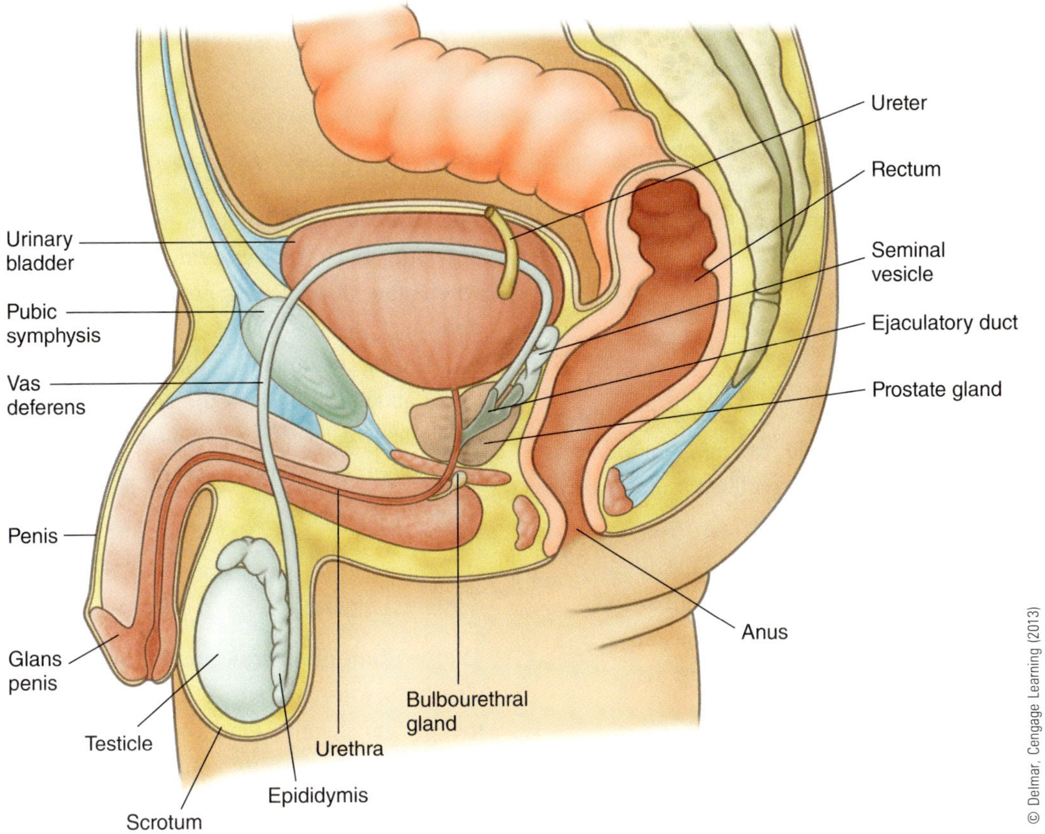

FIGURE 14.1 Organs and ducts of the male reproductive system shown in a lateral cross-section.

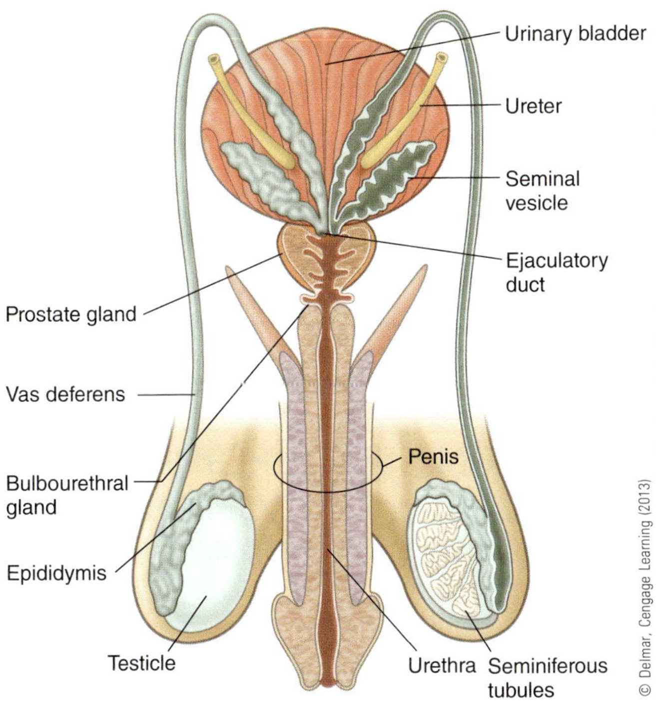

FIGURE 14.2 Structures of the male reproductive system as shown in an anterior cross-section view.

- The **spermatic cord** extends upward from the epididymis and is attached to each testicle. Each cord contains a vas deferens plus the arteries, veins, nerves, and lymphatic vessels required by each testicle.

Semen Formation

Sperm, also known as ***spermatozoa***, are the male gametes (reproductive cells). **Semen** (**SEE**-men) is the whitish fluid containing sperm that is ejaculated through the urethra at the peak of male sexual excitement. The term ***ejaculate*** means to expel suddenly.

- **Spermatogenesis** (**sper**-mah-toh-**JEN**-eh-sis) is the process of sperm formation (**spermat/o** means sperm, and **-genesis** means creation).
- The ideal temperature for sperm formation is 93.2°F. The scrotum aids in maintaining this temperature by adjusting how closely it holds the testicles to the body.
- Sperm are formed in the seminiferous tubules of the testicles.

- From here, the sperm move into the epididymis where they become motile and are temporarily stored. *Motile* means capable of spontaneous motion.
- From the epididymis, the sperm travel upward into the body and enter the vas deferens. Here, the seminal vesicles and the prostate gland add their secretions to form semen.

The Penis

The **penis** (**PEE**-nis) is the male sex organ that transports the sperm into the female vagina. The penis is composed of three columns of erectile tissue (Figures 14.1 and 14.2).

- During sexual stimulation, the erectile tissue fills with blood under high pressure. This causes the swelling, hardness, and stiffness known as an *erection*.
- The adjectives *penile* and *phallic* both mean relating to the penis (both **pen/i** and **phall/i** mean penis).
- The **glans penis** (glanz **PEE**-nis), also known as the *head of the penis*, is the sensitive region located at the tip of the penis (Figure 14.1).
- The **foreskin**, also known as the *prepuce*, is a retractable double-layered fold of skin and mucous membrane that covers and protects the glans penis.

The Vas Deferens, Seminal Vesicles, and the Ejaculatory Duct

- The **vas deferens** (vas **DEF**-er-enz), also known as the *ductus deferens*, are the long, narrow continuations of each epididymis. These structures lead upward and eventually join the urethra (Figures 14.1 and 14.2).
- The **seminal vesicles** (**SEM**-ih-nal) are glands that secrete a thick, yellow substance to nourish the sperm cells. This secretion forms 60% of the volume of semen. These glands are located at the base of the urinary bladder and open into the vas deferens as it joins the urethra.
- The **ejaculatory duct**, which begins at the vas deferens, passes through the prostate gland and empties into the urethra. During ejaculation, a reflex action caused by these ducts, semen passes into the urethra, which exits the body via the penis.

The Prostate Gland

The **prostate gland** (**PROS**-tayt) lies under the bladder and surrounds the end of the urethra in the region where the vas deferens enters the urethra (Figures 14.1 and 14.2).

During ejaculation, the prostate gland secretes a thick, alkaline fluid into the semen that aids the motility of the sperm. *Motility* means ability to move. Disorders and treatment of the prostate gland are discussed in Chapter 9.

The Bulbourethral Glands

The two **bulbourethral glands** (**bul**-boh-you-**REE**-thral), also known as *Cowper's glands*, are located just below the prostate gland. One of these glands is located on either side of the urethra, and they open into the urethra (Figures 14.1 and 14.2).

During sexual arousal, these glands secrete a fluid known as *pre-ejaculate*. This fluid helps flush out any residual urine or foreign matter in the urethra. It also lubricates the urethra for sperm to pass through. This fluid can contain sperm and is able to cause pregnancy even if ejaculation does not occur.

The Urethra

The **urethra** passes through the penis to the outside of the body. In the male, the urethra serves both the reproductive and the urinary systems. Disorders of the urethra are discussed in Chapter 9.

MEDICAL SPECIALTIES RELATED TO THE MALE REPRODUCTIVE SYSTEM

A **urologist** (you-**ROL**-oh-jist) is a physician who specializes in diagnosing and treating diseases and disorders of the genitourinary system of males and the urinary system of females (**ur** means urine, and **-ologist** means specialist). The term *genitourinary* refers to both the genital and urinary organs.

PATHOLOGY OF THE MALE REPRODUCTIVE SYSTEM

The Penis

- **Balanitis** (**bal**-ah-**NIGH**-tis) is an inflammation of the glans penis that is usually caused by poor hygiene in men who have not had the foreskin removed by circumcision (**balan** means glans penis, and **-itis** means inflammation).
- **Phimosis** (figh-**MOH**-sis) is a narrowing of the opening of the foreskin so it cannot be retracted (pulled back) to expose the glans penis. This condition can be present at birth or become apparent during childhood.
- **Erectile dysfunction** (ED), also known as ***impotence***, is the inability of the male to achieve or maintain a penile erection. A penis that is not erect is referred to as being ***flaccid***, or limp.
- **Peyronie's disease** (pay-roh-**NEEZ**), also known as ***penile curvature***, is a form of sexual dysfunction in which the penis is bent or curved during erection.
- **Priapism** (**PRYE**-ah-**piz**-em) is a painful erection that lasts 4 hours or more but is either not accompanied by sexual excitement or does not go away after sexual stimulation has ended. The condition can be caused by medications or by blood-related diseases such as sickle cell anemia or leukemia.
- **Premature ejaculation** is a condition in which the male reaches climax too soon, usually before or shortly after penetration of the female.

The Testicles and Related Structures

- **Andropause** (**AN**-droh-pawz), which is referred to as *ADAM* (*Androgen **D**ecline in the **A**ging **M**ale*), is marked by the decrease of the male hormone testosterone (**andr/o** means male or masculine, and **-pause** means stopping). It usually begins in the late 40s and progresses very gradually over several decades. ***Androgen*** is a male sex hormone.
- **Cryptorchidism** (krip-**TOR**-kih-dizm), also known as an ***undescended testicle***, is a developmental defect in which one or both of the testicles fail to descend into their normal position in the scrotum (**crypt** means hidden, **orchid** means testicle, and **-ism** means abnormal condition).
- **Epididymitis** (**ep**-ih-did-ih-**MY**-tis) is inflammation of the epididymis that is frequently caused by the spread of infection from the urethra or the bladder (**epididym** means epididymis, and **-itis** means inflammation) (Figure 14.3A).
- A **hydrocele** (**HIGH**-droh-seel) is a fluid-filled sac in the scrotum along the spermatic cord leading from the testicles (**hydr/o** means relating to water, and **-cele** means a hernia or swelling). Note: The term *hydrocele* is also used to describe the accumulation of fluid in any body cavity.
- A **spermatocele** (sper-**MAH**-toh-seel) is a cyst that develops in the epididymis and is filled with a milky fluid containing sperm (**spermat/o** means sperm, and **-cele** means hernia, tumor, or swelling).
- **Testicular cancer** is cancer that begins in the testicles. It is the most common cancer in American males between the ages of 15 and 34 years. This cancer is highly treatable when diagnosed early.
- **Testicular torsion** is a sharp pain in the scrotum caused by twisting of the vas deferens and blood vessels leading into the testicle. ***Torsion*** means twisting.
- **Testitis** (test-**TYE**-tis), also known as ***orchitis***, is inflammation of one or both testicles (**test** means testicle, and **-itis** means inflammation) (Figure 14.3B).
- A **varicocele** (**VAR**-ih-koh-**seel**) is a knot of widening varicose veins in one side of the scrotum (**varic/o** means varicose veins, and **-cele** means a hernia or swelling). ***Varicose veins*** are abnormally swollen veins (Figure 14.3C).

Sperm Count

A **normal sperm count** is 20 to 120 million or more sperm per milliliter (mL) of semen.

- **Azoospermia** (ay-**zoh**-oh-**SPER**-mee-ah) is the absence of sperm in the semen (**a-** means without, **zoo** means life, **sperm** means sperm, and **-ia** means abnormal condition).
- **Oligospermia** (**ol**-ih-goh-**SPER**-mee-ah) is a sperm count of below 20 million/mL (**olig/o** means few, **sperm** means sperm, and **-ia** means abnormal condition). This is also known as a ***low sperm count*** and is a common cause of ***male infertility***.

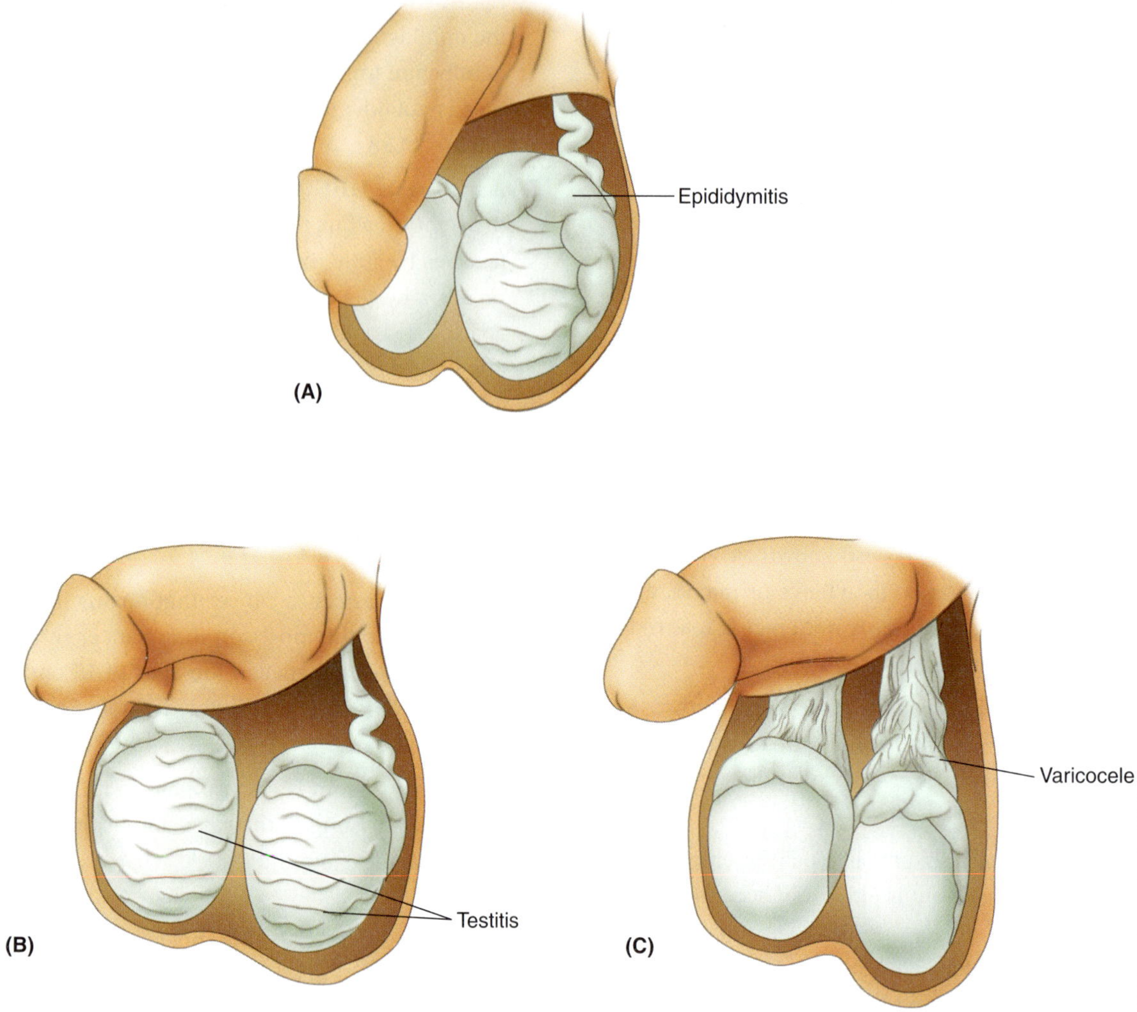

FIGURE 14.3 Pathology of the testicles. (A) Epididymitis of the left testicle. (B) Testitis of both testicles. (C) A varicocele affecting the left testicle.

- **Hematospermia** (**hee**-mah-toh-**SPER**-mee-ah) is the presence of blood in the seminal fluid (**hemat/o** means relating to blood, **sperm** means sperm, and **-ia** means abnormal condition). This condition can be caused by infections of the seminal vesicles, prostatitis, urethritis, or urethral strictures, which are discussed in Chapter 9.

StudyWARE CONNECTION

Watch the **Male Reproductive System** animation in the StudyWARE™ CD-ROM.

DIAGNOSTIC PROCEDURES OF THE MALE REPRODUCTIVE SYSTEM

- **Sperm count**, also known as a *sperm analysis*, is the testing of freshly ejaculated semen to determine the volume plus the number, shape, size, and motility of the sperm.
- **Testicular self-examination** is a self-help step in early detection of testicular cancer by detecting lumps, swelling, or changes in the skin of the scrotum.

TREATMENT PROCEDURES OF THE MALE REPRODUCTIVE SYSTEM

General Treatment Procedures

- **Circumcision** (**ser**-kum-**SIZH**-un) is the surgical removal of the foreskin of the penis. This optional procedure is usually performed within a few days of birth.

- An **orchidectomy** (**or**-kih-**DECK**-toh-mee), also spelled as *orchiectomy*, is the surgical removal of one or both testicles (**orchid** means testicle, and **-ectomy** means surgical removal).
- **Orchiopexy** (**or**-kee-oh-**PECK**-see) is the repair of an undescended testicle (**orchi/o** means testicle, and **-pexy** means surgical fixation). This is endoscopic surgery performed on infants before the age of 1 year to move the testicle into its normal position in the scrotum.
- A **varicocelectomy** (**var**-ih-koh-sih-**LECK**-toh-mee) is the removal of a portion of an enlarged vein to relieve a varicocele (**varic/o** means varicose vein, **cel** means swelling, and **-ectomy** means surgical removal).

Male Sterilization

Sterilization is any procedure rendering an individual (male or female) incapable of reproduction.

- **Castration** (kas-**TRAY**-shun), also known as *bilateral orchidectomy*, is the surgical removal or destruction of both testicles.
- A **vasectomy** (vah-**SECK**-toh-mee) is the male sterilization procedure in which a small portion of the vas deferens is surgically removed (**vas** means vas deferens, and **-ectomy** means surgical removal). This prevents sperm from entering the ejaculate but does not change the volume of semen created by the body (Figure 14.4).
- A **vasovasostomy** (**vay**-soh-vah-**ZOS**-toh-mee), also known as a *vasectomy reversal*, is a procedure performed as an attempt to restore fertility to a vasectomized male (**vas/o** means blood vessel, **vas** means the vas deferens, and **-ostomy** means surgically creating an opening).

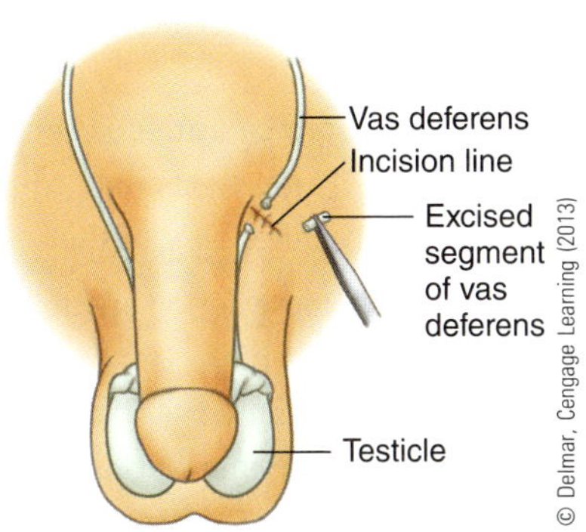

FIGURE 14.4 In a vasectomy, a portion of the vas deferens is removed to prevent sperm from entering the semen.

SEXUALLY TRANSMITTED DISEASES

Sexually transmitted diseases (STDs), which are also known as *venereal diseases* (VD) or sexually transmitted infections (STIs), are infections caused by either bacteria or a virus that affects both males and females. These conditions are commonly spread through sexual intercourse or other genital contact.

- A pregnant woman who is infected with one of these diseases can transmit it to her baby during birth. For this reason, all newborns receive an antibiotic ointment in each eye within an hour after birth to prevent *ophthalmia neonatorum*. This condition is a form of conjunctivitis that is caused by the bacteria responsible for chlamydia or gonorrhea.

There are more than 20 types of STDs. The following are several of the more common diseases.

Chlamydia

Chlamydia (klah-**MID**-ee-ah), which is caused by the bacterium *Chlamydia trachomatis*, is the most commonly reported STD in the United States. It is highly contagious and requires early treatment with antibiotics.

- In females, chlamydia can damage the reproductive organs. Even though symptoms are usually mild or absent, serious complications can cause irreversible damage, including infertility.
- In males, chlamydia is one of the causes of urethritis (see Chapter 9).

Other Sexually Transmitted Diseases

- **Bacterial vaginosis** (BV) (**vaj**-ih-**NOH**-sis) is a condition in women in which there is an abnormal overgrowth of certain bacteria in the vagina (**vagin** means vagina, and **-osis** means abnormal condition or disease). This condition can cause complications during pregnancy and an increased risk of HIV infection if exposed to the virus. Symptoms sometimes include a discharge, odor, pain, itching, or burning.

- **Genital herpes** (**HER**-peez) is caused by the *herpes simplex virus type 1 or 2*. Symptoms include itching or burning before the appearance of lesions (sores) on the genitals or rectum. This condition is highly contagious, even when visible lesions are not present. Antiviral drugs ease symptoms and can suppress future outbreaks; however, currently there is no cure.
- **Genital warts**, which are caused by **human papillomaviruses** (HPV), are highly contagious. In the male, this virus infects the urethra. In the female, it infects the external genitalia, cervix, and vagina. It also increases the risk of cervical cancer. An HPV vaccine is available to prevent the spread of this disease. It is recommended that it be administered to girls between the ages of 11 and 12 or before they become sexually active.
- **Gonorrhea** (**gon**-oh-**REE**-ah) is a highly contagious condition caused by the bacterium *Neisseria gonorrhoeae*. In women, this condition affects the cervix, uterus, and fallopian tubes. In men, it affects the urethra by causing painful urination and an abnormal discharge. It can also affect the mouth, throat, and anus of both men and women.
- The **human immunodeficiency virus** (HIV) is transmitted through exposure to infected body fluids, particularly through sexual intercourse with an infected partner. HIV and AIDS are discussed in Chapter 6.
- **Syphilis** (**SIF**-ih-lis), which is caused by the bacterium *Treponema pallidum*, has many symptoms that are difficult to distinguish from other STDs. Syphilis is highly contagious and is passed from person to person through direct contact with a ***chancre***, which is a sore caused by syphilis. This condition can be detected through the VDRL (**V**enereal **D**isease **R**esearch **L**aboratory) blood test before the lesions appear. The RPR test (**R**apid **P**lasma **R**eagin) is another blood test for syphilis.
- **Trichomoniasis** (**trick**-oh-moh-**NYE**-ah-sis), also known as ***trich***, is an infection caused by the parasite *Trichomonas vaginalis*. One of the most common symptoms in infected women is a thin, frothy, yellow-green, foul-smelling vaginal discharge. Infected men often do not have symptoms; however, when symptoms are present, they include painful urination or a clear discharge from the penis.

FUNCTIONS OF THE FEMALE REPRODUCTIVE SYSTEM

The primary function of the female reproductive system is the creation and support of new life.

- The ovaries produce mature eggs to be fertilized by the sperm.
- The uterus provides the environment and support for the developing child.
- After birth, the breasts produce milk to feed the child.

STRUCTURES OF THE FEMALE REPRODUCTIVE SYSTEM

The structures of the female reproductive system are described as being the external female genitalia and the internal female reproductive organs (Figure 14.5).

The External Female Genitalia

The ***external female genitalia*** are located posterior to the **mons pubis** (monz **PYOU**-bis), which is a rounded, fleshy prominence located over the pubic symphysis (Figure 14.6). These structures are known collectively as the **vulva** (**VUL**-vah) or the ***pudendum***. The vulva consists of the labia, clitoris, Bartholin's glands, and vaginal orifice.

- The **labia majora** and **labia minora** (**LAY**-bee-ah mah-**JOR**-ah and **LAY**-bee-ah mih-**NOR**-ah) are the vaginal lips that protect the other external genitalia and the urethral meatus (singular, *labium*). The ***urethral meatus***, which is the external opening of the urethra, is discussed in Chapter 9.
- The **clitoris** (**KLIT**-oh-ris) is an organ of sensitive, erectile tissue located anterior to the urethral meatus and the vaginal orifice.
- **Bartholin's glands** produce a mucus secretion to lubricate the vagina. These two small, round glands are located on either side of the vaginal orifice.
- The **vaginal orifice** is the exterior opening of the vagina. ***Orifice*** means opening. The **hymen** (**HIGH**-men) is a mucous membrane that partially covers this opening and can be torn either during the first instance of intercourse or other activity. This tissue can be absent in a woman who has not been sexually active.

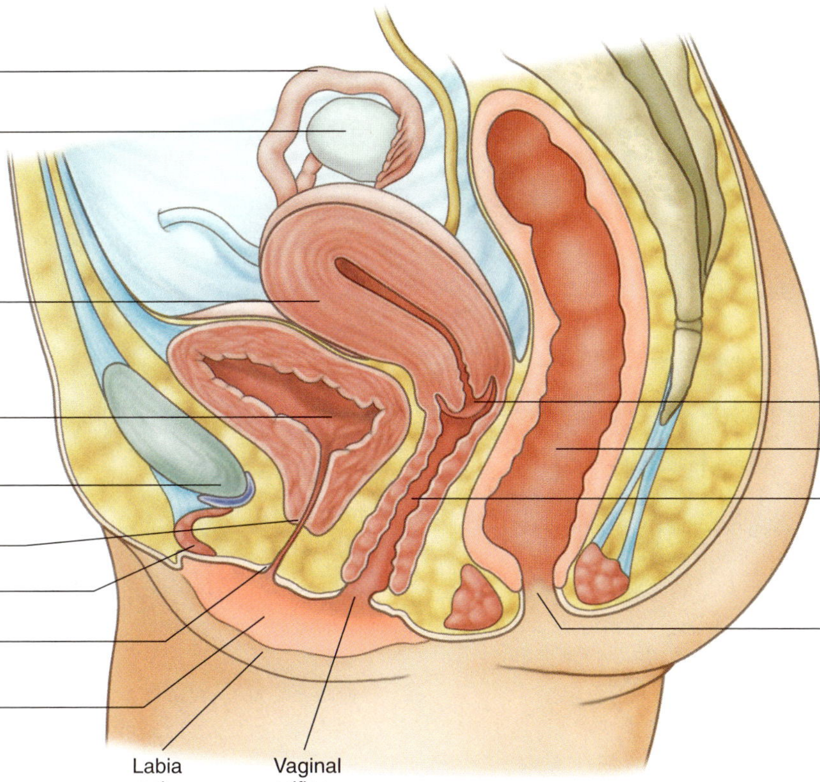

FIGURE 14.5 Structures of the female reproductive system shown in a lateral cross-section.

Breasts

Breasts are made up of fat, connective tissue, and the mammary glands (the word parts **mamm/o** and **mast/o** both mean breast). Each breast is fixed to the overlying skin and the underlying pectoral muscles by suspensory ligaments (Figure 14.7). Breast cancer, its diagnosis and treatment, are discussed in Chapter 6.

- **Mammary glands**, also known as the ***lactiferous glands***, are the milk-producing glands that develop during puberty.
- The **lactiferous ducts** (lack-**TIF**-er-us), also known as ***milk ducts***, carry milk from the mammary glands to the nipple (**lact** means milk, and **-iferous** means carrying or producing).
- Breast milk flows through the **nipple**, which is surrounded by the dark-pigmented area known as the **areola** (ah-**REE**-oh-lah).

The Internal Female Genitalia

The internal female genitalia are located within the pelvic cavity where they are protected by the bony pelvis. These structures include two ovaries, two fallopian tubes, the uterus, and the vagina (Figures 14.5 and 14.8).

The Ovaries

The **ovaries** (**OH**-vah-rees) are a pair of small, almond-shaped organs located in the lower abdomen, one on either side of the uterus.

- A **follicle** (**FOL**-lick-kul) is a fluid-filled sac containing a single ovum (egg). There are thousands of these sacs on the inside surface of the ovaries.
- The **ova** (**OH**-vah), also known as ***eggs***, are the female gametes (singular, *ovum*). These immature ova are present at birth. Normally, after puberty, one ovum matures and is released each month.
- The ovaries also produce the sex hormones estrogen and progesterone, which are discussed in Chapter 13.

The Fallopian Tubes

There are two **fallopian tubes** (fal-**LOH**-pee-an), which are also known as ***uterine tubes***. These tubes extend from the upper end of the uterus to a point near but not attached to an ovary.

- The **infundibulum** (**in**-fun-**DIB**-you-lum) is the funnel-shaped opening into the fallopian tube near the ovary.

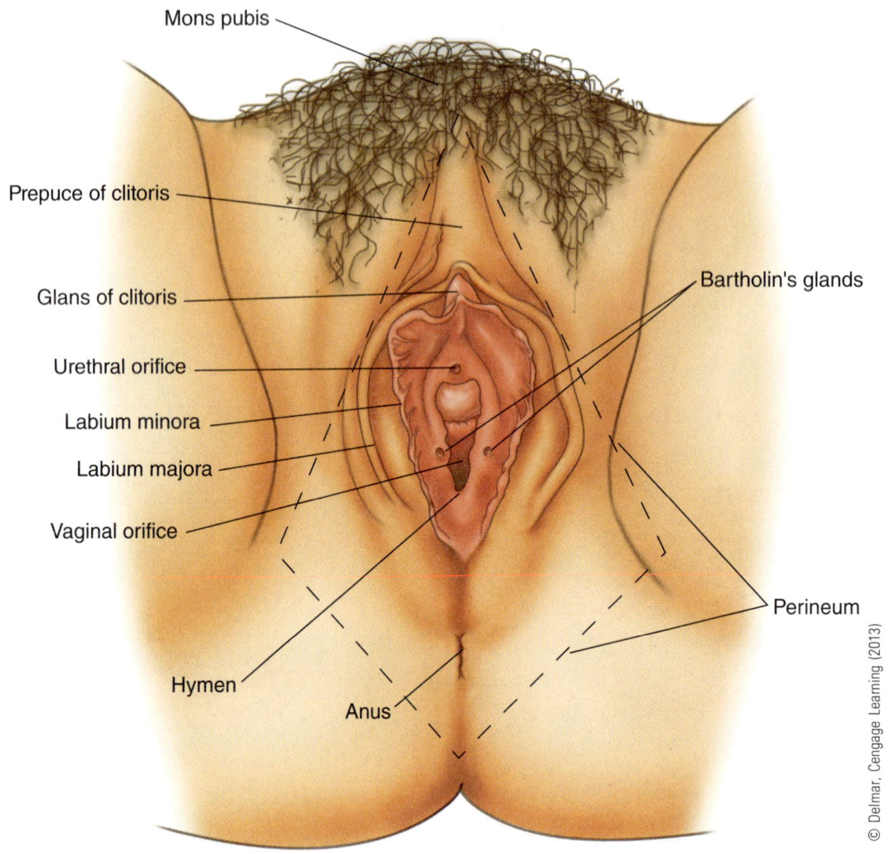

FIGURE 14.6 Female external genitalia.

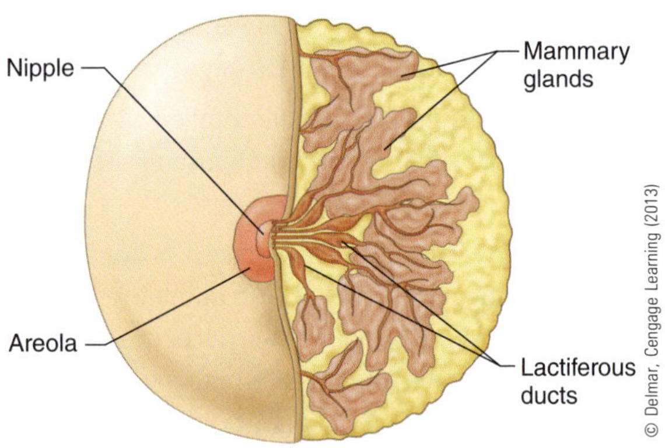

FIGURE 14.7 Structures of the breast.

- The **fimbriae** (**FIM**-bree-ee) are the fringed, finger-like extensions of this opening. Their role is to catch the mature ovum when it leaves the ovary (singular, *fimbria*).
- Each month, one of these tubes carries a mature ovum from the ovary to the uterus (Figure 14.8). These tubes also carry sperm upward from the uterus toward the descending mature ovum so that fertilization can occur.

The Uterus

The **uterus** (**YOU**-ter-us), formerly known as the ***womb***, is a pear-shaped organ with muscular walls and a mucous membrane lining filled with a rich supply of blood vessels (Figure 14.8).

- The uterus is located between the urinary bladder and the rectum and midway between the sacrum and the pubic bone.
- In its normal position, which is known as **anteflexion** (**an**-tee-**FLECK**-shun), the body of the uterus is bent forward (**ante-** means forward, **flex** means bend, and **-ion** means condition) (Figure 14.5).

The Parts of the Uterus

The body of the uterus consists of three major anatomic areas:

- The **fundus** (**FUN**-dus) is the bulging, rounded part above the entrance of the fallopian tubes. Because the fundus rises during pregnancy, measuring the fundal height in relation to the pubic bone helps determine the baby's growth.
- The **corpus** (**KOR**-pus), also known as the ***body of the uterus***, is the middle portion.

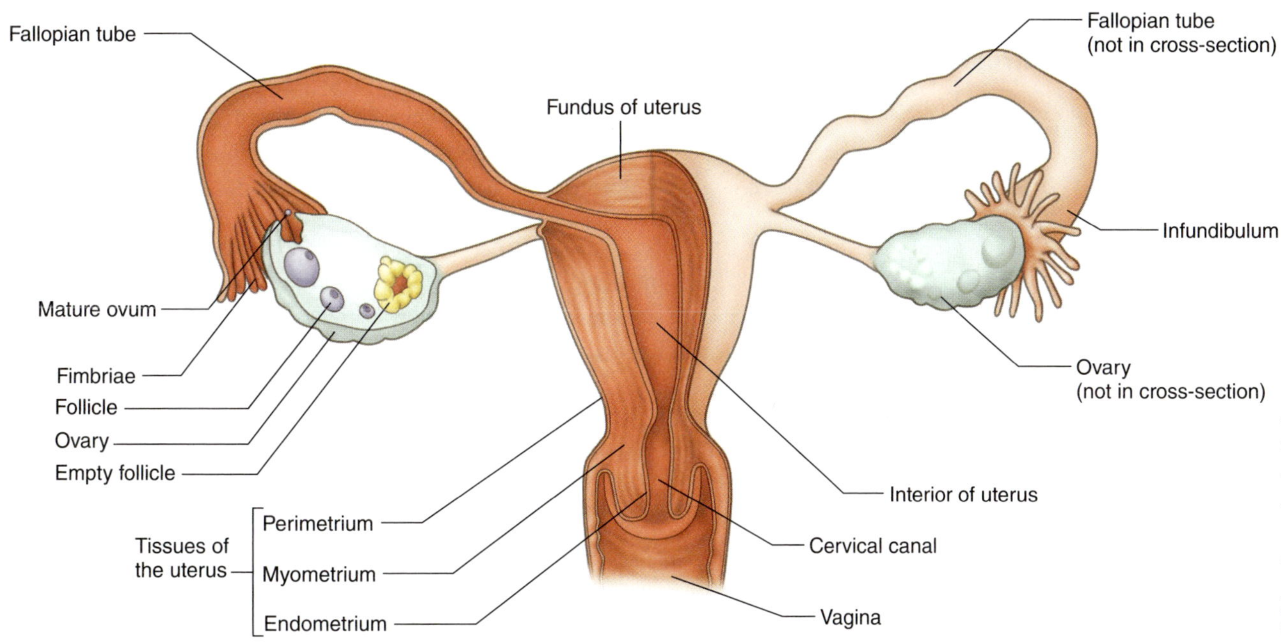

FIGURE 14.8 An anterior schematic view of the female reproductive organs. The left ovary, shown here in cross-section, contains developing ova in different stages of maturation. Also shown on the left is a mature ovum that has just been released.

- The **cervix** (**SER**-vicks), also known as the *cervix uteri*, is the lower, narrow portion that extends into the vagina. Within the cervix is the *cervical canal*, which ends at the *cervical os* at the vagina.

The Tissues of the Uterus

The uterus is composed of three major layers of tissue:

- The **perimetrium** (pehr-ih-**MEE**-tree-um), also known as the *uterine serosa*, is the tough, membranous outer layer (**peri-** means surrounding, **metri** means uterus, and **-um** is a singular noun ending). *Membranous* means pertaining to a thin layer of tissue.
- The **myometrium** (my-oh-**MEE**-tree-um) is the muscular middle layer (**my/o** means muscle, **metri** means uterus, and **-um** is a singular noun ending).
- The **endometrium** (en-doh-**MEE**-tree-um) is the inner layer, and it consists of specialized epithelial mucosa that is rich in blood vessels (**endo-** means within, **metri** means uterus, and **-um** is a singular noun ending). *Mucosa* means referring to mucous membrane.

Vagina

The **vagina** (vah-**JIGH**-nah) is the muscular tube lined with mucosa that extends from the cervix to the outside of the body. The word parts **colp/o** and **vagin/o** both mean vagina (Figures 14.7 and 14.8).

Menstruation

Menstruation (**men**-stroo-**AY**-shun), also known as *menses*, is the normal periodic discharge of the endometrial lining and unfertilized egg from uterus.

- **Menarche** (**MEN**-ar-kee) is the beginning of the menstrual function (**men** means menstruation, and **-arche** means beginning). This function begins after the maturation that occurs during puberty. In the United States the average age is 12.
- The average *menstrual cycle* consists of 28 days. These days are grouped into four phases and are summarized in Table 14.1.
- **Menopause** (**MEN**-oh-pawz) is the normal termination of the menstrual function in a woman during middle age (**men/o** means menstruation and **-pause** means stopping). Menopause is considered to be confirmed when a woman has gone 1 year without having a period.
- **Perimenopause** (pehr-ih-**MEN**-oh-pawz) is the term used to designate the transition phase between regular menstrual periods and no periods at all (**peri-** means surrounding, **men/o** means menstruation, and **-pause** means stopping). During this phase, which can last as long as 10 years, changes in hormone production can cause symptoms, including irregular menstrual cycles, hot flashes, mood swings, and disturbed sleep.

TABLE 14.1
Phases of the Menstrual Cycle

Approximately Days 1–5	*Menstrual phase*. These are the days when the endometrial lining of the uterus is sloughed off and discharged through the vagina as the menstrual flow.
Approximately Days 6–12	*Postmenstrual phase*. After the menstrual period, the pituitary gland secretes follicle-stimulating hormone (FSH), causing an ovum to mature. Estrogen, which is secreted by the ovaries, stimulates the lining of the uterus to prepare itself to receive a zygote (fertilized egg).
Approximately Days 13–14	*Ovulatory phase*. On approximately the 13th or 14th day of the cycle ovulation occurs. Ovulation is the release of a mature ovum. The mature egg leaves the ovary and travels slowly down the fallopian tube toward the uterus. During this time, the female is fertile and can become pregnant.
Approximately Days 15–28	*Premenstrual phase*. If fertilization does not occur, hormone levels change to cause the breakdown of the uterine endometrium and the beginning of a new menstrual cycle.

TERMS RELATED TO PREGNANCY AND CHILDBIRTH

Ovulation

Ovulation (**ov**-you-**LAY**-shun) is the release of a mature egg from a follicle on the surface of one of the ovaries that happens on approximately the 13th or 14th day of a woman's menstrual cycle.

- After the ovum (egg) is released, it is caught up by the fimbriae of the fallopian tube. Wave-like peristaltic actions move the ovum down the fallopian tube toward the uterus.
- It usually takes an ovum about 5 days to pass through the fallopian tube. If sperm are present at that time, one will fertilize the ovum within the fallopian tube.
- After the ovum has been released, the ruptured follicle enlarges, takes on a yellow fatty substance, and becomes the corpus luteum.
- The **corpus luteum** (**KOR**-pus **LOO**-tee-um) secretes the hormone progesterone during the second half of the menstrual cycle. This maintains the growth of the uterine lining in preparation for the fertilized egg.
- If the ovum is not fertilized, the corpus luteum dies, and the endometrium lining of the uterus sloughs off as the menstrual flow occurs.
- If the ovum is fertilized, the corpus luteum continues to secrete the hormones required to maintain the pregnancy.

Fertilization

- During **coitus** (**KOH**-ih-tus), also known as *sexual intercourse* or *copulation*, the male ejaculates approximately 100 million sperm into the female's vagina. The sperm travel upward through the vagina, into the uterus, and on into the fallopian tubes.
- **Conception** occurs when a sperm penetrates and fertilizes the descending ovum. This union, which is the beginning of a new life, forms a single cell known as a **zygote** (**ZYE**-goht).
- After fertilization occurs in the fallopian tube, the zygote travels to the uterus where it is implanted. *Implantation* is the embedding of the zygote into the lining of the uterus.
- From implantation through the 8th week of pregnancy, the developing child is known as an **embryo** (**EM**-bree-oh).
- From the 9th week of pregnancy to the time of birth, the developing child in utero is known as a **fetus** (**fet** means unborn child, and **-us** is a singular noun ending). *In utero* means within the uterus (Figure 14.9).

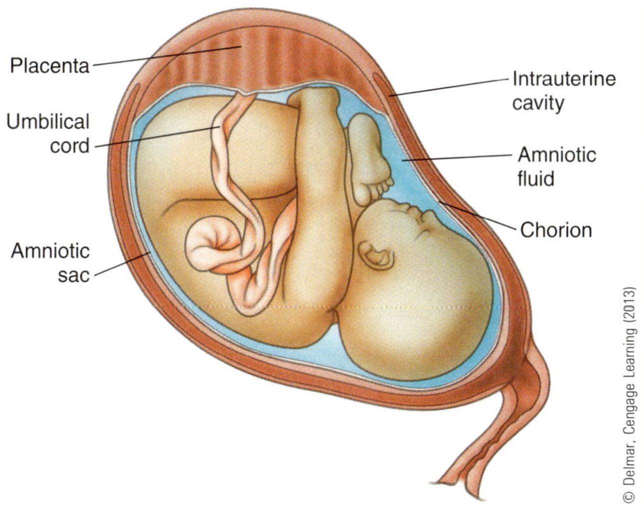

FIGURE 14.9 A normal pregnant uterus viewed in cross-section.

StudyWARE CONNECTION

Watch the **Female Reproductive System** animation in the StudyWARE™.

Multiple Births

If more than one egg is passing down the fallopian tube when sperm are present, the fertilization of more than one egg is possible.

- **Fraternal twins** result from the fertilization of separate ova by separate sperm cells. These develop into two separate embryos (Figure 14.10).
- **Identical twins** are formed by the fertilization of a single egg cell by a single sperm that divides to form two embryos. Each of these twins receives exactly the same genetic information from the parents.
- The term **multiples** is used to describe a birth involving more than two infants.

The Chorion and Placenta

- The **chorion** (**KOR**-ee-on) is the thin outer membrane that encloses the embryo. It contributes to the formation of the placenta (Figure 14.9).
- The **placenta** (plah-**SEN**-tah) is a temporary organ that forms within the uterus to allow the exchange of nutrients, oxygen, and waste products between the mother and fetus without allowing maternal blood and fetal blood to mix. The placental barrier does not, however, keep chemicals and/or drugs from reaching the fetus.

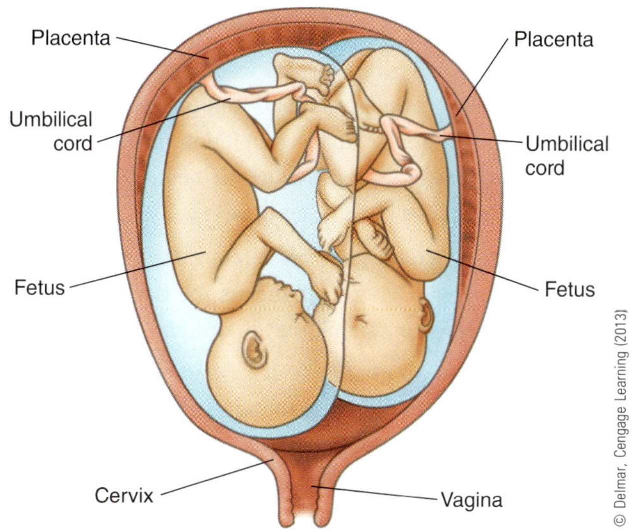

FIGURE 14.10 Fraternal twins in utero.

- The placenta also produces hormones necessary to maintain the pregnancy. These hormones are discussed in Chapter 13.
- After delivery of the newborn, the placenta and fetal membranes are expelled as the **afterbirth**.

The Amniotic Sac

The **amniotic sac** (**am**-nee-**OT**-ick), which is also known as the ***amnion***, is the innermost membrane that surrounds the embryo in the uterus (Figure 14.9). The common name for this structure is the ***bag of waters***.

- The developing embryo is surrounded by the **amniotic cavity**. This is the fluid-filled space between the embryo and the amniotic sac.
- **Amnionic fluid** (**am**-nee-**ON**-ick), also known as ***amniotic fluid***, is the liquid that protects the fetus and makes possible its floating movements.

The Umbilical Cord

The **umbilical cord** (um-**BILL**-ih-kal) is the tube that carries blood, oxygen, and nutrients from the placenta to the developing child. It also transports waste from the fetus to be disposed of through the mother's excretory system. This cord is cut soon after the birth of the infant and before the delivery of the placenta.

- After birth, the **navel**, also known as the ***belly button***, is formed where the umbilical cord was attached to the fetus.

Gestation

Gestation (jes-**TAY**-shun), which lasts approximately 280 days (40 weeks), is the period of development of the child in the mother's uterus. Upon completion of this developmental time, the fetus is described as being *at term* and should be ready for birth (Figure 14.11).

- The term **pregnancy**, which is often used interchangeably with *gestation*, means the condition of having a developing child in the uterus.
- The length of pregnancy is described according to the number of weeks of gestation (usually 40 weeks total). For descriptive purposes, pregnancy can also be divided into three **trimesters** of about 13 weeks each.
- The **due date**, or *estimated date of confinement*, is calculated from the first day of the last menstrual period (LMP). *Confinement* is an old-fashioned term describing the period of rest for the mother that followed childbirth.
- **Quickening** is the first movement of the fetus in the uterus that can be felt by the mother. This usually occurs during the 16th to 20th week of pregnancy.
- **Braxton Hicks contractions** are intermittent painless uterine contractions that occur with increasing frequently as the pregnancy progresses. These contractions are not true labor pains and are usually infrequent, irregular, and essentially painless.
- The fetus is described as being **viable** when it is capable of living outside the uterus. Viability depends on the developmental age, birth weight, and developmental stage of the lungs of the fetus.
- The term **antepartum** (**an**-tee-**PAHR**-tum) refers to the final stage of pregnancy just before the onset of labor.

The Mother

- A **nulligravida** (**null**-ih-**GRAV**-ih-dah) is a woman who has never been pregnant (**nulli-** means none, and **-gravida** means pregnant). Compare with *nullipara*.
- A **nullipara** (nuh-**LIP**-ah-rah) is a woman who has never borne a viable child (**nulli-** means none, and **-para** means to bring forth). Compare with *nulligravida*.
- A **primigravida** (**prye**-mih-**GRAV**-ih-dah) is a woman during her first pregnancy (**primi-** means first, and **-gravida** means pregnant). Compare with *primipara*.
- A **primipara** (prye-**MIP**-ah-rah) is a woman who has borne one viable child (**primi-** means first, and **-para** means to bring forth). Compare with *primigravida*.
- **Multiparous** (mul-**TIP**-ah-rus) means a woman who has given birth two or more times (**multi-** means many, and **-parous** means having borne one or more children).

Childbirth

Labor and delivery, also known as *childbirth* or *parturition*, occurs in three stages, shown in Figure 14.11. The stages of labor and delivery are:

1. Dilation
2. Delivery of the baby
3. Expulsion of the afterbirth

The First Stage

During the first (and longest) stage of labor, the changes that occur include the gradual **dilation** (dye-**LAY**-shun) and effacement of the cervix and the rupture of the amniotic sac. *Effacement* is the process by which the cervix prepares for delivery as it gradually softens, shortens, and becomes thinner (Figure 14.11B).

- **Fetal monitoring** is the use of an electronic device to record the fetal heart rate and the maternal uterine contractions during labor.

The Second Stage

The second stage, which begins when the cervix is dilated to 10 centimeters, is the delivery of the infant. As the uterine contractions become stronger and more frequent, the mother pushes to help expel the child through the *birth canal* (vagina). Normally, the baby's head presents first. **Cephalic presentation** or *crowning* describes when the baby is coming head first. The head can be seen at the vaginal opening (Figure 14.11C).

The Third Stage

The third stage is the expulsion of the placenta as the *afterbirth* (Figure 14.11D).

Postpartum

The term **postpartum** (pohst-**PAR**-tum) means after childbirth.

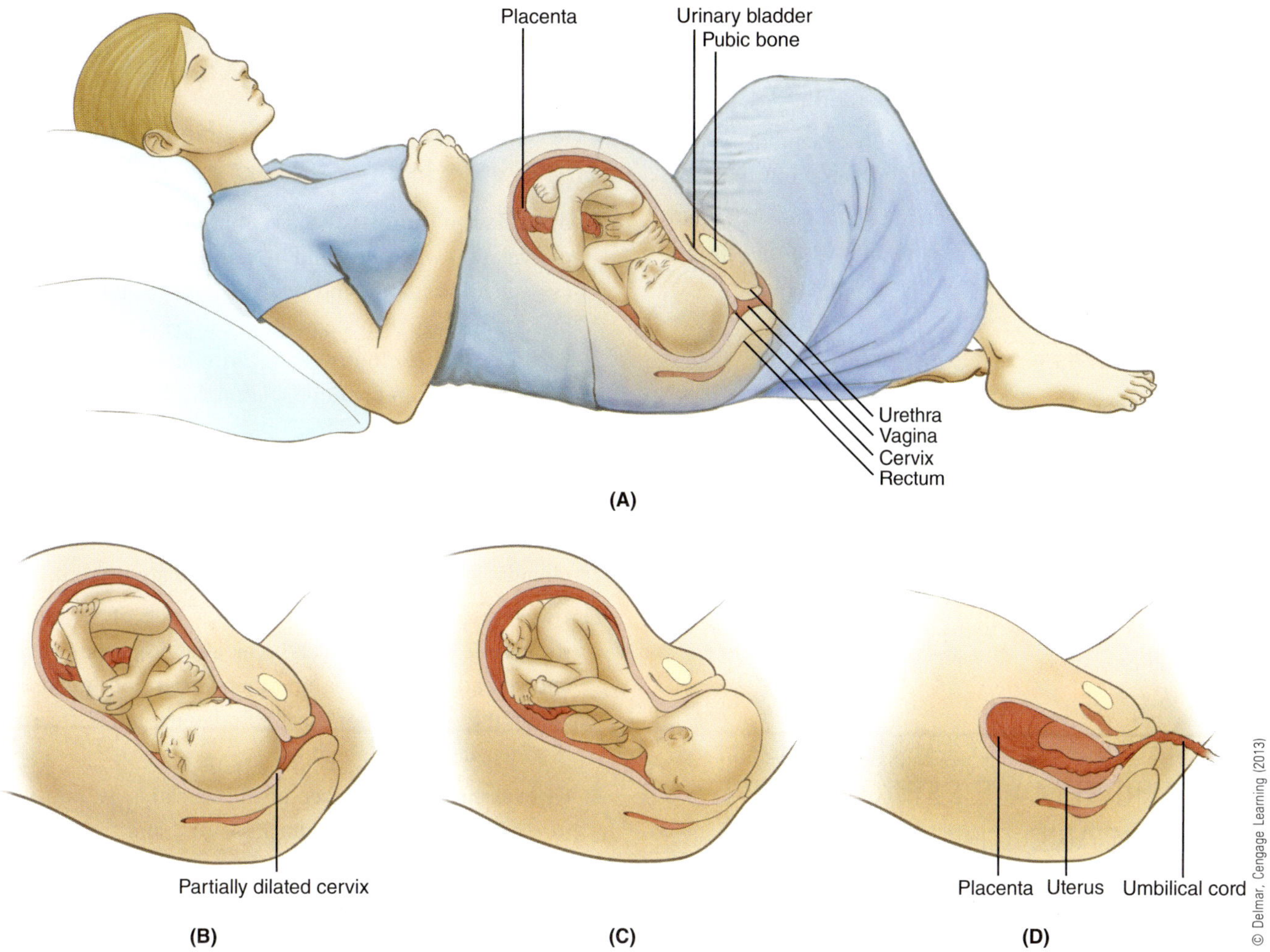

FIGURE 14.11 The stages of labor. (A) Position of the fetus before labor. (B) First state of labor, cervical dilation. (C) Second stage of labor, fetal delivery. (D) Third stage of labor, delivery of the afterbirth (placenta and fetal membranes).

The Mother

- **Puerperium** (**pyou**-er-**PEE**-ree-um) is the time from the delivery of the placenta through approximately the first 6 weeks after the delivery. By the end of this period, most of the changes in the mother's body due to pregnancy have resolved, and the body has reverted to the nonpregnant state.
- **Lochia** (**LOH**-kee-ah) is the postpartum vaginal discharge that typically continues for 4 to 6 weeks after childbirth (**loch** means childbirth, and **-ia** means pertaining to). It consists primarily of blood and mucus.
- **Uterine involution** is the return of the uterus to its normal size and former condition after delivery. ***Involution*** means the return of an enlarged organ to its normal size.
- **Colostrum** (kuh-**LOS**-trum) is a specialized form of milk that delivers essential nutrients and antibodies in a form that the newborn can digest. Colostrum is produced by the mammary glands in late pregnancy and during the first few days after giving birth.
- **Lactation** (lack-**TAY**-shun) is the process of forming and secreting milk from the breasts as nourishment for the infant. The breast milk develops a few days after giving birth to replace the colostrum.
- **Postpartum depression** is a mood disorder characterized by feelings of sadness and the loss of pleasure in normal activities that can occur shortly after giving birth. One cause of this depression is the rapid change in the hormone levels that occurs after giving birth. When the depression is severe, treatment is required.

The Baby

The newborn infant is known as a **neonate** (**NEE**-oh-nayt) during the first 4 weeks after birth.

- **Vernix** (**VER**-nicks) is a greasy substance that protects the fetus in utero and can still be present at birth.
- **Meconium** (meh-**KOH**-nee-um) is the greenish material that collects in the intestine of a fetus and forms the first stools of a newborn.

Apgar Scores

An **Apgar score** is a scale of 1 to 10 to evaluate a newborn infant's physical status at 1 and 5 minutes after birth.

- The newborn is evaluated by assigning numerical values (0 to 2) to each of five criteria: (1) heart rate, (2) respiratory effort, (3) muscle tone, (4) response stimulation, and (5) skin color.
- A total score of 8 to 10 indicates the best possible condition.

MEDICAL SPECIALTIES RELATED TO THE FEMALE REPRODUCTIVE SYSTEM AND CHILDBIRTH

- A **gynecologist** (**guy**-neh-**KOL**-oh-jist), or GYN, is a physician who specializes in diagnosing and treating diseases and disorders of the female reproductive system (**gynec** means female, and **-ologist** means specialist).
- An **obstetrician** (**ob**-steh-**TRISH**-un), or OB, is a physician who specializes in providing medical care to women during pregnancy, childbirth, and immediately thereafter. This specialty is referred to as ***obstetrics***.
- A ***midwife*** assists in labor and delivery. A certified nurse midwife (CNM) is an RN with specialized training in obstetrics and gynecology who provides primary care in normal pregnancies and deliveries.
- A **neonatologist** (**nee**-oh-nay-**TOL**-oh-jist) is a physician who specializes in diagnosing and treating disorders of the newborn (**neo-** means new, **nat** means born, and **-ologist** means specialist).
- An **infertility specialist**, also known as a ***fertility specialist*** helps infertile couples by diagnosing and treating problems associated with conception and maintaining pregnancy.

PATHOLOGY OF THE FEMALE REPRODUCTIVE SYSTEM

The Ovaries, Fallopian Tubes, and Ovulation

- **Anovulation** (**an**-ov-you-**LAY**-shun) is the absence of ovulation when it would be normally expected (**an-** means without, and **ovulation** means the release of a mature egg). This condition can be caused by stress, inadequate nutrition, or hormonal imbalances. Menstruation can continue, although ovulation does not occur.
- **Oophoritis** (**oh**-ahf-oh-**RYE**-tis) is inflammation of an ovary (**oophor** means ovary, and **-itis** means inflammation). This condition frequently occurs when salpingitis or pelvic inflammatory disease are present.
- **Ovarian cancer** originates within the cells of the ovaries. These cancer cells can break away from the ovary and spread (metastasize) to other tissues and organs within the abdomen or travel through the bloodstream to other parts of the body.
- **Ovariorrhexis** (oh-**vay**-ree-oh-**RECK**-sis) is the rupture of an ovary (**ovari/o** means ovary, and **-rrhexis** means to rupture).
- **Pelvic inflammatory disease** (PID) is any inflammation of the female reproductive organs that is not associated with surgery or pregnancy. This condition occurs most frequently as a complication of a sexually transmitted disease and can lead to infertility, ectopic pregnancy, and other serious disorders.
- **Polycystic ovary syndrome** (**pol**-ee-**SIS**-tick), also known as PCOS, is a condition caused by a hormonal imbalance in which the ovaries are enlarged by the presence of many cysts formed by incompletely developed follicles.
- **Pyosalpinx** (**pye**-oh-**SAL**-pinks) is an accumulation of pus in a fallopian tube (**py/o** means pus, and **-salpinx** means fallopian tube).
- **Salpingitis** (**sal**-pin-**JIGH**-tis) is an inflammation of a fallopian tube (**salping** means fallopian tube, and **-itis** means inflammation).

The Uterus

- **Endometriosis** (**en**-doh-**mee**-tree-**OH**-sis) is a condition in which patches of endometrial tissue escape the uterus and become attached to other structures in the pelvic cavity (**endo-** means within, **metri** means uterus, and **-osis** means abnormal condition). It is a leading cause of infertility.

- **Metrorrhea** (**mee**-troh-**REE**-ah) is an abnormal discharge, such as mucus or pus, from the uterus (**metr/o** means uterus, and **-rrhea** means flow or discharge).
- **Endometrial cancer** (**en**-doh-**MEE**-tree-al) involves a cancerous growth that begins in the lining of the uterus. One of the earliest symptoms of this cancer that frequently occurs after menopause is abnormal bleeding from the uterus.
- A **uterine fibroid**, also known as a ***myoma***, is a benign tumor composed of muscle and fibrous tissue that occurs in the wall of the uterus (Figure 14.12).
- A **uterine prolapse** (proh-**LAPS**), also known as a ***pelvic floor hernia***, is the condition in which the uterus slides from its normal position in the pelvic cavity and sags into the vagina. ***Prolapse*** means the falling or dropping down of an organ or internal part.

The Cervix

- **Cervical cancer** is the second-most common cancer in women and usually affects women between the ages of 45 and 65 years. It is caused by human papillomaviruses (HPV), which can now be prevented through vaccination and can be detected early through routine Pap tests.
- **Cervical dysplasia** (**SER**-vih-kal dis-**PLAY**-see-ah) is the presence of precancerous changes in the cells that make up the inner lining of the cervix. Without early detection and treatment, these cells can become malignant.
- **Cervicitis** (**ser**-vih-**SIGH**-tis) is an inflammation of the cervix that is usually caused by an infection (**cervic** means cervix, and **-itis** means inflammation).
- **Endocervicitis** (**en**-doh-**ser**-vih-**SIGH**-tis) is an inflammation of the mucous membrane lining of the cervix (**endo-** means within, **cervic** means cervix, and **-itis** means inflammation).

The Vagina

- **Colporrhexis** (**kol**-poh-**RECK**-sis) means tearing or laceration of the vaginal wall (**colp/o** means vagina, and **-rrhexis** means to rupture). A ***laceration*** is a torn, ragged wound or an accidental cut.

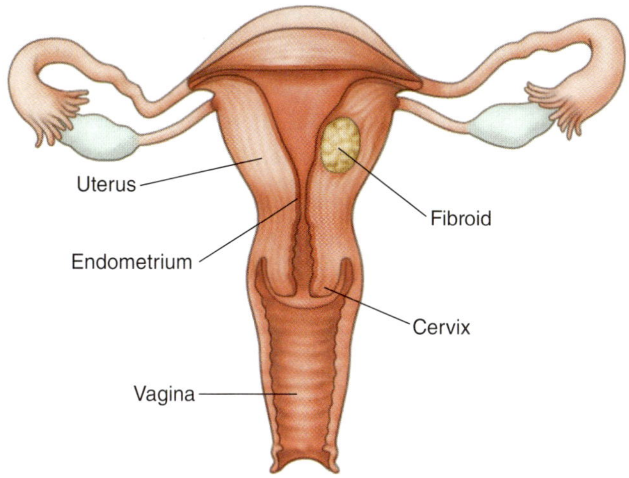

FIGURE 14.12 Uterine fibroid.

- **Dyspareunia** (**dis**-pah-**ROO**-nee-ah) is characterized by pain during sexual intercourse (**dys** means painful and **-pareunia** means sexual intercourse).
- **Leukorrhea** (**loo**-koh-**REE**-ah) is a profuse, whitish mucus discharge from the uterus and vagina (**leuk/o** means white, and **-rrhea** means flow or discharge). Women normally may have some vaginal discharge; however, leukorrhea describes a change and increase in this discharge that can be due to an infection, malignancy, or hormonal changes.
- **Vaginal candidiasis** (**kan**-dih-**DYE**-ah-sis), also known as a ***yeast infection***, is a vaginal infection caused by the yeast-like fungus *Candida albicans*. The growth of this fungus is usually controlled by bacteria normally present in the vagina. When these bacteria are not able to control fungal growth, symptoms occur that include burning, itching, and a "cottage cheese-like" vaginal discharge.
- **Vaginitis** (**vaj**-ih-**NIGH**-tis), also known as ***colpitis***, is an inflammation of the lining of the vagina (**vagin** and **colp** both mean vagina, and **-itis** means inflammation). The most common causes of a vaginal inflammation are bacterial vaginosis, trichomoniasis, and vaginal candidiasis (discussed in the section "Sexually Transmitted Diseases").

The External Genitalia

- **Pruritus vulvae** (proo-**RYE**-tus **VUL**-vee) is a condition of severe itching of the external female genitalia. ***Pruritus*** means itching.

- **Vulvodynia** (vul-voh-**DIN**-ee-ah) is a painful syndrome of unknown cause (**vulv/o** means vulva, and **-dynia** means pain). It is characterized by chronic burning, pain during sexual intercourse, itching, or stinging irritation of the vulva.
- **Vulvitis** (vul-**VYE**-tis) is an inflammation of the vulva (**vulv** means vulva, and **-itis** means inflammation). Possible causes include fungal or bacterial infections, chafing, skin conditions, or allergies to products such as soaps and bubble bath.

Breast Diseases

- **Breast cancer**, its diagnosis and treatment, are discussed in Chapter 6.
- A **fibroadenoma** (**figh**-broh-**ad**-eh-**NOH**-mah) is a round, firm, rubbery mass that arises from excess growth of glandular and connective tissue in the breast (Figure 14.13). These masses, which can grow to the size of a small plum, are benign and usually painless. Fibroadenomas often enlarge during pregnancy and shrink during menopause.
- **Fibrocystic breast disease** (**figh**-broh-**SIS**-tick) is the presence of single or multiple benign cysts in the breasts. This condition occurs more frequently in older women. A ***cyst*** is a closed sac containing fluid or semisolid material.
- **Galactorrhea** (gah-**lack**-toh-**REE**-ah) is the production of breast milk in a woman who is not breastfeeding (**galact/o** means milk, and **-rrhea** means flow or discharge). This condition is caused by a malfunction of the thyroid or pituitary gland.
- **Mastalgia** (mass-**TAL**-jee-ah), also known as ***mastodynia***, is pain in the breast (**mast** means breast, and **-algia** means pain).

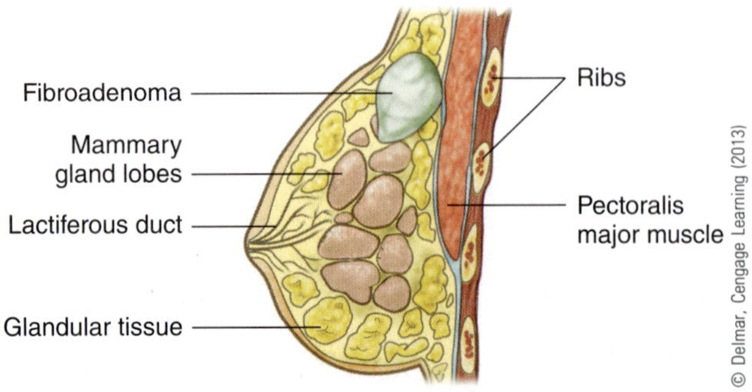

FIGURE 14.13 A fibroadenoma of the breast.

- **Mastitis** (mas-**TYE**-tis) is a breast infection that is caused by bacteria that enter the breast tissue, most frequently during breastfeeding (**mast** means breast, and **-itis** means inflammation).

Menstrual Disorders

- **Amenorrhea** (ah-**men**-oh-**REE**-ah) is an abnormal absence of menstrual periods for 90 days or more (**a-** means without, **men/o** means menstruation, and **-rrhea** means flow or discharge). This condition, which is normal only before puberty, during pregnancy, while breastfeeding, and after menopause, can be caused by stress, hormonal problems, poor nutrition, or excessive exercise.
- **Dysmenorrhea** (**dis**-men-oh-**REE**-ah) is pain caused by uterine cramps during a menstrual period (**dys-** means bad, **men/o** means menstruation, and **-rrhea** means flow or discharge). This pain, which occurs in the lower abdomen, can be sharp, intermittent, dull, or aching.
- **Dysfunctional uterine bleeding** (DUB) is a condition characterized by abnormal bleeding often due to an imbalance in hormone level changes.
- **Hypermenorrhea** (**high**-per-men-oh-**REE**-ah), also known as ***menorrhagia***, is an excessive amount of menstrual flow over a period of more than 7 days (**hyper-** means excessive, **men/o** means menstruation, and **-rrhea** means flow or discharge). Hypermenorrhea is the opposite of *hypomenorrhea.*
- **Hypomenorrhea** (**high**-poh-men-oh-**REE**-ah) is an unusually small amount of menstrual flow during a shortened regular menstrual period (**hypo-** means deficient, **men/o** means menstruation, and **-rrhea** means flow or discharge). Hypomenorrhea is the opposite of *hypermenorrhea.*
- **Menometrorrhagia** (**men**-oh-**met**-roh-**RAY**-jee-ah), also known as ***intermenstrual bleeding***, is excessive uterine bleeding at both the usual time of menstrual periods and at other irregular intervals (**men/o** means menstruation, **metr/o** means uterus, and **-rrhagia** means abnormal bleeding).
- **Oligomenorrhea** (**ol**-ih-goh-**men**-oh-**REE**-ah) is the term used to describe infrequent or very light menstruation in a woman with previously normal periods (**olig/o** means scanty, **men/o** means menstruation, and **-rrhea** means flow or discharge). Oligomenorrhea is the opposite of *polymenorrhea.*

- **Polymenorrhea** (**pol**-ee-**men**-oh-**REE**-ah) is the occurrence of menstrual cycles more frequently than is normal (**poly-** means many, **men/o** means menstruation, and **-rrhea** means flow or discharge). Polymenorrhea is the opposite of *oligomenorrhea*.
- **Premature menopause** is a condition in which the ovaries cease functioning before age 40 years due to disease, a hormonal disorder, or surgical removal. This causes infertility and often brings on menopausal symptoms.
- **Premenstrual syndrome** (PMS) is a group of symptoms experienced by some women within the 2-week period before menstruation. These symptoms can include bloating, swelling, headaches, mood swings, and breast discomfort.
- **Premenstrual dysphoric disorder** (PMDD) is a condition associated with severe emotional and physical problems that are closely linked to the menstrual cycle. Symptoms occur regularly in the second half of the cycle and end when menstruation begins or shortly thereafter.

PATHOLOGY OF PREGNANCY AND CHILDBIRTH

Pregnancy

- An **abortion** (ah-**BOR**-shun) is the interruption or termination of pregnancy before the fetus is viable. A ***spontaneous abortion***, also known as a ***miscarriage***, usually occurs early in the pregnancy and is due to an abnormality or genetic disorder.
- An ***induced abortion***, caused by human intervention, is achieved through the use of drugs or suctioning. When done for medical purposes, it is known as a ***therapeutic abortion***.
- An **ectopic pregnancy** (eck-**TOP**-ick), also known as an ***extrauterine pregnancy***, is a potentially dangerous condition in which a fertilized egg is implanted and begins to develop outside of the uterus. ***Ectopic*** means out of place, and Figure 14.14 illustrates some of these potential locations.
- **Gestational diabetes mellitus** is discussed in Chapter 13.
- **Infertility** is the inability of a couple to achieve pregnancy after 1 year of regular, unprotected intercourse, or the inability of a woman to carry a pregnancy to a live birth.

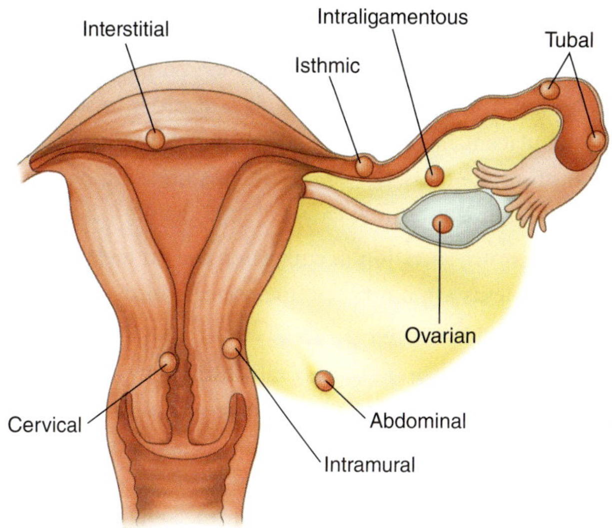

FIGURE 14.14 Potential sites of an ectopic pregnancy.

- **Preeclampsia** (**pree**-ee-**KLAMP**-see-ah), also known as ***pregnancy-induced hypertension*** or ***toxemia***, is a complication of pregnancy characterized by hypertension (high blood pressure), edema (swelling), and proteinuria (an abnormally high level of protein in the urine).
- **Eclampsia** (eh-**KLAMP**-see-ah), which is a more serious form of preeclampsia, is characterized by convulsions and sometimes coma. Treatment for this condition includes the delivery of the fetus.

The Rh Factor

The **Rh factor** defines the presence or absence of the Rh antigen on red blood cells. (See Chapter 5.) The Rh factor can cause difficulties when an Rh negative (Rh−) mother is pregnant with an Rh positive (Rh+) baby. If a small amount of the baby's blood enters the mother's bloodstream, she can develop antibodies in an allergic response.

- A man who is Rh+ can father a baby that is either Rh+ or Rh−, potentially causing a reaction if the mother is Rh−. (If both parents are Rh−, there is no danger of incompatibility.)
- The antibodies that develop in the mother's body during pregnancy can cause anemia and other problems for the baby, and also be a factor in subsequent pregnancies if the mother is not treated.
- Blood tests of both parents can identify this potential problem. If it exists, the mother is vaccinated with a blood product called ***Rh immunoglobulin*** (RhIg).

Childbirth

- **Abruptio placentae** (ah-**BRUP**-shee-oh plah-**SEN**-tee), or ***placental abruption***, is a disorder in which the placenta separates from the uterine wall before the birth of the fetus. ***Abruption*** means breaking off. This condition is a leading cause of fetal death.
- **Breech presentation** occurs when the buttocks or feet of the fetus are positioned to enter the birth canal first instead of the head.
- **Placenta previa** (plah-**SEN**-tah **PREE**-vee-ah) is the abnormal implantation of the placenta in the lower portion of the uterus. ***Previa*** means appearing before or in front of. Symptoms include painless, sudden-onset bleeding during the third trimester.
- A **premature infant**, also known as a ***preemie***, is a fetus born before the 37th week of gestation.
- A **stillbirth** is the birth of a fetus that died before, or during, delivery.

DIAGNOSTIC PROCEDURES OF THE FEMALE REPRODUCTIVE SYSTEM

- **Colposcopy** (kol-**POS**-koh-pee) is the direct visual examination of the tissues of the cervix and vagina (**colp/o** means vagina, and **-scopy** means direct visual examination). This examination is performed using a binocular magnifier known as a ***colposcope***.
- In an **endometrial biopsy**, a small amount of the tissue from the lining of the uterus is removed for microscopic examination. This test is most often used to determine the cause of abnormal vaginal bleeding.
- **Endovaginal ultrasound** (**en**-doh-**VAJ**-ih-nal) is performed to determine the cause of abnormal vaginal bleeding. This test is performed by placing an ultrasound transducer in the vagina so that the sound waves can create images of the uterus and ovaries.
- **Hysterosalpingography** (**hiss**-ter-oh-**sal**-pin-**GOG**-rah-fee) (HSG) is a radiographic examination of the uterus and fallopian tubes (**hyster/o** means uterus, **salping/o** means tube, and **-graphy** means the process of producing a picture or record). This test requires the instillation of radio-opaque contrast material into the uterine cavity and fallopian tubes to make them visible. ***Instillation*** means slowly pouring a liquid onto a body part or into a body cavity.
- **Hysteroscopy** (HYS) (**hiss**-ter-**OSS**-koh-pee) is the direct visual examination of the interior of the uterus and fallopian tubes (**hyster/o** means uterus, and **-scopy** means direct visual examination). This examination is performed by using the magnification of a ***hysteroscope***.
- A **Pap smear** is an exfoliative biopsy of the cervix. It is performed to detect conditions that can be early indicators of cervical cancer (Figure 14.15). As used here, ***exfoliative*** means that cells are scraped from the tissue and examined under a microscope. A ***speculum*** is used to enlarge the opening of the vagina during the examination of the cervix and vagina.

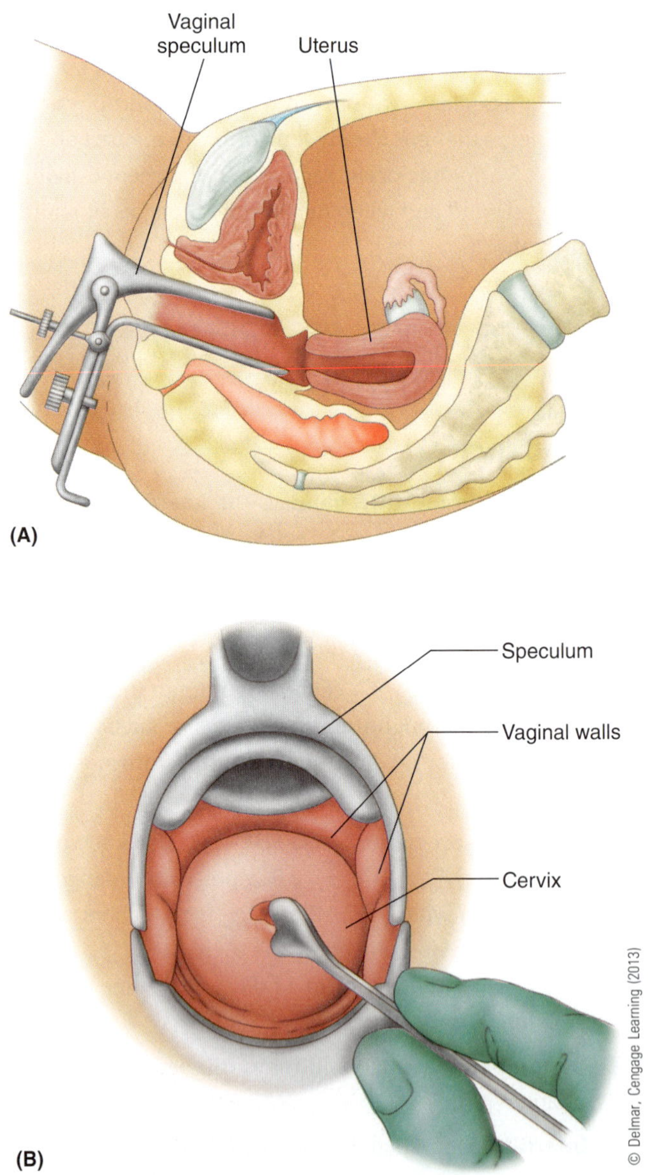

FIGURE 14.15 For a pap smear, a speculum is used to enlarge the vaginal opening (A) and a few cervical cells are removed for study under a microscope (B).

- *Ultrasound* and *laparoscopy*, which are also used to diagnose disorders of the reproductive system, are discussed further in Chapter 15.

Diagnostic Procedures Related to Pregnancy and Childbirth

- A **pregnancy test** is performed to detect an unusually high level of the *human chorionic gonadotropin* (HCG) hormone in either a blood or urine specimen, which is usually an indication of pregnancy. A home pregnancy test uses a urine specimen, whereas a pregnancy test based on a blood specimen at a doctor's office usually provides more reliable results.
- **Fetal ultrasound** testing is discussed in Chapter 15.
- **First trimester screening**, also known as *combined screening*, is performed between 11 and 13 weeks of pregnancy and involves an ultrasound and a finger-stick blood test. The combined results of these two measurements, plus the mother's age, detect if the fetus is at increased risk for Down syndrome, which is discussed in Chapter 2. Diagnostic tests, such as amniocentesis or chorionic villus sampling, are recommended for those at increased risk for this condition.
- **Chorionic villus sampling** (CVS) (**kor**-ee-**ON**-ick **VIL**-us) is the examination of cells retrieved from the chorionic villi, which are minute, vascular projections on the chorion. This test is performed between the 8th and 10th weeks of pregnancy to search for genetic abnormalities in the developing fetus.
- **Amniocentesis** (AMN) (**am**-nee-oh-sen-**TEE**-sis) is a surgical puncture with a needle to obtain a specimen of amniotic fluid (**amnio** means amnion and fetal membrane, and **-centesis** means a surgical puncture to remove fluid). This specimen, which is usually obtained after the 14th week of pregnancy, is used to evaluate fetal health and to diagnose certain congenital disorders.
- **Pelvimetry** (pel-**VIM**-eh-tree) is a radiographic study to measure the dimensions of the pelvis to evaluate its capacity to allow passage of the fetus through the birth canal (**pelvi** means pelvis, and **-metry** means to measure).

TREATMENT PROCEDURES OF THE FEMALE REPRODUCTIVE SYSTEM

Medications

- A **contraceptive** is a measure taken to lessen the likelihood of pregnancy.
- *Birth control pills* are a form of hormones that are administered as an oral contraceptive. Other forms of this type of contraceptive are available as an injection, a patch, and an inserted ring.
- A **diaphragm** is a barrier contraceptive that prevents the sperm from reaching and fertilizing the egg.
- An **intrauterine device** (IUD) is a molded plastic contraceptive inserted through the cervix into the uterus to prevent pregnancy (**intra-** means within, and **uterine** means uterus).
- A **condom** will also prevent pregnancy when used correctly. It is the only contraceptive method mentioned here that will also prevent the transmission of sexually transmitted diseases (STDs).
- **Hormone replacement therapy** (HRT) is the use of the female hormones estrogen and progestin to replace those the body no longer produces during and after perimenopause. *Progestin* is a synthetic form of the female hormone progesterone.

The Ovaries and Fallopian Tubes

- An **oophorectomy** (**oh**-ahf-oh-**RECK**-toh-mee), also known as an *ovariectomy*, is the surgical removal of one or both ovaries (**oophor** mean ovary, and **-ectomy** means surgical removal). If both ovaries are removed in a premenopausal woman, the patient experiences *surgical menopause*.
- A **salpingectomy** (**sal**-pin-**JECK**-toh-mee) is the surgical removal of one or both fallopian tubes (**salping** means tube, and **-ectomy** means surgical removal).
- A **salpingo-oophorectomy** (SO) (sal-**ping**-goh oh-**ahf**-oh-**RECK**-toh-mee) is the surgical removal of a fallopian tube and ovary (**salping/o** means tube, **oophor** means ovary, and **-ectomy** means surgical removal). A *bilateral salpingo-oophorectomy* is the removal of both of the fallopian tubes and ovaries.

- **Tubal ligation** is a surgical sterilization procedure in which the fallopian tubes are sealed or cut to prevent sperm from reaching a mature ovum.

The Uterus, Cervix, and Vagina

- A **colpopexy** (**KOL**-poh-**peck**-see), also known as *vaginofixation*, is the surgical fixation of a prolapsed vagina to a surrounding structure such as the abdominal wall (**colp/o** means vagina, and **-pexy** means surgical fixation in place).
- **Conization** (**kon**-ih-**ZAY**-shun), also known as a *cone biopsy*, is the surgical removal of a cone-shaped specimen of tissue from the cervix. This is performed as a diagnostic procedure or to remove abnormal tissue.
- **Colporrhaphy** (kol-**POR**-ah-fee) is the surgical suturing of a tear in the vagina (**colp/o** means vagina, and **-rrhaphy** means surgical suturing).
- **Dilation and curettage** (dye-**LAY**-shun and **kyou**-reh-**TAHZH**), commonly known as a *D & C*, is a surgical procedure in which the cervix is dilated and the endometrium of the uterus is scraped away. This can be performed as a diagnostic or a treatment procedure. *Dilation* means the expansion of an opening. *Curettage* is the removal of material from the surface by scraping with an instrument known as a curette.
- A **myomectomy** (**my**-oh-**MECK**-toh-mee) is the surgical removal of uterine fibroids (**myom** means muscle tumor, and **-ectomy** means surgical removal).

Hysterectomies

A **hysterectomy** (**hiss**-teh-**RECK**-toh-mee) is the surgical removal of the uterus (**hyster** means uterus, and **-ectomy** means surgical removal). The procedure is further described depending upon the structures that are removed (Figure 14.16).

- In a **total hysterectomy**, also known as a *complete hysterectomy*, the uterus and cervix are removed. This procedure can be performed through the vagina or laparoscopically through the abdomen.
- In a *partial* or *subtotal hysterectomy*, the uterus is removed and the cervix is left in place.
- A **radical hysterectomy**, also known as a *bilateral hysterosalpingo-oophorectomy*, is most commonly performed to treat uterine cancer (Figure 14.16B). This procedure includes the surgical removal of the ovaries and fallopian tubes, the uterus and cervix, plus nearby lymph nodes. If this surgery is performed before natural menopause, the patient immediately experiences *surgical menopause*.

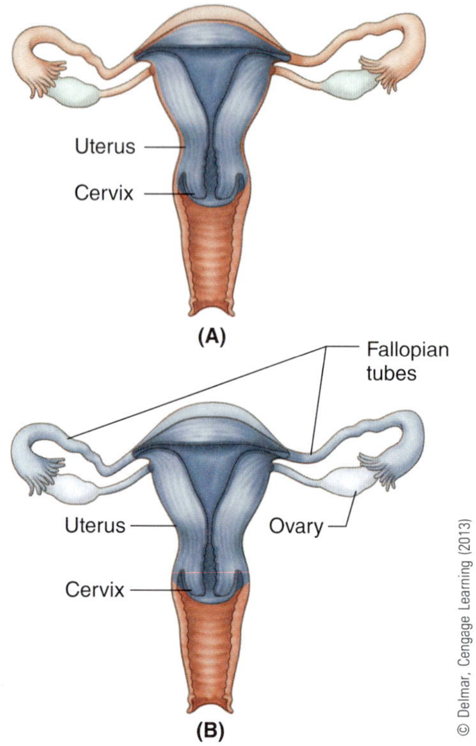

FIGURE 14.16 Types of hysterectomies, with the areas removed shown in blue. (A) In a total hysterectomy, the uterus and cervix are removed. (B) In a radical hysterectomy, the ovaries, fallopian tubes, uterus, and cervix are removed.

Mammoplasty

Mammoplasty (**MAM**-oh-**plas**-tee), also spelled *mammaplasty*, is a general term for a cosmetic operation on the breasts (**mamm/o** means breast, and **-plasty** means surgical repair).

- **Breast augmentation** is mammoplasty performed to increase breast size. *Augmentation* means the process of adding to make larger. Breast augmentation is the opposite of breast reduction.
- **Breast reduction** is mammoplasty performed to decrease and reshape excessively large, heavy breasts. Breast reduction is the opposite of breast augmentation.
- **Mastopexy** (**MAS**-toh-**peck**-see), also called a breast lift, is a mammoplasty to affix sagging breasts in a more elevated position (**mast/o** means breast, and **-pexy** means surgical fixation).

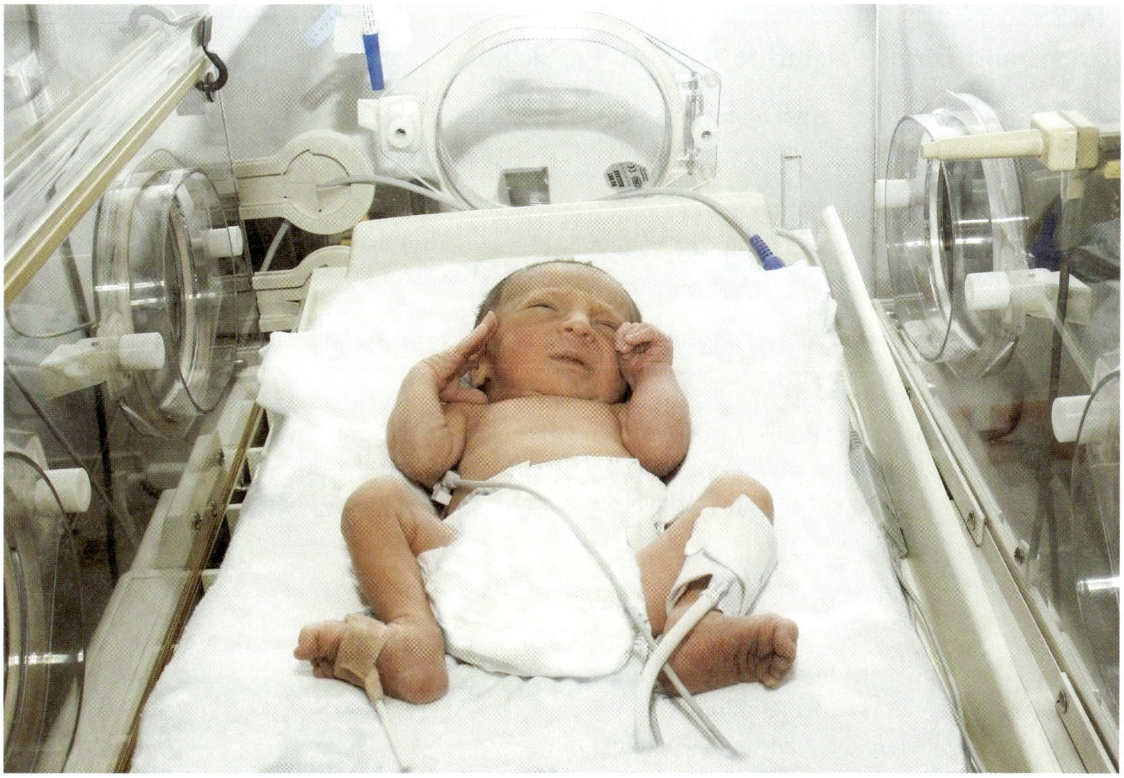

Reflekta/www.Shutterstock.com

FIGURE 14.17 An incubator provides a newborn infant with an environment of the controlled temperature, humidity, and oxygen.

- *Breast reconstruction* following a mastectomy is discussed in Chapter 6.

Treatment Procedures Related to Pregnancy and Childbirth

- A **cesarean section** (seh-**ZEHR**-ee-un **SECK**-shun), also known as a *C-section*, is the delivery of the child through an incision in the maternal abdominal and uterine walls. This is usually performed when a vaginal birth would be unsafe for either the mother or baby.
- *VBAC* is the acronym used to describe **v**aginal **b**irth **a**fter a **c**esarean.
- An **episiotomy** (eh-**piz**-ee-**OT**-oh-mee) is a surgical incision made into the perineum to enlarge the vaginal orifice to prevent tearing of the tissues as the infant moves out of the birth canal (**episi** means vulva, and **-otomy** means a surgical incision).
- An **episiorrhaphy** (eh-**piz**-ee-**OR**-ah-fee) is the surgical suturing to repair an episiotomy (**episi/o** means vulva, and **-rrhaphy** means surgical suturing).
- An **incubator** (**IN**-kyou-**bate**-or) is an apparatus for maintaining an environment of controlled temperature, humidity, and oxygen concentration for a premature or ill newborn (Figure 14.17).

Assisted Reproduction

The term **assisted reproductive technology** describes techniques used to aid an infertile couple in achieving a viable pregnancy.

- **Artificial insemination**, also called intrauterine insemination (IUI), is a technique in which sperm from a woman's partner or from a donor are introduced into the vagina or uterus during the ovulatory phase of her menstrual cycle.
- **In vitro fertilization** is a procedure in which mature ova are removed from the mother to be fertilized. The resulting embryos are transferred into the uterus with the hope that they will implant and continue to develop as in a normal pregnancy. *In vitro* means in an artificial environment such as a test tube.
- A *gestational carrier* is an option for a woman with ovaries but no uterus. Her egg is fertilized by her partner's sperm and placed inside another woman's uterus (the carrier).

TABLE 14.2
Abbreviations and Terms Related to Assisted Fertilization

AMA	**Advanced maternal age** is the term applied to women in their late 30s to late 40s. As one of these women age, the possibility of her becoming pregnant decreases.
AI	**Artificial insemination** is a technique in which sperm from a woman's partner or from a donor are introduced into the vagina or uterus during the ovulatory phase of her menstrual cycle.
ART	The term **assisted reproductive technology** describes techniques used to aid an infertile couple in achieving a viable pregnancy.
IVF	**In vitro fertilization** is a procedure in which mature ova are removed from the mother to be fertilized. The resulting embryos are transferred into the uterus with the hope that they will implant and continue to develop as a normal pregnancy. ***In vitro*** means in an artificial environment such as a test tube.

- A woman who volunteers to be inseminated with the sperm of a man who is not her partner in order to conceive and carry a child for the man and his partner is referred to as a *surrogate*.

ABBREVIATIONS RELATED TO THE REPRODUCTIVE SYSTEMS

Table 14.3 presents an overview of the abbreviations related to the terms introduced in this chapter. Note: To avoid errors or confusion, always be cautious when using abbreviations.

StudyWARE CONNECTION

For more practice and to test your mastery of this material, go to the StudyWARE™ to play interactive games and complete the quiz for this chapter.

Workbook Practice

Go to your workbook, and complete the exercises for this chapter.

Downloadable audio is available for selected medical terms in this chapter to enhance your learning of medical terminology.

TABLE 14.3
Abbreviations Related to the Reproductive Systems

amniocentesis = AMN	**AMN** = amniocentesis
bacterial vaginosis = BV	**BV** = bacterial vaginosis
cesarean section = CS	**CS** = cesarean section
hormone replacement therapy = HRT	**HRT** = hormone replacement therapy
human papillomaviruses = HPV	**HPV** = human papillomaviruses
hysterosalpingography = HSG	**HSG** = hysterosalpingography
hysteroscopy = HYS	**HYS** = hysteroscopy
intrauterine device = IUD	**IUD** = intrauterine device
labor and delivery = L & D	**L & D** = labor and delivery
neonatal intensive care unit = NICU	**NICU** = neonatal intensive care unit
pelvic inflammatory disease = PID	**PID** = pelvic inflammatory disease
premenstrual syndrome = PMS	**PMS** = premenstrual syndrome

CHAPTER 13

LEARNING EXERCISES

MATCHING WORD PARTS 1

Write the correct answer in the middle column.

Definition	Correct Answer	Possible Answers
14.1. cervix	____________	men/o
14.2. female	____________	gynec/o
14.3. menstruation	____________	-gravida
14.4. pregnant	____________	colp/o
14.5. vagina	____________	cervic/o

MATCHING WORD PARTS 2

Write the correct answer in the middle column.

Definition	Correct Answer	Possible Answers
14.6. egg	____________	vagin/o
14.7. ovary	____________	test/i
14.8. testicle	____________	ov/o
14.9. uterus	____________	ovari/o
14.10. vagina	____________	hyster/o

MATCHING WORD PARTS 3

Write the correct answer in the middle column.

Definition	Correct Answer	Possible Answers
14.11. breast	____________	salping/o
14.12. none	____________	-pexy

14.13. surgical fixation ______________________ **-para**

14.14. to give birth ______________________ **nulli-**

14.15. tube ______________________ **mast/o**

DEFINITIONS

Select the correct answer, and write it on the line provided.

14.16. The term that describes the inner layer of the uterus is ______________________.

corpus endometrium myometrium perimetrium

14.17. The term describing the single cells formed immediately after conception is ______________________.

embryo fetus gamete zygote

14.18. The mucus that lubricates the vagina is produced by the ______________________.

Bartholin's glands bulbourethral glands Cowper's glands hymen glands

14.19. The finger-like structures of the fallopian tube that catch the ovum are the ______________________.

fimbriae fundus infundibulum oviducts

14.20. The term ______________________ is used to designate the transition phase between regular menstrual periods and no periods at all.

menarche menopause perimenopause puberty

14.21. The medical term for the condition also known as a yeast infection is ______________________.

colporrhea leukorrhea pruritus vulvae vaginal candidiasis

14.22. Sperm are formed within the ______________________ of each testicle.

ejaculatory ducts epididymis seminiferous tubules urethra

14.23. During puberty, the term ______________________ describes the beginning of the menstrual function.

menarche menopause menses menstruation

14.24. In the female, the region between the vaginal orifice and the anus is known as the ______________________.

clitoris mons pubis perineum vulva

14.25. The release of a mature egg by the ovary is known as ____________.

coitus fertilization menstruation ovulation

MATCHING STRUCTURES

Write the correct answer in the middle column.

	Definition	Correct Answer	Possible Answers
14.26.	carry milk from the mammary glands	____________	vulva
14.27.	surrounds the testicles	____________	scrotum
14.28.	external female genitalia	____________	lactiferous ducts
14.29.	protects the tip of the penis	____________	foreskin
14.30.	sensitive tissue near the vaginal opening	____________	clitoris

WHICH WORD?

Select the correct answer, and write it on the line provided.

14.31. The term used to describe a woman during her first pregnancy is a ____________.

primigravida primipara

14.32. The fluid produced by the mammary glands during the first few days after giving birth is ____________.

colostrum meconium

14.33. The term ____________ describes an inflammation of the cervix that is usually caused by an infection.

cervicitis vulvitis

14.34. From implantation through the 8th week of pregnancy, the developing child is known as a/an ____________.

embryo fetus

14.35. A ____________ is a woman who has never borne a viable child.

nulligravida nullipara

SPELLING COUNTS

Find the misspelled word in each sentence. Then write that word, spelled correctly, on the line provided.

14.36. The prostrate gland secretes a thick fluid that aids the motility of the sperm. ____________

14.37. The normal periodic discharge from the uterus is known as menstration. ____________

14.38. The third stage of labor and delivery is the expulsion of the plasenta as the afterbirth. ____________

14.39. The term hemataspermia is the presence of blood in the seminal fluid. ____________

14.40. The surgical removal of the foreskin of the penis is known as cercumsion. ____________

ABBREVIATION IDENTIFICATION

In the space provided, write the words that each abbreviation stands for.

14.41. **AMA** ____________

14.42. **PID** ____________

14.43. **PMDD** ____________

14.44. **IUD** ____________

14.45. **VD** ____________

TERM SELECTION

Select the correct answer, and write it on the line provided.

14.46. An accumulation of pus in the fallopian tube is known as ____________.

oophoritis pelvic inflammatory disease pyosalpinx salpingitis

14.47. A ____________ is a knot of widening varicose veins in one side of the scrotum.

hydrocele phimosis priapism varicocele

14.48. The direct visual examination of the tissues of the cervix and vagina using a binocular magnifier is known as ____________.

colposcopy endovaginal ultrasound hysteroscopy laparoscopy

14.49. The term used to describe infrequent or very light menstruation in a woman with previously normal periods is ______________________.

amenorrhea hypomenorrhea oligomenorrhea polymenorrhea

14.50. The examination of cells retrieved from the edge of the placenta between the 8th and 10th weeks of pregnancy is known as ______________________.

amniocentesis chorionic villus sampling fetal monitoring pelvimetry

SENTENCE COMPLETION

Write the correct term or terms on the lines provided.

14.51. The dark-pigmented area surrounding the nipple is known as the ______________________.

14.52. A fluid-filled sac in the scrotum along the spermatic cord leading from the testicles is known as a/an ______________________.

14.53. The serious complication of pregnancy that is characterized by convulsions and sometimes coma is known as ______________________. The treatment for this condition is delivery of the fetus.

14.54. Surgical suturing of a tear in the vagina is known as ______________________.

14.55. The ______________________ is the tube that carries blood, oxygen, and nutrients from the placenta to the developing child.

WORD SURGERY

Divide each term into its component word parts. Write these word parts, in sequence, on the lines provided. When necessary use a slash (/) to indicate a combining vowel. (You may not need all of the lines provided.)

14.56. **Endocervicitis** is an inflammation of the mucous membrane lining of the cervix.

__________ __________ __________ __________

14.57. **Menometrorrhagia** is excessive uterine bleeding at both the usual time of menstrual periods and at other irregular intervals.

__________ __________ __________ __________

14.58. **Hysterosalpingography** is a radiographic examination of the uterus and fallopian tubes.

__________ __________ __________ __________

14.59. **Galactorrhea** is the production of breast milk in a woman who is not breastfeeding.

__________ __________ __________ __________

14.60. **Azoospermia** is the absence of sperm in the semen.

__________ __________ __________ __________

TRUE/FALSE

If the statement is true, write **True** on the line. If the statement is false, write **False** on the line.

14.61. ____________________ Peyronie's disease causes a sexual dysfunction in which the penis is bent or curved during erection.

14.62. ____________________ Braxton Hicks contractions are the first true labor pains.

14.63. ____________________ An Apgar score is an evaluation of a newborn infant's physical status at 1 and 5 minutes after birth.

14.64. ____________________ Breast augmentation is mammoplasty that is performed to reduce breast size.

14.65. ____________________ An ectopic pregnancy is a potentially dangerous condition in which a fertilized egg is implanted and begins to develop outside of the uterus.

CLINICAL CONDITIONS

Write the correct answer on the line provided.

14.66. Baby Ortega was born with cryptorchidism. When this testicle had not descended by the time he was 9 months old, a/an ____________________ was performed.

14.67. When she went into labor with her first child, Mrs. Hoshi's baby was in a breech presentation. Because of risks associated with this, her obstetrician delivered the baby surgically by performing a/an ____________________.

14.68. Dawn Grossman was diagnosed as having uterine fibroids that required surgical removal. Her gynecologist scheduled Dawn for a/an ____________________.

14.69. Rita Chen, who is 25 years old and knows that she is not pregnant, is concerned because she has not had a menstrual period for 3 months. Her doctor described this condition as ____________________.

14.70. Enrico Flores' physician removed a portion of each vas deferens. The medical term for this sterilization procedure is a/an ______________________.

14.71. Tiffany Thomas developed a thin, frothy, yellow-green, foul-smelling vaginal discharge. She was diagnosed as having ______________________, which is caused by the parasite *Trichomonas vaginalis.*

14.72. Mr. Wolford, who is age 65, has been reading a lot about the decrease of testosterone in older men. His physician told him that the medical term for this condition is ______________________.

14.73. Just before the delivery of her baby, Barbara Klein's obstetrician performed a/an ______________________ to prevent tearing of the tissues.

14.74. Jane Marsall's pregnancy was complicated by the abnormal implantation of the placenta in the lower portion of the uterus. The medical term for this condition is ______________________.

14.75. Immediately after birth, the Reicher baby was described as being a newborn or a/an ______________________.

WHICH IS THE CORRECT MEDICAL TERM?

Select the correct answer, and write it on the line provided.

14.76. The postpartum vaginal discharge during the first several weeks after childbirth is known as ______________________.

colostrum involution lochia meconium

14.77. Abdominal pain caused by uterine cramps during a menstrual period is known as ______________________.

dysmenorrhea hypermenorrhea menometrorrhagia polymenorrhea

14.78. The term that describes an inflammation of the glans penis is ______________________.

phimosis balanitis epididymitis testitis

14.79. An inflammation of the lining of the vagina is known as ______________________. The most common causes of this condition are bacterial vaginosis, trichomoniasis, and vaginal candidiasis.

cervical dysplasia cervicitis colporrhexis vaginitis

14.80. The term that describes a profuse whitish mucus discharge from the uterus and vagina is ______________. This type of discharge can be due to an infection, malignancy, or hormonal changes.

endocervicitis   leukorrhea   pruritus vulvae   vaginitis

CHALLENGE WORD BUILDING

These terms are *not* found in this chapter; however, they are made up of the following familiar word parts. If you need help in creating the term, refer to your medical dictionary.

endo-	**hyster/o**	**-cele**
	mast/o	**-dynia**
	metr/i	**-itis**
	oophor/o	**-pexy**
	orchid/o	**-plasty**
	vagin/o	**-rrhaphy**
	vulv/o	**-rrhexis**

14.81. The term meaning a hernia protruding into the vagina is ______________.

14.82. The term meaning the surgical repair of one or both testicles is ______________.

14.83. The term meaning an inflammation of the endometrium is ______________.

14.84. The term meaning the surgical repair of an ovary is a/an ______________.

14.85. The term meaning pain in the vagina is ______________.

14.86. The term meaning surgical suturing of the uterus is ______________.

14.87. The term meaning a hernia of the uterus, particularly during pregnancy, is a/an ______________.

14.88. The term meaning the surgical fixation of a displaced ovary is ______________.

14.89. The term meaning the rupture of the uterus, particularly during pregnancy, is ______________.

14.90. The term meaning an inflammation of the vulva and the vagina is ______________.

LABELING EXERCISES

Identify the numbered items on these accompanying figures.

14.91. ________________________ bladder

14.92. ________________________ gland

14.93. ________________________

14.94. ________________________

14.95. ________________________

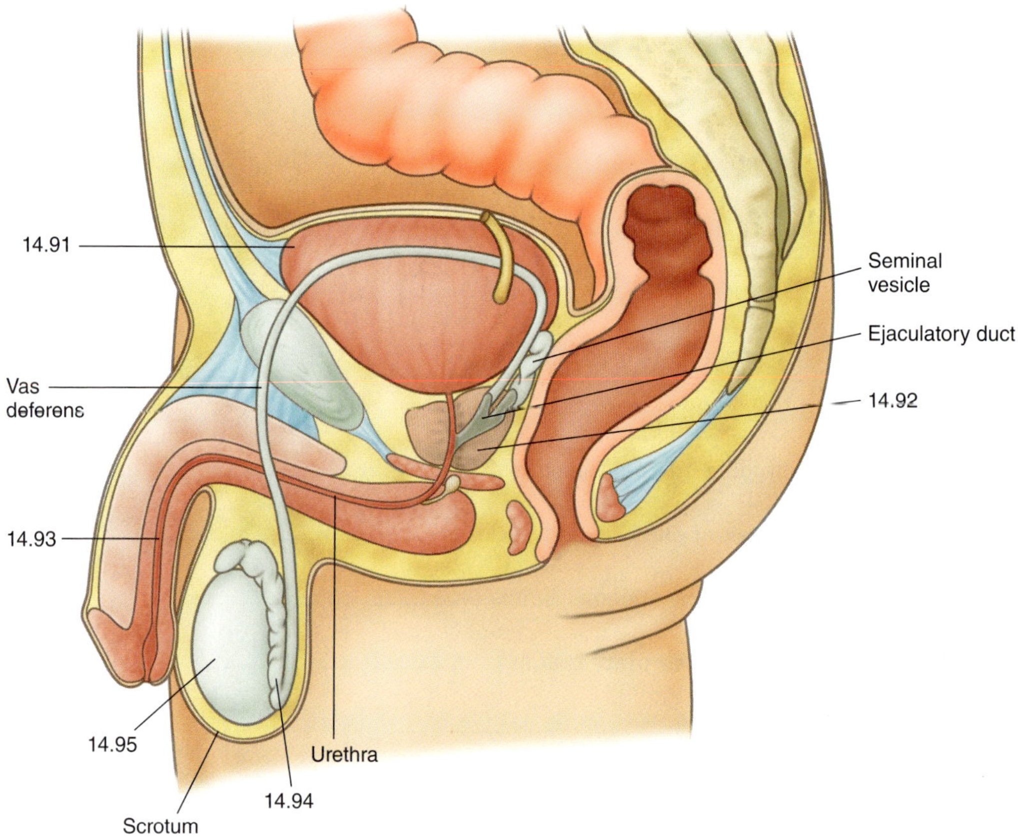

14.96. ______________________ or uterine tube

14.97. body of the ______________________

14.98 ______________________ bladder

14.99. ______________________

14.100. ______________________

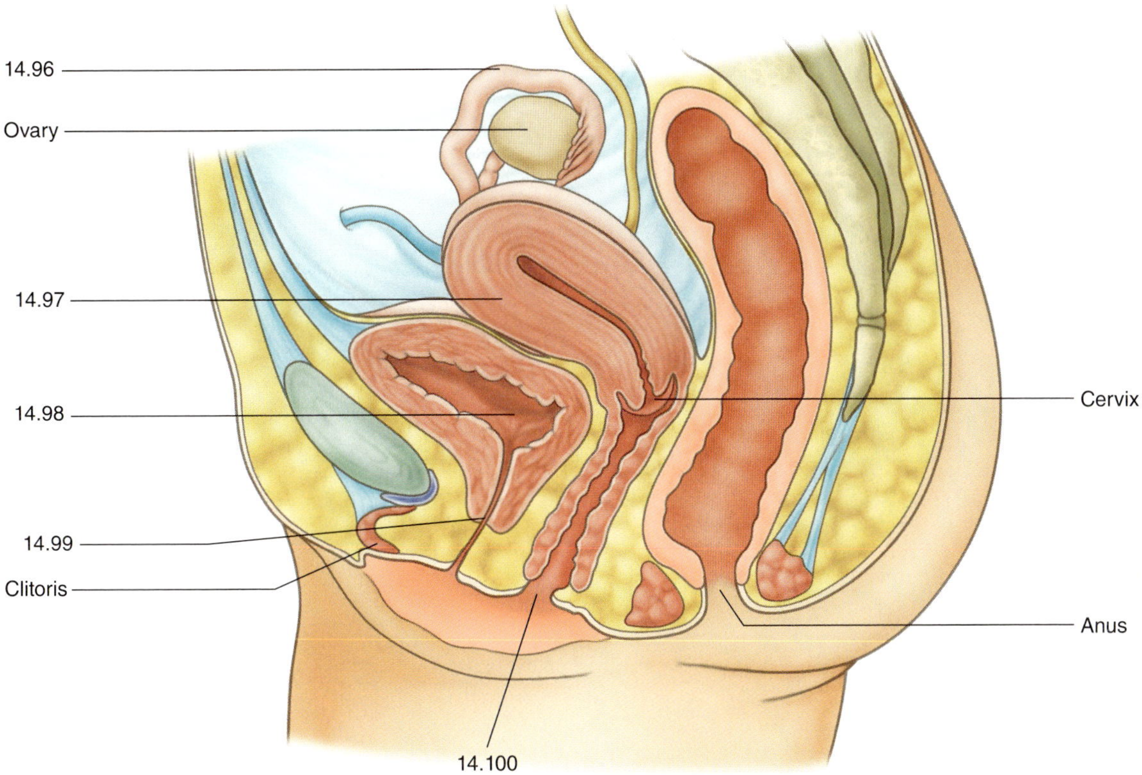

Appendix A

PREFIXES, COMBINING FORMS, AND SUFFIXES

Pertaining to

-ac pertaining to
-al pertaining to
-ar pertaining to
-ary pertaining to
-eal pertaining to
-ial pertaining to
-ical pertaining to
-ic pertaining to
-ine pertaining to
-ior pertaining to
-ory pertaining to
-ous pertaining to
-tic pertaining to

Abnormal Conditions

-ago abnormal condition, disease
-esis abnormal condition, disease
-ia abnormal condition, disease
-iasis abnormal condition, disease
-ion condition
-ism condition, state of
-osis abnormal condition, disease

Noun Endings

-a noun ending
-ae plural noun ending
-e noun ending
-i plural noun ending
-um singular noun ending
-us singular noun ending
-y noun ending

A

a-	no, not, without, away from, negative
-a	noun ending
ab-	away from, negative, absent
abdomin/o	abdomen
-able	capable of, able to
abort/o	premature expulsion of a nonviable fetus
abrad/o, **abras/o**	rub or scrape off
abrupt/o	broken away from
abs-	away from
abscess/o	collection of pus, going away
absorpt/o	suck up, suck in
-ac	pertaining to
acanth/o	spiny, thorny
acetabul/o	acetabulum (hip socket)
-acious	characterized by
acne/o	point or peak
acous/o, **acoust/o**	hearing, sound
acquir/o	get, obtain
acr/o	extremities (hands and feet), top, extreme point
acromi/o	acromion, point of shoulder blade
actin/o	light
acu/o	sharp, severe, sudden
acuit/o, **acut/o**	sharp, sharpness
acust/o, **-acusia**, **-acusis**	hearing, sense of hearing
ad-	toward, to, in the direction of
aden/o	gland
adenoid/o	adenoids
adhes/o	stick to, cling to
adip/o	fat
adnex/o	bound to
adren/o, **adrenal/o**	adrenal glands
aer/o	air, gas
aesthet/o	sensation, sense of perception
af-	toward, to
affect/o	exert influence on
agglutin/o	clumping, stick together
aggress/o	attack, step forward
-ago	abnormal condition, disease
agor/a	marketplace
-agra	excessive pain, seizure, attack of severe pain
-aise	comfort, ease
-al	pertaining to
alb/i, **alb/o**, **albin/o**	white
albumin/o	albumin, protein
alg/e, **algi/o**, **alg/o**, **algesi/o**	relationship to pain
-algesia, **-algesic**	painful, pain sense
-algia	pain, suffering, painful condition
align/o	bring into line or correct position
aliment/o	to nourish
all/o, **all-**	other, different from normal, reversal
alopec/o	baldness, mangy
alveol/o	alveolus, air sac, small sac
ambi-	both sides, around or about, double
ambly/o	dull, dim
ambul/o, **ambulat/o**	walk
ametr/o	out of proportion
-amine	nitrogen compound
amni/o	amnion, fetal membrane
amph-	around, on both sides, doubly
amput/o, **amputat/o**	cut away, cut off a part of the body
amyl/o	starch
an-	no, not, without
an-, **ana-**	up, apart, backward, excessive
an/o	anus, ring
-an	characteristic of, pertaining to
-ancy	state of
andr/o	male, masculine
aneurysm/o	aneurysm
angi/o	blood or lymph vessel
angin/o	angina, choking, strangling
anis/o	unequal
ankyl/o	crooked, bent, stiff
anomal/o	irregularity
ante-	before, in front of, forward
anter/o	before, front
anthrac/o	coal, coal dust
anti-	against
anxi/o, **anxiet/o**	anxiety, anxious, uneasy
aort/o	aorta
ap-	toward, to
-apheresis	removal
aphth/o	ulcer
apic/o	apex
ap-, **apo-**	separation, away from, opposed, detached
aplast/o	defective development, lack of development

aponeur/o aponeurosis (type of tendon)
apoplect/o a stroke
append/o, appendic/o appendix
aqu/i, aqu/o, aque/o water
-ar pertaining to
arachn/o spiderweb, spider
arc/o bow, arc, or arch
-arche beginning
areat/o occurring in patches or circumscribed areas
areol/o little open space
-aria connected with
arrect/o upright, lifted up, raised
arter/o, arteri/o artery
arthr/o joint
articul/o joint
-ary pertaining to
as- toward, to
asbest/o asbestos
-ase enzyme
aspir/o, aspirat/o to breathe in
asthen-, -asthenia weakness, lack of strength
asthmat/o gasping, choking
astr/o star, star-shaped
at- toward, to
atel/o incomplete, imperfect
ather/o plaque, fatty substance
athet/o uncontrolled
-ation state or action
atop/o strange, out of place
atres/i without an opening
atri/o atrium
attenuat/o diluted, weakened
aud-, audi/o, audit/o ear, hearing, the sense of hearing
aur/i, aur/o ear, hearing
auscult/a, auscult/o listen
aut/o self
-ax noun ending
ax/o axis, main stem
axill/o armpit

B

bacill/o rod-shaped bacterium (plural, *bacteria*)
bacteri/o bacteria (singular, *bacterium*)
balan/o glans penis
bar/o pressure, weight
bartholin/o Bartholin's gland
bas/o base, opposite of acid
bi- twice, double, two
bi/o life
bifid/o split, divided into two parts
bifurcat/o divide or fork into two branches
bil/i bile, gall
bilirubin/o bilirubin
bin- two
-blast embryonic, immature, formative element
blephar/o eyelid
borborygm/o rumbling sound
brachi/o arm
brachy- short
brady- slow
brev/i, brev/o short
bronch/i, bronchi/o, bronch/o bronchial tube, bronchus
bronchiol/o bronchiole, bronchiolus
brux/o grind
bucc/o cheek
burs/o bursa, sac of fluid near joint

C

cadaver/o dead body, corpse
calcane/o calcaneus, heel bone
calc/i calcium, lime, the heel
calci-, calc/o calcium
calcul/o stone, little stone
cali/o, calic/o cup, calyx
call/i, callos/o hard, hardened and thickened
calor/i heat
canalicul/o little canal or duct
canth/o corner of the eye
capill/o hair
capit/o head
capn/o carbon dioxide, sooty or smoky appearance
capsul/o little box
carb/o carbon
carbuncl/o carbuncle
carcin/o cancerous
cardi/o, card/o heart
cari/o rottenness, decay
carot/o stupor, sleep
carp/o wrist bones
cartilag/o cartilage, gristle

carunculo	bit of flesh
cat-, cata-, cath-	down, lower, under
catabol/o	a breaking down
cathart/o	cleansing, purging
cathet/o	insert, send down
caud/o	lower part of body, tail
caus/o, caust/o	burning, burn
cauter/o, caut/o	heat, burn
cav/i, cav/o	hollow, cave
cavern/o	containing hollow spaces
cec/o	cecum
-cele	hernia, tumor, swelling
celi/o, cel/o	abdomen, belly
cement/o	cementum, a rough stone
cent-	hundred
-centesis	surgical puncture to remove fluid
cephal/o	head
cera-	wax
cerebell/o	cerebellum
cerebr/o	cerebrum, brain
cerumin/o	cerumen, earwax
cervic/o	neck, cervix (neck of uterus)
cheil/o	lip or lips
cheir/o	hand
chem/i, chem/o, chemic/o	drug, chemical
chir/o	hand
chlor/o	green
chlorhydr/o	hydrochloric acid
chol/e	bile, gall
cholangi/o	bile duct
cholecyst/o	gallbladder
choledoch/o	common bile duct
cholesterol/o	cholesterol
chondr/i, chondr/o	cartilage
chord/o	spinal cord, cord
chori/o, chorion/o	chorion, membrane
choroid/o	choroid layer of eye
chrom/o, chromat/o	color
chron/o	time
chym/o	to pour, juice
cib/o	meal
cicatric/o	scar
-cidal	pertaining to killing
-cide	causing death
cili/o	eyelashes, microscopic hair-like projections
cine-	relationship to movement
circ/i	ring or circle
circulat/o	circulate, go around in a circle
circum-	around, about
circumcis/o	cutting around
circumscrib/o	confined, limited in space
cirrh/o	orange-yellow, tawny
cis/o	cut
-clasis, -clast	break down
claudicat/o	limping
claustr/o	barrier
clav/i	key
clavicul/o, cleid/o	clavicle, collar bone
clitor/o	clitoris
-clonus	violent action
clus/o	shut or close
-clysis	irrigation, washing
co-	together, with
coagul/o, coagulat/o	clotting, coagulation
coarct/o, coarctat/o	press together, narrow
cocc/i, cocc/o, -coccus	spherical bacteria
coccyg/o	coccyx, tailbone
cochle/o	spiral, snail, snail shell
coher/o, cohes/o	cling, stick together
coit/o	a coming together
col/o	colon, large intestine
coll/a	glue
colon/o	colon, large intestine
colp/o	vagina
column/o	pillar
com-	together, with
comat/o	deep sleep
comminut/o	break into pieces
communic/o	share, to make common
compatibil/o	sympathize with
con-	together, with
concav/o	hollow
concentr/o	condense, intensify, remove excess water
concept/o	become pregnant
conch/o	shell
concuss/o	shaken together, violently agitated
condyl/o	knuckle, knob
confus/o	confusion, disorder
coni/o	dust
conjunctiv/o	conjunctiva, joined together, connected
consci/o	aware, awareness
consolid/o	become firm or solid

constipat/o	pressed together, crowded together
constrict/o	draw tightly together
contact/o	touched, infected
contagi/o	infection, unclean, touching of something
contaminat/o	render unclean by contact, pollute
contine/o, continent/o	keep in, contain, hold back, restrain
contra-	against, counter, opposite
contracept/o	prevention of conception
contus/o	bruise
convalesc/o	recover, become strong
convex/o	arched, vaulted
convolut/o	coiled, twisted
convuls/o	pull together
copi/o	plentiful
copulat/o	joining together, linking
cor/o	pupil
cord/o	cord, spinal cord
cordi/o	heart
core/o	pupil
cori/o	skin, leather
corne/o	cornea
coron/o	coronary, crown
corp/u, corpor/o	body
corpuscul/o	little body
cort-	covering
cortic/o	cortex, outer region
cost/o	rib
cox/o	hip, hip joint
crani/o	skull
-crasia	a mixture or blending
creatin/o	creatinine
crepit/o, crepitat/o	crackling, rattling
crin/o, -crine	secrete
cris/o, critic/o	turning point
-crit	to separate
cry/o	cold
crypt/o	hidden
cubit/o	elbow
culd/o	cul-de-sac, blind pouch
cult/o	cultivate
-cusis	hearing
cusp/i	point, pointed flap
cutane/o	skin
cyan/o	blue
cycl/o	ciliary body of eye, cycle
-cyesis	pregnancy
cyst-, -cyst	bladder, bag
cyst/o	urinary bladder, cyst, sac of fluid
cyt/o, -cyte	cell
-cytic	pertaining to a cell
-cytosis	condition of cells

D

dacry/o	tear, lacrimal duct (tear duct)
dacryocyst/o	lacrimal sac (tear sac)
dactyl/o	fingers, toes
de-	down, lack of, from, not, removal
debrid/e	open a wound
deca-, deci-	ten, tenth
decidu/o	shedding, falling off
decubit/o	lying down
defec/o, defecat/o	to free from waste, clear
defer/o	carrying down or out
degenerat/o	gradual impairment, breakdown, diminished function
deglutit/o	swallow
deliri/o	wandering in the mind
delt/o	Greek letter delta, triangular shape
delus/o	delude, mock, cheat
-dema	swelling (fluid)
dem/i, dem/o	people, population
demi-	half
dendr/o	branching, resembling a tree
dent/i, dent/o	tooth, teeth
depilate/o	hair removal
depress/o	press down, lower, pressed or sunk down
dermat/o, derm/o	skin
desic/o	drying
-desis	to bind, tie together
deteriorat/o	worsening or gradual impairment
dextr/o	right side
di-	twice, twofold, double
dia-	through, between, apart, complete
diaphor/o	sweat
diaphragmat/o	diaphragm, wall across
diastole/o	standing apart, expansion
didym/o	testes, twins, double
diffus/o	pour out, spread apart
digest/o	divide, distribute
digit/o	finger or toe
dilat/o, dilatat/o	spread out, expand
-dilation	widening, stretching, expanding
dilut/o	dissolve, separate
diphther/o	membrane
dipl/o	double

dips/o, **-dipsia** thirst
dis- negative, apart, absence of
dislocat/o displacement
dissect/o cutting apart
disseminat/o widely scattered
dist/o far
distend/o, **distent/o** stretch apart, expand
diur/o, **diuret/o** tending to increase urine output
divert/i turning aside
domin/o controlling, ruling
don/o give
dors/i, **dors/o** back of body
-dote what is given
-drome to run, running
-duct opening
duct/o to lead, carry
duoden/i, **duoden/o** duodenum, first part of small intestine
-dural pertaining to dura mater
-dynia pain
dys- bad, difficult, painful

E

e- out of, from
-e noun ending
-eal pertaining to
ec- out, outside
ecchym/o pouring out of juice
ech/o sound
eclamps/o, **eclampt/o** flashing or shining forth
ectasia, **-ectasis** stretching, dilation, enlargement
ecto- out, outside
-ectomy surgical removal, cutting out, excision
-ectopy displacement
eczemat/o eruption
-edema swelling
edem-, **edemat/o** swelling, fluid, tumor
edentul/o without teeth
ef- out
effect/o bring about a response, activate
effus/o pouring out
ejaculat/o throw or hurl out
electr/o electricity, electric
eliminat/o expel from the body
em- in
emaciat/o wasted by disease
embol/o something inserted or thrown in
embry/o fertilized ovum, embryo
-emesis vomiting
emet/o vomit
-emia blood, blood condition
emmetr/o in proper measure
emolli/o make soft, soften
en- in, within, into
encephal/o brain
end-, **endo-** in, within, inside
endocrin/o secrete within
enem/o end in, inject
enter/o small intestine
ento- within
epi- above, upon, on
epidemi/o among the people, an epidemic
epididym/o epididymis
epiglott/o epiglottis
episi/o vulva
epithel/i, **epitheli/o** epithelium
equin/o pertaining to a horse
-er one who
erect/o upright
erg/o, **-ergy** work
erot/o sexual love
eruct/o, **eructat/o** belch forth
erupt/o break out, burst forth
erythem/o, **erythemat/o** flushed, redness
erythr/o red
es- out of, outside, away from
-esis abnormal condition, disease
eso- inward
esophag/o esophagus
-esthesia, **esthesi/o** sensation, feeling
esthet/o feeling, nervous sensation, sense of perception
estr/o female
ethm/o sieve
eti/o cause
eu- good, normal, well, easy
-eurysm widening
evacu/o, **evacuat/o** empty out
ex- out of, outside, away from
exacerbat/o aggravate, irritate
exanthemat/o rash
excis/o cutting out

excori/o, excoriat/o	abrade or scratch
excret/o	separate, discharge
excruciat/o	intense pain, agony
exhal/o, exhalat/o	breathe out
exo-	out of, outside, away from
exocrin/o	secrete out of
expector/o	cough up
expir/o, expirat/o	breathe out
exstroph/o	turned or twisted out
extern/o	outside, outer
extra-	on the outside, beyond, outside
extreme/o, extremit/o	extremity, outermost
extrins/o	from the outside, contained outside
exud/o, exudat/o	to sweat out

F

faci/o	face, form
-facient	making, producing
fasci/o	fascia, fibrous band
fascicul/o	little bundle
fatal/o	pertaining to fate, death
fauc/i	narrow pass, throat
febr/i	fever
fec/i, fec/o	dregs, sediment, waste
femor/o	femur, thigh bone
fenestr/a	window
fer/o	bear, carry
-ferent	carrying
-ferous	bearing, carrying, producing
fertil/o	fertile, fruitful, productive
fet/i, fet/o	fetus, unborn child
fibr/o	fibrous tissue, fiber
fibrill/o	muscular twitching
fibrin/o	fibrin, fibers, threads of a clot
fibros/o	fibrous connective tissue
fibul/o	fibula
-fic, fic/o	making, producing, forming
-fication	process of making
-fida	split
filtr/o, filtrat/o	filter, to strain through
fimbri/o	fringe
fiss/o, fissur/o	crack, split, cleft
fistul/o	tube or pipe
flat/o	flatus, breaking wind, rectal gas
flex/o	bend
flu/o	flow
fluor/o	glowing, luminous
foc/o	focus, point
foll/i	bag, sac
follicul/o	follicle, small sac
foramin/o	opening, foramen
fore-	before, in front of
-form, form/o	resembling, in the shape of
fove/o	pit
fract/o	break, broken
frigid/o	cold
front/o	forehead, brow
-fuge	to drive away
funct/o, function/o	perform, function
fund/o	bottom, base, ground
fung/i	fungus
furc/o	forking, branching
furuncul/o	furunculus, a boil, an infection
-fusion	pour

G

galact/o	milk
gamet/o	wife or husband, egg or sperm
gangli/o, ganglion/o	ganglion
gangren/o	eating sore, gangrene
gastr/o	stomach, belly
gastrocnemi/o	gastrocnemius, calf muscle
gemin/o	twin, double
gen-, gen/o, -gen	producing, forming
-gene	production, origin, formation
-genic, -genesis	creation, reproduction
genit/o	produced by, birth, reproductive organs
-genous	producing
ger/i	old age
germin/o	bud, sprout, germ
geront/o	old age
gest/o, gestat/o	bear, carry young or offspring
gigant/o	giant, very large
gingiv/o	gingival tissue, gums
glauc/o	gray
glen/o	socket or pit
gli/o	neurologic tissue, supportive tissue of nervous system
globin/o, -globulin	protein
globul/o	little ball
glomerul/o	glomerulus
glott/i, glott/o	back of the tongue
gluc/o	glucose, sugar

glute/o	buttocks
glyc/o, glycos/o	glucose, sugar
glycer/o	sweet
glycogen/o	glycogen, animal starch
-gnosia	knowledge, to know
-gog, -gogue	make flow
goitr/o	goiter, enlargement of the thyroid gland
gon/e, gon/o	seed
gonad/o	gonad, sex glands
goni/o	angle
grad/i	move, go, step, walk
-gram	a picture or record
granul/o	granule(s)
-graph	a picture or record, machine for recording record
-graphy	the process of producing a picture or record
gravid/o	pregnancy
-gravida	pregnant
gynec/o	woman, female
gyr/o	turning, folding

H

hal/o, halit/o	breath
hallucin/o	hallucination, to wander in the mind
hem/e	deep red iron-containing pigment
hem/o, hemat/o	blood, relating to the blood
hemi-	half
hemoglobin/o	hemoglobin
hepat/o	liver
hered/o, heredit/o	inherited, inheritance
herni/o	hernia
herpet/o	creeping
-hexia	habit
hiat/o	opening
hidr/o	sweat
hirsut/o	hairy, rough
hist/o, histi/o	tissue
holo-	all
hom/o	same, like, alike
home/o	sameness, unchanging, constant
hormon/o	hormone
humer/o	humerus (upper arm bone)
hydr/o, hydra-	relating to water
hygien/o	healthy
hymen/o	a membrane, hymen
hyper-	excessive, increased
hyp-	deficient, decreased
hypn/o	sleep
hypo-	deficient, decreased
hyster/o	uterus

I

-ia	abnormal condition, disease, plural of **-ium**
-ial	pertaining to
-ian	specialist
-iasis	abnormal condition, disease
iatr/o	physician, treatment
-iatrics	field of medicine, healing
-iatrist	specialist
-iatry	field of medicine
-ible	capable of, able to
-ic	pertaining to
ichthy/o	dry, scaly
-ician	specialist
icter/o	jaundice
idi/o	peculiar to the individual or organ, one, distinct
-iferous	bearing, carrying, producing
-ific	making, producing
-iform	shaped or formed like, resembling
-igo	attack, diseased condition
-ile	capable of
ile/o	ileum, small intestine
ili/o	ilium, hip bone
illusi/o	deception
im-	not
immun/o	immune, protection, safe
impact/o	pushed against, wedged against, packed
impress/o	pressing into
impuls/o	pressure or pushing force, drive, urging on
in-	in, into, not, without
incis/o	cutting into
incubat/o	incubation, hatching
indurat/o	hardened
-ine	pertaining to
infarct/o	filled in, stuffed
infect/o	infected, tainted
infer/o	below, beneath
infest/o	attack, assail, molest
inflammat/o	flame within, set on fire
infra-	below, beneath, inferior to
infundibul/o	funnel

ingest/o	carry or pour in
inguin/o	groin
inhal/o, **inhalat/o**	breathe in
inject/o	to force or throw in
innominat/o	unnamed, nameless
inocul/o	implant, introduce
insipid/o	tasteless
inspir/o, **inspirat/o**	breathe in
insul/o	island
insulin/o	insulin
intact/o	untouched, whole
inter-	between, among
intermitt/o	not continuous
intern/o	within, inner
interstiti/o	the space between things
intestin/o	intestine
intim/o	innermost
intoxic/o	put poison in
intra-	within, inside
intrins/o	contained within
intro-	within, into, inside
introit/o	entrance or passage
intussuscept/o	take up or receive within
involut/o	rolled up, curled inward
iod/o	iodine
-ion	action, process, state or condition
ion/o	ion, to wander
-ior	pertaining to
ipsi-	same
ir-	in
-is	noun ending
ir/i, **ir/o**, **irid/o**, **irit/o**	iris, colored part of eye
is/o	same, equal
isch/o	to hold back
ischi/o	ischium
-ism	condition, state of
iso-	equal
-ist	a person who practices, specialist
-isy	noun ending
-itis	inflammation
-ium	structure, tissue
-ive	performs, tends toward
-ize	to make, to treat

J

jejun/o	jejunum
jugul/o	throat
juxta-	beside, near, nearby

K

kary/o	nucleus, nut
kata-, **kath-**	down
kel/o	growth, tumor
kerat/o	horny, hard, cornea
ket/o, **keton/o**	ketones, acetones
kines/o, **kinesi/o**, **-kinesia**	movement
-kinesis	motion
klept/o	to steal
koil/o	hollow or concave
kraur/o	dry
kyph/o	bent, hump

L

labi/o	lip
labyrinth/o	maze, labyrinth, the inner ear
lacer/o, **lacerat/o**	torn, mangled
lacrim/o	tear, tear duct, lacrimal duct
lact/i, **lact/o**	milk
lactat/o	secrete milk
lamin/o	lamina
lapar/o	abdomen, abdominal wall
laps/o	slip, fall, slide
-lapse	to slide, fall, sag
laryng/o	larynx, throat
lat/i, **lat/o**	broad
later/o	side
lav/o, **lavat/o**	wash, bathe
lax/o, **laxat/o**	loosen, relax
leiomy/o	smooth (visceral) muscle
lent/i	the lens of the eye
lenticul/o	shaped like a lens, pertaining to a lens
-lepsy	seizure
lept/o	thin, slender
-leptic	to seize, take hold of
lepto-	small, soft
letharg/o	drowsiness, oblivion
leuk/o	white
lev/o, **levat/o**	raise, lift up
lex/o, **-lexia**	word, phrase
libid/o, **libidin/o**	sexual drive, desire, passion
ligament/o	ligament
ligat/o	binding or tying off
lingu/o	tongue
lipid/o, **lip/o**	fat, lipid
-listhesis	slipping

lith/o, **-lith**	stone, calculus
-lithiasis	presence of stones
lob/i, **lob/o**	lobe, well-defined part of an organ
loc/o	place
loch/i	childbirth, confinement
-logy	study of
longev/o	long-lived, long life
lord/o	curve, swayback, bent
lumb/o	lower back, loin
lumin/o	light
lun/o, **lunat/o**	moon
lunul/o	crescent
lup/i, **lup/o**	wolf
lute/o	yellow
lux/o	to slide
lymph/o	lymph, lymphatic tissue
lymphaden/o	lymph node or gland
lymphangi/o	lymph vessel
-lysis	breakdown, separation, setting free, destruction, loosening
-lyst	agent that causes lysis or loosening
-lytic	to reduce, destroy

M

macro-	large, abnormal size or length, long
macul/o	spot
magn/o	great, large
major/o	larger
mal-	bad, poor, evil
-malacia	abnormal softening
malign/o	bad, evil
malle/o	malleus, hammer
malleol/o	malleolus, little hammer
mamm/o	breast
man/i	madness, rage
man/i, **man/o**	hand
mandibul/o	mandible, lower jaw
-mania	obsessive preoccupation
manipul/o	use of hands
manubri/o	handle
masset/o	chew
mast/o	breast
mastic/o, **masticat/o**	chew
mastoid/o	mastoid process
matern/o	maternal, of a mother
matur/o	ripe
maxill/o	maxilla (upper jaw)
maxim/o	largest, greatest
meat/o	opening or passageway
medi/o	middle
mediastin/o	mediastinum, middle
medic/o	medicine, physician, healing
medicat/o	medication, healing
medull/o	medulla (inner section), middle, soft, marrow
mega-, **megal/o**	large, great
-megaly	enlargement
mei/o	less, meiosis
melan/o	black, dark
mellit/o	honey, honeyed
membran/o	membrane, thin skin
men/o	menstruation, menses
mening/o, **meningi/o**	membranes, meninges
menisc/o	meniscus, crescent
mens/o	menstruate, menstruation, menses
menstru/o, **menstruat/o**	occurring monthly
ment/o	mind, chin
mes-	middle
mesenter/o	mesentery
mesi/o	middle, median plane
meso-	middle
meta-	change, beyond, subsequent to, behind, after or next
metabol/o	change
metacarp/o	metacarpals, bones of the hand
metatars/o	bones of the foot between the tarsus and toes
-meter	measure, instrument used to measure
metr/i, **metr/o**, **metri/o**	uterus
-metrist	one who measures
-metry	to measure
micr/o, **micro-**	small
mictur/o, **micturit/o**	urinate
mid-	middle
midsagitt/o	from front to back, at the middle
milli-	one-thousandth
-mimetic	mimic, copy
mineral/o	mineral
minim/o	smallest, least
minor/o	smaller
mio-	smaller, less
-mission	to send
mit/o	a thread
mitr/o	a miter, having two points on top

mobil/o capable of moving
monil/i string of beads, genus of parasitic mold or fungus
mono- one, single
morbid/o disease, sickness
moribund/o dying
morph/o shape, form
mort/i, **mort/o**, **mort/u** death, dead
mortal/i pertaining to death, subject to death
mot/o, **motil/o** motion, movement
mu/o close, shut
muc/o, **mucos/o** mucus
multi- many, much
muscul/o muscle
mut/a genetic change
mut/o unable to speak, inarticulate
mutagen/o causing genetic change
my/o muscle
myc/e, **myc/o** fungus
mydri/o wide
mydrias/i dilation of the pupil
myel/o spinal cord, bone marrow
myocardi/o myocardium, heart muscle
myom/o muscle tumor
myos/o muscle
myring/o tympanic membrane, eardrum
myx/o, **myxa-** mucus

N

nar/i nostril
narc/o numbness, stupor
nas/i, **nas/o** nose
nat/i birth
natr/o sodium
nause/o nausea, seasickness
necr/o death
-necrosis tissue death
neo-, **ne/o** new, strange
nephr/o kidney
nerv/o, **neur/i**, **neur/o** nerve, nerve tissue
neutr/o neither, neutral
nev/o birthmark, mole
nid/o next
niter-, **nitro-** nitrogen
noct/i night
nod/o knot, swelling
nodul/o little knot
nom/o law, control
non- no
nor- chemical compound
norm/o normal or usual
nuch/o the nape
nucle/o nucleus
nucleol/o little nucleus, nucleolus
nulli- none
numer/o number, count
nunci/o messenger
nutri/o, **nutrit/o** nourishment, food, nourish, feed
nyct/o, **nyctal/o** night

O

ob- against
obes/o obese, extremely fat
obliqu/o slanted, sideways
oblongat/o oblong, elongated
obstetr/i, **obstetr/o** midwife, one who stands to receive
occipit/o back of the skull, occiput
occlud/o, **occlus/o** shut, close up
occult/o hidden, concealed
ocul/o eye
odont/o tooth
-oid like, resembling
-ole little, small
olfact/o smell, sense of smell
olig/o scanty, few
-ologist specialist
-ology the science or study of
-oma tumor, neoplasm
om/o shoulder
oment/o omentum, fat
omphal/o umbilical cord, the navel
onc/o tumor
-one hormone
onych/o fingernail or toenail
o/o, **oo/o** egg
oophor/o ovary
opac/o, **opacit/o** shaded, dark, impenetrable to light
-opaque obscure
oper/o, **operat/o** perform, operate, work
opercul/o cover or lid
ophthalm/o eye, vision
-opia vision condition
opisth/o backward
-opsia, **-opsis**, **-opsy** vision, view of

opt/i, **opt/o**, **optic/o** eye, vision
or/o mouth, oral cavity
orbit/o orbit, bony cavity or socket
orch/o, **orchid/o**, **orchi/o** testicles, testis, testes
-orexia appetite
organ/o organ
orgasm/o swell, be excited
orth/o straight, normal, correct
-ory pertaining to
os- mouth, bone
-ose full of, pertaining to, sugar
-osis abnormal condition, disease
osm/o pushing, thrusting
-osmia smell, odor
oss/e, **oss/i** bone
ossicul/o ossicle (small bone)
oste/o, **ost/o** bone
-ostomy the surgical creation of an artificial opening to the body surface
-ostosis condition of bone
ot/o ear, hearing
-otia ear condition
-otomy cutting, surgical incision
ov/i, **ov/o** egg, ovum
ovari/o ovary
ovul/o egg
ox/i, **ox/o**, **ox/y** oxygen
-oxia oxygen condition
oxid/o containing oxygen
oxy/o the presence of oxygen in a compound

P

pachy- heavy, thick
palat/o palate, roof of mouth
pall/o, **pallid/o** pale, lacking or drained of color
palliat/o cloaked, hidden
palpat/o touch, feel, stroke
palpebr/o eyelid
palpit/o throbbing, quivering
pan- all, entire, every
pancreat/o pancreas
papill/i, **papill/o** nipple-like
papul/o pimple
par-, **para-** beside, near, beyond, abnormal, apart from, opposite, along side of
par/o to bear, bring forth, labor
-para to give birth
paralys/o, **paralyt/o** disable
parasit/o parasite
parathyroid/o parathyroid glands
pares/i to disable
-paresis partial or incomplete paralysis
paret/o to disable
-pareunia sexual intercourse
pariet/o wall
parotid/o parotid gland
-parous having borne one or more children
paroxysm/o sudden attack
-partum, **parturit/o** childbirth, labor
patell/a, **patell/o** patella, kneecap
path/o, **-pathy** disease, suffering, feeling, emotion
paus/o cessation, stopping
-pause stopping
pector/o chest
ped/o child, foot
pedi/a child
pedicul/o louse (singular), lice (plural)
pelv/i, **pelv/o** pelvic bone, pelvic cavity, hip
pen/i penis
pend/o to hang
-penia deficiency, lack, too few
peps/i, **-pepsia**, **pept/o** digest, digestion
per- excessive, through
percept/o become aware, perceive
percuss/o strike, tap, beat
peri- surrounding, around
perine/o perineum
peristals/o, **peristalt/o** constrict around
peritone/o peritoneum
perme/o to pass or go through
pernici/o destructive, harmful
perone/o fibula
perspir/o perspiration
pertuss/i intensive cough
petechi/o skin spot
-pexy surgical fixation
phac/o lens of eye
phag/o eat, swallow
-phage a cell that destroys, eat, swallow
-phagia eating, swallowing
phak/o lens of eye
phalang/o phalanges, finger and toe
phall/i, **phill/o** penis

pharmac/o, **pharmaceut/o**	drug
pharyng/o	throat, pharynx
phas/o	speech
-phasia	speak or speech
phe/o	dusky
pher/o	to bear or carry
-pheresis	removal
phil/o, **-phil**, **-philia**	attraction to, like, love
phleb/o	vein
phlegm/o	thick mucus
phob/o, **-phobia**	abnormal fear
phon/o, **-phonia**	sound, voice
phor/o	carry, bear, movement
-phoresis	carrying, transmission
-phoria	to bear, carry, feeling, mental state
phot/o	light
phren/o	diaphragm, mind
-phthisis	wasting away
-phylactic	protective, preventive
-phylaxis	protection
physi/o, **physic/o**	nature, physical
-physis	to grow
phyt/o, **-phyte**	plant
pigment/o	pigment, color
pil/i, **pil/o**	hair
pineal/o	pineal gland
pinn/i	external ear, auricle
pituit/o, **pituitar/o**	pituitary gland
plac/o	flat plate or patch
placent/o	placenta, round flat cake
plak/o, **-plakia**	plaque, plate, thin flat layer or scale
plan/o	flat
plant/i, **plant/o**	sole of foot
plas/i, **plas/o**, **-plasia**	development, growth, formation
-plasm	formative material of cells
plasm/o	something molded or formed
-plastic	pertaining to formation
-plasty	surgical repair
ple/o	more, many
-plegia	paralysis, stroke
-plegic	one affected with paralysis
pleur/o	pleura, side of the body
plex/o	plexus, network
plic/o	fold or ridge
pne/o-	breath, breathing
-pnea	breathing
-pneic	pertaining to breathing
pneum/o, **pneumon/o**	lung, air
pod/o	foot
-poiesis	formation, to make
pol/o	extreme
poli/o	gray matter of brain and spinal cord
pollic/o	thumb
poly-	many
polyp/o	polyp, small growth
pont/o	pons (a part of the brain), bridge
poplit/o	back of the knee
por/o	pore, small opening
-porosis	lessening in density, porous condition
port/i	gate, door
post-	after, behind
poster/o	behind, toward the back
potent/o	powerful
pract/i, **practic/o**	practice, pursue an occupation
prandi/o, **-prandial**	meal
-praxia	action, condition concerning the performance of movements
-praxis	act, activity, practice use
pre-	before, in front of
precoc/i	early, premature
pregn/o	pregnant, full of
prematur/o	too early, untimely
preputi/o	foreskin, prepuce
presby/o	old age
press/o	press, draw
priap/o	penis
primi-	first
pro-	before, in behalf of
process/o	going forth
procreat/o	reproduce
proct/o	anus and rectum
prodrom/o	running ahead, precursor
product/o	lead forward, yield, produce
prolaps/o	fall downward, slide forward
prolifer/o	reproduce, bear offspring
pron/o, **pronat/o**	bent forward
pros-	before
prostat/o	prostate gland
prosth/o, **prosthet/o**	addition, appendage
prot/o, **prote/o**	first
protein/o	protein
proxim/o	near
prurit/o	itching
pseud/o	false

psor/i, psor/o itch, itching
psych/o mind
-ptosis droop, sag, prolapse, fall
-ptyal/o saliva
-ptysis spitting
pub/o pubis, part of hip bone
pubert/o ripe age, adult
pudend/o pudendum
puerper/i childbearing, labor
pulm/o, pulmon/o lung
pulpos/o fleshy, pulpy
puls/o beat, beating, striking
punct/o sting, prick, puncture
pupill/o pupil
pur/o pus
purpur/o purple
purul/o pus-filled
pustul/o infected pimple
py/o pus
pyel/o renal pelvis, bowl of kidney
pylor/o pylorus, pyloric sphincter
pyr/o, pyret/o fever, fire

Q

quadr/i, quadr/o four

R

rabi/o madness, rage
rachi/o spinal column, vertebrae
radi/o radiation, x-rays, radius (lateral lower arm bone)
radiat/o giving off rays or radiant energy
radicul/o nerve root
raph/o seam, suture
re- back, again
recept/o receive, receiver
recipi/o receive, take to oneself
rect/o rectum, straight
recticul/o network
recuperat/o recover, regain health
reduct/o bring back together
refract/o bend back, turn aside
regurgit/o flood or gush back
remiss/o give up, let go, relax
ren/o kidney
restor/o rebuild, put back, restore
resuscit/o revive
retent/o hold back
reticul/o network
retin/o retina, net
retract/o draw back or in
retro- behind, backward, back of
rhabd/o rod, rod-shaped
rhabdomy/o striated muscle
rheum/o, rheumat/o watery flow, subject to flow
rhin/o nose
rhiz/o root
rhonc/o snore, snoring
rhythm/o rhythm
rhytid/o wrinkle
rigid/o stiff
ris/o laugh
rotat/o rotate, revolve
-rrhage, -rrhagia bleeding, abnormal excessive fluid discharge
-rrhaphy surgical suturing
-rrhea flow or discharge
-rrhexis rupture
rube- red
rug/o wrinkle, fold

S

sacc/i, sacc/o sac
sacchar/o sugar
sacr/o sacrum
saliv/o saliva
salping/o uterine (fallopian) tube, auditory (eustachian) tube
-salpinx uterine (fallopian) tube
san/o sound, healthy, sane
sangu/i, sanguin/o blood
sanit/o soundness, health
saphen/o clear, apparent, manifest
sapr/o decaying, rotten
sarc/o flesh, connective tissue
scalp/o carve, scrape
scapul/o scapula, shoulder blade
schiz/o division, split
scirrh/o hard
scler/o sclera, white of eye, hard
-sclerosis abnormal hardening
scoli/o curved, bent
-scope instrument for visual examination
-scopic pertaining to visual examination

-scopy visual examination
scot/o darkness
scrib/o, **script/o** write
scrot/o bag or pouch
seb/o sebum
secret/o produce, separate out
sect/o, **secti/o** cut, cutting
segment/o pieces
sell/o saddle
semi- half
semin/i semen, seed, sperm
sen/i old
senesc/o grow old
senil/o old age
sens/i feeling, sensation
sensitiv/o sensitive to, affected by
seps/o infection
sept/o infection, partition
ser/o serum
seros/o serous
sial/o saliva
sialaden/o salivary gland
sigm/o Greek letter sigma
sigmoid/o sigmoid colon
silic/o glass
sin/o, **sin/u** hollow, sinus
sinistr/o left, left side
sinus/o sinus
-sis abnormal condition, disease
sit/u place
skelet/o skeleton
soci/o companion, fellow being
-sol solution
solut/o, **solv/o** loosened, dissolved
soma-, **somat/o** body
somn/i, **somn/o** sleep
son/o sound
sopor/o sleep
spad/o draw off, draw
-spasm, **spasmod/o** sudden involuntary contraction, tightening, cramping
spec/i look at, a kind or sort
specul/o mirror
sperm/o, **spermat/o** sperm, spermatozoa, seed
sphen/o sphenoid bone, wedge
spher/o round, sphere, ball
sphincter/o tight band
sphygm/o pulse
spin/o spine, backbone
spir/o to breathe
spirill/o little coil
spirochet/o coiled microorganism
splen/o spleen
spondyl/o vertebrae, vertebral column, backbone
spontane/o unexplained, of one's own accord
spor/o seed, spore
sput/o sputum, spit
squam/o scale
-stalsis contraction, constriction
staped/o, **stapedi/o** stapes (middle ear bone)
staphyl/o clusters, bunch of grapes
-stasis, **-static** control, maintenance of a constant level
steat/o fat, lipid, sebum
sten/o narrowing, contracted
-stenosis abnormal narrowing
ster/o solid structure
stere/o solid, three-dimensional
steril/i sterile
stern/o sternum, the breast bone
steth/o chest
-sthenia strength
stigmat/o point, spot
stimul/o goad, prick, incite
stol/o send or place
stom/o, **stomat/o** mouth, oral cavity
-stomosis, **-stomy** furnish with a mouth or outlet, new opening
strab/i squint, squint-eyed
strat/i layer
strept/o twisted chain
striat/o stripe, furrow, groove
stric- narrowing
strict/o draw tightly together, bind or tie
strid/o harsh sound
stup/e benumbed, stunned
styl/o pen, pointed instrument
sub- under, less, below
subluxat/o partial dislocation
sucr/o sugar
sudor/i sweat
suffoc/o, **suffocat/o** choke, strangle
sulc/o furrow, groove
super-, **super/o** above, excessive, higher than
superflu/o overflowing, excessive
supin/o lying on the back
supinat/o bend backward, place on the back
suppress/o press down

suppur/o, suppurate/o to form pus
supra- above, upper, excessive
supraren/o above or on the kidney, suprarenal gland
-surgery operative procedure
sutur/o stitch, seam
sym- with, together, joined together
symptomat/o falling together, symptom
syn- together, with, union, association
synaps/o, synapt/o point of contact
syncop/o to cut short, cut off
-syndesis surgical fixation of vertebrae
syndrom/o running together
synovi/o, synov/o synovial membrane, synovial fluid
syphil/i, syphil/o syphilis
syring/o tube
system/o, systemat/o body system
systol/o contraction

T

tachy- fast, rapid
tact/i touch
talip/o foot and ankle deformity
tars/o tarsus (ankle bone), instep, edge of the eyelid
tax/o coordination, order
techn/o, techni/o skill
tectori/o covering, rooflike
tele/o distant, far
tempor/o temporal bone, temple
ten/o, tend/o tendon, stretch out, extend, strain
tenac/i holding fast, sticky
tendin/o tendon
tens/o stretch out, extend, strain
termin/o end, limit
test/i, test/o testicle, testis
tetan/o rigid, tense
tetra- four
thalam/o thalamus, inner room
thanas/o, thanat/o death
the/o put, place
thec/o sheath
thel/o nipple
therap/o, therapeut/o treatment
therm/o heat
thio- sulfur
thora/o, thorac/o chest
-thorax chest, pleural cavity
thromb/o clot
thym/o thymus gland
-thymia a state of mind
-thymic pertaining to the mind, relating to the thymus gland
thyr/o, thyroid/o thyroid gland
tibi/o tibia (shin bone)
-tic pertaining to
tine/o gnawing worm, ringworm
tinnit/o ringing, buzzing, tinkling
-tion process, state or quality of
toc/o, -tocia, -tocin labor, birth
tom/o cut, section, slice
-tome instrument to cut
-tomy process of cutting
ton/o tension, tone, stretching
tone/o to stretch
tonsill/o tonsil, throat
top/o place, position, location
tors/o twist, rotate
tort/i twisted
tox/o, toxic/o poison, poisonous
trabecul/o little beam marked with cross bars or beams
trache/i, trache/o trachea, windpipe
trachel- neck
tract/o draw, pull, path, bundle of nerve fibers
tranquil/o quiet, calm, tranquil
trans- across, through
transfus/o pour across, transfer
transit/o changing
transvers/o across, crosswise
traumat/o injury
trem/o shaking, trembling
tremul/o fine tremor or shaking
treponem/o coiled, turning microbe
tri- three
trich/o hair
trigon/o trigone
-tripsy to crush
-trite instrument for crushing
trop/o, -tropia turn, change
troph/o, -trophy development, nourishment
-tropic having an affinity for
-tropin to stimulate, act on
tub/i, tub/o tube, pipe
tubercul/o little knot, swelling

tunic/o covering, cloak, sheath
turbinat/o coiled, spiral shaped
tuss/i cough
tympan/o tympanic membrane, eardrum
-type classification, picture

U

-ula small, little
-ule small one
ulcer/o sore, ulcer
uln/o ulna (medial lower arm bone)
ultra- beyond, excess
-um singular noun ending
umbilic/o navel
un- not
ungu/o nail
uni- one
ur/o urine, urinary tract
-uresis urination
ureter/o ureter
urethr/o urethra
urg/o press, push
-uria urination, urine
urin/o urine or urinary organs
urtic/o nettle, rash, hives
-us thing, singular noun ending
uter/i, **uter/o** uterus
uve/o iris, choroid, ciliary body, uveal tract
uvul/o uvula, little grape

V

vaccin/i, **vaccin/o** vaccine
vacu/o empty
vag/o vagus nerve, wandering
vagin/o vagina
valg/o bent or twisted outward
valv/o, **valvul/o** valve
var/o bent or twisted inward
varic/o varicose veins, swollen or dilated vein
vas/o vas deferens, vessel
vascul/o blood vessel, little vessel
vast/o vast, great, extensive
vect/o carry, convey
ven/o vein
vener/o sexual intercourse
venter- abdomen
ventilat/o expose to air, fan
ventr/o in front, belly side of body
ventricul/o ventricle of brain or heart, small chamber
venul/o venule, small vein
verg/o twist, incline
verm/i worm
verruc/o wart
-verse, **-version** to turn
vers/o, **vert/o** turn
vertebr/o vertebra, backbone
vertig/o, **vertigin/o** whirling round
vesic/o urinary bladder
vesicul/o seminal vesicle, blister, little bladder
vestibul/o entrance, vestibule
vi/o force
vill/i shaggy hair, tuft of hair
vir/o poison, virus
viril/o masculine, manly
vis/o seeing, sight
visc/o sticky
viscer/o viscera, internal organ
viscos/o sticky
vit/a, **vit/o** life
viti/o blemish, defect
vitre/o glassy, made of glass
voc/i voice
vol/o palm or sole
volv/o roll, turn
vulgar/i common
vulv/o vulva, covering

X

xanth/o yellow
xen/o strange, foreign
xer/o dry
xiph/i, **xiph/o** sword

Y

-y noun ending

Z

zo/o animal life
zygomat/o cheek bone, yoke
zygot/o joined together

Appendix B

ABBREVIATIONS AND THEIR MEANINGS

Reminder about abbreviations: An abbreviation can have several meanings, and a term can have several abbreviations. When in doubt, always verify the meaning of the abbreviation!

A

A2 or A_2	aortic valve closure
A	abnormal; adult; age; allergy; anaphylaxis; anesthesia; anterior; antibody; auscultation
a	accommodation; acid
aa	amino acid
AA	alopecia areata; asthma; asthmatic
AAA	abdominal aortic aneurysm
AAL	anterior axillary line
AAV	adeno-associated virus
A&B	apnea and bradycardia
A/B	acid-base ratio
AB, Ab, ab	abortion
AB, Abnl, abn	abnormal
Ab	antibody
ABC	aspiration, biopsy, cytology
Abd, Abdo	abdomen
ABE	acute bacterial endocarditis
ABG	arterial blood gases
ABP	arterial blood pressure
ABR	auditory brainstem response
abx	antibiotics
ac	acute
AC, ac	anticoagulant; before meals; air conduction
acc	accident; accommodation
ACD	absolute cardiac dullness; acid-citrate-dextrose; anterior chest diameter; area of cardiac disease
ACE	acute care of the elderly; aerobic chair exercises; angiotensin-converting enzyme
ACG	angiocardiogram; angiocardiography; apex cardiogram
ACH	adrenocortical hormone
ACL	anterior cruciate ligament
ACLS	advanced cardiac life support
ACT	activated coagulation time; anticoagulant therapy
ACTH	adrenocorticotropic hormone
ACU	acute care unit; ambulatory care unit
ACVD	acute cardiovascular disease
AD	admitting diagnosis; advanced directive; after discharge; Alzheimer's disease; right ear
ADC	AIDS dementia complex
ADD	attention-deficit disorder
ADE	acute disseminated encephalitis; adverse drug event
ADH	adhesion; antidiuretic hormone
ADHD	attention-deficit hyperactivity disorder
ADL	activities of daily life; activities of daily living
ad lib	as desired
adm	admission
ADR	adverse drug reaction
ADS	antibody deficiency syndrome

ADT	admission, discharge, transfer
AE, A/E	above elbow
AED	automated external defibrillation
AF	acid-fast; amniotic fluid; atrial flutter
AF, A fib, A-fib	atrial fibrillation
AFB	acid-fast bacilli
AFP	alpha-fetoprotein
AG, Ag	antigen
AH	abdominal hysterectomy
AHD	antihypertensive drug; arteriosclerotic heart disease; autoimmune hemolytic disease
AI	accidentally incurred; aortic insufficiency; artificial insemination
AIC, AICD	automated implantable cardioverter-defibrillator
AID	acute infectious disease; artificial insemination donor
AIDS	acquired immunodeficiency syndrome
AIH	artificial insemination husband
AIHA	autoimmune hemolytic anemia
AJ, aj	ankle jerk
AK	above knee
AKA	above-knee amputation
alb	albumin
ALD	aldosterone, assistive listening device
alk	alkaline
ALL	acute lymphoblastic leukemia; acute lymphocytic leukemia
ALND	axillary lymph node dissection
ALP	acute lupus pericarditis; alkaline phosphatase
ALS	advanced life support; amyotrophic lateral sclerosis; antilymphocytic serum
ALT, alt	alternative; altitude
alt dieb	alternate days; every other day
alt hor	alternate hours
alt noct	alternate nights
Am	amnion
AMA	advanced maternal age; against medical advice; American Medical Association
amb	ambulance; ambulatory
AMD	age-related macular degeneration
AMI	acute myocardial infarction
AML	acute myeloblastic leukemia; acute myelocytic leukemia; amyotrophic lateral sclerosis
AMN	amniocentesis
amp	amplification; ampule; amputate
AMS	altered mental status; automated multiphasic screening
amt	amount
AN	aneurysm; anorexia nervosa
ANA	antinuclear antibodies
ANAS	anastomosis
anat	anatomy
anes, anesth	anesthesia; anesthetic
ANLL	acute nonlymphocytic leukemia
ANS	anterior nasal spine; autonomic nervous system
ant, ANT	anterior
ANUG	acute necrotizing ulcerative gingivitis
AOD	arterial occlusive disease
AODM	adult-onset diabetes mellitus
AOM	acute otitis media
A & P	anatomy and physiology; anterior and posterior; auscultation and percussion
AP	abruptio placenta; angina pectoris; anteroposterior; anterior-posterior; appendectomy; appendicitis
APAP	acetaminophen
Aph	aphasia
APLD	aspiration percutaneous lumbar diskectomy
aPTT	activated partial thromboplastin time
aq	aqueous; water
AR	abnormal record; achievement ratio; alarm reaction; artificial respiration
ARD	acute respiratory disease
ARDS	acute respiratory distress syndrome; adult respiratory distress syndrome
ARF	acute renal failure; acute respiratory failure
ARI	acute respiratory infection
ARM	artificial rupture of membranes
ART	arthritis; assisted reproductive technology
AS	ankylosing spondylitis; aortic stenosis; astigmatism; left ear

ASA	acetylsalicylic acid (aspirin)
ASAP	as soon as possible
ASCVD	arteriosclerotic cardiovascular disease
ASD	atrial septal defect
ASH	asymmetrical septal hypertrophy
ASHD	arteriosclerotic heart disease
ASO	administrative services only; arteriosclerosis obliterans
ASS	anterior superior spine
AST	Aphasia Screening Test; aspartate aminotransferase
As tol	as tolerated
AT	Achilles tendon
ATP	adenosine triphosphate
atr	atrophy
AU	aures unitas; both ears
AUL	acute undifferentiated leukemia
aus, ausc, auscul	auscultation
A-V, AV	aortic valve; artificial ventilation; arteriovenous; atrioventricular
AVM	arteriovenous malfunction
AVN	atrioventricular node
AVR	aortic valve replacement
A & W	alive and well
ax, Ax	axilla; axillary
AZT	Aschheim-Zondek test

B

B	bruit
B/A	backache
BA	bronchial asthma
Ba	barium
BAC	blood alcohol concentration
BACT, Bact, bact	bacteria; bacterium
BaE	barium enema
BAO	basal acid output
bas	basophils
BBB	blood-brain barrier; bundle branch block
BBT	basal body temperature
BC	bone conduction
BCC	basal cell carcinoma
BD	bronchodilator
BDT	bone density testing
BE	barium enema; below elbow
BEAM	brain electrical activity map
BED	binge eating disorder
BFP	biologic false positive
bid, b.i.d.	bis in die; twice a day
BID	brought in dead
BIL, Bil, Bili	bilirubin
bil	bilateral
BIN, bin	twice a night
BK	below knee
BKA	below-knee amputation
Bld	blood
BM	bone marrow; bowel movement
BMB	bone marrow biopsy
BMD	Becker's muscular dystrophy; bone mineral density
BMI	body mass index
BMR	basal metabolic rate
BMT	barium meal test; bone marrow transplant
BNO	bladder neck obstruction
BNR	bladder neck resection
BOM	bilateral otitis media
BP	Bell's palsy; bedpan; bathroom privileges; blood pressure
BPD	borderline personality disorder
BPH	benign prostatic hyperplasia; benign prostatic hypertrophy
BPM, bpm	beats per minute, breaths per minute
BP&P	blood pressure and pulse
BPPV	benign paroxysmal positional vertigo
Br	bed rest; chronic bronchitis
BRBPR	bright red blood per rectum
BRO, Bronch	bronchoscope; bronchoscopy
BRP	bathroom privileges
BS	blood sugar; bowel sounds; breath sounds
BSE	breast self-examination
BSO	bilateral salpingo-oophorectomy
BT	bleeding time
BUN	blood urea nitrogen
BV	bacterial vaginosis; blood volume
Bx, bx	biopsy

C

C1 through C7	cervical vertebrae
C	centigrade; Celsius; cholesterol; convergence; cyanosis
C.	chlamydia
c	centimeter
$\bar{c}$	with

Ca	calcium
CA, Ca	cancer; cardiac arrest; carcinoma; chronological age
CAB	coronary artery bypass
CABG	coronary artery bypass graft
CAD	computer-assisted diagnosis; coronary artery disease
CAL	calcitonin
cal	calorie
CAM	complementary and alternative medicine
cap, caps	capsule
CAPD	continuous ambulatory peritoneal dialysis
card cath	cardiac catheterization
Cat	cataract
cath	catheter; catheterization; catheterize
caut	cauterization
CAVH	continuous arteriovenous hemofiltration
CBC, cbc	complete blood count
CBF	capillary blood flow; coronary blood flow
CBI	continuous bladder irrigation
CBR	complete bed rest
CBS	chronic brain syndrome
CC	chief complaint; colony count; cardiac cycle; cardiac cauterization; cardiac catheterization; creatinine clearance
cc	cubic centimeter (1/1,000 liter)
CCA	circumflex coronary artery
CCCR	closed chest cardiopulmonary resuscitation
CCE	cholecystectomy
CCPD	continuous cycle peritoneal dialysis
CCr	creatinine clearance
CCT	computerized cranial tomography
CCU	coronary care unit
CD	communicable disease; contact dermatitis; Crohn's disease
CDC	calculated date (day) of confinement; Centers for Disease Control and Prevention
CDE	common duct exploration
CDH	congenital dislocation of the hip
CEA	carotid endarterectomy
CEPH	cephalic
CF	complete fixation; counting fingers; cystic fibrosis
CFS	chronic fatigue syndrome
CGL	chronic granulomatous leukemia
C gl	with correction; with glasses
CH	chromosome
CHB	complete heart block
CHD	congenital heart defects; coronary heart disease
CHF	congestive heart failure
CHO	carbohydrate
chol	cholesterol
chole	cholecystectomy
chr	chromosome, chronic
CI	conjunctivitis; coronary insufficiency
cib	food
CID	cytomegalic inclusion disease
CIR, CIRR	cirrhosis
CIRC, circum	circumcision
CIS	carcinoma in situ
CIT	conventional insulin treatment
CK	creatine kinase
ck	check
CKD	chronic kidney disease
Cl, cl	clinic; chloride
CL	cholelithiasis; chronic leukemia; cirrhosis of the liver; cleft lip; corpus luteum
CLD	chronic liver disease
CLL	chronic lymphocytic leukemia
cl liq	clear liquid
cm	centimeter (1/100 meter)
cm^3	cubic centimeter
CME	cystoid macular edema
CMG	cystometrogram
CML	chronic myelocytic leukemia
CMM	cutaneous malignant melanoma
CMV	controlled mechanical ventilation; cytomegalovirus
CNS	central nervous system; cutaneous nerve stimulation
C/O, c/o	complains of
CO	carbon monoxide; coronary occlusion; coronary output
CO_2	carbon dioxide
COD	cause of death
COH	carbohydrate
COL	colonoscopy
COLD	chronic obstructive lung disease
comp	compound
cond	condition
contra	against

COPD chronic obstructive pulmonary disease
CP cardiopulmonary; cerebral palsy
CPA carotid phonoangiograph
CPAP continuous positive airway pressure
CPC clinicopathologic conference
CPD cephalopelvic disproportion
CPE cardio-pulmonary edema
CPK creatine phosphokinase
CPN chronic pyelonephritis
CPPB continuous positive-pressure breathing
CPR cardiopulmonary resuscitation
CPS cycles per second
CR closed reduction; complete response; conditioned reflex
CRC colorectal carcinoma
CRD chronic respiratory disease
creat creatinine
CRF chronic renal failure
CRP C-reactive protein
CRPS complex regional pain syndrome
CRYO cryosurgery
C & S culture and sensitivity
CS central supply; complete stroke; conditioned stimulus; Cushing's syndrome; cesarean section
CSAP cryosurgical ablation of the prostate
CSB Cheyne-Stokes breathing
C-section cesarean section
CSF cerebrospinal fluid
CSO craniostenosis
CSR central supply room; Cheyne-Stokes respiration
CT computerized tomography
CTCL cutaneous T-cell lymphoma
CTD cumulative trauma disorders
CTR carpal tunnel release
CTS carpal tunnel syndrome
cu cubic
CUC chronic ulcerative colitis
CUG cystourethrogram
CV cardiovascular
CVA cardiovascular accident; cerebrovascular accident
CVD cardiovascular disease
CVI chronic venous insufficiency
CVL central venous line
CVP central venous pressure; Cytoxan, vincristine, prednisone
CVS chorionic villus sampling
CWP childbirth without pain; coal workers' pneumoconiosis
Cx cervix
CX, CXR chest x-ray film
cysto cystoscopic examination; cystoscopy
cyt cytology; cytoplasm

D

D diopter; dorsal
d day
DAT diet as tolerated
db, dB decibel
D & C dilation and curettage
D/C, d/c, dc diarrhea/constipation, discharge, discontinue
DCC direct-current cardioversion
DCIS ductal carcinoma in situ
DCR direct cortical response
D/D, DD, DDx, Ddx differential diagnosis
D & E dilation and evacuation
debr debridement
Dg, dg diagnosis (see also DX; Diag)
del delivery
DES diethylstilbestrol
DEXA dual energy x-ray absorptiometry
DF dorsiflexion
DG, dg diagnosis
DGE delayed gastric emptying
DHFS dengue hemorrhagic fever shock syndrome
DI diabetes insipidus
Diag, diag diagnosis
DIC diffuse intravascular coagulation
diff differential diagnosis
diopt, Dptr diopter
DIP distal interphalangeal
diph diphtheria
disch discharge
DJD degenerative joint disease
DKA diabetic ketoacidosis
DL danger list
DLE discoid lupus erythematosus
DM dermatomyositis; diabetes mellitus; diastolic murmur
DMD Duchenne's muscular dystrophy
DNA deoxyribonucleic acid
DNR do not resuscitate

DNS deviated nasal septum
DOA dead on arrival
DOB date of birth
DOC date of conception
DOE dyspnea on exertion
DOMS delayed-onset muscle soreness
DOT directly observed therapy
DPT diphtheria-pertussis-tetanus
DQ developmental quotient
DR diabetic retinopathy; digital radiography; doctor
dr dram; dressing
DRD developmental reading disorder
DRE digital rectal examination
DRG diagnosis-related group
DRP diabetic retinopathy
D/S dextrose in saline
DS Down syndrome
DSA digital subtraction angiography
DSD dry sterile dressing
dsg dressing
DT diphtheria and tetanus toxoids
DT, DT's, DTs delirium tremens
DTP diphtheria, tetanus toxoids, and pertussis vaccine
DTR deep tendon reflex
du decubitus ulcer
DUB dysfunctional uterine bleeding
DVA distance visual acuity
DVI digital vascular imaging
DVT deep vein thrombosis
D/W dextrose in water
DX, Dx diagnosis
DXA dual x-ray absorptiometry

E

E encephalitis; enema; etiology
e epinephrine; estrogen
EBL estimated blood loss
EBP epidural blood patch
EBV Epstein-Barr virus
ECC endocervical curettage; extracorporeal circulation
ECCE extracapsular cataract extraction
ECG electrocardiogram; electrocardiography
ECHO echocardiogram; echocardiography
E coli *Escherichia coli*
ECT electroconvulsive therapy
Ecz, Ez eczema
ED effective dose; emergency department; epidural; erythema dose; erectile dysfunction
EDA epidural anesthesia
EDC estimated date (day) of confinement
EDD end-diastolic dimension
EDS Ehlers-Danlos syndrome
EDV end-diastolic volume
EECG electroencephalography
EEE Eastern equine encephalomyelitis
EEG electroencephalogram; electroencephalography
EENT eye, ear, nose, and throat
EFM electronic fetal monitor
EGD esophagogastroduodenoscopy
EIA enzyme immunoassay
EIB exercise-induced bronchospasm
Ej elbow jerk
EKG electrocardiogram; electrocardiography
ELISA enzyme-linked immunosorbent assay
elix elixir
EM electron microscope; emmetropia, erythema multiforme
emb embolism
EMG electromyogram; electromyography
EMP emphysema
EMR educable mentally retarded; electronic medical record; eye movement record
EMS early morning specimen; electromagnetic spectrum
EN, endo endoscopy
Endo endometriosis
ENG electronystagmography
ENT ear, nose, and throat
EOG electro-oculogram
EOM extraocular muscles; extraocular movement
EOS eosinophils
EP ectopic pregnancy; evoked potential
EPF early pregnancy factor; exophthalmos-producing factor
Epi, EPI epinephrine
epi, epil epilepsy
epid epidemic
epis episiotomy

EPO erythropoietin
EPR electron paramagnetic resonance; emergency physical restraint
EPS extrapyramidal symptoms; exophthalmos-producing substance
ER emergency room; epigastric region
ERCP endoscopic retrograde cholangiopancreatography
ERPF effective renal plasma flow
ERT estrogen replacement therapy; external radiation therapy
ERV expiratory reserve volume
ESD end-systolic dimension
ESPF end-stage pulmonary fibrosis
ESR erythrocyte sedimentation rate
EST electric shock therapy
ESRD end-stage renal disease
ESWL extracorporeal shock-wave lithotripsy
ESV end-systolic volume
ET embryo transfer; enterically transmitted; esotropia; eustachian tube
et and
ETF eustachian tube function
ETI endotracheal intubation
etiol etiology
ETT endotracheal intubation; exercise tolerance test
EU Ehrlich units; emergency unit; etiology unknown
EV esophageal varices
EWB estrogen withdrawal bleeding
ex excision; exercise
exam examination
exp expiration
ext extraction; external
Ez, Ecz eczema

F

F Fahrenheit
FA, FAG fluorescein angiography; fluorescent antibody; fructosamine test
FAS fetal alcohol syndrome
FB foreign body
FBS fasting blood sugar
FCD fibrocystic disease
FDP fibrin-fibrinogen degradation products
FECG fetal electrocardiogram
FEF forced expiratory flow
FESS functional endoscopic sinus surgery
fet fetus
FEV forced expiratory volume
FFA free fatty acids
FH family history
FHR fetal heart rate
FHS fetal heart sounds
FHT fetal heart tones
FIA fluorescent immunoassay; fluoroimmunoassay
Fluor fluoroscopy
FME full mouth extractions
fMRI functional magnetic resonance imaging
FMS fibromyalgia syndrome
FNA fine-needle aspiration
FOBT fecal occult blood test
FPG fasting plasma glucose
fr French (catheter size)
FRC functional residual capacity
FROM full range of motion
FS frozen section, fluoroscopy
FSH follicle-stimulating hormone
FSP fibrin-fibrinogen split products
FSS functional endoscopic sinus surgery
FT family therapy
FTND full-term normal delivery
FTT failure to thrive
FU, F/U follow-up; follow up
FUO fever of unknown origin
Fx fracture

G

G gingiva; glaucoma; glycogen
g gram (see also gm)
G, grav gravida (used to indicate the number of times a woman has been pregnant); pregnancy
GA gastric analysis; general anesthesia
ga gallium
GAD generalized anxiety disorder
GB gallbladder
GBM glomerular basement membrane
GBS gallbladder series; Guillain-Barré syndrome

G-Cs	glucocorticoids
GC	gonorrhea
GCG	glucagon
G&D	growth and development
GD	Graves' disease
GDM	gestational diabetes mellitus
GE	gastroenteritis
GER	gastroesophageal reflux
GERD	gastroesophageal reflux disease
GFR	glomerular filtration rate
GG	gamma globulin
GGT	gamma-glutamyl transferase
GH	growth hormone
GHb	glycohemoglobin
GI	gastrointestinal
GIFT	gamete intrafallopian transfer
GIT	gastrointestinal tract
glau, glc	glaucoma
GLTT	glucose tolerance test
gm	gram
GN	glomerulonephritis
GP	general practice
gr	grain
grav I	pregnancy one; primigravida
GS	general surgery
GSW	gunshot wound
GT	glucose tolerance
GTT	glucose tolerance test
gtt	drops
GU	genitourinary
GVHD	graft-versus host disease
GxT	graded exercise test
GYN, Gyn	gynecology

H

H	hydrogen; hypodermic; hyperopia
h, hr	hour
H & H	hemoglobin and hematocrit
H & L	heart and lungs
H & P	history and physical
HA	hemolytic anemia; histamine
HAA	hepatitis-associated antigen; hepatitis Australia antigen
halluc	hallucination
HASHD	hypertensive arteriosclerotic heart disease
HAV	hepatitis A virus
HB	heart block; hemoglobin; hepatitis B; His bundle
Hb	hemoglobin
HBE	His bundle electrocardiogram
HbF	fetal hemoglobin
HBGM	home blood glucose monitoring
HBOT	hyperbaric oxygen therapy
HBP	high blood pressure
HbS	sickle cell hemoglobin
HBV	hepatitis B virus
HCD	heavy-chain disease
HCG	human chorionic gonadotropin
HCl	hydrochloric acid
HCL	hairy cell leukemia
HCT, Hct, hct	hematocrit
HCV	hepatitis C virus
HCVD	hypertensive cardiovascular disease
HD	hearing distance; heart disease; hemodialysis; hip disarticulation; Hodgkin's disease; Huntington's disease
HDL	high-density lipoproteins
HDN	hemolytic disease of the newborn
HDS	herniated disk syndrome
HE	hereditary elliptocytosis; hyperextension
He	helium; hemorrhage
HEENT	head, eyes, ears, nose, throat
HEM	hematuria
HEM, hemo	hemophilia; hemodialysis
hemat	hematocrit
hemi	hemiplegia
HF	heart failure
HG	hypoglycemia
Hg	mercury
HgA1c	glycohemoglobin test
Hgb	hemoglobin
HH	hiatal hernia
HIE	hypoxic ischemic encephalopathy
Hi, his	histamine
HIS, Histo, histol	histology
HIV	human immunodeficiency virus
HL	Hodgkin's lymphoma
HLA	human leukocyte antigen
HLR	heart-lung resuscitation
HM	hand motion; Holter monitor
HMD	hyaline membrane disease
HMO	health maintenance organization
hmt	hematocrit
HNP	herniated nucleus pulposus
HO	hyperbaric oxygen

HOB head of bed
HP hemipelvectomy; hyperparathyroidism
HPN hypertension
HPO hypothalamic-pituitary-ovarian
HPS hantavirus pulmonary syndrome
HPV human papillomavirus
HR heart rate
HRT hormone replacement therapy
HS hamstring; heavy smoker; herpes simplex; hospital stay
hs, h.s. at bedtime; hour of sleep
HSG hysterosalpingogram, hysterosalpingography
HSV herpes simplex virus
HSV-1 oral herpes simplex virus type 1
HSV-2 herpes simplex virus type 2
HT Hashimoto's thyroiditis; hormone therapy
ht height; hematocrit
HTO high tibial osteotomy
HTN hypertension
HV hallux valgus; hospital visit
HVD hypertensive vascular disease
HVT hyperventilation
Hx history
hypo hypodermic
HYS hysteroscopy
HZ herpes zoster
Hz hertz

I

I intensity of magnetism; iodine
IABP intra-aortic balloon pump
IACP intra-aortic counterpulsation
IADH inappropriate antidiuretic hormone
IASD interatrial septal defect
IBC iron-binding capacity
IBD inflammatory bowel disease
IBS irritable bowel syndrome
IC inspiratory capacity; intermittent claudication; interstitial cystitis
ICCE intracapsular lens extraction
ICCU intensive coronary care unit
ICD implantable cardioverter defibrillator
ICF intracellular fluid
ICP intracranial pressure
ICS ileocecal sphincter; intercostal space
ICSI intracytoplasmic sperm injection
ICT indirect Coombs' test; insulin coma therapy
ict ind icterus index
ICU intensive care unit
I & D incision and drainage, irrigation and debridement
ID infectious disease; intradermal
IDC infiltrating ductal carcinoma; invasive ductal carcinoma
IDD insulin-dependent diabetes
IDDM insulin-dependent diabetes mellitus
IDK internal derangement of the knee
IDS immunity deficiency state
I/E inspiratory-expiratory ratio
IEMG integrated electromyogram
IF interferon; interstitial fluid
IFG impaired fasting glucose
Ig, IG immunoglobulin
IgA immunoglobulin A
IgD immunoglobulin D
IgE immunoglobulin E
IgG immunoglobulin G
IgM immunoglobulin M
IGT impaired glucose tolerance
IH infectious hepatitis; inguinal hernia
IHD ischemic heart disease
IL interleukin
ILC infiltrating lobular carcinoma; invasive lobular carcinoma
ILD interstitial lung diseases
IM infectious mononucleosis; intramuscular
IMAG internal mammary artery graft
IMF idiopathic myelofibrosis
IMI immunofluorescence
IMV intermittent mandatory ventilation
inf inferior; infusion; inflammation
Inflam, Inflamm inflammation
I & O intake and output
IO intestinal obstruction; intraocular
IOD iron-overload disease (hemochromatosis)
IOL intraocular lens
IOP intraocular pressure
IPF idiopathic pulmonary fibrosis
IPG impedance plethysmography

IPPB	intermittent positive-pressure breathing
IQ	intelligence quotient
irrig	irrigation
IS	impingement syndrome; intercostal space
ISG	immune serum globulin
isol	isolation
IT	immunotherapy
ITP	idiopathic thrombocytopenic purpura
IU	international unit
IUD	intrauterine device
IUP	intrauterine pressure
IV	intravenous; intravenously
IVC	inferior vena cava
IVCP	inferior vena cava pressure
IVD	intervertebral disk
IVDA	intravenous drug abuse
IVF	in vitro fertilization
IVFA	intravenous fluorescein angiography
IVP	intravenous pyelogram
IVSD	interventricular septal defect
IVU	intravenous urogram

J

j, jaund	jaundice
jct	junctions
JOD	juvenile-onset diabetes
JRA	juvenile rheumatoid arthritis
Jt	joint
JVP	jugular venous pressure; jugular venous pulse

K

K	potassium
KB	ketone bodies
KCF	key clinical findings
KCl	potassium chloride
KD	knee disarticulation
KE	kinetic energy
kg	kilogram
kj	knee jerk
KO	keep open
KOH	potassium hydrochloride
KS	Kaposi's sarcoma
KUB	kidneys, ureters, bladder
KVO	keep vein open

L

l	liter
L1 through L5	lumbar vertebrae
L & A	light and accommodation
LA	left atrium
lab	laboratory
lac	laceration
LAD	left anterior descending
LADA	latent autoimmune diabetes in adults
LAP	laparoscopy; leucine aminopeptidase
lap	laparotomy
lar, lx	larynx
laryn	laryngitis; laryngoscopy
laser	light amplification by stimulated emission of radiation
LASIK	laser in situ keratomileusis
lat	lateral
LAVH	laparoscopically assisted vaginal hysterectomy
LB	large bowel; low back
lb	pound
LBBB	left bundle branch block
LBP	low back pain
LBW	low birth weight
LBBX	left breast biopsy and examination
LCIS	lobular carcinoma in situ
L & D	labor and delivery
LDD	light-dark discrimination
LDL	low-density lipoproteins
LE	left eye; life expectancy; lower extremity; lupus erythematosus; lymphedema
LEP, LPT	leptin
LES	lower esophageal sphincter
lg	large
LH	luteinizing hormone
LHBD	left heart bypass device
LHF	left-sided heart failure
lig	ligament
liq	liquid
litho	lithotripsy
LLE	lower left extremity
LLL	left lower lobe
LLQ	left lower quadrant
LLSB	left lower sternal border
L/min	liters per minute
LMP	last menstrual period
LNMP	last normal menstrual period

LOC	levels of consciousness; loss of consciousness
LOM	limitation of motion; loss of motion
LOS	length of stay
LP	light perception; lumbar puncture; lumboperitoneal
LPF	low-power field
LPS	lipase
LR	light reaction
LRDKT	living related donor kidney transplant
LRT	lower respiratory tract
LSB	left sternal border
lt	left
LTB	laryngotracheobronchitis
LTC	long-term care
LTH	lactogenic hormone; luteotropic hormone
LUE	left upper extremity
LUL	left upper lobe
LUQ	left upper quadrant
LV	left ventricle
LVH	left ventricle hypertrophy
lymphs	lymphocytes

M

M	meter; murmur; myopia
MABS	monoclonal antibodies
MAO	maximal acid output; monoamine oxidase
MAR	multiple antibiotic resistant
MBC	maximal breathing capacity
MBD	minimal brain damage
mc	millicurie
mcg	microgram
MCH	mean corpuscular hemoglobin
MCHC	mean corpuscular hemoglobin concentration
MCT	mean circulation time
MCV	mean corpuscular volume
MD	macular degeneration; medical doctor; muscular dystrophy
MDS	myelodysplastic syndrome
MDR-TB	multidrug-resistant tuberculosis
ME	middle ear
MED	minimal effective dose; minimal erythema dose
men	meningitis; menstruation
men, mgtis	meningitis
mEq	milliequivalent
MET	metastasis
met	metastasize
M & F	mother and father
MFT	muscle function test
mg	milligram
MG	myasthenia gravis
mgm	milligram
MH	malignant hyperpyrexia; malignant hyperthermia; marital history
MHC	mental health care
MI	mitral insufficiency; myocardial infarction
MICU	medical intensive care unit; mobile intensive care unit
MID	multi-infarct dementia
MIDCAB	minimally invasive direct coronary artery bypass
MIP	maximal inspiratory pressure
ml, mL	milliliter
MLD	median lethal dose
MM	multiple myeloma; malignant melanoma
mm	millimeter
mm Hg	millimeters of mercury
MMR	measles, mumps, and rubella vaccination
MND	motor neuron disease
MNT	medical nutrition therapy
MO	morbid obesity
MODY	maturity-onset diabetes of the young
MOM	milk of magnesia
mono	monocytes
MP	metacarpal-phalangeal
MPD	myofascial pain dysfunction
MR	mental retardation; metabolic rate; mitral regurgitation
MRA	magnetic resonance angiography
MRD	medical record department
MRI	magnetic resonance imaging
MS	mitral stenosis; multiple sclerosis; musculoskeletal; morphine sulfate, magnesium sulfate
MSH	melanocyte-stimulating hormone
MTD	right eardrum
MTS	left eardrum
MTX	methotrexate
MV	mitral valve
MVP	mitral valve prolapse

MY, Myop, myop	myopia
myel	myelogram

N

N & M	nerves and muscles; night and morning
N & T	nose and throat
N & V	nausea and vomiting
NA	not applicable; numerical aperture
Na	sodium
NaCl	sodium chloride
NAD	no acute disease; no apparent distress
NB	newborn
N/C	no complaints
NCV	nerve conduction velocity
NED	no evidence of disease
NEG, neg	negative
Neph	nephron
neuro	neurology
NF	National Formulary; necrotizing fasciitis; neurofibromatosis
N/G	nasogastric (tube)
ng	Neisseria gonorrhoeae
NG	nasogastric tube
NGF	nerve growth factor
NGU	non-gonococcal urethritis
NHL	non-Hodgkin's lymphoma
NI	nuclear imaging
NICU	neurologic intensive care unit, neonatal intensive care unit
NIDDM	non-insulin-dependent diabetes mellitus
NK cell	natural killer cell
NKA	no known allergies
NLP	neurolinguistic programming
NM	nuclear medicine
nm	neuromuscular
NMR	nuclear magnetic resonance
No	number
noc, noct	night
NOFTT	nonorganic failure to thrive
NP	nasopharynx, nurse practitioner
NPC	no point of convergence
NPO	nothing by mouth
NR	no response
NREM	no rapid eye movements
NS	nephrotic syndrome; normal saline; not stated; not sufficient
NSAID	nonsteroidal anti-inflammatory drug
NSR	normal sinus rhythm
nst	nystagmus
NSU	nonspecific urethritis
Nt	neutralization
NTD	neural tube defect
NTG	nitroglycerin
NVA	near visual acuity
NVD	nausea, vomiting diarrhea; neck vein distention
NVS	neural vital signs
NYD	not yet diagnosed
ny	nystagmus

O

OA	osteoarthritis
OAB	overactive bladder
OB	obstetrics
OB-GYN	obstetrics and gynecology
obl	oblique
OBS	organic brain syndrome
Obs	obstetrics
OC	office call; oral contraceptive
OCC	occasional
OCD	obsessive-compulsive disorder; oral cholecystogram
OCT	oral contraceptive therapy
OD	overdose; right eye (oculus dexter)
od	once a day
OGN	obstetric-gynecologic-neonatal
OGTT	oral glucose tolerance test
oint	ointment
OJD	osteoarthritic joint disease
OM	otitis media
OME	otitis media with effusion
OMR	optic mark recognition
OOB	out of bed
O & P	ova and parasites
OP	oropharynx; osteoporosis; outpatient
OPA	oropharyngeal airway
OPD	outpatient department
Ophth	ophthalmic
OPT	outpatient
OPV	oral poliovirus vaccine
OR	operating room
ORIF	open reduction internal fixation
ORT	oral rehydration therapy
Orth	orthopedics

OS	left eye (oculus sinister)
os	mouth
OSA	obstructive sleep apnea
OT	occupational therapy; old tuberculin
OTC	over-the-counter
Oto	otology
OU	each eye (oculus unitas)
oz	ounce
OXT	oxytocin

P

P	percussion; phosphorus; physiology; posterior; presbyopia; progesterone; prolactin; pulse
P & A	percussion and auscultation
PA	pernicious anemia; physician's assistant; polyarteritis; posteroanterior; pulmonary artery
PA, pa	pathology
PAC	premature atrial contraction
PACAB	port-access coronary artery bypass
PAD	peripheral artery disease
PADP	pulmonary artery diastolic pressure
PAMP	pulmonary arterial mean pressure
Pap	Papanicolaou smear
PAR	perennial allergic rhinitis; postanesthetic recovery
PARA	prior pregnancies resulting in viable births, paraplegic
paren	parenteral (through the skin or mucous membrane)
PASP	pulmonary artery systolic pressure
PAT	paroxysmal atrial tachycardia
Path	pathology
Pb	presbyopia
PBC	primary biliary cirrhosis
PBI	protein-bound iodine
PBP	progressive bulbar palsy
PBT_4	protein-bound thyroxine
PC	pheochromocytoma; prostate cancer
p.c.	after meals
PCA	prostate cancer
PCKD, PKD	polycystic kidney disease
PCNL	percutaneous nephrolithotomy
PCO, PCOS	polycystic ovary syndrome
PCP	*Pneumocystis carinii* pneumonia, primary care physician or provider
PCT	plasmacrit time
PCU	progressive care unit
PCV	packed cell volume
PD	interpupillary distance; Parkinson's disease; peritoneal dialysis; postural drainage
PDA	patent ductus arteriosus
PDD	pervasive developmental disorder
PDL	periodontal ligament
PDT	photodynamic therapy
PE	physical examination; preeclampsia
PEA	pulseless electrical activity
Peds	pediatrics
PEEP	positive end-expiratory pressure
PEF	peak expiratory flow rate
PEG	pneumoencephalogram; pneumoencephalography
PEL	permissible exposure limit
per	by; through
PERLA	pupils equally reactive (responsive) to light and accommodation
PERRLA	pupils equal, round, react (respond) to light and accommodation
PET	positron emission tomography; preeclamptic toxemia
PFT	pulmonary function tests
PG	pregnant; prostaglandin
PGH	pituitary growth hormone
PGL	persistent generalized lymphadenopathy
PH	past history; personal history; public health
pH	acidity; hydrogen ion concentration
PHN	postherpetic neuralgia
PI	present illness
PICU	pulmonary intensive care unit; pediatric intensive care unit
PID	pelvic inflammatory disease
PIF	peak inspiratory flow
PIH	pregnancy-induced hypertension
PK	pyruvate kinase; pyruvate kinase deficiency
PKD	polycystic kidney disease
PKR	partial knee replacement
PKU	phenylketonuria
PL	light perception
pl	placenta
PLC	platelet count
PLMS	periodic limb movements in sleep
PLS	primary lateral sclerosis
PLTS	platelets

PM evening or afternoon; physical medicine; polymyositis; postmortem
PMA progressive muscular atrophy
PMDD premenstrual dysphoric disorder
PMH past medical history
PMI point of maximal impulse
PMN polymorphonuclear neutrophils
PMP past menstrual period; previous menstrual period
PMR physical medicine and rehabilitation; polymyalgia rheumatica
PMS premenstrual syndrome
PMT premenstrual tension
PMVS prolapsed mitral valve syndrome
PN peripheral neuropathy; postnatal
Pn, PNA, pneu pneumonia
PND paroxysmal nocturnal dyspnea; postnasal drip
PNH postnatal headache
Pno pneumothorax
PNP peripheral neuropathy
PNS parasympathetic nervous system; peripheral nervous system
PO, p.o. by mouth; orally; phone order; postoperative
POC products of conception
polys polymorphonuclear leukocytes
POMR problem-oriented medical record
POS polycystic ovary syndrome
pos positive
post-op postoperatively
PP placenta previa; postpartum; postprandial (after meals); pulse pressure
ppb parts per billion
PPBS postprandial blood sugar
PPD purified protein derivative
ppm parts per million
PPS postperfusion syndrome; postpolio syndrome; progressive systemic sclerosis
PPT partial prothrombin time
PPV positive-pressure ventilation
PR peripheral resistance; pulse rate
Pr presbyopia; prism
pr by rectum
PRA plasma renin activity
PRC packed red cells
PRE progressive restrictive exercise
preg pregnant
preop preoperative
prep prepare
PRK photo-refractive keratectomy
p.r.n. as needed
proct proctology
prog, progn prognosis
PROM passive range of motion; premature rupture of membranes
pro time prothrombin time
PRRE pupils round, regular, and equal
Prx prognosis
Ps psoriasis
PSA prostate-specific antigen
PSS progressive systemic sclerosis; physiologic saline solution
psych psychiatry
PT paroxysmal tachycardia; physical therapy; prothrombin time
pt patient; pint
PTA percutaneous transluminal angioplasty
PTE pulmonary thromboembolism
PTC percutaneous transhepatic cholangiography
PTCA percutaneous transluminal coronary angioplasty
PTD permanent and total disability
PTE parathyroid extract; pulmonary thromboemboliam
PTH parathyroid hormone; parathormone
PTSD post-traumatic stress disorder
PTT partial thromboplastin time; prothrombin time
PU peptic ulcer; pregnancy urine; prostatic urethra
PUD peptic ulcer disease; pulmonary disease
pul pulmonary
P & V pyloroplasty and vagotomy
PV peripheral vascular; plasma volume; polycythemia vera
PVC premature ventricular contraction
PVD peripheral vascular disease
PVE prosthetic valve endocarditis
PVOD peripheral vascular occlusive disease
PVS persistent vegetative state

PVT paroxysmal ventricular tachycardia
pvt private
PWB partial weight-bearing
PWP pulmonary wedge pressure
Px prognosis

Q

q every
qd, q.d. every day
qh, q.h every hour
q 2 h every 2 hours
QID, qid, q.i.d. four times a day
qm every morning
qn every night
qns quantity not sufficient
qod every other day
qoh every other hour
QOL quality of life
qs quantity sufficient
qt quart; quiet
q.q. each
quad quadrant, quadriplegia, quadriplegic

R

R rectal; respiration; right
RA refractory anemia; rheumatoid arthritis; right arm; right atrium
rad radiation absorbed dose
RAF rheumatoid arthritis factor
RAI radioactive iodine
RAIU radioactive iodine uptake determination
RAS reticular activating system
RAST radioallergosorbent
RAT radiation therapy
RBBB right bundle branch block
RBC red blood cell; red blood count
RBCV red blood cell volume
RBE relative biologic effects
RCA right coronary artery
RD respiratory distress; retinal detachment
RDA recommended daily allowance
RDS respiratory distress syndrome
RE right eye
reg regular
rehab rehabilitation
rem roentgen-equivalent-man
REM sleep rapid eye movement sleep
RER renal excretion rate
resp respiration
RF renal failure; respiratory failure; rheumatoid factor; rheumatic fever
RFS renal function study
RH right hand
RHD rheumatic heart disease
Rh neg Rhesus factor negative
Rh pos Rhesus factor positive
RIA radioimmunoassay
RICE rest, ice, compression, elevate
Rick rickettsia
RIST radioimmunosorbent
RK radial keratotomy
RL right leg
RLC residual lung capacity
RLD related living donor
RLE right lower extremity
RLL right lower lobe
RLQ right lower quadrant
RLS restless legs syndrome
RM respiratory movement
RMD repetitive motion disorder
RML right mediolateral
RMSF Rocky Mountain spotted fever
RNA ribonucleic acid
RND radical neck dissection
R/O rule out
ROA radiopaque agents
ROM range of motion; rupture of membranes
ROP retinopathy of prematurity
ROPS roll over protection structures
ROS review of systems
ROT right occipitis transverse
RP radiopharmaceuticals; Raynaud's phenomenon; relapsing polychondritis; retrograde pyelogram
RPF renal plasma flow
RPG retrograde pyelogram
rpm revolutions per minute
RPO right posterior oblique
RPR rapid plasma reagin
RQ respiratory quotient
R & R rate and rhythm
RR recovery room; respiratory rate
RSD repetitive stress disorder

RSDS reflex sympathetic dystrophy syndrome
RSHF right-sided heart failure
RSI repetitive stress injuries
RSR regular sinus rhythm
RSV right subclavian vein
RT radiation therapy; renal transplantation; respiratory therapy
rt right; routine
RTA renal tubular acidosis
rt lat right lateral
rtd retarded
RU roentgen unit; routine urinalysis
RUE right upper extremity
RUL right upper lobe
RUQ right upper quadrant
RV residual volume; right ventricle
RVG radionuclide ventriculogram
RVH right ventricular hypertrophy
RVS relative value schedule
RW ragweed
Rx prescription; take; therapy; treatment

S

s̄ without
S-A sinoatrial node
S & A sugar and acetone
SA salicylic acid; sinoatrial; sperm analysis; surgeon's assistant
SAAT serum aspartate aminotransferase
SAB spontaneous abortion
SACH self-assessed change in health
SAD seasonal affective disorder
SAH subarachnoid hemorrhage
SAL sensorineural activity level; sterility assurance level; suction-assisted lipectomy
Sal, Salm salmonella
SALP salpingectomy; salpingography; serum alkaline phosphatase
Salpx salpingectomy
SAM self-administered medication program
SARS severe acute respiratory syndrome
SAS short arm splint; sleep apnea syndrome; social adjustment scale; subarachnoid space
SB small bowl; spina bifida; stillbirth; suction biopsy
SBE subacute bacterial endocarditis
SBO small bowel obstruction
SC, sc, subq subcutaneous
SC Snellen chart; spinal cord
SCA sickle cell anemia
SCC squamous cell carcinoma
SCD sudden cardiac death, scleroderma
schiz schizophrenia
SCI spinal cord injury
SCID severe combined immune deficiency
SCT sickle cell trait
SD septal defect; shoulder disarticulation; spontaneous delivery; standard deviation; sudden death
SDAT senile dementia of Alzheimer's type
SDM standard deviation of the mean
SDS sudden death syndrome
sec second
SED sub-erythema dose
sed rate sedimentation rate
seg segmented neutrophils
SEM scanning electron microscopy
semi half
SES subcutaneous electric stimulation
sev sever; severed
SF scarlet fever; spinal fluid
SG serum globulin; skin graft
SGA small for gestational age
SH serum hepatitis; sex hormone; social history
sh shoulder
SI saturation index
SICU surgical intensive care unit
SIDS sudden infant death syndrome
sig let it be labeled
SIRS systemic inflammatory response syndrome
SIS saline infusion sonohysterography
SISI short increment sensitivity index
SLE slit-lamp examination; systemic lupus erythematosus
SLND sentinel lymph node dissection
SLPS serum lipase
SM simple mastectomy
sm small
SMA sequential multiple analysis

SMAC	sequential multiple analysis computer
SMG	senile macular degeneration
SMR	submucous resection
SMRR	submucous resection and rhinoplasty
SNR	signal-to-noise ratio
SNRI	serotonin and norepinephrine reuptake inhibitor
SNS	sensory nervous system; sympathetic nervous system
SO	salpingo-oophorectomy
SOAP	medical notation format: subjective, objective, assessment, plan; symptoms, observations, assessments, plan
SOB	shortness of breath
SOM	serous otitis media
SONO	sonography
SOP	standard operating procedure
sos	if necessary
spec	specimen
SPECT	single photon emission computerized tomography
SPF	skin protective factor; sun protective factor
sp gr	specific gravity
SPP	suprapubic prostatectomy
SPR	scanned projection radiography
SQ	subcutaneous
SR	sedimentation rate; stimulus response; system review
SRS	smoker's respiratory syndrome
ss	half
SS	signs and symptoms; Sjögren's syndrome; soap solution
SSE	soap suds enema
SSRI	selective serotonin reuptake inhibitor
SSU	sterile supply unit
ST	esotropia; sclerotherapy
staph	staphylococcus
stat	immediately
STD	sexually transmitted disease; skin test dose
STH	somatotropic hormone
STK	streptokinase
strab	strabismus
strep	streptococcus
STS	serologic test for syphilis
STSG	split thickness skin graft
subcu, sub-Q	subcutaneous
SUI	stress urinary incontinence
supp	suppository
surg	surgical; surgery
SVC	superior vena cava
SVD	spontaneous vaginal delivery
SVG	saphenous vein graft
SVN	small volume nebulizer
SX	symptom reduction
Sx	symptoms
Sz	seizure

T

T	temperature; thrombosis
T1 through T12	thoracic vertebrae
T3	triiodothyronine
T4	thyroxine
T & A	tonsillectomy and adenoidectomy
TA, TAB	therapeutic abortion
tab	tablet
TACT	target air-enema computed tomography
TAF	tumor angiogenesis factor
TAH	total abdominal hysterectomy
TAH-BSO	total abdominal hysterectomy with bilateral salpingo-oophorectomy
TAO	thromboangiitis obliterans
TB	tuberculosis
TBD	total body density
TBF	total body fat
TBG	thyroxine-binding globulin
TBI	thyroxine-binding index
TBW	total body weight
TCD	transcranial doppler
TCDB	turn, cough, deep breathe
TCP	time care profile
TD	total disability; transdermal
TDM	therapeutic drug monitoring
TDT	tone decay test
TE	tetanus; tonsillectomy
TEE	transesophageal echocardiography
temp	temperature
TEN	toxic epidermal necrolysis
TENS	transcutaneous electrical nerve stimulation
TES	treadmill exercise score
TFS	thyroid function studies
TGA	transposition of great arteries

THA	total hip arthroplasty
THR	total hip replacement
TIA	transient ischemic attack
TIA-IR	transient ischemic attack incomplete recovery
TIBC	total iron-binding capacity
TID, tid, t.i.d.	times interval difference; three times a day
tinct	tincture
TJA	total joint arthroplasty
TKA	total knee arthroplasty
TKO	to keep open
TKR	total knee replacement
TLC	tender loving care; total lung capacity
TLE	temporal lobe epilepsy
TM	temporomandibular; tympanic membrane
TMD	temporomandibular disease; temporomandibular disorder
TMJ	temporomandibular joint
TMs	tympanic membranes
Tn	normal intraocular tension
TND	term normal delivery
TNF	tumor necrosis factor
TNI	total nodal irradiation
TNM	tumor, nodes, metastases
TO	telephone order
top	topically
TP	testosterone propionate; total protein
TPA, tPA	tissue plasminogen activator; *treponema pallidum* agglutination
TPBF	total pulmonary blood flow
TPI	*Treponema pallidum* immobilization
TPN	total parenteral nutrition
TPR	temperature, pulse, respiration
TPUR	transperineal urethral resection
TR	tuberculin residue
tr	tincture
trach	trachea; tracheostomy
TRBF	total renal blood flow
TRH	thyrotropin-releasing hormone
Trich	trichomonas
TS	Tourette syndrome
TSD	Tay-Sachs disease
TSE	testicular self-examination
TSH	thyroid stimulating hormone
TSP	total serum protein
TSS	toxic shock syndrome
TST	thallium stress test; tuberculin skin test
TT	thrombin time
TTH	thyrotropic hormone
TULIP	transurethral ultrasound-guided laser-induced proctectomy
TUMT	transurethral microwave therapy
TUR	transurethral resection
TURP	transurethral resection of prostate; prostatectomy
TV	tidal volume; tricuspid valve
TVH	total vaginal hysterectomy
TW	tap water
TWE	tap water enema
Tx	traction; treatment

U

U	units
U/A, UA	urinalysis
UB	urinary bladder
UC	ulcerative colitis; urine culture; uterine contractions
UCD	usual childhood diseases
UCG	urinary chorionic gonadotropin; uterine chorionic gonadotropin
UCR	unconditioned reflex
UE	upper extremity
UFR	uroflowmeter; uroflowmetry
UG	upper gastrointestinal; urogenital
UGI	upper gastrointestinal
UK	unknown
UL	upper lobe
ULQ	upper left quadrant
umb	umbilical; umbilicus
UN	urea nitrogen
ung	ointment
UOQ	upper outer quadrant
UPP	urethral pressure profile
UR	upper respiratory
ur	urine
URD	upper respiratory disease
URI	upper respiratory infection
urol	urology
URQ	upper right quadrant
URT	upper respiratory tract
US	ultrasonic; ultrasonography
USP	United States Pharmacopeia
UTI	urinary tract infection

UV	ultraviolet
UVJ	ureterovesical junction

V

V	ventral; visual acuity
VA	vacuum aspiration; visual acuity
vag	vaginal
VAS	vasectomy
VB	viable birth
VBAC	vaginal birth after cesarean
VBP	ventricular premature beat
VC	acuity of color vision; vena cava; vital capacity
VCUG	voiding cystourethrogram
VD	venereal disease
VDG	venereal disease, gonorrhea
VDH	valvular disease of heart
VDRL	Venereal Disease Research Laboratory
VDS	venereal disease, syphilis
VE	visual efficiency
Vent, ventr	ventral
VEP	visual evoked potential
VER	visual evoked response
VF	ventricular fibrillation; visual field; vocal fremitus
V-fib	ventricular fibrillation
VG	ventricular gallop
VH	vaginal hysterectomy
VHD	valvular heart disease; ventricular heart disease
VI	volume index
vit cap	vital capacity
VLDL	very-low-density lipoprotein
VP	venipuncture; venous pressure
V & P	vagotomy and pyloroplasty
VPC	ventricular premature contraction
VPRC	volume of packed red cells
VS, vs	vital signs
VSD	ventricular septal defect
VSZ	varicella
VTAs	vascular targeting agents
VV	varicose veins
VVF	vesicovaginal fistula
VZV	varicella-zoster virus (chickenpox)

W

W	water
WA	while awake
WB	weight-bearing; whole blood
WBC	white blood cell; white blood count
W/C, w/c	wheelchair
wd	wound
WD, w/d	well-developed
WDWN	well-developed, well-nourished
wf	white female
w/n	well nourished
WNL	within normal limits
w/o	without
WR, W.r.	Wassermann reaction
wt	weight
w/v	weight by volume

X

X	xerophthalmia
x	multiplied by; times
XDP	xeroderma pigmentosum
XM	cross-match
XR	x-ray
XT	exotropia
XU	excretory urogram

Y

y/o	year(s) old
YOB	year of birth
yr	year

Z

Z	atomic number; no effect; zero
zyg	zygote

Appendix C

GLOSSARY OF PATHOLOGY AND PROCEDURES

A

abdominal computed tomography: a radiographic procedure that produces a detailed cross-section of the tissue structure within the abdomen.

abdominal ultrasound: a noninvasive test used to visualize internal organs by using very high frequency sound waves.

abdominocentesis (ab-**dom**-ih-noh-sen-**TEE**-sis)**:** the surgical puncture of the abdominal cavity to remove fluid.

ablation (ab-**LAY**-shun)**:** the removal of a body part or the destruction of its function.

abortion (ah-**BOR**-shun)**:** the interruption or termination of pregnancy before the fetus is viable.

abrasion (ah-**BRAY**-zhun)**:** an injury in which superficial layers of skin are scraped or rubbed away.

abruptio placentae (ab-**RUP**-shee-oh plah-**SEN**-tee)**:** a disorder in which the placenta separates from the uterine wall before the birth of the fetus.

abscess (**AB**-sess)**:** a closed pocket containing pus caused by a bacterial infection.

absence seizure: a brief disturbance in brain function in which there is a loss of awareness often described as a staring episode.

ACE inhibitors: medications administered to treat hypertension and congestive heart failure.

acetaminophen (ah-**seet**-ah-**MIN**-oh-fen)**:** analgesic that reduces pain and fever, but does not relieve inflammation.

Achilles tendinitis (**ten**-dih-**NIGH**-tis)**:** inflammation of the Achilles tendon caused by excessive stress being placed on that tendon.

acne vulgaris (**ACK**-nee vul-**GAY**-ris)**:** a chronic inflammatory disease that is characterized by pustular eruptions of the skin caused by an overproduction of sebum around the hair shaft.

acoustic neuroma (new-**ROH**-mah)**:** a brain tumor that develops adjacent to the cranial nerve running from the brain to the inner ear.

acquired immunity: immunity obtained by having had a contagious disease.

acquired immunodeficiency syndrome: the advanced stage of an HIV infection.

acromegaly (**ack**-roh-**MEG**-ah-lee)**:** enlargement of the extremities caused by excessive secretion of growth hormone after puberty.

acrophobia (**ack**-roh-**FOH**-bee-ah)**:** an excessive fear of heights.

actinic keratosis (ack-**TIN**-ick **kerr**-ah-**TOH**-sis)**:** a precancerous skin growth that occurs on sun-damaged skin.

activities of daily living (ADL)**:** include bathing, grooming, brushing teeth, eating, and dressing.

acupressure (**AK**-que-**presh**-ur)**:** a traditional Chinese touch therapy involving finger pressure applied to specific areas of the body.

acupuncture (**AK**-que-**punk**-tyour)**:** a traditional Chinese medical practice using very thin acupuncture needles inserted into specific points of the body.

acute necrotizing ulcerative gingivitis: an abnormal growth of bacteria in the mouth.

acute renal failure: sudden onset of kidney failure that may be caused by the kidneys not receiving enough blood to filter.

acute respiratory distress syndrome: a life-threatening condition in which inflammation in the lungs and fluid in the alveoli lead to low levels of oxygen in the blood.

addiction: compulsive, uncontrollable dependence on a substance, habit, or practice.

Addison's disease (**AD**-ih-sonz)**:** a condition that occurs when the adrenal glands do not produce enough cortisol or aldosterone.

adenectomy (**ad**-eh-**NECK**-toh-mee)**:** surgical removal of a gland.

adenitis (**ad**-eh-**NIGH**-tis)**:** inflammation of a gland.

adenocarcinoma (**ad**-eh-noh-**kar**-sih-**NOH**-mah)**:** carcinoma derived from glandular tissue.

adenoma (**ad**-eh-**NOH**-mah)**:** benign tumor that arises from, or resembles, glandular tissue.

adenomalacia (**ad**-eh-noh-mal-**LAY**-shee-ah)**:** abnormal softening of a gland.

adenosclerosis (**ad**-eh-noh-skleh-**ROH**-sis)**:** abnormal hardening of a gland.

adenosis (**ad**-eh-**NOH**-sis)**:** any disease or condition of a gland.

adhesion (ad-**HEE**-zhun)**:** a band of fibrous tissue that holds structures together abnormally.

adjuvant therapy (**AD**-jeh-vant)**:** cancer treatment used after the primary treatments have been completed to decrease the chance that a cancer will recur.

adrenalitis (ah-**dree**-nal-**EYE**-tis)**:** inflammation of the adrenal glands.

adverse drug reaction: an undesirable reaction that accompanies the principal response for which the drug was taken.

aerophagia (**ay**-er-oh-**FAY**-jee-ah)**:** excessive swallowing of air while eating or drinking.

age spots: discolorations caused by sun exposure.

agoraphobia (**ag**-oh-rah-**FOH**-bee-ah)**:** an excessive fear of environments where the person fears a panic attack might occur.

airborne transmission: occurs through contact with contaminated respiratory droplets spread by a cough or sneeze.

airway inflammation: the swelling and clogging of the bronchial tubes with mucus.

airway obstruction: occurs when food or a foreign object partially or completely blocks the airway and prevents air from entering or leaving the lungs.

albinism (**AL**-bih-niz-um)**:** a genetic condition characterized by a deficiency or absence of pigment in the skin, hair, and irises.

albuminuria (**al**-byou-mih-**NEW**-ree-ah)**:** the presence of the protein albumin in the urine.

alcoholism (**AL**-koh-hol-izm)**:** chronic alcohol dependence with specific signs and symptoms upon withdrawal.

aldosteronism (al-**DOSS**-teh-roh-**niz**-em)**:** an abnormality of electrolyte balance caused by excessive secretion of aldosterone.

allergen (**AL**-er-jen)**:** a substance that produces an allergic response in an individual.

allergic reaction: occurs when the body's immune system reacts to a harmless allergen as if it were a dangerous invader.

allergic rhinitis (rye-**NIGH**-tis)**:** an allergic reaction to airborne allergens.

allergy: an overreaction by the body to a particular antigen.

allogenic bone marrow transplant (**al**-oh-**JEN**-ick)**:** a transplant in which the recipient receives bone marrow from a compatible donor.

allopathic medicine (**ah**-low-**PAH**-thick)**:** conventional medical practices and systems of health care.

alopecia (**al**-oh-**PEE**-shee-ah)**:** the partial or complete loss of hair, most commonly on the scalp.

alopecia areata: an autoimmune disorder that attacks the hair follicles, causing well-defined bald areas on the scalp or elsewhere on the body.

alopecia totalis: an uncommon condition characterized by the loss of all the hair on the scalp.

alopecia universalis: the total loss of hair on all parts of the body.

alternative medicine: a general term for practices and systems of health care used in place of allopathic medicine.

Alzheimer's disease (**ALTZ**-high-merz)**:** a group of disorders involving the parts of the brain that control thought, memory, and language.

amblyopia (**am**-blee-**OH**-pee-ah)**:** dimness of vision or the partial loss of sight, especially in one eye, without detectable disease of the eye.

amenorrhea (ah-**men**-oh-**REE**-ah *or* ay-**men**-oh-**REE**-ah)**:** the abnormal absence of menstrual periods for three months or more.

ametropia (**am**-eh-**TROH**-pee-ah)**:** any error of refraction in which images do not focus properly on the retina.

amnesia (am-**NEE**-zee-ah)**:** a memory disturbance marked by a total or partial inability to recall past experiences.

amniocentesis (**am**-nee-oh-sen-**TEE**-sis)**:** a surgical puncture to remove amniotic fluid to evaluate fetal health and to diagnose certain congenital disorders.

amyotrophic lateral sclerosis (ah-**my**-oh-**TROH**-fick)**:** a rapidly progressive neurological disease that attacks the nerve cells responsible for controlling voluntary muscles.

anal fissure: a small crack-like sore in the skin of the anus that can cause severe pain during a bowel movement.

analgesic (**an**-al-**JEE**-zick)**:** a medication that relieves pain without affecting consciousness.

anaphylaxis (**an**-ah-fih-**LACK**-sis)**:** a severe, systemic response to an allergen.

anaplasia (**an**-ah-**PLAY**-zee-ah)**:** a change in the structure of cells and in their orientation to each other.

anastomosis (ah-**nas**-toh-**MOH**-sis)**:** a surgical connection between two hollow or tubular structures.

andropause (**AN**-droh-pawz)**:** marked by the decrease of the male hormone testosterone, gradually beginning in the late 40s and progressing very gradually over several decades.

anemia (ah-**NEE**-mee-ah)**:** a disorder characterized by lower than normal levels of red blood cells in the blood.

anesthesia (**an**-es-**THEE**-zee-ah)**:** the absence of normal sensation, especially sensitivity to pain.

anesthetic (**an**-es-**THET**-ick)**:** medication used to induce anesthesia.

aneurysm (**AN**-you-rizm)**:** a localized weak spot or balloon-like enlargement of the wall of an artery.

aneurysmectomy (**an**-you-riz-**MECK**-toh-mee)**:** the surgical removal of an aneurysm.

aneurysmorrhaphy (**an**-you-riz-**MOR**-ah-fee)**:** surgical suturing of an aneurysm.

angina (an-**JIGH**-nah)**:** episodes of severe chest pain due to inadequate blood flow to the myocardium.

angiogenesis (**an**-jee-oh-**JEN**-eh-sis)**:** the process through which the tumor supports its growth by creating its own blood supply.

angiogram (**AN**-jee-oh-**gram**)**:** the film produced by angiography.

angiography (**an**-jee-**OG**-rah-fee)**:** a radiographic study of the blood vessels after the injection of a contrast medium.

angioplasty (**AN**-jee-oh-**plas**-tee)**:** mechanically widening a narrowed or obstructed blood vessel.

angiostenosis (**an**-jee-oh-steh-**NOH**-sis)**:** abnormal narrowing of a blood vessel.

anhidrosis (**an**-high-**DROH**-sis)**:** the abnormal condition of lacking sweat in response to heat.

anisocoria (**an**-ih-so-**KOH**-ree-ah)**:** a condition in which the pupils are unequal in size.

ankylosing spondylitis (**ang**-kih-**LOH**-sing **spon**-dih-**LYE**-tis)**:** a form of rheumatoid arthritis that primarily causes inflammation of the joints between the vertebrae.

ankylosis (**ang**-kih-**LOH**-sis)**:** the loss or absence of mobility in a joint due to disease, injury, or a surgical procedure.

anomaly (ah-**NOM**-ah-lee)**:** a deviation from what is regarded as normal.

anorexia (**an**-oh-**RECK**-see-ah)**:** the loss of appetite for food, especially when caused by disease.

anorexia nervosa (**an**-oh-**RECK**-see-ah ner-**VOH**-sah)**:** an eating disorder characterized by a false perception of body appearance that leads to a refusal to maintain a normal body weight.

anoscopy (ah-**NOS**-koh-pee)**:** the visual examination of the anal canal and lower rectum.

anovulation (**an**-ov-you-**LAY**-shun)**:** the absence of ovulation when it would normally be expected.

anoxia (ah-**NOCK**-see-ah)**:** the absence of oxygen from the body's tissues or organs despite adequate flow of blood.

antacids: medications to relieve indigestion or help peptic ulcers heal by neutralizing stomach acids.

anthracosis (**an**-thrah-**KOH**-sis)**:** the form of pneumoconiosis caused by coal dust in the lungs.

anthrax (an-thraks)**:** a contagious disease that can be transmitted through livestock.

antiangiogenesis: cancer treatment that disrupts the blood supply to the tumor.

antiarrhythmic (**an**-tih-ah-**RITH**-mick)**:** medication administered to control irregularities of the heartbeat.

antibiotic-resistant bacteria: develops when an antibiotic fails to kill all of the bacteria it targets. When this occurs, the surviving bacteria become resistant to that particular drug.

antibiotics: medications capable of inhibiting growth or killing pathogenic bacteria.

antibody (**AN**-tih-**bod**-ee)**:** a disease-fighting protein created by the immune system in response to the presence of a specific antigen.

anticoagulant (**an**-tih-koh-**AG**-you-lant)**:** medication that slows coagulation and prevents new clots from forming.

anticonvulsant (**an**-tih-kon-**VUL**-sant)**:** medication that prevents seizures.

antidepressant: medications administered to prevent or relieve depression.

antiemetic (**an**-tih-ee-**MET**-ick)**:** medication administered to prevent or relieve nausea and vomiting.

antifungal (**an**-tih-**FUNG**-gul)**:** an agent that destroys or inhibits the growth of fungi.

antigen (**AN**-tih-jen)**:** any substance that the body regards as being foreign.

antihistamines: medications administered to block and control allergic reactions.

antihypertensive (**an**-tih-**high**-per-**TEN**-siv)**:** medication administered to lower blood pressure.

anti-inflammatory: medication administered to relieve inflammation and pain.

antineoplastic (**an**-tih-nee-oh-**PLAS**-tick)**:** medication that blocks the development, growth, or proliferation of malignant cells.

antipsychotic drug (**an**-tih-sigh-**KOT**-ick)**:** administered to treat symptoms of severe disorders of thinking and mood that are associated with neurological and psychiatric illnesses.

antipyretic (**an**-tih-pye-**RET**-ick)**:** medication administered to prevent or reduce fever.

antispasmodic: medication administered to suppress smooth muscle contractions.

antithyroid drug: a medication administered to slow the ability of the thyroid gland to produce thyroid hormones.

antitussive (**an**-tih-**TUSS**-iv)**:** medication administered to prevent or relieve coughing.

antiviral drug (**an**-tih-**VYE**-ral)**:** medication administered to treat viral infections or to provide temporary immunity.

anuria (ah-**NEW**-ree-ah)**:** the absence of urine formation by the kidneys.

anxiety disorders: mental conditions characterized by excessive, irrational dread of everyday situations, or fear that is out of proportion to the real danger in a situation.

anxiolytic drug (**ang**-zee-oh-**LIT**-ick)**:** medication administered to temporarily relieve anxiety and reduce tension.

Apgar score: an evaluation of a newborn infant's physical status.

aphasia (ah-**FAY**-zee-ah)**:** loss of the ability to speak, write, and/or comprehend the written or spoken word.

aphonia (ah-**FOH**-nee-ah)**:** the loss of the ability of the larynx to produce normal speech sounds.

aphthous ulcers (**AF**-thus **UL**-serz)**:** gray-white pits with a red border in the soft tissues lining the mouth.

aplasia (ah-**PLAY**-zee-ah)**:** the defective development or congenital absence of an organ or tissue.

aplastic anemia (ay-**PLAS**-tick ah-**NEE**-mee-ah)**:** a condition marked by the absence of all formed blood elements.

apnea (**AP**-nee-ah *or* ap-**NEE**-ah)**:** the absence of spontaneous respiration.

appendectomy (**ap**-en-**DECK**-toh-mee)**:** surgical removal of the appendix.

appendicitis (ah-**pen**-dih-**SIGH**-tis)**:** inflammation of the appendix.

arrhythmia (ah-**RITH**-mee-ah)**:** a loss of the normal rhythm of the heartbeat.

arterial blood gas analysis: a test to measure the pH, oxygen, and carbon dioxide levels of arterial blood.

arterial stick: the puncture of an artery to obtain arterial blood.

arteriectomy (**ar**-teh-ree-**ECK**-toh-mee)**:** surgical removal of part of an artery.

arteriomalacia (ar-**tee**-ree-oh-mah-**LAY**-shee-ah)**:** abnormal softening of the walls of an artery or arteries.

arterionecrosis (ar-**tee**-ree-oh-neh-**KROH**-sis)**:** tissue death of an artery or arteries.

arteriosclerosis (ar-**tee**-ree-oh-skleh-**ROH**-sis)**:** abnormal hardening of the walls of an artery or arteries.

arteriostenosis (ar-**tee**-ree-oh-steh-**NOH**-sis)**:** abnormal narrowing of an artery or arteries.

arteriovenous malformation (ar-**tee**-ree-oh-**VEE**-nus)**:** an abnormal connection between the arteries and veins in the brain; may cause a hemorrhagic stroke.

arthralgia (ar-**THRAL**-jee-ah)**:** pain in one or more joints.

arthritis (ar-**THRIGH**-tis)**:** an inflammatory condition of one or more joints.

arthrocentesis (**ar**-throh-sen-**TEE**-sis)**:** surgical puncture of the joint space to remove synovial fluid for analysis.

arthrodesis (**ar**-throh-**DEE**-sis)**:** a surgical procedure to stiffen a joint.

arthrolysis (ar-**THROL**-ih-sis)**:** surgical loosening of an ankylosed joint.

arthroplasty (**AR**-throh-**plas**-tee)**:** surgical repair of a damaged joint; also the surgical replacement of a joint with an artificial joint.

arthrosclerosis (**ar**-throh-skleh-**ROH**-sis)**:** stiffness of the joints, especially in the elderly.

arthroscopic surgery (**ar**-throh-**SKOP**-ick)**:** a minimally invasive procedure for the treatment of the interior of a joint.

arthroscopy (ar-**THROS**-koh-pee)**:** visual examination of the internal structure of a joint using an arthroscope.

artificial insemination: a technique in which sperm from a woman's partner or donor are introduced into the vagina or uterus during the ovulatory phase of her menstrual cycle.

artificial pacemaker: electronic device used primarily as treatment for bradycardia or atrial fibrillation.

asbestosis (**ass**-beh-**STOH**-sis)**:** the form of pneumoconiosis caused by asbestos particles in the lungs.

ascites (ah-**SIGH**-teez)**:** an abnormal accumulation of serous fluid in the peritoneal cavity.

asphyxia (ass-**FICK**-see-ah)**:** the loss of consciousness that occurs when the body cannot get the oxygen it needs to function.

aspiration pneumonia (**ass**-pih-**RAY**-shun)**:** pneumonia caused by a foreign substance, such as vomit, being inhaled into the lungs.

aspirin: medication that may be recommended in a very small daily dose to reduce the risk of a heart attack or stroke by slightly reducing the ability of the blood to clot.

assisted reproductive technology: techniques used to aid an infertile couple in achieving a viable pregnancy.

assistive listening device: a device that transmits, processes, or amplifies sound, and can be used with or without a hearing aid.

asthma (**AZ**-mah)**:** a chronic inflammatory disease of the bronchial tubes.

astigmatism (ah-**STIG**-mah-tizm)**:** a condition in which the eye does not focus properly because of uneven curvatures of the cornea.

asystole (ay-**SIS**-toh-lee)**:** complete lack of electrical activity in the heart.

ataxia (ah-**TACK**-see-ah)**:** the lack of muscle coordination during voluntary movement.

atelectasis (**at**-ee-**LEK**-tah-sis)**:** incomplete expansion of part or all of the lung.

atherectomy (**ath**-er-**ECK**-toh-mee)**:** surgical removal of plaque buildup from the interior lining of an artery.

atheroma (**ath**-er-**OH**-mah)**:** a deposit of fatty plaque on or within the arterial wall.

atherosclerosis (**ath**-er-**oh**-skleh-**ROH**-sis)**:** hardening and narrowing of the arteries due to a buildup of cholesterol plaque.

atonic (ah-**TON**-ick)**:** lacking normal muscle tone or strength.

atresia (at-**TREE**-zee-ah)**:** describes the congenital absence of a normal opening or the failure of a structure to be tubular.

atrial fibrillation: rapid irregular twitching of the muscular wall of the atria.

atrophy (**AT**-roh-fee)**:** weakness or wearing away of body tissues and structures caused by pathology or by disuse over a long period of time.

attention-deficit/hyperactivity disorder (ADHD)**:** a condition characterized by a short attention span and impulsive behavior inappropriate for the child's developmental age.

audiological evaluation: the measurement of the ability to hear and understand speech sounds based on their pitch and loudness.

audiometry (**aw**-dee-**OM**-eh-tree)**:** the use of an audiometer to measure hearing acuity.

auscultation (**aws**-kul-**TAY**-shun)**:** listening for sounds within the body, usually done with a stethoscope.

autism (**AW**-tizm)**:** a subgroup of autistic spectrum disorders.

autistic spectrum disorders (aw-**TIS**-tic)**:** a group of conditions in which a young child has difficulty developing normal social relationships and communication skills, may compulsively follow repetitive routines, and has narrowly focused, intense interests.

autoimmune disorder (**aw**-toh-ih-**MYOUN**)**:** a condition in which the immune system produces antibodies against the body's own tissues.

autologous bone marrow transplant (aw-**TOL**-uh-guss)**:** a transplant utilizing the patient's own bone marrow that was harvested before treatment began.

automated external defibrillator (dee-**fib**-rih-**LAY**-ter)**:** electronic equipment that externally shocks the heart to restore a normal cardiac rhythm.

automated implantable cardioverter defibrillator (**KAR**-dee-oh-**ver**-ter dee-**fib**-rih-**LAY**-ter)**:** a double-action pacemaker that regulates the heartbeat and acts as an automatic defibrillator.

autopsy (**AW**-top-see)**:** postmortem (after death) examination.

Ayurvedic medicine (**ay**-uhr-**VEH**-dick)**:** traditional Hindu system of medicine.

azoospermia (ay-**zoh**-oh-**SPER**-mee-ah)**:** the absence of sperm in the semen.

B

bacilli (bah-**SILL**-eye)**:** rod-shaped spore-forming bacteria.

bacteria (back-**TEER**-ree-ah)**:** one-celled microscopic organisms.

bacterial endocarditis: inflammation of the lining or valves of the heart caused by bacteria in the bloodstream.

bacterial pneumonia: pneumonia caused by *Streptococcus pneumoniae.*

bacterial vaginosis (**vaj**-ih-**NOH**-sis)**:** a condition in women in which there is an abnormal overgrowth of certain bacteria in the vagina.

bactericide (back-**TEER**-ih-sighd)**:** a substance that causes the death of bacteria.

bacteriuria (back-**tee**-ree-**YOU**-ree-ah)**:** the presence of bacteria in the urine.

balanitis (**bal**-ah-**NIGH**-tis)**:** inflammation of the glans penis.

barbiturates (bar-**BIT**-you-raytz)**:** a class of drugs whose major action is a calming or depressed effect on the central nervous system.

bariatric surgery: performed to treat morbid obesity by restricting the amount of food that can enter the stomach and be digested.

bariatrics (**bayr**-ee-**AT**-ricks)**:** the branch of medicine for the prevention and control of obesity and associated diseases.

barium: a radiopaque contrast medium used primarily to visualize the gastrointestinal tract.

barotrauma (**bar**-oh-**TRAW**-mah)**:** pressure-related ear condition.

Barrett's esophagus: a condition that occurs when the cells in the epithelial tissue of the esophagus are damaged by chronic acid exposure.

basal cell carcinoma: a malignant tumor of the basal cell layer of the epidermis.

behavioral therapy: therapy that focuses on changing behavior by identifying problem behaviors, replacing them with appropriate behaviors, and using rewards or other consequences to make the changes.

Bell's palsy: temporary paralysis of the seventh cranial nerve that causes paralysis only on the affected side of the face.

benign: something that is not life-threatening and does not recur.

benign prostatic hyperplasia (high-per-**PLAY**-zee-ah)**:** abnormal enlargement of the prostate gland often found in men over 50.

beta-blockers: medications administered to reduce the workload of the heart by slowing the heartbeat.

binaural testing (bye-**NAW**-rul *or* bin-**AW**-rahl)**:** involves both ears.

biofeedback: treatment that teaches a person to control bodily functions through cognitive control techniques to decrease stress.

bioimpedance spectroscopy (**BYE**-oh-im-**pee**-dens)**:** a noninvasive method of diagnosing lymphedema by measuring the limb's resistance to an electrical current.

biopsy (**BYE**-op-see)**:** the removal of a small piece of living tissue for examination to confirm or establish a diagnosis.

BiPAP machine: noninvasive ventilation device like a CPAP machine; however, it can be set at a higher pressure for inhaling and a lower pressure for exhaling.

bipolar disorder: a mental condition characterized by cycles of severe mood changes shifting from highs and severe lows.

bladder retraining: behavioral training in which the patient learns to urinate on a schedule with increasingly longer time intervals between scheduled urination.

bladder ultrasound: the use of a handheld ultrasound transducer to measure the amount of urine remaining in the bladder after urination.

blepharoplasty (**BLEF**-ah-roh-**plas**-tee)**:** surgical reduction of the upper and lower eyelids.

blindness: the inability to see.

blood dyscrasia (dis-**KRAY**-zee-ah)**:** any pathologic condition of the cellular elements of the blood.

bloodborne transmission: the spread of a disease through contact with blood or other body fluids that are contaminated with blood.

blood urea nitrogen (you-**REE**-ah)**:** a blood test performed to determine the amount of urea present in the blood.

body mass index (BMI)**:** a number that shows body weight adjusted for height.

bolus (**BOH**-lus)**:** a single dose of a drug usually injected into a blood vessel over a short period of time.

bone density testing: a diagnostic test to determine losses or changes in bone density.

bone marrow biopsy: a diagnostic test to determine why blood cells are abnormal or to find a donor match for a bone marrow transplant.

bone marrow transplant: cancer treatment in which abnormal bone marrow is destroyed and replaced with new stem cells.

bone scan: a specialized nuclear scan that identifies new areas of bone growth or breakdown.

borborygmus (**bor**-boh-**RIG**-mus)**:** the rumbling noise caused by the movement of gas in the intestine.

Botox: a formulation of botulinum toxin that is administered by injection to temporarily improve the appearance of frown lines between the eyebrows.

bowel incontinence (in-**KON**-tih-nents)**:** the inability to control the excretion of feces.

brachytherapy (**brack**-ee-**THER**-ah-pee)**:** the use of radioactive materials in contact with or implanted into the tissues to be treated.

bradycardia (**brad**-ee-**KAR**-dee-ah)**:** an abnormally slow resting heart rate, usually at a rate of less than 60 beats per minute.

bradykinesia (**brad**-ee-kih-**NEE**-zee-ah)**:** extreme slowness in movement.

bradypnea (**brad**-ihp-**NEE**-ah)**:** an abnormally slow rate of respiration, usually of less than 10 breaths per minute.

brain tumor: an abnormal growth within the skull.

brand name: medication sold under the name given the drug by the manufacturer.

Braxton Hicks contractions: intermittent painless uterine contractions that are not true labor pains.

breast augmentation: mammoplasty performed to increase breast size.

breast cancer: a carcinoma that develops from the cells of the breast and can spread to adjacent lymph nodes and other body sites.

breast reduction: mammoplasty performed to decrease and reshape excessively large, heavy breasts.

breast self-examination: a self-care procedure for the early detection of breast cancer.

breech presentation: a birth complication in which the buttocks or feet of the fetus are positioned to enter the birth canal first instead of the head.

bronchiectasis (**brong**-kee-**ECK**-tah-sis)**:** permanent dilation of the bronchi caused by chronic infection and inflammation.

bronchodilator (**brong**-koh-dye-**LAY**-tor)**:** a medication that relaxes and expands the bronchial passages into the lungs.

bronchopneumonia (**brong**-koh-new-**MOH**-nee-ah)**:** a localized form of pneumonia often affects the bronchioles.

bronchorrhea (**brong**-koh-**REE**-ah)**:** an excessive discharge of mucus from the bronchi.

bronchoscopy (brong-**KOS**-koh-pee)**:** the visual examination of the bronchi using a bronchoscope.

bronchospasm (**brong**-koh-spazm)**:** a contraction of the smooth muscle in the walls of the bronchi and bronchioles that tighten and squeeze the airway shut.

bruit (**BREW**-ee)**:** an abnormal sound or murmur heard during auscultation of an artery.

bruxism (**BRUCK**-sizm)**:** involuntary grinding or clenching of the teeth that usually occurs during sleep.

bulimia nervosa (byou-**LIM**-ee-ah *or* boo-**LEE**-meeah)**:** an eating disorder characterized by frequent episodes of binge eating followed by compensatory behaviors, such as self-induced vomiting.

bulla (**BULL**-ah)**:** a large blister that is usually more than 0.5 cm in diameter.

burn: an injury to body tissues caused by heat, flame, electricity, sun, chemicals, or radiation.

burn, first-degree: a burn in which there are no blisters and only superficial damage to the epidermis.

burn, second-degree: a burn in which there are blisters and damage to both the epidermis and the dermis.

burn, third-degree: a burn in which there is damage to the epidermis, dermis, subcutaneous layers, and possibly also the muscle below.

bursitis (ber-**SIGH**-tis)**:** inflammation of a bursa.

C

cachexia (kah-**KEKS**-eeh-ah)**:** physical wasting away due to the loss of weight and muscle mass that occurs in patients with diseases such as advanced cancer or AIDS.

calcium channel blocker agents: medications that cause the heart and blood vessels to relax by decreasing the movement of calcium into the cells of these structures.

calciuria (**kal**-sih-**YOU**-ree-ah)**:** the presence of calcium in the urine.

callus (**KAL**-us)**:** a bulging deposit that forms around the area of the break in a bone; also a thickening of the skin that is caused by repeated rubbing.

cancer: a class of diseases characterized by the uncontrolled division of cells and the ability of these cells to invade other tissues.

candidiasis (**kan**-dih-**DYE**-ah-sis)**:** a yeast infection.

capillary hemangioma (**KAP**-uh-**ler**-ee hee-**man**-jee-**OH**-mah)**:** a soft, raised, pink, or red vascular birthmark.

capillary puncture: technique used to obtain a small amount of blood for a blood test.

capsule endoscopy: a tiny video camera in a capsule that the patient swallows that transmits images of the walls of the small intestine.

carbuncle (**KAR**-bung-kul)**:** a cluster of connected furuncles (boils).

carcinoma (**kar**-sih-**NOH**-mah)**:** a malignant tumor that occurs in epithelial tissue.

carcinoma in situ: a malignant tumor in its original position that has not yet disturbed or invaded the surrounding tissues.

cardiac arrest: an event in which the heart abruptly stops beating or develops an arrhythmia that prevents it from pumping blood.

cardiac catheterization (**KAR**-dee-ack **kath**-eh-ter-eye-**ZAY**-shun)**:** a diagnostic procedure in which a catheter is passed into a vein or artery and guided into the heart.

cardiocentesis (**kar**-dee-oh-sen-**TEE**-sis)**:** the puncture of a chamber of the heart for diagnosis or therapy.

cardiomegaly (**kar**-dee-oh-**MEG**-ah-lee)**:** abnormal enlargement of the heart.

cardiomyopathy (**kar**-dee-oh-my-**OP**-pah-thee)**:** all diseases of the heart muscle.

cardioplegia (**kar**-dee-oh-**PLEE**-jee-ah)**:** paralysis of the heart muscle.

cardiopulmonary resuscitation: an emergency procedure for life support consisting of artificial respiration and manual external cardiac compression.

carditis (kar-**DYE**-tis)**:** an inflammation of the heart.

carotid endarterectomy (**end**-ar-ter-**ECK**-toh-mee)**:** surgical removal of the lining of a portion of a clogged carotid artery.

carotid ultrasonography: an ultrasound study of the carotid artery that is performed to predict or diagnose an ischemic stroke.

carpal tunnel release: the surgical enlargement of the carpal tunnel or cutting of the carpal ligament to relieve pressure on nerves and tendons.

carpal tunnel syndrome: swelling that creates pressure on the median nerve as it passes through the carpal tunnel.

castration (kas-**TRAY**-shun)**:** surgical removal or destruction of both testicles.

cataract (**KAT**-ah-rakt)**:** the loss of transparency of the lens of the eye.

catatonic behavior (**kat**-ah-**TON**-ick)**:** marked by a lack of responsiveness, stupor, and a tendency to remain in a fixed posture.

causalgia (kaw-**ZAL**-jee-ah)**:** persistent, severe, burning pain that usually follows an injury to a sensory nerve.

cauterization (**kaw**-ter-eye-**ZAY**-zhun)**:** the destruction of tissue by burning.

celiac disease (**SEE**-lee-ak)**:** an inherited autoimmune disorder characterized by a severe reaction to foods containing gluten.

cellulitis (**sell**-you-**LYE**-tis)**:** an acute, rapidly spreading bacterial infection within the connective tissues of the skin.

centesis (sen-**TEE**-sis)**:** a surgical puncture to remove fluid for diagnostic purposes or to remove excess fluid.

cephalalgia (**sef**-ah-**LAL**-jee-ah)**:** pain in the head.

cephalic presentation: when the baby is born head first.

cerebral contusion (**SER**-eh-bral kon-**TOO**-zhun)**:** bruising of brain tissue as the result of a head injury that causes the brain to bounce against the skull.

cerebral palsy (**SER**-eh-bral *or* **seh**-**REE**-bral **PAWL**-zee)**:** a condition characterized by poor muscle control, spasticity, and other neurologic deficiencies.

cerebrovascular accident (**ser**-eh-broh-**VAS**-kyou-lar)**:** damage to the brain that occurs when the blood flow to the brain is disrupted.

cervical cancer: cancer that develops in the cervix.

cervical dysplasia (**SER**-vih-kal dis-**PLAY**-see-ah)**:** the presence of precancerous changes in the cells that make up the inner lining of the cervix.

cervical radiculopathy (rah-**dick**-you-**LOP**-ah-thee)**:** nerve pain caused by pressure on the spinal nerve roots in the neck region.

cervicitis (**ser**-vih-**SIGH**-tis)**:** inflammation of the cervix.

cesarean section (seh-**ZEHR**-ee-un **SECK**-shun)**:** the delivery of the child through an incision in the maternal abdominal and uterine walls.

chalazion (kah-**LAY**-zee-on)**:** a nodule or cyst, usually on the upper eyelid caused by obstruction of a sebaceous gland.

cheilosis (kee-**LOH**-sis)**:** a disorder of the lips characterized by crack-like sores at the corners of the mouth.

chemabrasion (keem-ah-**BRAY**-shun)**:** the use of chemicals to remove the outer layers of skin.

chemoprevention: the use of natural or synthetic substances such as drugs or vitamins to reduce the risk of developing cancer or to reduce the chance that cancer will occur.

chemotherapy: the use of chemical agents and drugs in combinations selected to destroy malignant cells and tissues.

chest x-ray: a valuable tool for diagnosing pneumonia, lung cancer, pneumothorax, pleural effusion, tuberculosis, and emphysema.

Cheyne-Stokes respiration (**CHAYN**-**STOHKS**)**:** an irregular pattern of breathing characterized by alternating rapid or shallow respiration followed by slow respiration or apnea.

chiropractic manipulative therapy: a system of mechanical spinal adjustments made by a chiropractor to correct biomechanical problems in the skeleton.

chlamydia (klah-**MID**-ee-ah)**:** a sexually transmitted disease caused by the bacteria *Chlamydia trachomatis.*

chloasma (kloh-**AZ**-mah)**:** a pigmentation disorder characterized by brownish spots on the face.

cholangiography (koh-**LAN**-jee-**og**-rah-fee)**:** a radiographic examination of the bile ducts with the use of a contrast medium.

cholangitis (**koh**-lan-**JIGH**-tis)**:** an acute inflammation of the bile duct characterized by pain in the upper-right quadrant of the abdomen, fever, and jaundice.

cholecystectomy (**koh**-luh-sis-**TECK**-toh-mee)**:** the surgical removal of the gallbladder.

cholecystitis (**koh**-luh-sis-**TYE**-tis)**:** inflammation of the gallbladder that is usually associated with gallstones.

choledocholithotomy (koh-**led**-oh-koh-lih-**THOT**-oh-mee)**:** an incision in the common bile duct for the removal of gallstones.

cholelithiasis (**koh**-lee-luh-**THIGH**-ah-sis)**:** the presence of gallstones in the gallbladder or bile ducts.

cholesteatoma (koh-**les**-tee-ah-**TOH**-mah)**:** destructive epidermal cyst in the middle ear made up of epithelial cells and cholesterol.

cholesterol (koh-**LES**-ter-ol)**:** a fatty substance that travels through the blood and is found in all parts of the body.

cholesterol-lowering drugs: medications, such as statins, that are administered to reduce the undesirable cholesterol levels in the blood.

chondroma (kon-**DROH**-mah)**:** a slow-growing benign tumor derived from cartilage cells.

chondromalacia (**kon**-droh-mah-**LAY**-shee-ah)**:** abnormal softening of the cartilage.

chondroplasty (**KON**-droh-**plas**-tee)**:** surgical repair of damaged cartilage.

chorionic villus sampling (**kor**-ee-**ON**-ick **VIL**-us)**:** examination of cells retrieved from the chorionic villi between the 8th and 10th weeks of pregnancy.

chronic bronchitis: a disease in which the airways have become inflamed due to recurrent exposure to an inhaled irritant.

chronic fatigue syndrome: a disorder of unknown cause that affects many body systems, with symptoms similar to those of fibromyalgia syndrome.

chronic kidney disease: the progressive loss of renal function over months or years.

chronic obstructive pulmonary disease: a group of lung diseases in which the bronchial airflow is obstructed, making it hard to breathe.

chronic venous insufficiency: a condition in which venous circulation is inadequate due to partial vein blockage or leakage of venous valves.

cicatrix (sick-**AY**-tricks)**:** a normal scar resulting from the healing of a wound.

cineradiography (**sin**-eh-**ray**-dee-**OG**-rah-fee)**:** the recording of fluoroscopy images.

circumcision (**ser**-kum-**SIZH**-un)**:** surgical removal of the foreskin of the penis.

cirrhosis (sih-**ROH**-sis)**:** a chronic degenerative disease of the liver characterized by scarring.

claustrophobia (**klaws**-troh-**FOH**-bee-ah)**:** abnormal fear of being in small or enclosed spaces.

cleft lip: a birth defect resulting in a deep groove of the lip running upward to the nose.

cleft palate: failure of the palate to close during the early development of the fetus that involves the upper lip, hard palate, and/or soft palate.

clinical trials: testing new treatments that have not yet received FDA approval on patients who agree to be part of the research.

closed-angle glaucoma: a type of glaucoma in which the opening between the cornea and iris narrows so that fluid cannot reach the trabecular meshwork.

closed fracture: a fracture in which the bone is broken but there is no open wound in the skin.

closed reduction: the attempted realignment of the bone involved in a fracture or joint dislocation.

clostridium difficile (klos-**TRID**-ee-um dif-us-**SEEL**)**:** a bacterial infection common to older adults in hospitals or long-term care facilities.

clubbing: abnormal curving of the nails that is often accompanied by enlargement of the fingertips.

cluster headaches: intensely painful headaches that affect one side of the head and often occur in groups or clusters.

cochlear implant (**KOCK**-lee-ar)**:** an electronic device that bypasses the damaged portions of the ear and directly stimulates the auditory nerve.

cognition (kog-**NISH**-un)**:** the mental activities associated with thinking, learning, and memory.

cognitive therapy: treatment that focuses on changing cognitions or thoughts that are affecting a person's emotions and actions.

colectomy (koh-**LECK**-toh-mee)**:** surgical removal of all or part of the colon.

collagen replacement therapy: a form of soft-tissue augmentation used to soften facial lines or scars, or to make lips appear fuller.

Colles' fracture: a fracture at the lower end of the radius that occurs when a person tries to break a fall by landing on his or her hands.

colonoscopy (**koh**-lun-**OSS**-koh-pee)**:** direct visual examination of the inner surface of the colon from the rectum to the cecum.

colorectal carcinoma: a common form of cancer that often first manifests itself in polyps in the colon.

colostomy (koh-**LAHS**-toh-mee)**:** the surgical creation of an artificial excretory opening between the colon and the body surface.

colotomy (koh-**LOT**-oh-mee)**:** a surgical incision into the colon.

colpopexy (**KOL**-poh-**peck**-see)**:** surgical fixation of the vagina to a surrounding structure.

colporrhaphy (kol-**POR**-ah-fee)**:** surgical suturing of a tear in the vagina.

colporrhexis (**kol**-poh-**RECK**-sis)**:** tearing or laceration of the vaginal walls.

colposcopy (kol-**POS**-koh-pee)**:** direct visual examination of the tissues of the cervix and vagina.

coma (**KOH**-mah)**:** a deep state of unconsciousness marked by the absence of spontaneous eye movements, no response to painful stimuli, and no vocalization.

comedo (**KOM**-eh-doh)**:** a noninfected lesion formed by the buildup of sebum and keratin in a hair follicle.

comminuted fracture (**KOM**-ih-**newt**-ed)**:** a fracture in which the bone is splintered or crushed.

communicable disease (kuh-**MEW**-nih-kuh-bul)**:** any condition that is transmitted from one person to another by either direct or indirect contact with contaminated objects.

community-acquired pneumonia: a type of pneumonia that results from contagious infection outside of a hospital or clinic.

compartment syndrome: the compression of nerves and blood vessels due to swelling within the enclosed space created by the fascia that separates groups of muscles.

complementary medicine: practices and systems of health care used to supplement allopathic medicine.

complete blood cell count: a series of blood tests performed as a group to evaluate several blood conditions.

compression fracture: a fracture in which the bone is pressed together on itself.

computed tomography (toh-**MOG**-rah-fee)**:** an imaging technique that uses a thin, fan-shaped x-ray beam to produce multiple cross-sectional views of the body.

concussion (kon-**KUSH**-un)**:** a violent shaking up or jarring of the brain.

conductive hearing loss: a hearing loss in which sound waves are prevented from passing from the air to the fluid-filled inner ear.

congenital disorder (kon-**JEN**-ih-tahl)**:** an abnormal condition that exists at the time of birth.

congenital heart defects: structural abnormalities caused by the failure of the heart to develop normally before birth.

conization (**kon**-ih-**ZAY**-shun *or* **koh**-nih-**ZAY**-shun)**:** surgical removal of a cone-shaped section of tissue from the cervix.

conjunctivitis (kon-**junk**-tih-**VYE**-tis)**:** inflammation of the conjunctiva, usually caused by an infection or allergy.

Conn's syndrome (**KONS**)**:** a disorder of the adrenal glands caused by the excessive production of aldosterone.

conscious: the state of being awake, alert, aware, and responding appropriately.

constipation: having a bowel movement fewer than three times per week.

contact dermatitis: a localized allergic response caused by contact with an irritant or allergen.

contraceptive: a measure taken or a device used to lessen the likelihood of pregnancy.

contracture (kon-**TRACK**-chur)**:** the permanent tightening of fascia, muscles, tendons, ligaments, or skin that occurs when normally elastic connective tissues are replaced with nonelastic fibrous tissues.

contraindication: a factor in the patient's condition that makes the use of a medication or specific treatment dangerous or ill advised.

contrast medium: a substance used to make visible structures that are otherwise hard to see.

contusion (kon-**TOO**-zhun)**:** an injury to underlying tissues without breaking the skin, characterized by discoloration and pain.

conversion disorder: a condition characterized by a serious temporary or ongoing change in function, such as paralysis or blindness, triggered by psychological factors rather than any physical cause.

corneal abrasion: an injury, such as a scratch or irritation, to the outer layers of the cornea.

corneal transplant: the surgical replacement of a scarred or diseased cornea with clear corneal tissue from a donor.

corneal ulcer: a pitting of the cornea caused by an infection or injury.

coronary artery bypass graft: a surgical procedure in which a piece of vein from the leg is implanted on the heart to replace a blocked coronary artery.

coronary artery disease: atherosclerosis of the coronary arteries that reduces the blood supply to the heart muscle.

coronary thrombosis (**KOR**-uh-**nerr**-ee throm-**BOH**-sis)**:** damage to the heart muscle caused by a thrombus blocking a coronary artery.

corticosteroid drug: steroid hormones produced by the adrenal cortex, and their synthetically produced equivalents.

cortisone (**KOR**-tih-sohn)**:** the synthetic equivalent of natural corticosteroids that are administered to suppress inflammation and to act as an immunosuppressant.

costochondritis (**kos**-toh-kon-**DRIGH**-tis)**:** an inflammation of the cartilage that connects a rib to the sternum.

Coumadin: the brand name for *warfarin*, an anticoagulant administered to prevent blood clots from forming or growing larger.

cover test: an exam of how the two eyes work together, used to assess binocular vision.

CPAP machine (continuous positive airway pressure): a noninvasive ventilation device used in the treatment of sleep apnea.

cramp: a painful localized muscle spasm.

cranial hematoma (**hee**-mah-**TOH**-mah)**:** a collection of blood trapped in the tissues of the brain.

craniectomy (**kray**-nee-**EK**-toh-mee)**:** surgical removal of a portion of the skull.

cranioplasty (**KRAY**-nee-oh-**plas**-tee)**:** surgical repair of the skull.

craniosacral therapy (**kray**-nee-oh-**SAK**-ral)**:** the use of gentle touch to help the body release tension in order to correct restrictions resulting from stress on the CNS.

craniostenosis (**kray**-nee-oh-steh-**NOH**-sis)**:** a malformation of the skull due to the premature closure of the cranial sutures.

craniotomy (**kray**-nee-**OT**-oh-mee)**:** a surgical incision or opening into the skull.

C-reactive protein: a blood test that detects high levels of inflammation within the body.

creatinuria (kree-**at**-ih-**NEW**-ree-ah)**:** an increased concentration of creatinine in the urine.

crepitation (**krep**-ih-**TAY**-shun)**:** the grating sound heard when the ends of a broken bone move together.

cretinism (**CREE**-tin-izm)**:** a congenital form of hypothyroidism.

Crohn's disease: a chronic autoimmune disorder that can occur anywhere in the digestive tract; however, it is most often found in the ileum and in the colon.

crossmatch tests: tests performed to determine the compatibility of blood donor and recipient before a transfusion.

croup (**KROOP**)**:** an acute respiratory infection in children and infants characterized by obstruction of the larynx, hoarseness, and swelling around the vocal cords resulting in a barking cough and stridor.

crust: a collection of dried serum and cellular debris.

cryosurgery: the destruction or elimination of abnormal tissue cells through the application of extreme cold by using liquid nitrogen.

cryptorchidism (krip-**TOR**-kih-dizm)**:** a developmental defect in which one or both testicles fail to descend into the scrotum.

curettage (**kyou**-reh-**TAHZH**)**:** the removal of material from the surface by scraping.

Cushing's syndrome (**KUSH**-ingz **SIN**-drohm)**:** a condition caused by prolonged exposure to high levels of cortisol.

cyanosis (**sigh**-ah-**NOH**-sis)**:** bluish discoloration of the skin and mucous membranes caused by a lack of adequate oxygen in the blood.

cyst: an abnormal sac containing fluid, gas, or a semisolid material.

cystalgia (sis-**TAL**-jee-ah)**:** pain in the urinary bladder.

cystectomy (sis-**TECK**-toh-mee)**:** the surgical removal of all or part of the urinary bladder.

cystic fibrosis (**SIS**-tick figh-**BROH**-sis)**:** a life-threatening genetic disorder in which the lungs and pancreas are clogged with large quantities of abnormally thick mucus.

cystitis (sis-**TYE**-tis)**:** inflammation of the bladder.

cystocele (**SIS**-toh-seel)**:** a hernia of the bladder through the vaginal wall.

cystography (sis-**TOG**-rah-fee)**:** a radiographic examination of the bladder after instillation of a contrast medium via a urethral catheter.

cystolith (**SIS**-toh-lith)**:** a stone located within the urinary bladder.

cystopexy (**SIS**-toh-**peck**-see)**:** the surgical fixation of the bladder to the abdominal wall.

cystorrhaphy (sis-**TOR**-ah-fee)**:** surgical suturing of a wound or defect in the bladder.

cystoscopy (sis-**TOS**-koh-pee)**:** the visual examination of the urinary bladder using a cystoscope.

cytomegalovirus (**sigh**-toh-**meg**-ah-loh-**VYE**-rus)**:** a type of herpesvirus found in most body fluids.

cytotoxic drug (**sigh**-toh-**TOK**-sick)**:** medication that kills or damages cells.

D

dacryoadenitis (**dack**-ree-oh-ad-eh-**NIGH**-tis)**:** an inflammation of the lacrimal gland that can be caused by a bacterial, viral, or fungal infection.

deafness: the complete or partial loss of the ability to hear.

debridement (dah-**BREED**-ment)**:** the removal of dirt, foreign objects, damaged tissue, and cellular debris from a wound to prevent infection and to promote healing.

decibel: commonly used as the measurement of the loudness of sound.

deep brain stimulation: a neurosurgical procedure used in the treatment of dystonia, tremors, and Parkinson's disease.

deep tendon reflexes: testing of reflexes to diagnose disruptions of the nerve supply to the involved muscles.

deep vein thrombosis: the condition of having a thrombus attached to the interior wall of a deep vein.

defibrillation (dee-**fib**-rih-**LAY**-shun)**:** the use of electrical shock to restore the heart's normal rhythm.

dehydration: a condition in which fluid loss exceeds fluid intake and disrupts the body's normal electrolyte balance.

delirium (deh-**LEER**-ee-um)**:** an acute condition of confusion, disorientation, disordered thinking and memory, agitation, and hallucinations.

delirium tremens (deh-**LEER**-ee-um **TREE**-mens)**:** a disorder involving sudden and severe mental changes or seizures caused by abruptly stopping the use of alcohol.

delusion (dih-**LOO**-zhun)**:** a false personal belief that is maintained despite obvious proof or evidence to the contrary.

dementia (dih-**MEN**-shee-ah)**:** a slowly progressive decline in mental abilities including memory, thinking, and judgment that is often accompanied by personality changes.

dental calculus (**KAL**-kyou-luhs)**:** hardened dental plaque on the teeth.

dental caries (**KAYR**-eez)**:** an infectious disease that destroys the enamel and dentin of the tooth.

dental plaque (**PLACK**)**:** a soft deposit consisting of bacteria and bacterial by-products that builds up on the teeth.

dental prophylaxis (**proh**-fih-**LACK**-sis)**:** the professional cleaning of the teeth to remove plaque and calculus.

depression: a common mood disorder characterized by lethargy and sadness, as well as a loss of interest or pleasure in normal activities.

dermabrasion (**der**-mah-**BRAY**-zhun)**:** a form of abrasion involving the use of a revolving wire brush or sandpaper.

dermatitis (**der**-mah-**TYE**-tis)**:** inflammation of the skin.

dermatoplasty (**DER**-mah-toh-**plas**-tee)**:** the replacement of damaged skin with healthy tissue taken from a donor site on the patient's body.

dermatosis (**der**-mah-**TOH**-sis)**:** a general term used to denote skin lesions or eruptions of any type that are not associated with inflammation.

developmental disorder: disorder that can result in an anomaly or malformation such as the absence of a limb or the presence of an extra toe.

diabetes insipidus (**dye**-ah-**BEE**-teez in-**SIP**-ih-dus)**:** a condition caused by insufficient production of the antidiuretic hormone or by the inability of the kidneys to respond to this hormone.

diabetes mellitus (**dye**-ah-**BEE**-teez **MEL**-ih-tus)**:** a group of metabolic disorders characterized by hyperglycemia resulting from defects in insulin secretion, insulin action, or both.

diabetic coma: a diabetic emergency caused by very high blood sugar.

diabetic retinopathy (**ret**-ih-**NOP**-ah-thee)**:** damage to the retina as a complication of uncontrolled diabetes.

dialysis (dye-**AL**-ih-sis)**:** a procedure to remove waste products from the blood of patients whose kidneys no longer function.

diaphragmatic breathing: a relaxation technique used to relieve anxiety.

diarrhea (**dye**-ah-**REE**-ah)**:** the abnormally frequent flow of loose or watery stools.

digital rectal examination: a manual examination performed on men to palpate the prostate gland to detect prostate enlargement and look for indicators of prostate cancer.

digital subtraction angiography: a diagnostic technique that combines angiography with computerized components to clarify the view of the area of interest by removing soft tissue and bone from the images.

digitalis (**dij**-ih-**TAL**-is)**:** medication that strengthens the heart muscle contractions, slows the heart rate, and helps eliminate fluid from body tissues.

dilation and curettage (dye-**LAY**-shun and **kyou**-reh-**TAHZH**)**:** a surgical procedure in which the cervix is dilated and the endometrium of the uterus is scraped away.

diphtheria (dif-**THEE**-ree-ah)**:** an acute bacterial infection of the throat and upper respiratory tract.

diplopia (dih-**PLOH**-pee-ah)**:** the perception of two images of a single object.

dislocation: the total displacement of a bone from its joint.

dissociative disorders: conditions that occur when normal thought is separated from consciousness.

dissociative identity disorder: a mental illness characterized by the presence of two or more distinct personalities, each with its own characteristics, which appear to exist within the same individual.

diuresis (**dye**-you-**REE**-sis)**:** the increased output of urine.

diuretics (**dye**-you-**RET**-icks)**:** medications administered to increase urine secretion to rid the body of excess salt and water.

diverticulectomy (**dye**-ver-**tick**-you-**LECK**-toh-mee)**:** surgical removal of a diverticulum.

diverticulitis (**dye**-ver-tick-you-**LYE**-tis)**:** inflammation or infection of one or more diverticula in the wall of the colon.

diverticulosis (**dye**-ver-**tick**-you-**LOH**-sis)**:** the chronic presence of an abnormal number of diverticula in the wall of the colon.

diverticulum (**dye**-ver-**TICK**-you-lum)**:** a small pouch or sac occurring in the lining or wall of a tubular organ.

Doppler echocardiogram: an ultrasonic diagnostic procedure that measures the speed and direction of the blood flow within the heart.

dorsal recumbent position: position where the patient is lying on the back, face up, with the knees bent.

Down syndrome: a genetic variation that is associated with characteristic facial appearance, learning disabilities, and physical abnormalities such as heart valve disease.

drug abuse: the excessive use of illegal drugs or the misuse of prescription drugs.

drug interaction: the result of drugs reacting with each other, often in ways that are unexpected or potentially harmful.

drug overdose: the accidental or intentional use of an illegal drug or prescription medicine in an amount higher than what is safe or normal.

drug-screening urine test: a rapid method of identifying the presence in the body of one or more drugs of abuse.

dual x-ray absorptiometry (ab-**sorp**-shee-**OM**-eh-tree)**:** a low-exposure radiographic measurement of the spine and hips to measure bone density.

ductal carcinoma in situ: breast cancer at its earliest stage before the cancer has broken through the wall of the milk duct.

duplex ultrasound: a diagnostic procedure to image the structures of the blood vessels and the flow of blood through these vessels.

dysentery (**DIS**-en-**ter**-ee)**:** a bacterial infection spread through food or water contaminated by human feces.

dysfunctional uterine bleeding: a condition characterized by abnormal bleeding.

dyskinesia (**dis**-kih-**NEE**-zee-ah)**:** distortion or impairment of voluntary movement.

dyslexia (dis-**LECK**-see-ah)**:** a learning disability characterized by substandard reading achievement due to the inability of the brain to process symbols.

dysmenorrhea (**dis**-men-oh-**REE**-ah)**:** pain caused by uterine cramps during a menstrual period.

dyspareunia (**dis**-pah-**ROO**-nee-ah)**:** pain during sexual intercourse.

dyspepsia (dis-**PEP**-see-ah)**:** pain or discomfort in digestion.

dysphagia (dis-**FAY**-jee-ah)**:** difficulty in swallowing.

dysphonia (dis-**FOH**-nee-ah)**:** difficulty in speaking, which may include any impairment in vocal quality.

dysplasia (dis-**PLAY**-see-ah)**:** abnormal development or growth of cells, tissues, or organs.

dysplastic nevi (dis-**PLAS**-tick **NEE**-vye)**:** atypical moles that can develop into skin cancer.

dyspnea (**DISP**-nee-ah)**:** difficult or labored breathing.

dysthymia (dis-**THIGH**-mee-ah)**:** a low-grade chronic depression present on a majority of days for more than two years.

dystonia (dis-**TOH**-nee-ah)**:** a condition of abnormal muscle tone.

dysuria (dis-**YOU**-ree-ah)**:** difficult or painful urination.

E

ear tubes: tiny ventilating tubes placed through the eardrum to provide ongoing drainage for fluids and to relieve pressure that can build up after childhood ear infections.

ecchymosis (**eck**-ih-**MOH**-sis)**:** a large, irregular area of purplish discoloration due to bleeding under the skin.

echocardiography (**eck**-oh-**kar**-dee-**OG**-rah-fee)**:** an ultrasonic diagnostic procedure used to evaluate the structures and motion of the heart.

echoencephalography (**eck**-oh-en-**sef**-ah-**LOG**-rah-fee)**:** the use of ultrasound imaging to create a detailed visual image of the brain for diagnostic purposes.

eclampsia (eh-**KLAMP**-see-ah)**:** during pregnancy, a more serious form of preeclampsia characterized by convulsions and sometimes coma.

E. coli: infection caused by the bacteria *Escherichia coli,* transmitted through improperly cooked, contaminated foods.

ectopic pregnancy (eck-**TOP**-ick)**:** the condition in which a fertilized egg is implanted and begins to develop outside of the uterus.

ectropion (eck-**TROH**-pee-on)**:** the eversion of the edge of an eyelid.

eczema (**ECK**-zeh-mah)**:** a form of recurring dermatitis characterized by itching, redness, and dryness.

edema (eh-**DEE**-mah)**:** swelling caused by an abnormal accumulation of fluid in cells, tissues, or cavities of the body.

electrocardiogram (ee-**leck**-troh-**KAR**-dee-oh-**gram**)**:** a record of the electrical activity of the myocardium.

electrocardiography (ee-**leck**-troh-kar-dee-**OG**-rah-fee)**:** the noninvasive process of recording the electrical activity of the myocardium.

electroconvulsive therapy (ee-**leck**-troh-kon-**VUL**-siv)**:** a procedure in which small amounts of electric current is passed through the brain, deliberately triggering a brief seizure in order to reverse symptoms of certain mental illnesses.

electrodessication (ee-**leck**-troh-des-ih-**KAY**-shun)**:** a surgical technique in which tissue is destroyed using an electric spark.

electroencephalography (ee-**leck**-troh-en-**sef**-ah-**LOG**-rah-fee)**:** the process of recording the electrical activity of the brain through the use of electrodes attached to the scalp.

electrolysis: the use of electric current to destroy hair follicles for the removal of undesired hair.

electromyography (ee-**leck**-troh-my-**OG**-rah-fee)**:** a diagnostic test that measures the electrical activity within muscle fibers in response to nerve stimulation.

ELISA: the acronym for enzyme-linked immunosorbent assay, a blood test that is used to screen for the presence of HIV antibodies.

embolism (**EM**-boh-lizm)**:** the sudden blockage of a blood vessel by an embolus.

embolus (**EM**-boh-lus)**:** a foreign object, such as a blood clot, quantity of air or gas, or a bit of tissue or tumor, that is circulating in the blood.

emesis (**EM**-eh-sis)**:** the reflex ejection of the stomach contents outward through the mouth.

emphysema (**em**-fih-**SEE**-mah)**:** the progressive, long-term loss of lung function, usually due to smoking.

empyema (**em**-pye-**EE**-mah)**:** an accumulation of pus in a body cavity.

encephalitis (**en**-sef-ah-**LYE**-tis)**:** inflammation of the brain.

encephalocele (en-**SEF**-ah-loh-**seel**)**:** a congenital herniation of brain substance through a gap in the skull.

endemic (en-**DEM**-ick)**:** refers to the ongoing presence of a disease within a population, group, or area.

endocarditis (**en**-doh-kar-**DYE**-tis)**:** inflammation of the inner lining of the heart.

endocervicitis (**en**-doh-**ser**-vih-**SIGH**-tis)**:** inflammation of the mucous membrane lining of the cervix.

endometrial biopsy: a diagnostic test in which a small amount of the tissue lining the uterus is removed for microscopic examination.

endometrial cancer (**en**-doh-**MEE**-tree-al)**:** a cancerous growth that begins in the lining of the uterus.

endometriosis (**en**-doh-**mee**-tree-**OH**-sis)**:** a condition in which patches of endometrial tissue escape the uterus and become attached to other structures in the pelvic cavity.

endoscope (**EN**-doh-**skope**)**:** a small, flexible tube with a light and lens on the end.

endoscopic surgery: a surgical procedure performed through very small incisions with the use of an endoscope and specialized instruments.

endoscopy (en-**DOS**-koh-pee)**:** the visual examination of the interior of a body cavity or organ.

endotracheal intubation (**en**-doh-**TRAY**-kee-al **in**-too-**BAY**-shun)**:** the passage of a tube through the mouth into the trachea to establish or maintain an open airway.

endovaginal ultrasound (**en**-doh-**VAJ**-ih-nal)**:** a diagnostic test utilizing ultrasound to image the uterus and fallopian tubes to determine the cause of abnormal vaginal bleeding.

end-stage renal disease: the final stage of chronic kidney disease.

enema: the placement of a solution into the rectum and colon to empty the lower intestine through bowel activity.

enteritis (**en**-ter-**EYE**-tis)**:** inflammation of the small intestine caused by eating or drinking substances contaminated with viral or bacterial pathogens.

entropion (en-**TROH**-pee-on)**:** the inversion of the edge of an eyelid.

enucleation (ee-**new**-klee-**AY**-shun)**:** the removal of the eyeball, leaving the eye muscles intact.

enuresis (**en**-you-**REE**-sis)**:** the involuntary discharge of urine.

epicondylitis (**ep**-ih-**kon**-dih-**LYE**-tis)**:** inflammation of the tissues surrounding the elbow.

epidemic (**ep**-ih-**DEM**-ick)**:** a sudden and widespread outbreak of a disease within a specific population group or area.

epididymitis (**ep**-ih-did-ih-**MY**-tis)**:** inflammation of the epididymis.

epidural anesthesia (**ep**-ih-**DOO**-ral **an**-es-**THEE**-zee-ah)**:** regional anesthesia produced by injecting medication into the epidural space of the lumbar or sacral region of the spine.

epilepsy (**EP**-ih-**lep**-see)**:** a chronic neurologic condition characterized by recurrent episodes of seizures of varying severity.

episiorrhaphy (eh-**piz**-ee-**OR**-ah-fee)**:** surgical suturing to repair an episiotomy.

episiotomy (eh-**piz**-ee-**OT**-oh-mee)**:** a surgical incision made into the perineum to enlarge the vaginal orifice to prevent tearing of the tissues as the infant moves out of the birth canal.

epispadias (**ep**-ih-**SPAY**-dee-as)**:** a congenital abnormality of the urethral opening. In the male this opening is located on the upper surface of the penis; in the female the urethral opening is in the region of the clitoris.

epistaxis (**ep**-ih-**STACK**-sis)**:** bleeding from the nose.

erectile dysfunction: the inability of the male to achieve or maintain a penile erection.

ergonomics (er-goh-**NOM**-icks)**:** the study of the human factors that affect the design and operation of tools and the work environment.

erosion (eh-**ROH**-zhun)**:** the wearing away of a surface.

eructation (eh-ruk-**TAY**-shun)**:** the act of belching or raising gas orally from the stomach.

erythema (**er**-ih-**THEE**-mah)**:** redness of the skin due to capillary dilation.

erythrocyte sedimentation rate (eh-**RITH**-roh-site)**:** a blood test based on the speed with which the red blood cells separate from the plasma and settle to the bottom of a specialized test tube.

erythroderma (eh-**rith**-roh-**DER**-mah)**:** abnormal redness of the entire skin surface.

esophageal varices (eh-**sof**-ah-**JEE**-al **VAYR**-ih-seez)**:** enlarged and swollen veins at the lower end of the esophagus.

esophagogastroduodenoscopy (eh-**sof**-ah-goh-**gas**-troh-**dew**-oh-deh-**NOS**-koh-pee)**:** the endoscopic examination of the upper GI tract.

esotropia (**es**-oh-**TROH**-pee-ah)**:** strabismus characterized by an inward deviation of one or both eyes.

etiology (**ee**-tee-**OL**-oh-jee)**:** the study of the causes of diseases.

eupnea (youp-**NEE**-ah)**:** easy or normal breathing.

exanthem (eck-**ZAN**-thum)**:** a widespread rash, usually in children.

exfoliative cytology (ecks-**FOH**-lee-**ay**-tiv sigh-**TOL**-oh-jee)**:** a biopsy technique in which cells are scraped from the tissue and examined under a microscope.

exfoliative dermatitis (ecks-**FOH**-lee-**ay**-tiv **DER**-mah-**TYE**-tis)**:** a condition in which there is widespread scaling of the skin.

exophthalmos (**eck**-sof-**THAL**-mos)**:** an abnormal protrusion of the eyeball out of the orbit.

exotropia (**eck**-soh-**TROH**-pee-ah)**:** strabismus characterized by the outward deviation of one eye relative to the other.

expectoration (eck-**SPEK**-toh-**ray**-shun)**:** the act of coughing up and spitting out saliva, mucus, or other body fluid.

external fixation: a fracture treatment procedure in which pins are placed through the soft tissues and bone so that an external appliance can be used to hold the pieces of bone firmly in place during healing.

extracorporeal shockwave lithotripsy: the destruction of kidney stones using high-energy ultrasonic waves traveling through water or gel.

extraoral radiography: dental radiograph where the film is placed and exposed outside of the mouth.

exudate (**ECKS**-you-dayt)**:** fluid, such as pus, that leaks out of an infected wound.

F

factitious disorder (fack-**TISH**-us)**:** a condition in which a person acts as if he or she has a physical or mental illness when he or she is not really sick.

factitious disorder by proxy: a form of child abuse in which the mentally ill parent will falsify an illness in a child by making up or inducing symptoms and then seeking medical treatment, even surgery, for the child.

fasciitis (**fas**-ee-**EYE**-tis)**:** inflammation of a fascia.

fascioplasty (**FASH**-ee-oh-**plas**-tee)**:** surgical repair of a fascia.

fasciotomy (**fash**-ee-**OT**-oh-mee)**:** a surgical incision through a fascia to relieve tension or pressure.

fasting blood sugar: a blood test to measure the glucose levels after the patient has not eaten for 8 to 12 hours.

fat embolus (**EM**-boh-lus)**:** the release of fat cells from yellow bone marrow into the bloodstream when a long bone is fractured.

female pattern baldness: a condition in which the hair thins in the front and on the sides of the scalp and sometimes on the crown.

fenestration (fen-es-TRAY-shun): a surgical procedure in which a new opening is created in the labyrinth to restore lost hearing.

fetal alcohol syndrome: condition characterized by growth abnormalities, mental retardation, brain damage, and socialization difficulties, caused by the mother's consumption of alcohol during pregnancy.

fetal monitoring: the use of an electronic device to record the fetal heart rate and the maternal uterine contractions during labor.

fetal ultrasound: a noninvasive procedure used to image and evaluate fetal development during pregnancy.

fever: a body temperature of 100° F or higher.

fibrillation (fih-brih-LAY-shun): a rapid and uncontrolled heart beat.

fibroadenoma (figh-broh-ad-eh-NOH-mah): round, rubbery, firm mass that arises from excess growth of glandular and connective tissue in the breast.

fibrocystic breast disease (figh-broh-SIS-tick): the presence of single or multiple benign cysts in the breasts.

fibromyalgia syndrome (figh-broh-my-AL-jee-ah): a debilitating chronic condition characterized by fatigue, muscle, joint, or bone pain, and a wide range of other symptoms.

fibrous dysplasia (dis-PLAY-see-ah): a bone disorder of unknown cause that destroys normal bone structure and replaces it with fibrous (scar-like) tissue.

first trimester screening: performed between 11 and 13 weeks of pregnancy and involves an ultrasound and a finger-stick blood test.

fissure (FISH-ur): a groove or crack-like sore of the skin; also normal folds in the contours of the brain.

fistula (FIS-tyou-lah): an abnormal passage between two internal organs or leading from an organ to the surface of the body.

flatulence (FLAT-you-lens): passage of gas out of the body through the rectum.

floaters: particles of cellular debris that float in the vitreous fluid and cast shadows on the retina.

fluorescein angiography (flew-oh-RES-ee-in an-jee-OG-rah-fee): a radiographic study of the blood vessels in the retina of the eye following the intravenous injection of a fluorescein dye as a contrast medium.

fluorescein staining (flew-oh-RES-ee-in): the application of a fluorescent dye to the surface of the eye via eye drops or a strip applicator.

fluoroscopy (floo-or-OS-koh-pee): the visualization of body parts in motion by projecting x-ray images on a luminous fluorescent screen.

Foley catheter: the most common type of indwelling catheter.

folliculitis (foh-lick-you-LYE-tis): inflammation of the hair follicles.

food-borne and waterborne transmission: caused by eating or drinking contaminated food or water that has not been properly treated to remove contamination or kill pathogens that are present.

fracture: a broken bone.

fructosamine test (fruck-TOHS-ah-meen): a blood test that measures average glucose levels over the past three weeks.

functional disorder: a condition that produces symptoms for which no physiological or anatomical cause can be identified.

functional endoscopic sinus surgery: a surgical procedure performed using an endoscope in which chronic sinusitis is treated by enlarging the opening between the nose and sinus.

functional MRI: detects changes in blood flow in the brain when the patient is asked to perform a specific task.

fungus (FUNG-gus): a simple parasitic organism.

furuncles (FYOU-rung-kulz): large, tender, swollen areas caused by a staphylococcal infection around hair follicles or sebaceous glands.

G

galactorrhea (gah-lack-toh-REE-ah): the production of breast milk in women who are not breast feeding.

gallstone: a hard deposit that forms in the gallbladder and bile ducts.

Gamma knife surgery: a type of radiation treatment for brain tumors.

ganglion cyst: a harmless fluid-filled swelling that occurs most commonly on the outer surface of the wrist.

gangrene (GANG-green): tissue death caused by a loss of circulation to the affected tissues.

gastralgia (gas-TRAL-jee-ah): pain in the stomach.

gastrectomy (gas-TRECK-toh-mee): surgical removal of all or a part of the stomach.

gastritis (gas-TRY-tis): inflammation of the stomach lining.

gastroduodenostomy (gas-troh-dew-oh-deh-NOS-toh-mee): the establishment of an anastomosis between the upper portion of the stomach and the duodenum.

gastrodynia (**gas**-troh-**DIN**-ee-ah)**:** pain in the stomach.

gastroenteritis (**gas**-troh-en-ter-**EYE**-tis)**:** inflammation of the mucous membrane lining the stomach and intestines.

gastroesophageal reflux disease (gas-troh-eh-**sof**-ah-**JEE**-al **REE**-flucks)**:** the upward flow of acid from the stomach into the esophagus.

gastrorrhea (**gas**-troh-**REE**-ah)**:** the excessive secretion of gastric juice or mucus in the stomach.

gastrosis (gas-**TROH**-sis)**:** any disease of the stomach.

gastrostomy tube (gas-**TROS**-toh-mee)**:** a surgically placed feeding tube from the exterior of the body directly into the stomach.

generalized anxiety disorder: a mental condition characterized by chronic, excessive worrying.

generic drug: medication named for its chemical structure that is not protected by a brand name or trademark.

genetic disorder: a pathological condition caused by an absent or defective gene.

genital herpes (**HER**-peez)**:** a sexually transmitted disease caused by the herpes simplex virus type 1 or 2.

genital warts: a sexually transmitted disease caused by the human papillomavirus.

gestational diabetes mellitus (jes-**TAY**-shun-al **dye**-ah-**BEE**-teez mel-**EYE**-tus *or* **MEL**-ih-tus)**:** the form of diabetes that occurs during some pregnancies.

gigantism (jigh-**GAN**-tiz-em)**:** abnormal growth of the entire body caused by excessive secretion of the growth hormone before puberty.

gingivectomy (**jin**-jih-**VECK**-toh-mee)**:** surgical removal of diseased gingival tissue.

gingivitis (**jin**-jih-**VYE**-tis)**:** inflammation of the gums; the earliest stage of periodontal disease.

glaucoma (glaw-**KOH**-mah)**:** a group of diseases characterized by increased intraocular pressure that causes damage to the optic nerve and retinal nerve fibers.

glomerulonephritis (gloh-**mer**-you-loh-neh-**FRY**-tis)**:** a type of nephritis caused by inflammation of the glomeruli.

glycosuria (**glye**-koh-**SOO**-ree-ah)**:** the presence of glucose in the urine.

goiter (**GOI**-ter)**:** an abnormal, nonmalignant enlargement of the thyroid gland.

gonorrhea (**gon**-oh-**REE**-ah)**:** a highly contagious sexually transmitted disease caused by the bacterium *Neisseria gonorrhoeae.*

gouty arthritis (**GOW**-tee ar-**THRIGH**-tis)**:** a type of arthritis characterized by deposits of uric acid in the joints.

granulation tissue: the tissue that normally forms during the healing of a wound that will become the scar tissue.

granuloma (**gran**-you-**LOH**-mah)**:** a general term used to describe a small, knot-like swelling of granulation tissue in the epidermis.

Graves' disease (**GRAYVZ** dih-**ZEEZ**)**:** an autoimmune disorder in which the immune system stimulates the thyroid to make excessive amounts of thyroid hormone.

greenstick fracture: a type of fracture in which the bone is bent and only partially broken.

guided imagery: a type of treatment in which a patient follows verbal prompts to envision a peaceful location and distance himself from current pain or stress.

Guillain-Barré syndrome (gee-**YAHN**-bah-**RAY**)**:** inflammation of the myelin sheath of peripheral nerves, characterized by rapidly worsening muscle weakness that may lead to temporary paralysis.

gynecomastia (**guy**-neh-koh-**MAS**-tee-ah)**:** the condition of excessive mammary development in the male.

H

halitosis (hal-ih-**TOH**-sis)**:** an unpleasant odor coming from the mouth.

hallucination (hah-**loo**-sih-**NAY**-shun)**:** a sensory perception experienced in the absence of an external stimulation.

hallux valgus (**HAL**-ucks **VAL**-guss)**:** an abnormal enlargement of the joint at the base of the great toe.

hamstring injury: a strain or tear on any of the three hamstring muscles that straighten the hip and bend the knee.

Hashimoto's disease (hah-shee-**MOH**-tohz)**:** an autoimmune disorder in which the body's own antibodies attack and destroy the cells of the thyroid gland.

hearing aid: an electronic device that is worn to correct a hearing loss.

heart failure: a chronic condition in which the heart is unable to pump out all of the blood it receives.

heart murmur: an abnormal blowing or clicking sound heard when listening to the heart or neighboring large blood vessels.

heel spurs: a calcium deposit in the plantar fascia near its attachment to the heel.

hemangioma (hee-**man**-jee-**OH**-mah)**:** a benign tumor made up of newly formed blood vessels.

hemarthrosis (**hem**-ar-**THROH**-sis)**:** blood within a joint.

hematemesis (**hee**-mah-**TEM**-eh-sis)**:** the vomiting of blood.

hematochezia (hee-**mat**-oh-**KEE**-zee-uh)**:** the flow of bright red blood in the stool.

hematocrit (hee-**MAT**-oh-krit) (**Hct** or **HCT**)**:** a blood test that measures the percentage by volume of red blood cells in a whole blood sample.

hematoma (**hee**-mah-**TOH**-mah)**:** a swelling of clotted blood trapped in the tissues.

hematospermia (**hee**-moh-**SPER**-mee-ah)**:** the presence of blood in the seminal fluid.

hematuria (**hee**-mah-**TOO**-ree-ah)**:** the presence of blood in the urine.

hemianopia (**hem**-ee-ah-**NOH**-pee-ah)**:** blindness in one half of the visual field.

hemiparesis (**hem**-ee-pah-**REE**-sis)**:** slight paralysis or weakness affecting only one side of the body.

hemiplegia (**hem**-ee-**PLEE**-jee-ah)**:** total paralysis affecting only one side of the body.

Hemoccult test (**HEE**-moh-kult)**:** a laboratory test for hidden blood in the stools.

hemochromatosis (**hee**-moh-**kroh**-mah-**TOH**-sis)**:** a genetic disorder in which the intestines absorb too much iron.

hemodialysis (**hee**-moh-dye-**AL**-ih-sis)**:** a process by which waste products are filtered directly from the patient's blood.

hemoglobin A1c testing (HbA1c)**:** a blood test that measures the average blood glucose level over the previous three to four months.

hemolytic anemia (**hee**-moh-**LIT**-ick ah-**NEE**-meeah)**:** condition characterized by an inadequate number of circulating red blood cells due to their premature destruction by the spleen.

hemophilia (**hee**-moh-**FILL**-ee-ah)**:** a group of hereditary bleeding disorders in which a blood-clotting factor is missing.

hemoptysis (hee-**MOP**-tih-sis)**:** expectoration of blood or bloodstained sputum.

hemorrhage (**HEM**-or-idj)**:** the loss of a large amount of blood in a short time.

hemorrhagic stroke (**hem**-oh-**RAJ**-ick)**:** damage to the brain that occurs when a blood vessel in the brain leaks.

hemorrhoidectomy (**hem**-oh-roid-**ECK**-toh-mee)**:** the surgical removal of hemorrhoids.

hemorrhoids (**HEM**-oh-roids)**:** a condition that occurs when a cluster of enlarged veins, muscles, and tissues slip near or through the anal opening.

hemostasis (**hee**-moh-**STAY**-sis)**:** to stop or control bleeding.

hemothorax (**hee**-moh-**THOH**-racks)**:** a collection of blood in the pleural cavity.

hepatectomy (**hep**-ah-**TECK**-toh-mee)**:** the surgical removal of all or part of the liver.

hepatitis (**hep**-ah-**TYE**-tis)**:** inflammation of the liver.

hepatomegaly (**hep**-ah-toh-**MEG**-ah-lee)**:** abnormal enlargement of the liver.

hernia (**HER**-nee-ah)**:** the protrusion of a part or structure through the tissues normally containing it.

herniated disk (**HER**-nee-**ayt**-ed)**:** the breaking apart of a intervertebral disk that results in pressure on spinal nerve roots.

herpes labialis (**HER**-peez **lay**-bee-**AL**-iss)**:** blister-like sores on the lips caused by HSV-1.

herpes zoster (**HER**-peez **ZOS**-ter)**:** an acute viral infection characterized by painful skin eruptions that follow the underlying route of an inflamed nerve.

Hertz (Hz)**:** a measure of sound frequency that determines how high or low a pitch is.

hiatal hernia (high-**AY**-tal **HER**-nee-ah)**:** the protrusion of part of the stomach through an opening in the diaphragm.

high-density lipoprotein cholesterol: the form of cholesterol that does not contribute to plaque buildup.

hip resurfacing: an alternative to total hip replacement, a metal cap is placed over the head of the femur to allow it to move smoothly over a metal lining in the acetabulum.

hirsutism (**HER**-soot-izm)**:** excessive bodily and facial hair in women, usually occurring in a male pattern.

Hodgkin's lymphoma (**HODJ**-kinz lim-**FOH**-mah)**:** a malignancy of the lymphatic system that is distinguished from non-Hodgkin's lymphoma by the presence of *Reed-Sternberg cells.*

holistic (**hoe**-**LISS**-tick)**:** a treatment approach that takes into consideration the whole body and its environment, including the mind, body, and spirit.

Holter monitor: a portable electrocardiograph worn by an ambulatory patient to continuously monitor the heart rates and rhythms over a 24- or 48-hour period.

home blood glucose monitoring: test performed by the patient using a drop of blood to measure the current blood sugar level.

homeopathy (**hoh**-mee-**OP**-ah-thee)**:** the belief that the body can stimulate its own healing responses when the right substance is given in minute doses.

homeostasis (**hoh**-mee-oh-**STAY**-sis)**:** the processes through which the body maintains a constant internal environment.

hordeolum (hor-**DEE**-oh-lum)**:** a pus-filled lesion on the eyelid resulting from an infection in a sebaceous gland.

horizontal recumbent position: lying on the back with the *face up*.

hormone replacement therapy: the use of the female hormones estrogen and progestin to replace those the body no longer produces during and after perimenopause.

hospital-acquired pneumonia: a type of pneumonia contracted during a stay in the hospital when a patient's defenses are impaired.

human growth hormone: a synthetic version of the growth hormone that is administered to stimulate growth when the natural supply of growth hormone is insufficient for normal development.

human immunodeficiency virus: a bloodborne pathogen that damages or kills the T cells of the immune system, causing it to progressively fail.

human papillomavirus: a virus that causes genital warts and cervical cancer.

Huntington's disease: a genetic disorder that causes nerve degeneration with symptoms that most often appear in midlife.

hydrocele (**HIGH**-droh-seel)**:** a fluid-filled sac in the scrotum along the spermatic cord leading from the testicles.

hydrocephalus (high-droh-**SEF**-ah-lus)**:** a condition in which excess cerebrospinal fluid accumulates within the ventricles of the brain.

hydronephrosis (**high**-droh-neh-**FROH**-sis)**:** the dilation of one or both kidneys.

hydroureter (**high**-droh-**YOUR**-eh-ter)**:** the distention of the ureter with urine that cannot flow because the ureter is blocked.

hyperbaric oxygen therapy (**high**-per-**BARE**-ik)**:** use of inhaled oxygen in a special chamber with increased air pressure to promote healing and fight infection.

hypercalcemia (**high**-per-kal-**SEE**-mee-ah)**:** abnormally high concentrations of calcium circulating in the blood.

hypercapnia (**high**-per-**KAP**-nee-ah)**:** the abnormal buildup of carbon dioxide in the blood.

hyperemesis (**high**-per-**EM**-eh-sis)**:** extreme, persistent vomiting that can cause dehydration.

hyperesthesia (**high**-per-es-**THEE**-zee-ah)**:** a condition of abnormal and excessive sensitivity to touch, pain, or other sensory stimuli.

hyperglycemia (**high**-per-glye-**SEE**-mee-ah)**:** an abnormally high concentration of glucose in the blood.

hypergonadism (**high**-per-**GOH**-nad-izm)**:** the excessive secretion of hormones by the sex glands.

hyperhidrosis (**high**-per-high-**DROH**-sis)**:** a condition of excessive sweating in one area or over the whole body.

hyperinsulinism (**high**-per-**IN**-suh-lin-izm)**:** a condition marked by excessive secretion of insulin.

hyperkinesia (**high**-per-kye-**NEE**-zee-ah)**:** abnormally increased muscle function or activity.

hyperlipidemia (**high**-per-**lip**-ih-**DEE**-mee-ah)**:** the general term used to describe elevated levels of cholesterol and other fatty substances in the blood.

hypermenorrhea (**high**-poh-men-oh-**REE**-ah)**:** an excessive amount of menstrual flow over a period of more than seven days.

hyperopia (**high**-per-**OH**-pee-ah)**:** a vision defect in which light rays focus beyond the retina; also known as farsightedness.

hyperparathyroidism (**high**-per-**par**-ah-**THIGH**-roid-izm)**:** the overproduction of the parathyroid hormone that causes hypercalcemia.

hyperpituitarism (**high**-per-pih-**TOO**-ih-tah-rizm)**:** the excess secretion of growth hormone that causes acromegaly and gigantism.

hyperplasia (**high**-per-**PLAY**-zee-ah)**:** the enlargement of an organ or tissue because of an abnormal increase in the number of cells.

hyperpnea (**high**-perp-**NEE**-ah)**:** breathing that is deeper and more rapid than is normal at rest.

hyperproteinuria (**high**-per-**proh**-tee-in-**YOU**-ree-ah)**:** the presence of abnormally high concentrations of protein in the urine.

hypertension: the elevation of arterial blood pressure to a level that is likely to cause damage to the cardiovascular system.

hyperthermia (**high**-per-**THER**-mee-ah)**:** an extremely high fever.

hyperthyroidism (**high**-per-**THIGH**-roid-izm)**:** the overproduction of thyroid hormones.

hypertrophy (high-**PER**-troh-fee)**:** a general increase in the bulk of a body part or organ due to an increase in the size, but not in the number, of cells in the tissues.

hyperventilation (**high**-per-**ven**-tih-**LAY**-shun)**:** an abnormally rapid rate of deep respiration that is usually associated with anxiety.

hypnosis: a type of therapy in which a patient is placed in a susceptible state and then given suggestions directed toward their treatment goal.

hypnotherapy: the use of hypnosis to produce an altered state of focused attention in which the patient may be more willing to believe and act on suggestions.

hypnotic: medication that depresses the central nervous system and usually produces sleep.

hypocalcemia (**high**-poh-kal-**SEE**-mee-ah)**:** a condition characterized by abnormally low levels of calcium in the blood.

hypochondriasis (**high**-poh-kon-**DRY**-ah-sis)**:** a condition characterized by fearing that one has a serious illness despite appropriate medical evaluation and reassurance.

hypoglycemia (**high**-poh-glye-**SEE**-mee-ah)**:** an abnormally low concentration of glucose in the blood.

hypogonadism (**high**-poh-**GOH**-nad-izm)**:** the condition of deficient secretion of hormones by the sex glands.

hypomenorrhea (**high**-poh-men-oh-**REE**-ah)**:** an unusually small amount of menstrual flow during a shortened regular menstrual period.

hypoparathyroidism (**high**-poh-**par**-ah-**THIGH**-roidizm)**:** a condition caused by an insufficient or absent secretion of parathyroid hormone.

hypoperfusion (**high**-poh-per-**FYOU**-zhun)**:** a deficiency of blood passing through an organ or body part.

hypophysectomy (high-**pof**-ih-**SECK**-toh-mee)**:** the removal of abnormal tissue from the pituitary gland.

hypoplasia (**high**-poh-**PLAY**-zee-ah)**:** the incomplete development of an organ or tissue.

hypopnea (**high**-poh-**NEE**-ah)**:** shallow or slow respiration.

hypoproteinemia (**high**-poh-**proh**-tee-in-**EE**-mee-ah)**:** the presence of abnormally low concentrations of protein in the blood.

hypospadias (**high**-poh-**SPAY**-dee-as)**:** the congenital abnormality of the urethral opening. In the male the urethral opening is on the underside of the penis; in the female the urethra opens into the vagina.

hypotension (**high**-poh-**TEN**-shun)**:** lower than normal arterial blood pressure.

hypothermia (**high**-poh-**THER**-mee-ah)**:** an abnormally low body temperature.

hypothyroidism (**high**-poh-**THIGH**-roid-izm)**:** a deficiency of thyroid secretion.

hypotonia (**high**-poh-**TOH**-nee-ah)**:** a condition in which there is diminished tone of the skeletal muscles.

hypoxemia (**high**-pock-**SEE**-mee-ah)**:** a condition of having low oxygen levels in the blood.

hypoxia (high-**POCK**-see-ah)**:** the condition of having deficient oxygen levels in the body tissues and organs; less severe than anoxia.

hysterectomy (**hiss**-teh-**RECK**-toh-mee)**:** the surgical removal of the uterus.

hysterosalpingography (**hiss**-ter-oh-**sal**-pin-**GOG**-rah-fee)**:** a radiographic examination of the uterus and fallopian tubes.

hysteroscopy (**hiss**-ter-**OSS**-koh-pee)**:** the direct visual examination of the interior of the uterus and fallopian tubes.

I

iatrogenic illness (eye-**at**-roh-**JEN**-ick)**:** an unfavorable response due to prescribed medical treatment.

ichthyosis (**ick**-thee-**OH**-sis)**:** a group of hereditary disorders characterized by dry, thickened, and scaly skin.

idiopathic disorder (**id**-ee-oh-**PATH**-ick)**:** an illness without known cause.

idiosyncratic reaction (**id**-ee-oh-sin-**KRAT**-ick)**:** an unexpected reaction to a drug that is peculiar to the individual.

ileal conduit (**ill**-ee-al **KON**-doo-it)**:** use of a small piece of intestine to convey urine to the ureters and to a stoma in the abdomen.

ileectomy (**ill**-ee-**ECK**-toh-mee)**:** the surgical removal of the ileum.

ileostomy (**ill**-ee-**OS**-toh-mee)**:** the surgical creation of an artificial excretory opening between the ileum and the outside of the abdominal wall.

ileus (**ILL**-ee-us)**:** the partial or complete blockage of the small and/or large intestine.

iliotibial band syndrome (**ill**-ee-oh-**TIB**-ee-al)**:** an overuse injury caused by this band rubbing against bone, often in the area of the knee.

immobilization: the act of holding, suturing, or fastening a bone in a fixed position with strapping or a cast.

immunity: the state of being resistant to a specific disease.

immunodeficiency disorder (**im**-you-noh-deh-**FISH**-en-see)**:** a condition that occurs when immune system response is compromised.

immunoglobulins (**im**-you-noh-**GLOB**-you-lins)**:** antibodies that bind with specific antigens in the antigen-antibody response.

immunosuppressant (**im**-you-noh-soo-**PRES**-ant)**:** a substance that prevents or reduces the body's normal immune response.

immunosuppression (**im**-you-noh-sup-**PRESH**-un)**:** treatment to repress or interfere with the ability of the immune system to respond to stimulation by antigens.

immunotherapy (ih-**myou**-noh-**THER**-ah-pee)**:** a disease treatment that involves either stimulating or repressing the immune response.

impacted cerumen: an accumulation of earwax that forms a solid mass by adhering to the walls of the external auditory canal.

impetigo (**im**-peh-**TYE**-goh)**:** a highly contagious bacterial skin infection characterized by isolated pustules that become crusted and rupture.

impingement syndrome (im-**PINJ**-ment)**:** inflammation of tendons that get caught in the narrow space between the bones within the shoulder joint.

impulse control disorders: a group of psychiatric disorders characterized by failure to resist an impulse despite potential negative consequences.

incision: a cut made with a surgical instrument.

incontinence (in-**KON**-tih-nents)**:** the inability to control the excretion of urine and/or feces.

incubator (**IN**-kyou-**bate**-or)**:** an apparatus for maintaining a controlled environment for a premature or ill newborn.

indirect contact transmission: refers to situations in which a susceptible person is infected by contact with a contaminated surface.

indwelling catheter: a catheter that remains inside the body for a prolonged time based on need.

infection (in-**FECK**-shun)**:** invasion of the body by a pathogenic organism.

infectious disease (in-**FECK**-shus)**:** an illness caused by living pathogenic organisms such as bacteria and viruses.

infectious mononucleosis (**mon**-oh-**new**-klee-**OH**-sis)**:** an infection caused by the Epstein-Barr virus that is characterized by fever, a sore throat, and enlarged lymph nodes.

infectious myringitis (**mir**-in-**JIGH**-tis)**:** a contagious inflammation that causes painful blisters on the eardrum.

infestation: the dwelling of microscopic parasites on external surface tissue.

infiltrating ductal carcinoma: breast cancer that starts in the milk duct, breaks through the wall of that duct, and invades the fatty breast tissue.

infiltrating lobular carcinoma: breast cancer that starts in the milk glands, breaks through the wall of the gland, and invades the fatty tissue of the breast.

inflammation (**in**-flah-**MAY**-shun)**:** a localized response to an injury or to the destruction of tissues.

inflammatory bowel disease: the general name for diseases that cause inflammation and swelling in the intestines.

inflammatory breast cancer (IBC)**:** a rare but aggressive form of breast cancer.

influenza (**in**-flew-**EN**-zah)**:** a highly contagious viral respiratory infection that occurs in seasonal epidemics.

inguinal hernia (**ING**-gwih-nal **HER**-nee-ah)**:** the protrusion of a small loop of bowel through a weak place in the lower abdominal wall or groin.

inhalation administration: the administration of medication in the form of vapor and gases taken in through the nose or mouth and absorbed into the bloodstream through the lungs.

insomnia: the prolonged or abnormal inability to sleep.

insulinoma (**in**-suh-lin-**OH**-mah)**:** a benign tumor of the pancreas that causes hypoglycemia by secreting additional insulin.

insulin shock: a diabetic emergency caused by very low blood sugar.

integrative medicine: a health care model based on both allopathic and alternative medicine.

intermittent catheter: inserted as needed to drain urine from the bladder.

intermittent claudication (**klaw**-dih-**KAY**-shun)**:** pain in the leg muscles that occurs during exercise and is relieved by rest.

internal fixation: fracture treatment in which pins or a plate are placed directly into the bone to hold the broken pieces in place.

interstitial cystitis (**in**-ter-**STISH**-al sis-**TYE**-tis)**:** a chronic inflammation within the walls of the bladder.

interstitial lung diseases (**in**-ter-**STISH**-al)**:** a group of diseases that cause inflammation and scarring of the alveoli and their supporting structures.

interventional radiology: the use of radiographic imaging to guide a procedure or confirm placement of an inserted object.

intestinal obstruction: the partial or complete blockage of the small and/or large intestine caused by a physical obstruction.

intracranial pressure: the amount of pressure inside the skull.

intradermal injection: the administration of medication by injection into the middle layers of the skin.

intramuscular injection: the administration of medication by injection directly into muscle tissue.

intraocular lens: a surgically implanted replacement for a natural lens that has been removed.

intraoral radiography: the placement of x-ray film within the mouth with the camera positioned next to the cheek.

intrauterine device: a molded plastic contraceptive inserted through the cervix into the uterus to prevent pregnancy.

intravenous fluids (**in**-trah-**VEE**-nus)**:** fluids administered into a vein to combat the effects of dehydration.

intravenous injection: the administration of medication by injection directly into a vein.

intravenous pyelogram (**PYE**-eh-loh-**gram**)**:** a radiographic study of the kidneys and ureters.

intussusception (**in**-tus-sus-**SEP**-shun)**:** the telescoping of one part of the small intestine into the opening of an immediately adjacent part.

in vitro fertilization: a procedure in which mature ova are removed from the mother to be fertilized.

iridectomy (**ir**-ih-**DECK**-toh-mee)**:** the surgical removal of a portion of the tissue of the iris.

iritis (eye-**RYE**-tis)**:** inflammation of the uvea primarily affecting structures in the front of the eye.

iron-deficiency anemia: a decrease in the red cells of the blood that is caused by too little iron.

irrigation and debridement: a procedure using pressurized fluid to clean out wound debris.

irritable bowel syndrome: a common condition of unknown cause with symptoms that can include intermittent cramping, abdominal pain, bloating, constipation, and/or diarrhea.

ischemia (iss-**KEE**-mee-ah)**:** a condition in which there is an insufficient supply of oxygen in the tissues due to restricted blood flow to a part of the body.

ischemic colitis (iss-**KEE**-mick koh-**LYE**-tis)**:** a condition that occurs when part of the large intestine is partially or completely deprived of blood.

ischemic heart disease (iss-KEE-mick): a group of cardiac disabilities resulting from an insufficient supply of oxygenated blood to the heart.

ischemic stroke: damage that occurs when the flow of blood to the brain is blocked by the narrowing or blockage of a carotid artery.

J

jaundice (**JAWN**-dis)**:** a yellow discoloration of the skin, mucous membranes, and eyes.

juvenile rheumatoid arthritis: an autoimmune disorder affecting children aged 16 years or less, with symptoms that include stiffness, pain, joint swelling, skin rash, fever, slowed growth, and fatigue.

K

Kaposi's sarcoma (**KAP**-oh-seez sar-**KOH**-mah)**:** a cancer that causes patches of abnormal tissue to grow under the skin; in the lining of the mouth, nose, and throat; or in other organs.

Kegel exercises: a series of pelvic muscle exercises used to strengthen the muscles of the pelvic floor.

keloid (**KEE**-loid)**:** an abnormally raised or thickened scar that expands beyond the boundaries of the original incision.

keratitis (**ker**-ah-**TYE**-tis)**:** inflammation of the cornea.

keratosis (**kerr**-ah-**TOH**-sis)**:** any skin growth, such as a wart or a callus, in which there is overgrowth and thickening of the skin.

ketonuria (**kee**-toh-**NEW**-ree-ah)**:** the presence of ketones in the urine.

knee-chest position: position in which the patient is lying face down with the hips bent so that the knees and chest rest on the table.

koilonychia (**koy**-loh-**NICK**-ee-ah)**:** a malformation of the nails in which the outer surface is concave or scooped out like the bowl of a spoon.

KUB (kidney-ureter-bladder)**:** a radiographic study without the use of a contrast medium, used to detect bowel obstructions and nephroliths.

kyphosis (kye-**FOH**-sis)**:** an abnormal increase in the outward curvature of the thoracic spine as viewed from the side.

L

labyrinthectomy (**lab**-ih-rin-**THECK**-toh-mee)**:** the surgical removal of all or a portion of the labyrinth.

labyrinthitis (**lab**-ih-rin-**THIGH**-tis)**:** inflammation of the labyrinth that can result in vertigo and deafness.

laceration (**lass**-er-**AY**-shun)**:** a torn or jagged wound or an accidental cut.

laminectomy (**lam**-ih-**NECK**-toh-mee)**:** the surgical removal of a lamina from a vertebra.

laparoscopic adrenalectomy (ah-**dree**-nal-**ECK**-tohmee)**:** a minimally invasive procedure to surgically remove one or both adrenal glands.

laparoscopy (**lap**-ah-**ROS**-koh-pee)**:** the visual examination of the interior of the abdomen with the use of a laparoscope.

laryngectomy (**lar**-in-**JECK**-toh-mee)**:** the surgical removal of the larynx.
laryngitis (**lar**-in-**JIGH**-tis)**:** inflammation of the larynx.
laryngoscopy (**lar**-ing-**GOS**-koh-pee)**:** the visual examination of the larynx and vocal cords using a laryngoscope.
laryngospasm (lah-**RING**-goh-spazm)**:** the sudden spasmodic closure of the larynx.
laryngotomy (**lar**-ing-**OT**-oh-mee)**:** a surgical incision into the larynx.
laser: an acronym for *light amplification by stimulated emission of radiation,* used to treat skin conditions and other disorders of the body.
laser angioplasty (**AN**-jee-oh-**plas**-tee)**:** removing plaque deposit in an artery using beams of light from a laser on the end of a catheter.
laser iridotomy (**ir**-ih-**DOT**-oh-mee)**:** uses a focused beam of light to create a hole in the iris of the eye.
laser trabeculoplasty (trah-**BECK**-you-loh-**plas**-tee)**:** treatment of open-angle glaucoma by creating openings in the trabecular meshwork to allow fluid to drain properly.
LASIK (laser-assisted in situ keratomileusis)**:** treatment of vision conditions that are caused by the shape of the cornea.
latent autoimmune diabetes in adults: a condition in which type 1 diabetes develops in adults.
laxatives: medications or foods given to stimulate bowel movements.
learning disabilities: disorders found in children of normal intelligence who have difficulties in learning specific skills such as processing language or grasping mathematical concepts.
lensectomy (len-**SECK**-toh-mee)**:** the surgical removal of a cataract-clouded lens.
lesion (**LEE**-zhun)**:** a pathologic change of tissues due to disease or injury.
lethargy (**LETH**-ar-jee)**:** a lowered level of consciousness marked by listlessness, drowsiness, and apathy.
leukemia (loo-**KEE**-mee-ah)**:** a type of cancer characterized by a progressive increase in the number of abnormal white blood cells found in blood-forming tissues, other organs, and in the circulating blood.
leukopenia (**loo**-koh-**PEE**-nee-ah)**:** a decrease in the number of white blood cells circulating in the blood.
leukoplakia (**loo**-koh-**PLAY**-kee-ah)**:** an abnormal white precancerous lesion that develops inside the mouth in response to chronic irritation.
leukorrhea (**loo**-koh-**REE**-ah)**:** a profuse whitish mucus discharge from the uterus and vagina.
levels of consciousness: terms used to describe the measurement of response to arousal and stimulus.
light therapy: exposure to daylight or specific wavelengths of light in order to counteract seasonal affective disorder.
lipectomy (lih-**PECK**-toh-mee)**:** the surgical removal of fat from beneath the skin.
lipedema (lip-eh-**DEE**-mah)**:** a chronic abnormal condition characterized by the accumulation of fat and fluid in the tissues just under the skin of the hips and legs.
lipid panel: a blood test that measures the amounts of total cholesterol, high-density lipoprotein, low-density lipoprotein, and triglycerides.
lipoma (lih-**POH**-mah)**:** a benign, slow-growing fatty tumor located between the skin and the muscle layer.
liposuction (**LIP**-oh-**suck**-shun *or* **LYE**-poh-suckshun)**:** the surgical removal of fat beneath the skin with the aid of suction.
lithotomy (lih-**THOT**-oh-mee)**:** a surgical incision for the removal of a stone from the bladder.
lithotomy position (lih-**THOT**-oh-mee)**:** an examination position in which the patient is lying on the back with the feet and legs raised and supported in stirrups.
liver transplant: an option for a patient whose liver has failed for a reason other than liver cancer.
lobar pneumonia: a type of pneumonia that affects larger areas of the lungs, often including one or more sections, or lobes, of a lung.
lobectomy (loh-**BECK**-toh-mee)**:** the surgical removal of a lobe of an organ.
localized allergic response: includes redness, itching, and burning where the skin has come into contact with an allergen.
lordosis (lor-**DOH**-sis)**:** an abnormal increase in the forward curvature of the lumbar spine.
low-density lipoprotein cholesterol: the form of cholesterol that contributes to plaque buildup in the arteries.
lumbago (lum-**BAY**-goh)**:** pain of the lumbar region of the spine.
lumbar puncture: the process of obtaining a sample of cerebrospinal fluid by inserting a needle into the subarachnoid space of the lumbar region to withdraw fluid.
lumbar radiculopathy: nerve pain in the lower back.
lumpectomy: surgical removal of only the cancerous tissue with the surrounding margin of normal tissue.
lung cancer: a condition in which cancer cells form in the tissues of the lung.
Lyme disease: a bacterial infection caused by a spirochete belonging to the genus *Borrelia.*

lymphadenitis (lim-**fad**-eh-**NIGH**-tis)**:** inflammation of the lymph nodes.

lymphadenopathy (lim-**fad**-eh-**NOP**-ah-thee)**:** any disease process affecting a lymph node or nodes.

lymphangioma (lim-**fan**-jee-**OH**-mah)**:** a benign tumor formed by an abnormal collection of lymphatic vessels.

lymphedema (**lim**-feh-**DEE**-mah)**:** swelling of the tissues due to an abnormal accumulation of lymph fluid within the tissues.

lymph node dissection: a surgical procedure in which all of the lymph nodes in a major group are removed to determine or slow the spread of cancer.

lymphoma (lim-**FOH**-mah)**:** a general term applied to malignancies affecting lymphoid tissues.

lymphoscintigraphy (**lim**-foh-sin-**TIH**-grah-fee)**:** a diagnostic test that is performed to detect damage or malformations of the lymphatic vessels.

M

macular degeneration (**MACK**-you-lar)**:** a gradually progressive condition in which the macula at the center of the retina is damaged, resulting in the loss of central vision.

macule (**MACK**-youl)**:** a discolored, flat spot that is less than 1 cm in diameter.

magnetic resonance angiography: a specialized MRI study using a contrast medium to locate problems with blood vessels throughout the body.

magnetic resonance imaging (MRI)**:** an imaging technique that uses a combination of radio waves and a strong magnetic field to create signals that are sent to a computer and converted into images of any plane through the body.

malabsorption (**mal**-ab-**SORP**-shun)**:** a condition in which the small intestine cannot absorb nutrients from the food that passes through it.

malaise (mah-**LAYZ**)**:** a feeling of general discomfort, often the first indication of an infection or disease.

malaria (mah-**LAY**-ree-ah)**:** a disease caused by a parasite that lives in certain mosquitoes and is transferred to humans by the bite of an infected mosquito.

male pattern baldness: a common hair-loss pattern in men.

malignant melanoma (mel-ah-**NOH**-mah)**:** a type of skin cancer that occurs in the melanocytes.

malingering (mah-**LING**-ger-ing)**:** a condition characterized by the intentional creation of false or grossly exaggerated physical or psychological symptoms.

malnutrition: a lack of proper food or nutrients in the body, due to a shortage of food, poor eating habits, or the inability of the body to digest, absorb, and distribute these nutrients.

mammography (mam-**OG**-rah-fee)**:** a radiographic examination of the breast to detect the presence of tumors or precancerous cells.

mammoplasty (**MAM**-oh-**plas**-tee)**:** a cosmetic operation on the breasts.

manic behavior: an abnormally elevated mood state, including inappropriate elation, increased irritability, severe insomnia, poor judgment, and inappropriate social behavior.

Mantoux PPD skin test: a test for diagnosing tuberculosis.

mastalgia (mass-**TAL**-jee-ah)**:** pain in the breast.

mastectomy (mas-**TECK**-toh-mee)**:** surgical removal of the entire breast and nipple.

mastitis (mas-**TYE**-tis)**:** a breast infection that is caused by bacteria that enter the breast tissue, most frequently during breastfeeding.

mastoidectomy (**mas**-toy-**DECK**-toh-mee)**:** the surgical removal of mastoid cells.

mastoiditis (**mas**-toy-**DYE**-tis)**:** inflammation of any part of the mastoid bone cells.

mastopexy (**MAS**-toh-**peck**-see)**:** surgery to affix sagging breasts in a more elevated position.

maxillofacial surgery (mack-**sill**-oh-**FAY**-shul)**:** specialized surgery of the face and jaws to correct deformities, treat diseases, and repair injuries.

measles: an acute, highly contagious infection transmitted by respiratory droplets of the rubeola virus.

measles, mumps, and rubella vaccination (MMR)**:** childhood immunization that can prevent these three viral conditions.

meatotomy (**mee**-ah-**TOT**-oh-mee)**:** a surgical incision made in the urethral meatus to enlarge the opening.

megaloblastic anemia (**MEG**-ah-loh-**blas**-tick ah-**NEE**-mee-ah)**:** a blood disorder characterized by anemia in which red blood cells are larger than normal.

melanin (**MEL**-ah-nin)**:** the pigment that determines the color of the skin.

melena (meh-**LEE**-nah)**:** the passage of black, tarry, and foul-smelling stools.

Ménière's disease (men-**YEHRS**)**:** a rare chronic disorder in which the amount of fluid in the inner ear increases intermittently, causing vertigo, fluctuating hearing loss, and tinnitus.

meningioma (meh-**nin**-jee-**OH**-mah)**:** a common, slow-growing and usually benign tumor of the meninges.

meningitis (men-in-JIGH-tis): inflammation of the meninges of the brain and spinal cord.

meningocele (meh-NING-goh-seel): the congenital herniation of the meninges through a defect in the skull or spinal column.

menometrorrhagia (men-oh-met-roh-RAY-jee-ah): excessive uterine bleeding occurring both during the menses and at other irregular intervals.

mental retardation/intellectual disability: significant below-average intellectual and adaptive functioning present from birth or early infancy.

metastasis (meh-TAS-tah-sis): the new cancer site that results from the spreading process.

metastasize (meh-TAS-tah-sighz): the process by which cancer spreads from one place to another.

metered dose inhaler: a medical device that administers a specific amount of a medication such as a bronchodilator in aerosol form.

methicillin-resistant *Staphylococcus aureus* (MRSA): one of several types of bacteria that are now resistant to most antibiotics.

metrorrhea (mee-troh-REE-ah): an abnormal discharge, such as mucus or pus, from the uterus.

migraine (MY-grayn): a headache characterized by throbbing pain on one side of the head and may be preceded by a warning aura.

mindfulness meditation: treatment for stress focused on maintaining a calm, constant awareness and acceptance of thoughts and emotions.

minimally invasive coronary artery bypass: a bypass procedure performed with the aid of a fiberoptic camera through small openings between the ribs.

miosis (mye-OH-sis): the contraction of the pupil.

modified radical mastectomy: the surgical removal of the entire breast and axillary lymph nodes under the adjacent arm.

Mohs surgery: a technique used to treat various types of skin cancer by removing layers of cancerous tissue until a healthy margin is achieved.

monaural testing (mon-AW-rahl): involves one ear.

monochromatism (mon-oh-KROH-mah-tizm): the inability to distinguish certain colors in a normal manner.

monoclonal antibodies: artificially produced antibodies used to enhance a patient's immune response to certain malignancies.

mood-stabilizing drugs: used to treat mood instability and bipolar disorders.

morbid obesity: the condition of weighing two or more times the ideal weight or having a body mass index value greater than 40.

multiparous (mul-TIP-ah-rus): a woman who has given birth two or more times.

multiple sclerosis (skleh-ROH-sis): a progressive autoimmune disorder characterized by inflammation that causes demyelination of the myelin sheath.

mumps: an acute viral infection characterized by the swelling of the parotid glands.

muscle biopsy: removal of a plug of tissue with a biopsy needle for examination.

muscle tone: the state of balanced muscle tension that makes normal posture, coordination, and movement possible.

muscular dystrophy (DIS-troh-fee): a group of more than 30 genetic diseases that are characterized by progressive weakness and degeneration of the skeletal muscles without affecting the nervous system.

myalgia (my-AL-jee-ah): tenderness or pain in the muscles.

myasthenia gravis (my-as-THEE-nee-ah GRAH-vis): a chronic autoimmune disease that affects the neuromuscular junction and produces serious weakness of voluntary muscles.

mycosis (my-KOH-sis): any abnormal condition or disease caused by a fungus.

mydriasis (mih-DRY-ah-sis): the dilation of the pupil.

mydriatic drops (mid-ree-AT-ick): medication placed into the eyes to produce temporary paralysis forcing the pupils to remain wide open even in the presence of bright light.

myelitis (my-eh-LYE-tis): inflammation of the spinal cord; inflammation of bone marrow.

myelodysplastic syndrome (my-eh-loh-dis-PLAS-tick): a group of bone marrow disorders that are characterized by the insufficient production of one or more types of blood cells.

myelography (my-eh-LOG-rah-fee): a radiographic study of the spinal cord after the injection of a contrast medium through a lumbar puncture.

myeloma (my-eh-LOH-mah): a type of cancer that occurs in blood-making cells of the red bone marrow.

myelopathy (my-eh-LOP-ah-thee): any pathologic change or disease in the spinal cord.

myelosis (my-eh-LOH-sis): a tumor of the spinal cord.

myocardial infarction (my-oh-KAR-dee-al in-FARK-shun): the occlusion of one or more coronary arteries caused by plaque buildup.

myocarditis (**my**-oh-kar-**DYE**-tis)**:** inflammation of the myocardium.
myocele (**MY**-oh-seel)**:** the herniation of muscle substance through a tear in the fascia surrounding it.
myoclonus (**my**-oh-**KLOH**-nus *or* my-**OCK**-loh-nus)**:** the sudden, involuntary jerking of a muscle or group of muscles.
myofascial pain syndrome: a chronic pain disorder that affects muscles and fascia throughout the body.
myofascial release: a specialized soft-tissue manipulation technique used to ease the pain of conditions such as fibromyalgia, myofascial pain syndrome, movement restrictions, temporomandibular joint disorders, and carpal tunnel syndrome.
myolysis (my-**OL**-ih-sis)**:** the degeneration of muscle tissue.
myoma (my-**OH**-mah)**:** a benign tumor made up of muscle tissue.
myomectomy (**my**-oh-**MECK**-toh-mee)**:** the surgical removal of uterine fibroids.
myoparesis (**my**-oh-**PAR**-eh-sis)**:** weakness or slight muscular paralysis.
myopathy (my-**OP**-ah-thee)**:** any pathologic change or disease of muscle tissue.
myopia (my-**OH**-pee-ah)**:** a defect in which light rays focus in front of the retina; also known as nearsightedness.
myoplasty (**MY**-oh-**plas**-tee)**:** the surgical repair of a muscle.
myorrhaphy (my-**OR**-ah-fee)**:** surgical suturing of a muscle.
myorrhexis (**my**-oh-**RECK**-sis)**:** the rupture or tearing of a muscle.
myosarcoma (**my**-oh-sahr-**KOH**-mah)**:** a malignant tumor derived from muscle tissue.
myotomy (my-**OT**-oh-mee)**:** a surgical incision into a muscle.
myringotomy (**mir**-in-**GOT**-oh-mee)**:** a small surgical incision in the eardrum to relieve pressure from excess pus or fluid, or to create an opening for the placement of ear tubes.
myxedema (**mick**-seh-**DEE**-mah)**:** a severe form of adult hypothyroidism caused by extreme deficiency of thyroid secretion.

N

narcolepsy (**NAR**-koh-**lep**-see)**:** a sleep disorder consisting of sudden and uncontrollable brief episodes of falling asleep during the day.
nasogastric intubation (**nay**-zoh-**GAS**-trick **in**-too-**BAY**-shun)**:** the placement of a tube through the nose and into the stomach.
natural immunity: disease resistance without administration of an antigen or exposure to disease, either present at birth or passed on from mother to child through breast milk.
naturopathy (**nay**-cher-**AH**-pah-thee)**:** a form of alternative medicine emphasizing the healing power of nature and support of the body's own healing ability.
nausea (**NAW**-see-ah)**:** the urge to vomit.
nebulizer (**NEB**-you-lye-zer)**:** an electronic device that pumps air or oxygen through a liquid medicine to turn it into a mist that is inhaled via a face mask or mouthpiece.
necrotizing fasciitis (**NECK**-roh-**tiz**-ing **fas**-ee-**EYE**-tis) (NF)**:** a severe infection caused by group A strep bacteria.
needle breast biopsy: a technique in which an x-ray-guided needle is used to remove small samples of tissue from the breast.
neobladder (**NEE**-oh-**blad**-er)**:** bladder replacement using part of the small intestine.
neoplasm (**NEE**-oh-plazm)**:** an abnormal growth of body tissue in which the multiplication of cells is uncontrolled, abnormal, rapid, and progressive; also known as a tumor.
nephritis (neh-**FRY**-tis)**:** inflammation of the kidney or kidneys.
nephrolith (**NEF**-roh-lith)**:** a stone located in the kidney.
nephrolithiasis (**nef**-roh-lih-**THIGH**-ah-sis)**:** the presence of stones in the kidney.
nephrolysis (neh-**FROL**-ih-sis)**:** the surgical freeing of a kidney from adhesions.
nephropathy (neh-**FROP**-ah-thee)**:** any disease of the kidney.
nephropexy (**NEF**-roh-**peck**-see)**:** the surgical fixation of nephroptosis.
nephroptosis (**nef**-rop-**TOH**-sis)**:** the prolapse of a kidney into the pelvic area when the patient stands.
nephropyosis (**nef**-roh-pye-**OH**-sis)**:** suppuration of the kidney.
nephrostomy (neh-**FROS**-toh-mee)**:** the placement of a catheter to maintain an opening between the pelvis of one or both kidneys to the exterior of the body.
nephrotic syndrome (neh-**FROT**-ick)**:** a group of conditions in which excessive amounts of protein are lost in the urine.
neuritis (new-**RYE**-tis)**:** inflammation of a nerve accompanied by pain and sometimes loss of function.

neurodegenerative disease (**new**-roh-deh-**JEN**-er-ah-tiv)**:** an umbrella term for disorders in which there is a progressive loss of the structure or functions of neurons.

neurogenic bladder (new-roh-**JEN**-ick)**:** a urinary problem caused by interference with the normal nerve pathways associated with urination.

neuromuscular blocker: a medication that causes temporary paralysis by blocking the transmission of nerve stimuli to the muscles.

neuromuscular therapy: a form of massage that uses soft-tissue manipulation focusing on applying pressure to trigger points to treat injuries and alleviate pain.

neuroplasty (**NEW**-roh-**plas**-tee)**:** the surgical repair of a nerve or nerves.

neurorrhaphy (new-**ROR**-ah-fee)**:** surgically suturing together the ends of a severed nerve.

neurotomy (new-**ROT**-oh-mee)**:** the surgical division or dissection of a nerve.

nevus (**NEE**-vye)**:** a small, dark skin growth that develops from melanocytes in the skin.

nitroglycerin: a vasodilator that is prescribed to prevent or relieve the pain of angina.

nocturia (nock-**TOO**-ree-ah)**:** frequent and excessive urination during the night.

nocturnal enuresis (nock-**TER**-nal **en**-you-**REE**-sis): urinary incontinence during sleep.

nocturnal myoclonus (nock-**TER**-nal **my**-oh-**KLOH**-nus *or* my-**OCK**-loh-nus)**:** jerking of the limbs that can occur normally as a person is falling asleep.

nodule: a solid, raised skin lesion that is larger than 0.5 cm in diameter and deeper than a papule.

noise-induced hearing loss: nerve deafness caused by repeated exposure to extremely loud noises.

nonalcoholic fatty liver disease (NAFLD)**:** describes the accumulation of fat in the liver of people who drink little or no alcohol.

nonalcoholic steatohepatitis (NASH)**:** a more serious form of *nonalcoholic fatty liver disease,* consists of fatty accumulations plus liver-damaging inflammation.

non-Hodgkin's lymphoma (non-**HODJ**-kinz lim-**FOH**-mah)**:** the term used to describe all lymphomas *other than* Hodgkin's lymphoma.

non-steroidal anti-inflammatory drugs: medications administered to control pain by reducing inflammation and swelling.

normal sperm count: 20 to 120 million or more sperm per mL of semen.

nosocomial infection (**nos**-oh-**KOH**-mee-al)**:** a disease acquired in a hospital or clinical setting.

nuclear scan: a diagnostic procedure that uses nuclear medicine technology to gather information about the structure and function of organs or body systems.

nulligravida (**null**-ih-**GRAV**-ih-dah)**:** a woman who has never been pregnant.

nullipara (nuh-**LIP**-ah-rah)**:** a woman who has never borne a viable child.

nyctalopia (**nick**-tah-**LOH**-pee-ah)**:** a condition in which an individual with normal daytime vision has difficulty seeing at night.

nystagmus (nis-**TAG**-mus)**:** an involuntary, constant, rhythmic movement of the eyeball.

O

obesity (oh-**BEE**-sih-tee)**:** an excessive accumulation of fat in the body.

oblique fracture: a fracture that occurs at an angle across the bone.

obsessive-compulsive disorder: a mental condition characterized by obsessions and/or compulsions.

occupational therapy: activities to promote recovery and rehabilitation to assist patients in performing the activities of daily living.

ocular prosthesis: a replacement for an eyeball that is either congenitally missing or has been surgically removed.

oligomenorrhea (**ol**-ih-goh-**men**-oh-**REE**-ah)**:** light or infrequent menstruation in a woman with previously normal periods.

oligospermia (**ol**-ih-goh-**SPER**-mee-ah)**:** a sperm count of below 20 million/mL.

oliguria (**ol**-ih-**GOO**-ree-ah)**:** scanty urination.

onychia (oh-**NICK**-ee-ah)**:** inflammation of the matrix of the nail.

onychocryptosis (**on**-ih-koh-krip-**TOH**-sis)**:** ingrown toenail.

onychomycosis (**on**-ih-koh-my-**KOH**-sis)**:** a fungal infection of the nail.

onychophagia (**on**-ih-koh-**FAY**-jee-ah)**:** nail biting or nail eating.

oophorectomy (**oh**-ahf-oh-**RECK**-toh-mee)**:** the surgical removal of one or both ovaries.

oophoritis (**oh**-ahf-oh-**RYE**-tis)**:** inflammation of an ovary.

open-angle glaucoma: the most common form of glaucoma.

open fracture: a fracture in which the bone is broken and there is an open wound in the skin.

ophthalmoscope (ahf-**THAL**-moh-skope)**:** an instrument used to examine the interior of the eye.

ophthalmoscopy (**ahf**-thal-**MOS**-koh-pee)**:** the visual examination of the fundus of the eye with ophthalmoscope.

opportunistic infection (**op**-ur-too-**NIHS**-tick)**:** caused by a pathogen that does not normally produce an illness in healthy humans.

oral administration: medication taken by mouth to be absorbed through the walls of the stomach or small intestine.

oral glucose tolerance test (**GLOO**-kohs)**:** a test performed to confirm a diagnosis of diabetes mellitus and to aid in diagnosing hypoglycemia.

oral or maxillofacial surgeon (mack-**sill**-oh-**FAY**-shul)**:** a physician specializing in surgery of the face and jaws to correct deformities, treat diseases, and repair injuries.

oral rehydration therapy: treatment in which a solution of electrolytes is administered in a liquid preparation to counteract dehydration.

oral thrush: a type of stomatomycosis caused by the fungus *Candida albicans*.

orbitotomy (**or**-bih-**TOT**-oh-mee)**:** a surgical incision into the orbit.

orchidectomy (**or**-kih-**DECK**-toh-mee)**:** the surgical removal of one or both testicles.

orchiopexy (**or**-kee-oh-**PECK**-see)**:** the repair of an undescended testicle.

organic disorder (or-**GAN**-ick)**:** a disorder that produces symptoms caused by detectable physical changes in the body.

orthostatic hypotension (**or**-thoh-**STAT**-ick **high**-poh-**TEN**-shun)**:** low blood pressure that occurs upon standing up.

orthotic (or-**THOT**-ick)**:** a mechanical appliance, such a leg brace or splint, that is specially designed to control, correct, or compensate for impaired limb function.

ossification (**oss**-uh-fih-**KAY**-shun)**:** the normal process of bone formation.

ostealgia (**oss**-tee-**AL**-jee-ah)**:** pain in a bone.

ostectomy (oss-**TECK**-toh-mee)**:** the surgical removal of bone.

osteitis (**oss**-tee-**EYE**-tis)**:** inflammation of bone.

osteoarthritis (**oss**-tee-oh-ar-**THRIGH**-tis)**:** the type of arthritis most commonly associated with aging.

osteochondroma (**oss**-tee-oh-kon-**DROH**-mah)**:** a benign bony projection covered with cartilage.

osteoclasis (**oss**-tee-**OCK**-lah-sis)**:** the surgical fracture of a bone to correct a deformity.

osteomalacia (**oss**-tee-oh-mah-**LAY**-shee-ah)**:** abnormal softening of bones in adults.

osteomyelitis (**oss**-tee-oh-**my**-eh-**LYE**-tis)**:** inflammation of the bone marrow and adjacent bone.

osteonecrosis (**oss**-tee-oh-neh-**KROH**-sis)**:** the death of bone tissue due to an insufficient blood supply.

osteopathic manipulative therapy: mechanical spinal adjustment used in conjunction with conventional medical therapies by an osteopath.

osteopenia (**oss**-tee-oh-**PEE**-nee-ah)**:** thinner than average bone density.

osteophytes (**OSS**-tee-oh-**fites**)**:** are also known as bone spurs.

osteoplasty (**OSS**-tee-oh-**plas**-tee)**:** the surgical repair of a bone or bones.

osteoporosis (**oss**-tee-oh-poh-**ROH**-sis)**:** a marked loss of bone density and an increase in bone porosity that is frequently associated with aging.

osteoporotic hip fracture (**oss**-tee-oh-pah-**ROT**-ick)**:** a fracture of a hip weakened by osteoporosis that can occur spontaneously or as the result of a fall.

osteorrhaphy (**oss**-tee-**OR**-ah-fee)**:** surgical suturing or wiring together of bones.

osteosarcoma (**oss**-tee-oh-sar-**KOH**-mah)**:** a hard tissue sarcoma that usually involves the upper shaft of long bones, pelvis, or knee.

osteotomy (**oss**-tee-**OT**-oh-mee)**:** the surgical cutting of a bone.

ostomy (**OSS**-toh-mee)**:** a surgical procedure to create an artificial opening between an organ and the body surface.

otalgia (oh-**TAL**-gee-ah)**:** pain in the ear.

otitis (oh-**TYE**-tis)**:** inflammation of the ear.

otitis media (oh-**TYE**-tis **MEE**-dee-ah)**:** inflammation of the middle ear.

otomycosis (**oh**-toh-my-**KOH**-sis)**:** a fungal infection of the external auditory canal.

otoplasty (**OH**-toh-**plas**-tee)**:** the surgical repair, restoration or alteration of the pinna of the ear.

otopyorrhea (**oh**-toh-**pye**-oh-**REE**-ah)**:** the flow of pus from the ear.

otorrhagia (**oh**-toh-**RAY**-jee-ah)**:** bleeding from the ear.

otorrhea (**oh**-toh-**REE**-ah)**:** any discharge from the ear.

otosclerosis (**oh**-toh-skleh-**ROH**-sis)**:** ankylosis of the bones of the middle ear resulting in a conductive hearing loss.

otoscope (**OH**-toh-skope)**:** an instrument used to visually examine the external ear canal and tympanic membrane.

ovarian cancer: cancer that begins within the cells of the ovaries.

ovariorrhexis (oh-**vay**-ree-oh-**RECK**-sis)**:** the rupture of an ovary.

overactive bladder: a condition that occurs when the muscles of the bladder contract involuntarily even though the bladder is not full.

overflow incontinence: continuous leaking from the bladder either because it is full or because it does not empty completely.

over-the-counter drug: medication that can be purchased without a written prescription.

overuse injuries: injuries that occur when minor tissue injuries have not been given time to heal.

overuse tendinitis (ten-dih-**NIGH**-tis**):** inflammation of tendons caused by excessive or unusual use of a joint.

P

Paget's disease (PAJ-its**):** a bone disease of unknown cause, characterized by excessive breakdown of bone tissue followed by abnormal bone formation.

palatoplasty (PAL-ah-toh-**plas**-tee**):** surgical repair of a cleft palate or lip.

palliative (PAL-ee-**ay**-tiv *or* **PAL**-ee-ah-tiv**):** a substance that eases the pain or severity of a disease but does not cure it.

palpation (pal-**PAY**-shun**):** an examination technique in which the examiner's hands are used to feel the texture, size, consistency, and location of certain body parts.

palpitation (pal-pih-**TAY**-shun**):** a pounding or racing heart with or without irregularity in rhythm.

pancreatectomy (pan-kree-ah-**TECK**-toh-mee**):** surgical removal of all or part of the pancreas.

pancreatitis (pan-kree-ah-**TYE**-tis**):** inflammation of the pancreas.

pandemic (pan-**DEM**-ick**):** an outbreak of a disease occurring over a large geographic area, possibly worldwide.

panic attack: an unexpected, sudden experience of fear in the absence of danger, accompanied by physical symptoms such as shortness of breath and chest pain.

panic disorder: a condition characterized by having more than one panic attack, resulting in persistent fear of the attacks.

papilledema (pap-ill-eh-**DEE**-mah**):** swelling and inflammation of the optic nerve at the point of entrance into the eye through the optic disk.

papilloma (pap-ih-**LOH**-mah**):** a benign, superficial wart-like growth on the epithelial tissue or elsewhere in the body, such as in the bladder.

Pap smear: an exfoliative biopsy of the cervix.

papule (**PAP**-youl**):** a small, raised red lesion that is less than 0.5 cm in diameter.

paradoxical drug reaction: the result of medical treatment that yields the exact opposite of normally expected results.

paralysis (pah-**RAL**-ih-sis**):** the loss of sensation and voluntary muscle movements in a muscle through disease or injury to its nerve supply.

paraplegia (par-ah-**PLEE**-jee-ah**):** paralysis of both legs and the lower part of the body.

parasite (**PAR**-ah-sight**):** a plant or animal that lives on or within another living organism at the expense of that organism.

parathyroidectomy (par-ah-**thigh**-roi-**DECK**-toh-mee**):** surgical removal of one or more of the parathyroid glands.

parenteral administration (pah-**REN**-ter-al**):** the administration of medication by injection through a hypodermic syringe.

paresthesia (par-es-**THEE**-zee-ah**):** a burning or prickling sensation that is usually felt in the hands, arms, legs, or feet.

Parkinson's disease: a chronic, degenerative central nervous system disorder characterized by fine muscle tremors, rigidity, and a slow or shuffling gait.

paronychia (par-oh-**NICK**-ee-ah**):** an infection of the skin fold around a nail.

paroxysmal supraventricular tachycardia (par-ock-**SIZ**-mal **soo**-prah-ven-**TRICK**-you-lar tack-ee-**KAR**-dee-ah**):** an episode that begins and ends abruptly during which there are very rapid and regular heartbeats that originate in the atria or AV node.

partial knee replacement (PKR**):** a procedure in which only part of the knee is replaced.

pathogen (**PATH**-oh-jen**):** a disease-producing microorganism.

pathologic fracture: occurs when a weakened bone breaks under normal strain.

peak flow meter: a handheld device used to measure how quickly a person with asthma can expel air.

pediculosis (pee-**dick**-you-**LOH**-sis**):** an infestation with lice.

pelvic inflammatory disease: any inflammation of the female reproductive organs not associated with surgery or pregnancy.

pelvimetry (pel-**VIM**-eh-tree**):** a radiographic study to measure the dimensions of the pelvis to determine its capacity to allow passage of the fetus through the birth canal.

peptic ulcers (UL-serz): sores that affect the mucous membranes of the digestive system.

percussion (per-**KUSH**-un)**:** a diagnostic procedure to determine the density of a body area that uses the sound produced by tapping the surface with the fingers.

percutaneous diskectomy (per-kyou-**TAY**-nee-us dis-**KECK**-toh-mee)**:** a procedure to treat a herniated intervertebral disk.

percutaneous nephrolithotomy (per-kyou-**TAY**-nee-us **nef**-roh-lih-**THOT**-oh-mee)**:** surgical removal of a kidney stone through a small incision in the back.

percutaneous transluminal coronary angioplasty: a treatment procedure to open a partially blocked coronary artery by flattening the plaque deposit and stretching the lumen.

percutaneous vertebroplasty (per-kyou-**TAY**-nee-us **VER**-tee-broh-**plas**-tee)**:** treatment of osteoporosis-related compression fractures by injecting bone cement to stabilize compression fractures within the spinal column.

perfusion (per-**FYOU**-zuhn)**:** the flow of blood through an organ.

pericardiocentesis (pehr-ih-**kar**-dee-oh-sen-**TEE**-sis)**:** the puncture of the pericardial sac for the purpose of removing fluid.

pericarditis (pehr-ih-kar-**DYE**-tis)**:** inflammation of the pericardium.

periodontal disease: inflammation of the tissues that surround and support the teeth.

periorbital edema (pehr-ee-**OR**-bih-tal eh-**DEE**-mah): swelling of the tissues surrounding the eye or eyes.

periosteotomy (pehr-ee-**oss**-tee-**OT**-oh-mee)**:** an incision through the periosteum to the bone.

periostitis (pehr-ee-oss-**TYE**-tis)**:** inflammation of the periosteum.

peripheral arterial occlusive disease: an example of a peripheral vascular disease caused by atherosclerosis. Impaired circulation to the extremities and vital organs causes changes in the skin color and temperature, plus intermittent claudication.

peripheral neuropathy (new-**ROP**-ah-thee)**:** a disorder of the peripheral nerves that carry information to and from the brain and spinal cord, producing pain, loss of sensation, and inability to control muscles.

peripheral vascular disease: disorders of blood vessels outside the heart and brain.

peritoneal dialysis (pehr-ih-toh-**NEE**-al dye-**AL**-ih-sis)**:** dialysis in which the lining of the peritoneal cavity acts as the filter to remove waste from the blood.

peritonitis (pehr-ih-toh-**NIGH**-tis)**:** inflammation of the peritoneum.

pernicious anemia (per-**NISH**-us ah-**NEE**-mee-ah)**:** anemia caused by a lack of a protein that helps the body absorb vitamin B12 from the gastrointestinal tract.

PERRLA: an abbreviation meaning **P**upils are **E**qual, **R**ound, **R**esponsive to **L**ight and **A**ccomodation.

persistent vegetative state: a type of coma in which the patient exhibits alternating sleep and wake cycles; however, the individual is unconscious even when appearing to be awake.

personality disorder: a chronic pattern of inner experience and behavior that causes serious problems with relationships and work.

pertussis (per-**TUS**-is)**:** a contagious bacterial infection of the upper respiratory tract that is characterized by recurrent bouts of a paroxysmal cough.

petechiae (pee-**TEE**-kee-ee)**:** very small pinpoint hemorrhages less than 2 mm in diameter.

Peyronie's disease (pay-roh-**NEEZ**)**:** a form of sexual dysfunction in which the penis is bent or curved during erection.

phacoemulsification (fack-koh-ee-**mul**-sih-fih-**KAY**-shun)**:** the use of ultrasonic vibration to shatter and remove the lens clouded by a cataract.

pharyngitis (far-in-**JIGH**-tis)**:** inflammation of the pharynx.

phenylketonuria (fen-il-**kee**-toh-**NEW**-ree-ah)**:** a genetic disorder in which an essential digestive enzyme is missing.

pheochromocytoma (fee-oh-**kroh**-moh-sigh-**TOH**-mah)**:** a benign tumor of the adrenal gland that causes the release of excess epinephrine and norepinephrine.

phimosis (figh-**MOH**-sis)**:** narrowing of the opening of the foreskin so that it cannot be retracted to expose the glans penis.

phlebitis (fleh-**BYE**-tis)**:** inflammation of a vein.

phlebography (fleh-**BOG**-rah-fee)**:** a radiographic test that provides an image of veins after a contrast dye is injected.

phlebotomy (fleh-**BOT**-oh-mee)**:** the puncture of a vein for the purpose of drawing blood.

phlegm (FLEM): thick mucus secreted by the tissues lining the respiratory passages.

phobia (FOH-bee-ah)**:** a persistent irrational fear of a specific thing or situation strong enough to cause significant distress, interfere with functioning, and lead to avoidance of the thing or situation that causes this reaction.

photocoagulation: the use of lasers to treat some forms of wet macular degeneration by sealing leaking or damaged blood vessels.

photodynamic therapy (**foh**-toh-dye-**NAH**-mik)**:** a technique used to treat damaged and precancerous skin, as well as various types of cancer.

photophobia (**foh**-toh-**FOH**-bee-ah)**:** excessive sensitivity to light.

photopsia (foh-**TOP**-see-ah)**:** presence of what appear to be flashes of light.

physical therapy: treatment to prevent disability or to restore function through the use of exercise, heat, massage, or other techniques.

pica (**PYE**-kah)**:** an abnormal craving or appetite for nonfood substances such as dirt that lasts for at least one month.

pigmented birthmarks: irregularities in skin color, such as moles.

pinealectomy (**pin**-ee-al-**ECK**-toh-mee)**:** the surgical removal of the pineal gland.

pinealoma (pin-ee-ah-**LOH**-mah)**:** a tumor of the pineal gland.

pituitary adenoma (**ad**-eh-**NOH**-mah)**:** a slow-growing, benign tumor of the pituitary gland that may or may not cause excess hormone secretion.

placebo (plah-**SEE**-boh)**:** an inactive substance that is given for its suggestive effects.

placenta previa (plah-**SEN**-tah **PREE**-vee-ah)**:** abnormal implantation of the placenta in the lower portion of the uterus.

plantar fasciitis (**PLAN**-tar **fas**-ee-**EYE**-tis)**:** inflammation of the plantar fascia causing foot or heel pain when walking or running.

plaque (**PLACK**)**:** a fatty deposit within the blood vessels; also a soft buildup of bacterial debris on the exterior of the teeth; also a scaly, solid, raised area of closely spaced papules on the skin.

plasmapheresis (**plaz**-mah-feh-**REE**-sis)**:** the removal of whole blood from the body, separation of its cellular elements, and reinfusion of these cellular elements suspended in saline or a plasma substitute.

platelet count: a blood screening test that measures the number of platelets in a specified amount of blood.

pleural effusion (eh-**FEW**-zhun)**:** the excess accumulation of fluid in the pleural space that prevents the lung from fully expanding.

pleurisy (**PLOOR**-ih-see)**:** inflammation of the pleura that produces sharp chest pain with each breath.

pleurodynia (**ploor**-oh-**DIN**-ee-ah)**:** pain in the pleura or in the side.

pneumoconiosis (**new**-moh-**koh**-nee-**OH**-sis)**:** any fibrosis of the lung tissues caused by dust in the lungs after prolonged environmental or occupational contact.

pneumocystis pneumonia (**new**-moh-**SIS**-tis new-**MOH**-nee-ah)**:** the form of pneumonia caused by an opportunistic infection with the fungus *Pneumocystis carinii*.

pneumonectomy (**new**-moh-**NECK**-toh-mee)**:** the surgical removal of all or part of a lung.

pneumonia (new-**MOH**-nee-ah)**:** a serious infection or inflammation of the lungs in which the alveoli and air passages fill with pus and other liquid.

pneumorrhagia (**new**-moh-**RAY**-jee-ah)**:** bleeding from the lungs.

pneumothorax (**new**-moh-**THOR**-racks)**:** the accumulation of air in the pleural space resulting in a pressure imbalance that causes the lung to fully or partially collapse.

poliomyelitis (**poh**-lee-oh-**my**-eh-**LYE**-tis)**:** a highly contagious viral infection of the brainstem and spinal cord that sometimes leads to paralysis.

polyarteritis (**pol**-ee-**ar**-teh-**RYE**-tis)**:** a form of vasculitis involving several medium and small arteries at the same time.

polycystic kidney disease (**pol**-ee-**SIS**-tick)**:** a genetic disorder characterized by the growth of numerous fluid-filled cysts in the kidneys.

polycystic ovary syndrome (**pol**-ee-**SIS**-tick)**:** condition caused by a hormonal imbalance in which the ovaries are enlarged by the presence of many cysts formed by incompletely developed follicles.

polycythemia (**pol**-ee-sy-**THEE**-mee-ah)**:** an abnormal increase in the number of red cells in the blood due to excess production of these cells by the bone marrow.

polydipsia (**pol**-ee-**DIP**-see-ah)**:** excessive thirst.

polymenorrhea (**pol**-ee-**men**-oh-**REE**-ah)**:** abnormally frequent menstruation.

polymyalgia rheumatica (pol-ee-my-**AL**-jah roo-**MA**-tih-kah)**:** a geriatric inflammatory disorder of the muscles and joints characterized by pain and stiffness.

polymyositis (**pol**-ee-**my**-oh-**SIGH**-tis)**:** muscle disease characterized by the simultaneous inflammation and weakening of voluntary muscles in many parts of the body.

polyp (**POL**-ip)**:** a mushroom-like growth from the surface of a mucous membrane.

polyphagia (**pol**-ee-**FAY**-jee-ah)**:** excessive hunger.

polysomnography (**pol**-ee-som-**NOG**-rah-fee)**:** the diagnostic measurement of physiological activity during sleep.

polyuria (**pol**-ee-**YOU**-ree-ah)**:** excessive urination.

port-wine stain: a flat vascular birthmark made up of dilated blood capillaries.
positron emission tomography: an imaging technique that combines tomography with radionuclide tracers to produce enhanced images of selected body organs or areas.
post-traumatic stress disorder: the development of characteristic symptoms after a major traumatic event.
prediabetes: a condition in which the blood sugar level is higher than normal, but not high enough to be classified as type 2 diabetes.
preeclampsia (**pree**-ee-**KLAMP**-see-ah)**:** a complication of pregnancy characterized by hypertension, edema, and proteinuria.
pregnancy test: a diagnostic test to is determine if a woman is pregnant.
premature ejaculation: a condition in which the male reaches climax too soon, usually before or shortly after penetration.
premature infant: a neonate born before the 37th week of gestation.
premature menopause: a condition in which the ovaries cease functioning before age 40.
premenstrual dysphoric disorder: a condition associated with severe emotional and physical problems linked to the menstrual cycle.
premenstrual syndrome: a group of symptoms experienced by some women within the two-week period before menstruation.
prenatal influences: the mother's health, behavior, and the prenatal medical care she does or does not receive before delivery.
presbycusis (**pres**-beh-**KOO**-sis)**:** a gradual sensorineural hearing loss that occurs as the body ages.
presbyopia (**pres**-bee-**OH**-pee-ah)**:** condition of common changes in the eyes that occur with aging.
prescription drug: a medication that can legally be dispensed only by a pharmacist with an order from a licensed professional.
pressure sore: an open ulcerated wound that is caused by prolonged pressure on an area of skin.
priapism (**PRYE**-ah-**piz**-em)**:** a painful erection that lasts four hours or more, but is not accompanied by sexual excitement.
primary bone cancer: a relatively rare malignant tumor that originates in a bone.
primary lymphedema: a hereditary disorder in which swelling due to an abnormal accumulation of lymph within the tissues may appear at any time in life.
primigravida (**prye**-mih-**GRAV**-ih-dah)**:** a woman during her first pregnancy.
primipara (prye-**MIP**-ah-rah)**:** a woman who has borne one viable child.
proctopexy (**PROCK**-toh-**peck**-see)**:** surgical fixation of a prolapsed rectum to an adjacent tissue or organ.
professional palpation of the breast: performed to feel the texture, size, and consistency of the breast.
prolactinoma (proh-**lack**-tih-**NOH**-mah)**:** a benign tumor of the pituitary gland that causes it to produce too much prolactin.
prone position: position where the patient lies face down on the abdomen.
prophylaxis (**proh**-fih-**LACK**-sis)**:** treatment, such as vaccination, intended to prevent a disease or stop it from spreading.
prostate cancer: cancer beginning in the prostate.
prostatectomy (**pros**-tah-**TECK**-toh-mee)**:** surgical removal of all or part of the prostate gland.
prostate-specific antigen: a diagnostic blood test that is used to screen for prostate cancer.
prostatism (**PROS**-tah-tizm)**:** a disorder resulting from compression or obstruction of the urethra due to benign prostatic hyperplasia.
prostatitis (**pros**-tah-**TYE**-tis)**:** inflammation of the prostate gland.
prosthesis (pros-**THEE**-sis)**:** a substitute for a diseased or missing body part.
proteinuria (**proh**-tee-in-**YOU**-ree-ah)**:** the presence of an abnormal amount of protein in the urine.
prothrombin time (proh-**THROM**-bin)**:** a blood test used to diagnose conditions associated with abnormalities of clotting time and to monitor anticoagulant therapy.
proton pump inhibitors: medications that decrease the amount of acid produced by the stomach.
pruritus vulvae (proo-**RYE**-tus **VUL**-vee)**:** severe itching of the external female genitalia.
psoriasis (soh-**RYE**-uh-sis)**:** a common skin disorder characterized by flare-ups in which red papules covered with silvery scales occur on the elbows, knees, scalp, back, or buttocks.
psychoanalysis (**sigh**-koh-ah-**NAL**-ih-sis)**:** treatment based on the idea that mental disorders have underlying causes stemming from childhood and can only be overcome by gaining insight into one's feelings and patterns of behavior.
psychotic disorder (sigh-**KOT**-ick)**:** a condition characterized by the loss of contact with reality and deterioration of normal social functioning.

psychotropic drug (sigh-koh-TROP-pick): a drug that acts primarily on the central nervous system, where it produces temporary changes affecting the mind, emotions, and behavior.

ptosis (TOH-sis): drooping of the upper eyelid that is usually due to paralysis.

pulmonary edema (eh-DEE-mah): an accumulation of fluid in the lung tissues.

pulmonary embolism (EM-boh-lizm): the sudden blockage of a pulmonary artery by foreign matter or by an embolus that has formed in the leg or pelvic region.

pulmonary fibrosis (figh-BROH-sis): the progressive formation of scar tissue in the lung, resulting in decreased lung capacity and increased difficulty in breathing.

pulmonary function tests: a group of tests that measure volume and flow of air by utilizing a spirometer.

pulse oximeter (ock-SIM-eh-ter): an external monitor that measures the oxygen saturation level in the blood.

puncture wound: a deep hole made by a sharp object such as a nail.

purpura (PUR-pew-rah): the appearance of multiple purple discolorations on the skin caused by bleeding underneath the skin.

purulent (PYOU-roo-lent): producing or containing pus.

pustule (PUS-tyoul): a small, circumscribed lesion containing pus.

pyelitis (pye-eh-LYE-tis): inflammation of the renal pelvis.

pyelonephritis (pye-eh-loh-neh-FRY-tis): inflammation of the renal pelvis and of the kidney.

pyeloplasty (PYE-eh-loh-plas-tee): the surgical repair of the ureter and renal pelvis.

pyelotomy (pye-eh-LOT-oh-mee): a surgical incision into the renal pelvis.

pyoderma (pye-oh-DER-mah): any acute, inflammatory, pus-forming bacterial skin infection such as impetigo.

pyosalpinx (pye-oh-SAL-pinks): an accumulation of pus in the fallopian tube.

pyothorax (pye-oh-THOH-racks): the presence of pus in the pleural cavity between the layers of pleural membrane.

pyrosis (pye-ROH-sis): the burning sensation caused by the return of acidic stomach contents into the esophagus.

pyuria (pye-YOU-ree-ah): the presence of pus in the urine.

Q

Qi Gong (CHEE-gong): a Chinese system of movement, breathing techniques, and meditation.

quadriplegia (kwad-rih-PLEE-jee-ah): paralysis of all four extremities.

R

rabies (RAY-beez): an acute viral infection transmitted to humans by the bite or saliva of an infected animal.

radial keratotomy (ker-ah-TOT-oh-mee): a surgical procedure to treat myopia.

radiation therapy: the treatment of cancers through the use of x-rays.

radical hysterectomy: the surgical removal of the ovaries and fallopian tubes, the uterus and cervix, plus nearby lymph nodes.

radical mastectomy: the surgical removal of an entire breast and many of the surrounding tissues.

radiculitis (rah-dick-you-LYE-tis): inflammation of the root of a spinal nerve that causes pain and numbness radiating down the affected limb.

radioactive iodine treatment: oral administration of radioactive iodine to destroy thyroid cells.

radioactive iodine uptake test: test using radioactive iodine administered orally to measure thyroid function.

radiograph: the image produced by the use of radiant energy to visualize conditions such as bone fractures; also known as x-rays.

radiography: the use of x-radiation to visualize hard-tissue internal structures.

radiology (ray-dee-OL-oh-jee): the use of radiant energy and radioactive substances in medicine for diagnosis and treatment.

radiolucent (ray-dee-oh-LOO-sent): a substance that allows x-rays to pass through and appears black or dark gray on the resulting film.

radiopaque (ray-dee-oh-PAYK): a substance that does not allow x-rays to pass through and appears white or light gray on the resulting film.

rale (RAHL): an abnormal crackle-like lung sound heard while breathing in.

range of motion testing: a diagnostic procedure to evaluate joint mobility and muscle strength.

Raynaud's disease (ray-NOHZ): a peripheral arterial occlusive disease in which intermittent attacks are triggered by cold or stress.

rectal administration: the insertion of medication into the rectum as either suppositories or liquid solutions.

rectocele (**RECK**-toh-seel)**:** a bulging of the front wall of the rectum into the vagina.

recumbent (ree-**KUM**-bent)**:** any position in which the patient is lying down.

red blood cell count: a blood test that is performed to determine the number of erythrocytes in the blood.

refraction: an examination procedure to determine an eye's refractive error so that the best corrective lenses can be prescribed.

refractive disorder: a focusing problem caused when the lens and cornea do not bend light so that it focuses properly on the retina.

regurgitation (ree-**gur**-jih-**TAY**-shun)**:** the return of swallowed food into the mouth.

renal colic (**REE**-nal **KOLL**-ick)**:** acute pain in the kidney area that is caused by blockage during the passage of a kidney stone.

renal failure: the inability of one or both of the kidneys to perform their functions.

renal transplantation: the grafting of a donor kidney into the body to replace the recipient's failed kidneys.

repetitive stress disorders: a variety of muscular conditions that result from repeated motions performed in the course of normal activities.

respiratory failure (RF)**:** a condition in which the level of oxygen in the blood becomes dangerously low or the level of carbon dioxide becomes dangerously high.

restenosis: the condition when an artery that has been opened by angioplasty closes again.

restless legs syndrome (RLS)**:** a neurological disorder characterized by uncomfortable feelings in the legs, producing a strong urge to move them.

retinal detachment: the separation of all of the light-sensitive retina from the choroid.

retinal tear: the separation of some of the light-sensitive retina from the choroid.

retinitis pigmentosa (**ret**-ih-**NIGH**-tis pig-men-**TOH**-sah)**:** a progressive degeneration of the retina that affects night and peripheral vision.

retinoids (**RET**-ih-noydz)**:** a class of chemical compounds derived from vitamin A that are used in skin care and treatment.

retinopathy (**ret**-ih-**NOP**-ah-thee)**:** any disease of the retina.

retinopexy (**RET**-ih-noh-**peck**-see)**:** treatment to reattach the detached area in a retinal detachment.

retrograde ejaculation: when an orgasm results in semen flowing backward into the bladder instead of out through the penis.

retrograde urography: a radiograph of the urinary system taken after a contrast medium has been placed in the urethra and caused to flow upward through the urinary tract.

revision surgery: the replacement of a worn or failed implant.

Reye's syndrome: a potentially serious or deadly disorder in children that is characterized by vomiting and confusion, sometimes following a viral illness for which the child was treated with aspirin.

rheumatoid arthritis (**ROO**-mah-toyd ar-**THRIGH**-tis)**:** a chronic autoimmune disorder in which the synovial membranes, and other body tissues, are inflamed and thickened.

rhinitis (rye-**NIGH**-tis)**:** inflammation of the nose.

rhinophyma (**rye**-noh-**FIGH**-muh)**:** hyperplasia of the tissues of the nose.

rhinorrhea (**rye**-noh-**REE**-ah)**:** the watery flow of mucus from the nose.

rhonchi (**RONG**-kye)**:** a coarse rattling sound somewhat like snoring, usually caused by secretions in the bronchial airways.

rhytidectomy (**rit**-ih-**DECK**-toh-mee)**:** the surgical removal of excess skin and fat from the face to eliminate wrinkles.

rickets (**RICK**-ets)**:** a deficiency disease occurring in children involving defective bone growth due to vitamin D deficiency.

rickettsia (rih-**KET**-see-ah)**:** a small bacterium that lives in lice, fleas, ticks, and mites.

rosacea (roh-**ZAY**-shee-ah)**:** a chronic condition of unknown cause that produces tiny red pimples, and broken blood vessels.

rotator cuff tendinitis (**ten**-dih-**NIGH**-tis)**:** inflammation of the tendons of the rotator cuff.

rubella (roo-**BELL**-ah)**:** a viral infection characterized by a low-grade fever, swollen glands, inflamed eyes, and a fine, pink rash.

ruptured rotator cuff: develops when rotator cuff tendinitis is left untreated or if the overuse continues. This occurs as the irritated tendon weakens and tears.

S

salmonellosis (**sal**-moh-nel-**LOH**-sis)**:** an infectious disease transmitted by feces, either through direct contact or by eating contaminated raw or undercooked food.

salpingectomy (**sal**-pin-**JECK**-toh-mee)**:** surgical removal of one or both fallopian tubes.

salpingitis (**sal**-pin-**JIGH**-tis)**:** inflammation of a fallopian tube.

salpingo-oophorectomy (sal-**ping**-goh oh-**ahf**-oh-**RECK**-toh-mee)**:** the surgical removal of a fallopian tube and ovary.

sarcoma (sar-**KOH**-mah)**:** a malignant tumor that arises from connective tissues.

sarcopenia (**sar**-koh-**PEE**-nee-ah)**:** the loss of muscle mass, strength, and function that comes with aging.

scabies (**SKAY**-beez)**:** a skin infection caused by an infestation of itch mites.

scales: flakes or dry patches made up of excess dead epidermal cells.

schizophrenia (**skit**-soh-**FREE**-nee-ah)**:** a psychotic disorder characterized by withdrawal from reality, illogical patterns of thinking, delusions, and hallucinations.

sciatica (sigh-**AT**-ih-kah)**:** inflammation of the sciatic nerve that results in pain, burning, and tingling along the course of the affected nerve.

scleral buckle (**SKLER**-al)**:** a silicone band or sponge used to repair a detached retina.

scleritis (skleh-**RYE**-tis)**:** inflammation of the sclera of the eye.

scleroderma (**sklehr**-oh-**DER**-mah)**:** an autoimmune disorder in which the connective tissues become thickened and hardened, causing the skin to become hard and swollen.

sclerotherapy (**sklehr**-oh-**THER**-ah-pee)**:** treatment of spider veins by injecting a saline sclerosing solution into the vein.

scoliosis (**skoh**-lee-**OH**-sis)**:** an abnormal lateral curvature of the spine.

scotoma (skoh-**TOH**-mah)**:** an abnormal area of diminished vision surrounded by an area of normal vision.

seasonal affective disorder: a seasonal bout of depression associated with the decrease in hours of daylight during winter months.

sebaceous cyst (seh-**BAY**-shus)**:** a closed sac associated with a sebaceous gland that is found just under the skin.

seborrhea (**seb**-oh-**REE**-ah)**:** overactivity of the sebaceous glands that results in the production of an excessive amount of sebum.

seborrheic dermatitis (**seb**-oh-**REE**-ick **der**-mah-**TYE**-tis)**:** inflammation that causes scaling and itching of the upper layers of the skin or scalp.

seborrheic keratosis (**seb**-oh-**REE**-ick **kerr**-ah-**TOH**-sis)**:** a benign skin growth that has a waxy or "pasted-on" look.

secondary bone cancer: tumors that have metastasized to bones from other organs such as the breasts and lungs.

secondary lymphedema: swelling of the tissues due to an abnormal accumulation of lymph within the tissues that is the result of damage to lymphatic vessels.

sedative: medication that depresses the central nervous system to produce calm and diminished responsiveness without producing sleep.

seizure (**SEE**-zhur)**:** a sudden surge of electrical activity in the brain that affects how a person feels or acts for a short time.

sensorineural hearing loss: hearing loss that develops when the auditory nerve or hair cells in the inner ear are damaged.

septicemia (**sep**-tih-**SEE**-mee-ah)**:** caused by the presence of bacteria in the blood, symptoms include fever, tachypnea, and tachycardia.

septoplasty (**SEP**-toh-**plas**-tee)**:** the surgical repair or alteration of parts of the nasal septum.

septic shock: a serious condition that occurs when an overwhelming bacterial infection affects the body.

serum bilirubin test: a blood test that measures the ability of the liver to take up, process, and secrete bilirubin into the bile.

sexually transmitted diseases: infections caused by either a bacteria or a virus transmitted through sexual intercourse or other genital contact.

shaken baby syndrome: describes the results of a child being violently shaken by someone.

shin splint: pain caused by the muscle tearing away from the tibia.

short stature: condition resulting from the failure of the bones of the limbs to grow to an appropriate length compared to the size of the head and trunk.

sickle cell anemia: a genetic disorder that causes abnormal hemoglobin, resulting in red blood cells that assume an abnormal sickle shape.

sigmoidoscopy (**sig**-moi-**DOS**-koh-pee)**:** the endoscopic examination of the interior of the rectum, sigmoid colon, and possibly a portion of the descending colon.

sign: objective evidence of disease, such as a fever.

silicosis (**sill**-ih-**KOH**-sis)**:** the form of pneumoconiosis caused by inhaling silica dust in the lungs.

Sims' position: an examination position in which the patient is lying on the left side with the right knee and thigh drawn up with the left arm placed along the back.

single photon emission computed tomography: a type of nuclear imaging test that produces 3D computer-reconstructed images showing perfusion through tissues and organs.

singultus (sing-**GUL**-tus)**:** myoclonus of the diaphragm that causes the characteristic hiccup sound with each spasm.

sinusitis (**sigh**-nuh-**SIGH**-tis)**:** an inflammation of the sinuses.

skeletal muscle relaxant: administered to relax certain muscles and to relieve the stiffness, pain, and discomfort caused by strains, sprains, or other muscle injuries.

skin cancer: a harmful, malignant growth on the skin, which can have many causes, including repeated severe sunburns or long-term exposure to the sun.

skin tags: benign small flesh-colored or light-brown polyps that hang from the body by fine stalks.

sleep apnea (AP-nee-ah): a potentially serious disorder in which breathing repeatedly stops during sleep for long enough periods to cause a measurable decrease in blood oxygen levels.

sleep deprivation: a sufficient lack of restorative sleep over a cumulative period so as to cause physical or psychiatric symptoms and affect routine performance or tasks.

sleep hyperhidrosis: the occurrence of hyperhidrosis during sleep.

slit-lamp ophthalmoscopy (**ahf**-thal-**MOS**-koh-pee)**:** a diagnostic procedure in which a narrow beam of light is focused to permit the ophthalmologist to examine the structures at the front of the eye including the cornea, iris, and lens.

smoke inhalation: damage to the lungs in which particles from a fire coat the alveoli and prevent normal exchange of gases.

SOAP note: an acronym for subjective, objective, assessment, and plan.

social phobia: excessive fear of social situations where the person fears negative evaluation by others or embarrassing himself in front of others.

somatoform disorders (soh-**MAT**-oh-**form**)**:** conditions that are characterized by physical complaints or concerns about one's body that are out of proportion to any physical findings or disease.

somnambulism (som-**NAM**-byou-lizm)**:** the condition of walking or performing some other activity without awakening.

spasm: a sudden, involuntary contraction of one or more muscles.

spasmodic torticollis (spaz-**MOD**-ick **tor**-tih-**KOL**-is)**:** a stiff neck due to spasmodic contraction of the neck muscles that pull the head toward the affected side.

speculum (**SPECK**-you-lum)**:** an instrument used to enlarge the opening of any canal or cavity to facilitate inspection of its interior.

spermatocele (sper-**MAH**-toh-seel)**:** a cyst that develops in the epididymis and is filled with a milky fluid containing sperm.

sperm count: the testing of freshly ejaculated semen to determine the volume plus the number, shape, size, and motility of the sperm.

sphygmomanometer (**sfig**-moh-mah-**NOM**-eh-ter)**:** an instrument used to measure blood pressure.

spina bifida (**SPY**-nah **BIF**-ih-dah)**:** a congenital defect that occurs during early pregnancy in which the spinal canal fails to close completely around the spinal cord.

spinal anesthesia: regional anesthesia produced by injecting medication into the subarachnoid space.

spinal cord injury: paralysis resulting from damage to the spinal cord that prevents nerve impulses from being transmitted below the level of the injury.

spinal fusion: a technique to immobilize part of the spine by joining together two or more vertebrae.

spiral fracture: a fracture in which the bone has been twisted apart.

spirochetes (**SPY**-roh-keets)**:** long, slender spiral-shaped bacteria that have flexible walls and are capable of movement.

spirometer (spih-**ROM**-eh-ter)**:** a recording device that measures the amount of air inhaled or exhaled (volume) and the length of time required for each breath.

splenomegaly (**splee**-noh-**MEG**-ah-lee)**:** an abnormal enlargement of the spleen.

splenorrhagia (**splee**-noh-**RAY**-jee-ah)**:** bleeding from the spleen.

spondylolisthesis (**spon**-dih-loh-liss-**THEE**-sis)**:** the forward slipping movement of the body of one of the lower lumbar vertebrae on the vertebra below it.

spondylosis (**spon**-dih-**LOH**-sis)**:** a degenerative disorder that can cause the loss of normal spinal structure and function.

sprain: an injury to a joint, such as ankle, knee, or wrist, that usually involves a wrenched or torn ligament.

sputum (**SPYOU**-tum)**:** phlegm ejected through the mouth that can be examined for diagnostic purposes.

squamous cell carcinoma (**SKWAY**-mus)**:** a malignant tumor of the scaly squamous cells of the epithelium that can quickly spread to other body systems.

staging: the process of classifying tumors by how far the disease has progressed, the potential for its responding to therapy, and the patient's prognosis.

stapedectomy (stay-peh-**DECK**-toh-mee**):** the surgical removal of the top portion of the stapes bone and the insertion of a prosthetic device that conducts sound vibrations to the inner ear.

staphylococci (staf-ih-loh-**KOCK**-sigh**):** a group of about 30 species of bacteria that form irregular groups or clusters resembling grapes.

steatorrhea (stee-at-oh-**REE**-ah**):** the presence of excess fat in the stool.

stent: a wire-mesh tube that is implanted in a coronary artery to provide support to the arterial wall.

sterilization: any procedure rendering an individual (male or female) incapable of reproduction.

stethoscope (STETH-oh-skope**):** an instrument used to listen to sounds within the body.

stillbirth: the birth of a fetus that died before or during delivery.

stimulant: a substance that works by increasing activity in certain areas of the brain to increase concentration and wakefulness.

stomatitis (stoh-mah-**TYE**-tis**):** inflammation of the mucosa of the mouth.

stomatomycosis (stoh-mah-toh-my-**KOH**-sis**):** any disease of the mouth due to a fungus.

stone: an abnormal mineral deposit that has formed within the body.

stool samples: specimens of feces that are examined for content and characteristics.

strabismus (strah-**BIZ**-mus)**:** a disorder in which the eyes point in different directions or are not aligned correctly because the eye muscles are unable to focus together.

strain: an injury to the body of a muscle or the attachment of a tendon.

strangulated hernia: a condition that occurs when a portion of the intestine is constricted inside the hernia and its blood supply is cut off.

streptococci (**strep**-toh-**KOCK**-sigh)**:** bacteria that form a chain. Many are harmless; however, other members of this group are responsible for illnesses including strep throat.

stress fracture: a small crack in a bone that often develops from chronic, excessive impact.

stress incontinence: the inability to control the voiding of urine under physical stress such as running, sneezing, laughing, or coughing.

stress test: the use of electrocardiography to assess cardiovascular health and function during and after stress such as exercise on a treadmill.

stridor (STRYE-dor**):** an abnormal, high-pitched, musical breathing sound caused by a blockage in the throat or larynx.

stupor (STOO-per**):** an unresponsive state from which a person can be aroused only briefly despite vigorous, repeated attempts.

subconjunctival hemorrhage: bleeding between the conjunctiva and the sclera.

subcutaneous injection: the administration of medication by injection into the fatty layer just below the skin.

sublingual administration: the placement of medication under the tongue where it is allowed to dissolve slowly.

subluxation (**sub**-luck-**SAY**-shun)**:** the partial displacement of a bone from its joint.

substance abuse: the addictive use of tobacco, alcohol, medications, or illegal drugs.

sudden cardiac death: results when treatment of cardiac arrest is not provided within a few minutes.

sudden infant death syndrome: the sudden and unexplainable death of an apparently healthy sleeping infant between the ages of two and six months.

sunscreen: blocks the harmful ultraviolet B rays, measured in terms of the strength of the sun protection factor (SPF).

supplemental oxygen: administered when the patient is unable to maintain an adequate oxygen saturation level in the blood from breathing normal air.

suppuration (sup-you-**RAY**-shun**):** the formation or discharge of pus.

suprapubic catheterization (**soo**-prah-**PYOU**-bick)**:** the placement of a catheter into the bladder through a small incision made through the abdominal wall just above the pubic bone.

surgical biopsy (**BYE**-op-see)**:** the removal of a small piece of tissue for examination to confirm a diagnosis.

symptom (SIMP-tum**):** subjective evidence of a disease, such as pain or a headache.

syncope (SIN-koh-pee**):** the brief loss of consciousness caused by the decreased flow of blood to the brain.

syndrome (SIN-drohm**):** a set of signs and symptoms that occur together as part of a specific disease process.

syndrome of inappropriate antidiuretic hormone: overproduction of the antidiuretic hormone ADH, leading to bloating, water retention, and electrolyte imbalance.

synovectomy (sin-oh-**VECK**-toh-mee)**:** the surgical removal of a synovial membrane from a joint.

synovial sarcoma (sih-**NOH**-vee-al sar-**KOH**-mah)**:** a tumor of the tissues surrounding a synovial joint.

synovitis (sin-oh-**VYE**-tiss)**:** inflammation of the synovial membrane that results in swelling and pain of the affected joint.

synthetic immunoglobulins: a post-exposure preventive measure against certain viruses including rabies and some types of hepatitis.

synthetic interferon: medication administered to treat multiple sclerosis, hepatitis C, and some cancers.

synthetic thyroid hormones: medications administered to replace lost thyroid function.

syphilis (**SIF**-ih-lis)**:** a sexually transmitted disease that is caused by the bacterium *Treponema pallidum.*

systemic lupus erythematosus: an autoimmune disorder characterized by a red, scaly rash on the face and upper trunk that also attacks the connective tissue in other body systems.

T

tachycardia (**tack**-ee-**KAR**-dee-ah)**:** an abnormally rapid resting heartbeat usually at a rate of more than 100 beats per minute.

tachypnea (**tack**-ihp-**NEE**-ah)**:** an abnormally rapid rate of respiration usually of more than 20 breaths per minute.

talipes (**TAL**-ih-peez)**:** any congenital deformity of the foot involving the ankle bones.

targeted therapy: a developing form of anti-cancer drug therapy that uses drugs or other substances to identify and attack specific cancer cells without harming normal cells.

tarsorrhaphy (tahr-**SOR**-ah-fee)**:** the partial or complete suturing together of the upper and lower eyelids.

Tay-Sachs disease: a fatal genetic disorder in which harmful quantities of a fatty substance build up in tissues and nerve cells in the brain.

teletherapy (**tel**-eh-**THER**-ah-pee)**:** radiation therapy administered at a distance from the body that is precisely targeted with the use of three-dimensional computer imaging.

temporal arteritis (**TEM**-poh-**ral ar**-teh-**RYE**-tis)**:** a form of vasculitis with abnormally large cells, that can cause headache, visual impairment, or other symptoms.

tendinitis (**ten**-dih-**NIGH**-itis)**:** inflammation of the tendons caused by excessive or unusual use of the joint.

tenodesis (ten-**ODD**-eh-sis)**:** surgical suturing of the end of a tendon to bone.

tenolysis (ten-**OL**-ih-sis)**:** the release of a tendon from adhesions.

tenorrhaphy (ten-**OR**-ah-fee)**:** surgical suturing of the divided ends of a tendon.

tenosynovitis (**ten**-oh-**sin**-oh-**VYE**-tis)**:** inflammation of the sheath around a tendon.

testicular cancer: cancer that begins in the testicles.

testicular self-examination: a self-help step in early detection of testicular cancer by detecting lumps, swelling, or changes in the skin of the scrotum.

testicular torsion: a sharp pain in the scrotum caused by twisting of the vas deferens and blood vessels leading into the testicle.

testitis (test-**TYE**-tis)**:** inflammation of one or both testicles.

tetanus (**TET**-ah-nus)**:** an acute and potentially fatal infection of the central nervous system caused by a toxin produced by the tetanus bacteria.

thalamotomy (**thal**-ah-**MOT**-oh-mee)**:** a surgical incision into the thalamus.

thalassemia (thal-ah-**SEE**-mee-ah)**:** an inherited blood disorder that causes mild or severe anemia due to reduced hemoglobin and fewer red blood cells than normal.

thallium stress test (**THAL**-ee-um)**:** performed to evaluate blood flow to the heart during exercise by injecting a small amount of thallium into the blood.

therapeutic ultrasound: the use of high-frequency sound waves to treat muscle injuries by generating heat deep within muscle tissue.

thoracentesis (**thoh**-rah-sen-**TEE**-sis)**:** the surgical puncture of the chest wall with a needle to obtain fluid from the pleural cavity.

thoracotomy (**thoh**-rah-**KOT**-toh-mee)**:** a surgical incision into the chest walls to open the pleural cavity for biopsy or treatment.

thrombocytopenia (**throm**-boh-**sigh**-toh-**PEE**-nee-ah)**:** a condition in which there is an abnormally small number of platelets circulating in the blood.

thrombocytosis (**throm**-boh-sigh-**TOH**-sis)**:** an abnormal increase in the number of platelets in the circulating blood.

thrombolytic (**throm**-boh-**LIT**-ick)**:** medication that dissolves or causes a thrombus to break up.

thrombosis (throm-**BOH**-sis)**:** the abnormal condition of having a thrombus.

thrombotic occlusion (throm-**BOT**-ick ah-**KLOO**-zhun)**:** the blocking of an artery by a thrombus.

thrombus (**THROM**-bus)**:** a blood clot attached to the interior wall of an artery or vein.

thymectomy (thigh-**MECK**-toh-mee)**:** the surgical removal of the thymus gland.

thymitis (thigh-**MY**-tis)**:** inflammation of the thymus gland.

thyroid carcinoma: cancer of the thyroid gland.

thyroid scan: a specialized nuclear scan to evaluate thyroid function.

thyroid-stimulating hormone assay: a diagnostic test to measure the circulating blood level of thyroid-stimulating hormone.

thyroid storm: a relatively rare, life-threatening condition caused by exaggerated hyperthyroidism.

tinea (**TIN**-ee-ah)**:** a fungal infection that can grow on the skin, hair, or nails.

tinnitus (tih-**NIGH**-tus)**:** a condition of ringing, buzzing, or roaring sound in one or both ears.

tissue plasminogen activator (plaz-**MIN**-oh-jen)**:** a thrombolytic administered to some patients having a heart attack or stroke to dissolve damaging blood clots.

tolerance: acquired unresponsiveness to a specific antigen or decline in effective response to a drug usually due to repeated use.

tomotherapy: combination of tomography with radiation therapy to precisely target tumors.

tonic-clonic seizure: a type of seizure involving the whole body.

tonometry (toh-**NOM**-eh-tree)**:** the measurement of intraocular pressure.

tonsillectomy (**ton**-sih-**LECK**-toh-mee)**:** the surgical removal of the tonsils.

tonsillitis (**ton**-sih-**LYE**-tis)**:** inflammation of the tonsils.

topical application: liquid or ointment rubbed into the skin on the area to be treated.

topical steroids: steroids used in treatment of various skin disorders and diseases.

total hemoglobin test: a blood test that measures the amount of hemoglobin found in whole blood.

total hip replacement (THR)**:** surgery performed to restore a damaged hip to full function by removing the head of the femur and replacing it with a metal ball.

total hysterectomy: the removal of the uterus and cervix, either through the vagina or laparoscopically through the abdomen.

total knee replacement: surgical placement of an artificial joint during which all parts of the knee are replaced.

total parenteral nutrition (pah-**REN**-ter-al)**:** a specialized solution administered intravenously to patients who cannot or should not get their nutrition through eating.

Tourette syndrome (tuh **RET**)**:** a complex neurological disorder characterized by involuntary tics, grunts, and compulsive utterances.

toxoplasmosis (**tock**-soh-plaz-**MOH**-sis)**:** a parasite most commonly transmitted from animals (pets) to humans by contact with contaminated feces.

tracheorrhagia (**tray**-kee-oh-**RAY**-jee-ah)**:** bleeding from the mucous membranes of the trachea.

tracheostomy (**tray**-kee-**OS**-toh-mee)**:** the surgical creation of a stoma into the trachea in order to insert a tube to facilitate breathing.

tracheotomy (**tray**-kee-**OT**-oh-mee)**:** an emergency procedure in which an incision is made into the trachea to gain access to the airway below a blockage.

traction: a pulling force exerted on a limb in a distal direction in an effort to return the bone or joint to normal alignment.

traditional Chinese medicine: a system of ancient Chinese medicinal treatments, including acupuncture, to prevent, diagnose, and treat disease.

transcutaneous electronic nerve stimulation: a method of pain control by wearing a device that delivers small electrical impulses to the nerve endings through the skin.

transdermal: the administration of medication through the unbroken skin so that it is absorbed continuously to produce a systemic effect.

transesophageal echocardiography (**trans**-eh-**sof**-ah-**JEE**-al **eck**-oh-**kar**-dee-**OG**-rah-fee)**:** an ultrasonic imaging technique that is performed from inside the esophagus to evaluate heart structures.

transfusion reaction: a serious and potentially fatal complication of a blood transfusion in which a severe immune response occurs because the patient's blood and the donated blood do not match.

transient ischemic attack: a temporary interruption in the blood supply to the brain.

transurethral prostatectomy: the removal of excess tissue from an enlarged prostate gland with the use of a resectoscope.

transverse fracture: a fracture that occurs straight across the bone.

trauma (**TRAW**-mah)**:** wound or injury.

traumatic brain injury: a blow to the head or a penetrating head injury that damages the brain.

triage (tree-**AHZH**)**:** the medical screening of patients to determine their relative priority of need and the proper place of treatment.

trichomoniasis (**trick**-oh-moh-**NYE**-ah-sis)**:** a sexually transmitted infection caused by the parasite *Trichomonas vaginalis.*

trichomycosis axillaris (**try**-koh-my-**KOH**-sis **ak**-sih-**LAH**-ris)**:** superficial bacterial infection of the hair shafts in areas with extensive sweat glands such as the armpits.

trigeminal neuralgia (try-**JEM**-ih-nal new-**RAL**-jee-ah)**:** inflammation of the fifth cranial nerve characterized by sudden, intense, brief attacks of sharp pain on one side of the face.

trismus (**TRIZ**-mus)**:** any restriction to the opening of the mouth caused by trauma, surgery, or radiation associated with the treatment of oral cancer.

tubal ligation: a surgical procedure performed for the purpose of female sterilization.

tuberculin skin testing: a screening test for tuberculosis in which the skin of the arm is injected with a harmless antigen extracted from the TB bacteria.

tuberculosis (too-**ber**-kew-**LOH**-sis)**:** an infectious disease caused by *Mycobacterium tuberculosis* that usually attacks the lungs.

tumor: an abnormal growth of body tissue in which the multiplication of cells is uncontrolled, abnormal, rapid, and progressive; also known as a neoplasm.

tympanometry (**tim**-pah-**NOM**-eh-tree)**:** the use of air pressure in the ear canal to test for disorders of the middle ear.

tympanoplasty (**tim**-pah-noh-**PLAS**-tee)**:** the surgical correction of a damaged middle ear that is performed either to cure chronic inflammation or to restore function.

type 1 diabetes: an autoimmune insulin deficiency disorder caused by the destruction of pancreatic islet beta cells.

type 2 diabetes: an insulin resistance disorder in which, although insulin is being produced, the body does not use it effectively.

U

ulcer (**UL**-ser)**:** an open lesion of the skin or mucous membrane resulting in tissue loss around the edges.

ulcerative colitis (**UL**-ser-**ay**-tiv koh-**LYE**-tis)**:** a chronic condition of unknown cause in which repeated episodes of inflammation in the rectum and large intestine cause ulcers and irritation.

ultrasonic bone density testing: a screening test for osteoporosis or other conditions that cause a loss of bone mass.

ultrasonography (**ul**-trah-son-**OG**-rah-fee)**:** the imaging of deep body structures by recording the echoes of sound wave pulses that are above the range of human hearing; also known as ultrasound.

unconscious: a state of being unaware and unable to respond to any stimuli including pain.

upper GI series and **lower GI series:** radiographic studies to examine the digestive system. A contrast medium is used to make these structures visible.

upper respiratory infection: a term used to describe the common cold.

uremia (you-**REE**-mee-ah)**:** a toxic condition in which urea and other waste products normally excreted in the urine are retained in the blood.

ureterectasis (you-**reh**-ter-**ECK**-tah-sis)**:** the distention of a ureter.

ureterectomy (**you**-reh-ter-**ECK**-toh-mee)**:** the surgical removal of a ureter.

ureterolith (you-**REE**-ter-oh-**lith**)**:** a stone located anywhere along the ureter.

ureteroplasty (you-**REET**-er-oh-**plas**-tee)**:** the surgical repair of a ureter.

ureterorrhagia (you-**ree**-ter-oh-**RAY**-jee-ah)**:** the discharge of blood from the ureter.

ureterorrhaphy (you-**reet**-eh-**ROAR**-ah-fee)**:** surgical suturing of a ureter.

ureteroscopy (you-**reet**-eh-**ROS**-koh-pee)**:** a treatment for a stone lodged in the ureter.

urethral catheterization: the insertion of a tube through the urethra and into the bladder.

urethritis (**you**-reh-**THRIGH**-tis)**:** inflammation of the urethra.

urethropexy (you-**REE**-throh-**peck**-see)**:** surgical fixation of the urethra to nearby tissue.

urethrorrhagia (you-**ree**-throh-**RAY**-jee-ah)**:** bleeding from the urethra.

urethrorrhea (you **ree** throh **REE** ah)**:** abnormal discharge from the urethra.

urethrostenosis (you-**ree**-throh-steh-**NOH**-sis)**:** abnormal narrowing of the urethra.

urethrotomy (**you**-reh-**THROT**-oh-mee)**:** a surgical incision into the urethra.

urinalysis (**you**-rih-**NAL**-ih-sis)**:** the examination of urine to determine the presence of abnormal elements.

urinary catheterization (**kath**-eh-ter-eye-**ZAY**-shun)**:** the insertion of a tube into the bladder in order to obtain a sterile specimen or drain urine.

urinary hesitancy: difficulty in starting a urinary stream.

urinary incontinence: the inability to control the voiding of urine.

urinary retention: the inability to completely empty the bladder when attempting to urinate.

urinary tract infection: an infection involving the structures of the urinary system that usually begins in the bladder.

urticaria (**ur**-tih-**KARE**-ree-ah)**:** itchy wheals caused by an allergic reaction.

uterine fibroid: a benign tumor composed of muscle and fibrous tissue that occurs in the wall of the uterus.

uterine prolapse (proh-**LAPS**)**:** the condition in which the uterus slides from its normal position in the pelvic cavity and sags into the vagina.

uveitis (**you**-vee-**EYE**-tis)**:** inflammation of the uvea causing swelling and irritation.

V

vaginal candidiasis (**kan**-dih-**DYE**-ah-sis)**:** a vaginal infection caused by *Candida albicans.*

vaginitis (**vaj**-ih-**NIGH**-tis)**:** inflammation of the lining of the vagina.

valvoplasty (**VAL**-voh-**plas**-tee)**:** the surgical repair or replacement of a heart valve.

valvular prolapse (**VAL**-voo-lar proh-**LAPS**)**:** the abnormal protrusion of a heart valve that results in the inability of the valve to close completely.

valvular stenosis (steh-**NOH**-sis)**:** a condition in which there is narrowing, stiffening, thickening, or blockage of one or more valves of the heart.

valvulitis (**val**-view-**LYE**-tis)**:** an inflammation of a heart valve.

varicella (**var**-ih-**SEL**-ah)**:** a highly contagious infection caused by the herpes virus *Varicella zoster*; also known as chickenpox.

varicocele (**VAR**-ih-koh-**seel**)**:** a knot of varicose veins in one side of the scrotum.

varicocelectomy (**var**-ih-koh-sih-**LECK**-toh-mee)**:** the removal of a portion of an enlarged vein to relieve a varicocele.

varicose veins (**VAR**-ih-kohs **VAYNS**)**:** abnormally swollen veins usually occurring in the superficial veins of the legs.

vascular birthmarks: birthmarks caused by blood vessels close to the skin's surface.

vascular dementia: a form of dementia caused by a restriction of blood to the brain.

vasculitis (**vas**-kyou-**LYE**-tis)**:** inflammation of a blood or lymph vessel.

vasectomy (vah-**SECK**-toh-mee)**:** the male sterilization procedure in which a small portion of the vas deferens is surgically removed.

vasoconstrictor (**vas**-oh-kon-**STRICK**-tor)**:** medication that causes blood vessels to narrow.

vasodilator (**vas**-oh-dye-**LAYT**-or)**:** medication that causes blood vessels to expand.

vasovasostomy (**vay**-soh-vah-**ZOS**-toh-mee)**:** a procedure performed as an attempt to restore fertility to a vasectomized male.

vector-borne transmission: the spread of certain disease due to the bite of a vector (insects or animals that are capable of transmitting a disease).

ventilator: a mechanical device for artificial respiration that is used to replace or supplement the patient's natural breathing function.

ventricular fibrillation (ven-**TRICK**-you-lar **fih**-brih-**LAY**-shun)**:** rapid, irregular, and useless contractions of the ventricles.

ventricular tachycardia (ven-**TRICK**-you-lar **tack**-ee-**KAR**-dee-ah)**:** a very rapid heartbeat that begins within the ventricles.

verrucae (veh-**ROO**-kee)**:** small, hard skin lesions caused by the human papillomavirus.

vertigo (**VER**-tih-goh)**:** a sense of whirling, dizziness, and the loss of balance, often combined with nausea and vomiting.

vesicle (**VES**-ih-kul)**:** a small blister, less than 0.5 cm in diameter, containing watery fluid.

vesicovaginal fistula (**ves**-ih-koh-**VAJ**-ih-nahl **FIS**-tyou-lah)**:** an abnormal opening between the bladder and vagina.

vestibular rehabilitation therapy (ves-**TIB**-you-lar)**:** a form of physical therapy designed to treat a wide variety of balance disorders.

video-assisted thoracic surgery (VATS)**:** the use of a thoracoscope to view the inside of the pleural cavity through very small incisions.

viral (**VYE**-ral)**:** pertaining to a virus.

viral pneumonia: caused by several different types of viruses, accounts for approximately a third of all pneumonias.

viruses (**VYE**-rus-ez)**:** very small infectious agents that live only by invading other cells.

viscosupplementation (**vis**-ko-**sup**-leh-men-**TAY**-shun)**:** injections to add fluid to a joint.

visual acuity (ah-**KYOU**-ih-tee)**:** the ability to distinguish object details and shape at a distance.

visual field testing: a diagnostic test to determine losses in peripheral vision.

vitiligo (**vit**-ih-**LYE**-goh)**:** a skin condition resulting from the destruction of melanocytes due to unknown causes, resulting in irregular patches of white skin.

vitrectomy (vih-**TRECK**-toh-mee)**:** the removal of the vitreous humor and its replacement with a clear solution.

voiding cystourethrography (**sis**-toh-you-ree-**THROG**-rah-fee)**:** a diagnostic procedure in which a fluoroscope is used to examine the flow of urine from the bladder and through the urethra.

volvulus (**VOL**-view-lus)**:** twisting of the intestine on itself, causing an obstruction.

vulvitis (vul-**VYE**-tis)**:** inflammation of the vulva.

vulvodynia (vul-voh-**DIN**-ee-ah)**:** a painful syndrome of unknown cause characterized by chronic burning, pain during sexual intercourse, itching, or stinging irritation of the vulva.

W

walking pneumonia: a milder but longer-lasting form of pneumonia caused by the bacteria *Mycoplasma pneumoniae.*

Weber and Rinne tests: hearing tests that use a tuning fork to distinguish between conductive and sensorineural hearing losses.

wedge resection: a surgery in which a small wedge-shaped piece of cancerous lung tissue is removed, along with a margin of healthy tissue around the cancer.

western blot test: a blood test to confirm the diagnosis of HIV.

West Nile virus: a viral infection that causes flu-like symptoms, transmitted to humans by mosquito bites.

wheal (**WHEEL**)**:** a small bump that itches.

white blood cell count: a blood test to determine the number of leukocytes in the blood.

white blood cell differential: a blood test to determine what percentage of the total white blood cell count is composed of each of the five types of leukocytes.

Wilms tumor: a rare type of malignant tumor of the kidney that occurs in young children.

X

xeroderma (zee-roh-**DER**-mah)**:** excessively dry skin.

xerophthalmia (**zeer**-ahf-**THAL**-mee-ah)**:** drying of eye surfaces, including the conjunctiva.

xerostomia (**zeer**-oh-**STOH**-mee-ah)**:** the lack of adequate saliva due to diminished secretions by the salivary glands.

Y

yeast: a type of fungus.